Pioneers in Neuropsychopharmacology I.

Selected Writings
of
Joel Elkes

Edited by
Thomas A. Ban

Introductions by
Floyd E. Bloom and Philip B. Bradley

Animula, Budapest

© Collegium Internationale Neuro-Psychopharmacologicum, 2001
Second Edition 2010

ISBN 963 86115 6 1

Library of Congress Cataloging-in-Publication Data

Thomas A. Ban (ed.)
Selected Papers of Joel Elkes
p.   cm.
ISBN 963 861156 1 (hard)

1. Elkes, Joel (1913–

Publisher: CINP
CINP Central Office
Glenfinnan Suite, Braeview House
9/11 Braeview Place, East Kilbride
G74 3XH, Scotland, UK
E-mail: cinp@cinp.org
Website: www.cinp.org

Selected Writings

of

Joel Elkes

To the women in my life:

Sally Ruth – wife
Sara – sister
Anna – daughter
Laura – granddaughter

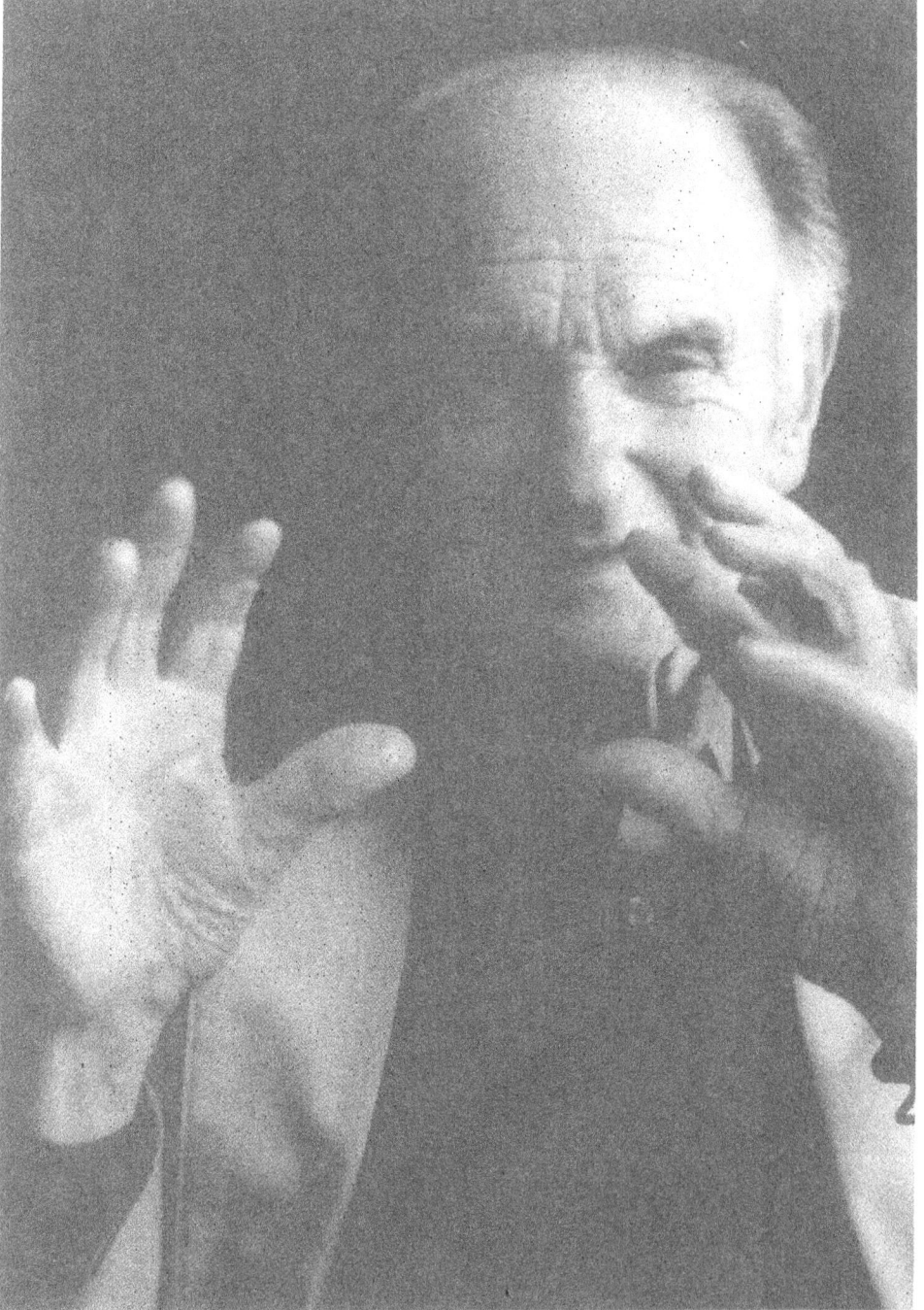

Joel Elkes, 2001
Photograph by Jonas Howard

TABLE OF CONTENTS

PART FOUR: REVIEWS

PART FIVE: SCHIZOPHRENIC DISORDER
AS A DISORDER OF CHEMICALLY MEDIATED
INFORMATION PROCESSING IN THE BRAIN

PART SIX: A PERSPECTIVE (1978)

PART SEVEN: HUMANIZING THE EDUCATION OF
PHYSICIANS. THE BEHAVIORAL SCIENCES
IN THE SERVICE OF MEDICINE

PART EIGHT: FIVE LECTURES

PAINTINGS

In Studio (ca 1965)
The Rocks at Joggins (1990)
Patterns in Rocks (1989)
Pool and Rocks (1989)
A Conversation (1988)
Shre Colors, afternoon (1990)
On my Walk (1990)
Tree Forms (1992)
Pool and rocks II (1989)
After the rain (1991)
Forms of Shore (1990)
Dusk: Point Prim, P.E.I. (1990)
Rocks, afternoon (1991)
Afternoon Light (1988)
A Play of Light, afternoon (1992)
The Light and the Dark (1992)

ACKNOWLEDGEMENTS

The author wishes to thank the Trustees of the Fetzer Institute and its President, Dr. Thomas Innui, for the opportunity afforded him to review old papers while in residence at the Institute in the Summer of 2000 and 2001; and Mrs. Christee Khan for meticulous secretarial assistance.

The author also wishes to express his warm thanks to the authors, editors and publishers of his sources as follows: Academic Press, ACNP Newsletter, Advances, American College of Neuropsychopharmacology, American Journal of Psychiatry, American Psychiatric Association, Animula, Blackwell Science Ltd., Blackwell Scientific Publications, BMJ Publishing Group, P.B. Bradley, Brain, British Medical Journal, Butterworth, Collegium Internationale Neuro-Psychopharmacologicum, Comprehensive Psychiatry, Leah Dickstein, Elsevier Science, Experimental Cell Research, Fetzer Institute, Journal of Mental Science, Bernard Lerer, National Institute for Psychobiology in Israel, Neuropsychopharmacology, Oxford University Press, Eugene S. Paykel, Pergamon Press, Proceedings of The Royal Society London, Psychiatric Annals, Oakley Ray, W.B. Saunders, Seminars in Psychiatry, Slack Inc., Springer Verlag, The British Journal of Psychiatry, The Johns Hopkins Medical Journal, The Johns Hopkins University Press, The Royal Society, The University of Birmingham, Charles C. Thomas Publishers Ltd., University of Birmingham Gazette, and John Wiley & Sons Ltd.

FOREWORD

I. INTRODUCTION

At the XXIst International Congress of the Collegium Internationale Neuro-Psychophar-macologicum (CINP) held in Glasgow, Scotland in 1998, Dr. Joel Elkes was one of the recipi-ents of the CINP–Pfizer Pioneer in Neuropsychopharmacology Award. It was for the first time that this honor was extended to three "exceptional individuals." The other two recipients were Pierre Deniker from France, and Heinz E. Lehmann from Canada.

In this first volume of a CINP series, dedicated to the "pioneers," the selected writings of Joel Elkes are presented. Elkes "made his mark with his visionary approach of linking basic research and clinical psy-chiatry" (1). By recognizing the importance of neurochemical trans-mission in the central nervous system far ahead of his peers, and defin-ing what a "neurotransmitter" is (2), he was instrumental in opening the path for the detection of molecular changes responsible for behav-ioral effects. Furthermore, by adopting "behavioral pharmacology" as a tool for examining psychiatric concepts, he triggered a re-evaluation of the frame of reference of mental illness. In 1966 Elkes wrote (3):

Dr. Joel Elkes after receiving the CINP-Pfizer Pioneers in Neuropsychopharmacology Award

"It is one of the overriding merits of 'behavioral pharmacol-ogy' that it is forcing many issues which have lain dormant in the behavioral sciences, and in clinical psychiatry; and that it compels a re-examination of both instruments, and point of references in neurobiology and psychiatry. The subject to be sure, is peculiarly suited to the role. It ranges from behavior to the neural substrate of behavior, from the silent transactions of 'thought,' to the physics, chemistry and mathematics of the cerebral machinery. Its evolution is marked by two mutually complementary processes, pro-ceeding simultaneously. First, the resolution of the area into the disciplines which com-pound it; and secondly, and more important, the fusion of disciplines, thus defined, into the elements of a new science. A pharmacology preoccupied with tissues and organs is gradu-ally giving way to a pharmacology of the behavior of the total organism; and although old rules obtain, new rules are in the making, and the game itself is assuming strange an unex-pected ways."

Elkes, through his professional activities put the behavioral sciences in the service of medi-cine, and art in the service of healing. With his exceptional ability "to make people aware that their work involves more than the routine drudgery of science, that they are also working on issues of fundamental concern to humanity," Elkes, "can deliver a unique message to that place in the listener's heart where 'meaning' and 'hope' meet" (4).

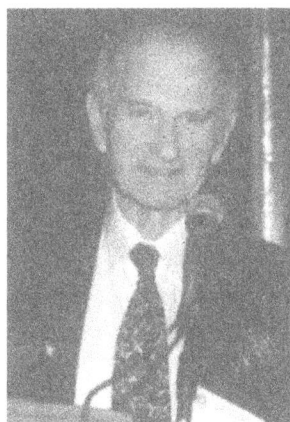

II. BIOGRAPHICAL

Joel Elkes was born in Koenigsberg, the capital of eastern Prussia on November 12, 1913. His father, a prestigious physician in nearby Lithuania, and the elected leader of the Kovno ghetto during the German occupation of the country, died in Dachau in October 1943. His mother, the daughter of a moderately prosperous grain merchant in Koenigsberg, survived the holocaust, and died in 1965 in Israel.

Joel spent his first five years in Russia. His father was a medical officer in the Russian army during the first World War and the family was traveling with him and his regiment through the vicissitudes of the Russian revolution. He was about five years old in 1918, when the family settled in Kovno, near Kalvaria, the birthplace of his father.

Joel grew up in Kovno. His parents spoke German at home, and he attended a "gymnasium" (high school) in which every subject was taught in modern Hebrew. Nevertheless, he could write in Lithuanian as a "mature poet," as one of his teachers noted (5). His school was founded by a group of idealists determined to give Jewish children a good education and prepare them for a cunstructive life in Palestine (Israel). Moshe Schwabe, the head of the school, was a professor of Greek in Germany, his native country. He was to become the rector of the Hebrew University of Jerusalem.

Joel finished high school with high honors. He excelled in literature and biology, but his favorite subject was physics. When recently asked about his early interests he mused and said: "To find out how the world is held together," and "to visualize the forces which keep it together." It was structure, particles, forces, fields, which have fascinated him all through the years (5).

After "Schwabe's Gymnasium" Joel studied in Koenigsberg for a year, to get a matriculation from a German school. It was a challenge to catch up with his peers in German literature and French language, but by the time of graduation he was at the top of his class. It was in the late 1920s, just a few years prior to Hitler's rise to power, and he was the only jew in the school.

After Koenigsberg, Joel spent four months in Lausanne, Switzerland, attending lectures at the university on elementary biology, embryology, and especially physics -which remained the center of his interest, even after he reached the decision to enter medical school. Then, in October 1930, he left Kovno for England with a letter of recommendation from the British Ambassador to Lithuania, that helped him to get admitted to study medicine at St. Mary's Hospital in London. The dean of the medical school was Sir Charles Wilson, who was to become Lord Moran (Churchill's personal physician), and the faculty included Sir Almroth Wright, who developed the typhus vaccine, Alexander Fleming, who discovered penicillin, and many others, including Aleck Bourne, eminent obstetrician, who was to become his father in-law.

In the mid-1930s Alastair Frazer, a senior lecturer in physiology, invited Joel to work with him in his laboratory. Frazer was studying the absorption of fat from the alimentary canal and was concerned with chylomicrons flooding the circulation from the thoracic duct after a fatty meal. Joel developed a microelectrophoretic cell to study the mobility of chylomicrons in an electric field. His research in physiology led to a paper on the composition of particles seen in normal human blood under ground illumination. It was published in the *Journal of Physiology* in 1939 (6), and its conclusions were incorporated by Starling in his prestigious *Principles of Human Physiology*, before he finished medical school.

In spite of his success in research, the pressures were growing and Joel, on the advice of his counselor, who was no lesser a person than John Bowlby, entered psychoanalysis. It began as a personal analysis, but continued as a training analysis which qualified him some years later for becoming a scientific associate in the Academy of Psychoanalysis (USA).

Joel also had financial difficulties. His earnings from tutoring were insufficient to support him and his sister, who had been left to his care in 1937. He had been cut off from the money he received from his father at the start of the second World War. The financial crisis was resolved with the help of Alastair Frazer, who found him a job in the newly established Transfusion Service, where he met Charmian Bourne, the daughter of his professor, who was to become his first wife.

Joel graduated from medicine in 1941, and subsequently worked as a rotating intern in orthopedic surgery, ophtalmology and internal medicine. He was enjoying clinical work and thinking of taking the necessary examinations for opening an office in London to practice medicine. This did not happen. Instead, he accepted an invitation from Alastair Frazer to join him as his research assistant. Frazer had just been appointed chairman of the Department of Pharmacology at the University of Birmingham.

On the 18th of December, 1944, Joel married Charmian Bourne, who was in general practice at the time. Their first and only child, Anna, was born on the 12th of April 1946. By that time he was in charge of a mental disease research unit in Frazer's department. To further his knowledge in psychiatry he spent about a year in the United States (as a Smith Kline and French, and Fulbright Fellow), working in Samuel Wortis' Institute at New York University, at the Pratt Diagnostic Center, and at Norwich State Hospital in Connecticut.

Upon return to Birmingham in 1951, he was appointed Head of the first Department of Experimental Psychiatry in the world. The department embodied Joel's vision of bridging basic research and clinical psychiatry. He became professor of psychiatry at a time when there were only three other chairs of psychiatry in the United Kingdom (4). The department received support from the Rockefeller Foundation and from the Medical Research Council of England. In spite of his lack of formal training in psychiatry Joel became a Charter Fellow of the Royal College of Psychiatrists of Great Britain.

In 1957 Joel moved with his family to the United States. He was invited by Seymour Kety and Robert Cohen, to set up and direct the Clinical Neuropharmacological Research Center of the National Institute of Mental Health (NIMH) at St. Elizabeths Hospital. Subsequently, from 1963 to 1974, he was Chairman of the Department of Psychiatry at Johns Hopkins University, and Director of the Phipps Psychiatric Clinic, succeeding Seymour Kety. He was elected Distinguished Service Professor at Hopkins at the time of his retirement. The end of his tenure were marred by his divorce from Charmian.

During the 1970s and 1980s Joel continued with his professional activities; first as Samuel Mc.Laughlin Professor at McMaster University (Hamilton, Ontario, Canada) and, then at the University of Louisville (Kentucky, USA). He married Josephine Rhodes, and while living in Canada he returned to painting, a long standing hobby. His summer home in Prince Edward Island, Canada, offered plenty of opportunity for this. It was also in their summer home on Prince Edward Island he completed his memoir on his father, Elkhanan Elkes (7).

While chairing departments and directing clinics and laboratories, Joel remained faithful to his long standing heritage of "Schwabe's Gymnasium." He played an important role in founding the Israel Center for Psychobiology, and developing it to become the National Institute of Psychobiology of Israel. He was Founding Director of this cooperative, inter-institutional, and deeply influential body for the support of the neurosciences and psychobiology in the country. He also served as Trustee of both, the Hebrew University of Jerusalem and Haifa University, where, in 1982, he was instrumental in convening a working conference on "Mankind 2000." Around his seventieth birthday, in 1984, an international symposium on psychopharmacology was held in his honor at the University of Louisville. Its theme, significantly, was "The Visible Brain." Visualizing by modern methods the regional neurochemistry of the brain had been Joel's preoccupation for many years. Four years later, in 1988, the Neuroscience Laboratories of the Department of Psychiatry and Behavioral Sciences at Johns Hopkins University were named after him. In 1989, together with Abba Eban, Zubin Mehta, and Senator Inouye, he received an honorary degree from the Hebrew Univesity.

On the 30th of October, 1989, Joel spoke for the first time of his father, Dr. Elkhanan Elkes to an audience in Leicester University in the UK. Also in 1989, Joel was elected Fellow and Senior Scholar of the Fetzer Institute in Kalamazoo, Michigan.

In the early 1990s Joel was still active in Louisville. In 1992, he delivered a Distinguished Psychiatrist Lecture at the Annual Meeting of the American Psychiatric Association in New Orleans (8), and in the same year, at an international meeting he was the recipient of the International Hans Selye Award.

From the mid 1990s, Joel spent summers at the Fetzer Institute in a cottage which bears his name, and the winters in his home in Sarasota (Florida) where he spends some of his time painting. Josephine died in 1999. Today, in his late eighties, Joel moves and acts, thinks and speaks like a much younger man. He is an accomplished artist. His paintings are in watercolor and charcoal.

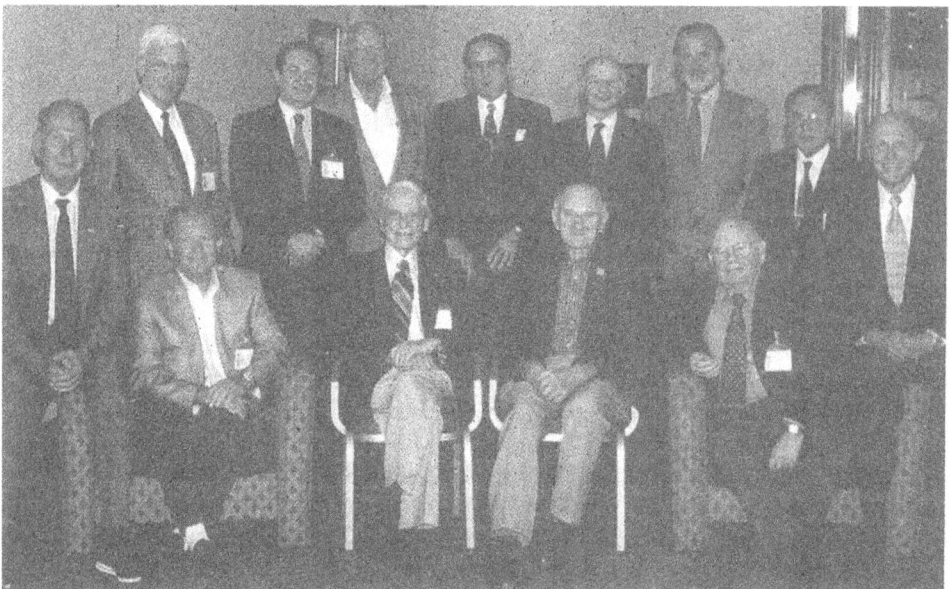

Past Presidents' and Congress Organizers' Luncheon. Tuesday, July 14, 1998. XXIth CINP Congress, Glasgow, Scotland. Front row (left to right): Leo Hollister, Julien Mendlewicz, Heinz Lehmann, Joel Elkes, Alec Coppen, William Bunney. Back row: Hanns Hippius, Giorgio Racagni, Oakley Ray, Claude de Montigny, Eugene Paykel, Gregor Laakmann, Tomoji Yanagita.

III. PROFESSIONAL ACTIVITIES

Joel Elkes' professional activities, while broad in range, have shown an inner consistency and durability over the years. Seen in retrospect, most of the themes recur and are intervowen in his writings, and are reflected in the planning of the working environments of the institutions which he founded and directed. Some ideas, while formulated early, had to await their time; others were taken up by students and collaborators and developed in new environments.

Elkes has consistently tried to maintain a transdisciplinary conversation in the groups he led. The science of which he is recognized founder – neuropsychopharmacology – made this a mandatory requirement from its earliest beginnings. For like few fields, it ranges from neurochemistry and cellular neurobiology to behavior and subjective experience, providing a conceptual link between brain, mind, behavior, and the social field; and between the neurosciences and psychiatry. He pointed out these connections, including the susceptibility of drug effects to social cues, in several papers, including the first World Health Organization (WHO) "Technical Report" that he wrote (*Ataractic and Hallucinogenic Drugs in Psychiatry*) (8). Psychopharmacology has provided him with a template, and early guideposts, to human biology, his real field of interest.

Well over 40 years passed since the publication of the WHO report, and during these years Elkes has become increasingly involved with the body's "inner pharmacy," and with the "autopharmacology" of the regulatory processes of the body. By the 1970s he felt that the neurosciences, including neurochemistry, neuroendocrinology, neuroimmunology, and cognitive psychology were ripe for quantitative inquiries into the more sparsely described states of health, wellbeing, successful coping, and personal competence; and by the 1980s he became keenly aware of the need for translation of this new knowledge for the benefit of the health professions and the general public, i.e., of the need for new educational experiments to bring this new knowledge into the mainstream of medical education and clinical practice.

Elkes' professional interests can be divided into five closely connected areas. In the following, his activities in these five areas are briefly reviewed.

III.1 Neurochemistry and psychopharmacology

Elkes began his scientific life in physical chemistry (9) and crystallography (10). With his first Ph.D. student, J. B. Finean, he was first to present, in the late 1940s, X-ray diffraction diagrams of the living myelin sheet (10, 11). This led him, by way of neuropharmacology and neurochemistry into work on the influence of drugs on electrochemical events in the brain, yielding ultimately to the field which later became known as "psychopharmacology." He tried to develop psychopharmacology with the help of devoted collegues, starting in the animal laboratory but rapidly extending into the clinic. In recognition of his activities, the "Department of Experimental Psychiatry" was created for him by the University of Birmingham in the early 1950s. It comprised experimental animal laboratories and a strong clinical arm, the "Uffculme Clinic," with an outpatient facility, a day hospital, a 40 bed unit, a patient's club, and a domiciliary visiting service (12).

It was during his "Birmingham period," that Elkes developed his concepts of the operation of regional chemical fields within the brain, and the existence of families of neuroregulatory compounds which, between them, govern and modulate states of excitation and inhibition. It was also in Birmingham that he was mapping the cholinesterases in various areas of the brain, and observing the effect of the inhibition of the cholinesterase enzyme on the emergence of various inborn reflexes (13, 14); in collaboration with Philip Bradley he studied the effects of physostigmine, atropine, hyoscyamine, amphetamine, and lysergic acid diethylamide on the electrical activity of the brain in conscious animal with the employment of a newly developed electrode technique (15); and in collaboration with Charmian Elkes, his late first wife, he was exploring the effects of amobarbital, amphetamine, and mephenesin on catatonic stupor (16). It was also with Charmian Elkes that he conducted the first blind controlled clinical trial of chlorpromazine in chronic psychotic patients (17).

Elkes' research in the Department of Experimental Psychiatry attracted attention in the United States and, as indicated before, in 1957 he was invited to the United States to create NIMH's Clinical Neuropharmacology Research Center (CNRC) in the William A. White Building at St. Elizabeths Hospital. By the late 1950s research in the CNRC ranged from the micropipette studies of Salmoiraghi and Bloom, the early dopamine studies of Weil-Malherbe, and the tryptamine studies of Szara, to the clinical drug trials of Freyhan, Hordern and Lofft. Within a period of merely six years Elkes succeeded in contributing to NIMH's influential, intramural research program in neuroscience.

Elkes was also active in developing the necessary means for communication in the new field, i.e., platforms (meetings) and organs (journals). As early as in the mid-1950s he organized, in collaboration with Drs. S. Kety, H. Waelsch, J. Folch, D. Richter and G.W. Harris, the first International Neurochemical Symposium in Oxford, followed by a symposium on regional neurochemistry. In 1957 he was the convener of the first working group of the World Health Organization (WHO) on psychotropic drugs, and represented neuropharmacology, together with the Nobel Laureate, Daniel Bovet, at the founding meeting of the International Brain Research Organization (IBRO). He also participated in 1960 in the writing of the constitution of IBRO; in the organization of the first congress of the Collegium Internationale Neuro-Psychopharmacologicum (CINP); and in the founding of the American College of Neuropsychopharmacology (ACNP). In his memorable lecture as Founding President of the ACNP he defined the place of neuropsychopharmacology and gave an identity to the "new science" by saying:

"It is not uncommon for any one of us to be told that Psychopharmacology is not a science, and that it would do well to emulate the precision of older and more established disciplines. Such statements betray a lack of understanding for the special demands made by Psychopharmacology upon the fields which compound it. For my own part, I draw comfort and firm conviction from the history of our group. For I know of no other branch of science which, like a good plough on a spring day, has tilled as many areas in neurobiology. To have, in a mere decade, questioned the concept of synaptic transmission in the central nervous system; to have emphasized compartmentalization and regionalization of chemical process in the unit cell and in the brain; to have focussed on the interaction of hormone and chemical process within the brain; to have given us tools for the study of the chemical basis of learning and temporary connection formation; to have emphasized the dependence of pharmacological response on its situational and social setting; to have compelled a hard look at the semantics of psychiatric diagnosis, description and communication; to have resuscitated that oldest of old remedies, the placebo response, for careful scrutiny; to have provided potential methods for the study of language in relation to the functional state of the brain; and to have encouraged the Biochemist, Physiologist, Psychologist, Clinician, and the Mathematician and Communication Engineer to join forces at bench level, is no mean achievement for a young science. That a chemical text should carry the imprint of experience, and partake in its growth, in no way invalidates study of symbols, and the rules among symbols, which keep us going, changing, evolving, and human. Thus, though moving cautiously, psycho~pharmacology is still protesting; yet in so doing it is, for the first time, compelling the physical and chemical sciences to look behavior in the face, and thus enriching both these sciences and behavior. If there be discomfiture in this encounter, it is hardly surprising; for it is in this discomfiture that there may well lie the germ of a new science." (See full text in Part One, Chapter 4).

An annual international award for distinguished work in psychopharmacology carries his name in the college.

Elkes was one of the founding editors of two major journals: *Psychopharmacologia* (now *Journal of Psychopharmacology*), and *Journal of Psychiatric Research.*

In the early 1960s he wrote the section on "Behavioral Pharmacology in Relation to Psychiatry" for Springer's International Handbook of Psychiatry. (See full text in Part Four, Chapter 15.) In this much quoted paper Elkes argues that pharmacology has the role of a conduit to psychobiology, an attitude he later also reflected in his closing chapter of Clark and del Giudice's Principles of Psychopharmacology. (See full text in Part Six, Chapter 17.)

In 1963 Elkes moved from the NIMH to Johns Hopkins University to become Chairman of the Department of Psychiatry. As Psychiatrist-in-Chief, and Henry Phipps Professor of Psychiatry, he supported his residents and fellows to develop the necessary skills to further experimental and clinical neuropsychopharmacologic research; and as Chairman of the department, he created research laboratories in psychopharmacology, neuroendocrinology, behavioral medicine, and in the clinical sciences.

III.2 Clinical psychiatry and behavioral medicine

Elkes believes that modern psychiatry provides a natural bridge between the behavioral sciences and medicine as a whole, including preventive medicine, and to facilitate the use of this natural bridge he changed the name of his department at Johns Hopkins from "Psychiatry" to "Psychiatry and Behavioral Sciences." It was one of the first, if not the first departments so to change its name in the world. The behavioral sciences thus represented a counterpoint to his interests in the neurosciences and neurobiology. What later was to become known as "behavioral medicine" grew at Hopkins under his direction as an organic continuation through the work of Curt Richter, Horsley Gantt and Jerome Frank in the great tradition in psychobiology, pioneered by Adolf Meyer. During his tenure at Johns Hopkins Elkes developed a program, rather than a center for "Behavioral Medicine." He also founded the first society for "Biofeedback and Self Regulation" in the USA.

To continue and expand what he started at Johns Hopkins, he developed at McMaster, a major program of "Brain and Behavior," and a "Division of Behavioral Medicine." He did the same in Louisville where he created with his second wife, Josephine Rhodes and some other colleagues, the Genesis Center for the management of chronic illness. He served as director of the program which was engaged in research on the effect of group counseling in chronic disease, particularly in rheumatoid arthritis, pain and cancer.

III.3 Study of subjective phenomena: the role of language in psychiatry

Elkes has had a central interest in the subject of personal awareness and the transforms of mental life, including the play of phantasy and imagination in daily living. The concepts of psychopharmacology led him to source, to physiology to the way the brain "does it naturally," without the aid of chemical prostheses. Awareness, self-observation, focussing on inner speech, became to him a valid area of inquiry. As a student he was deeply interested in states of consciousness, meditation, autoregulation, and also in the interaction of mental events with muscle activity, and bodily function. These subjects led him to an interest in the limitations of language in the description of subjective, behaviorally silent states of mind.

When invited to speak on psychopharmacology in his Harvey Lecture, delivered in 1961, he chose instead to speak on "Subjective and Objective Observations in Psychiatry" and the role of language in the description of subjective phenomena. (See full text in Part Eight, Chapter 24). He spoke in his presentation on the serial and parallel processing of information by the brain. He also argued for the establishment of "Inner Space Laboratories." Similarly, he examined information processing in relation to levels of neuronal organization in schizophrenia. (See full text in Part Five, Chapter 16). In his Salmon Lectures, delivered in 1963 he spoke on "Chemistry, Awareness, and the Imagination." (See abstracts in Part Eight, Chapters 22 and 23). And in his Bronowski Memorial Lecture, delivered in 1978, he examined the role of "Awareness" in daily life. (See Part Eight, Chapter 25). Elkes regards the day as an opportunity for experiment and the body/mind as an ever present portable laboratory, accessible to anyone who wishes to use it. Such ideas may seem a litte strange within the traditional medical framework; yet, there is a mounting body of evidence connecting imagery and states of consciousness with somatic function. He believes that the methods for somatic, (including biochemical and immunological) monitoring of mental events have now reached a degree of refinement compatible with good experimental design.

III.4 Social psychiatry and community planning

Stimulated by "The Peckham Experiment," an experimental health center in a working-class neighborhood in London in the late 1930s. (See more details in Part Nine, Chapter 27), Elkes organized his early treatment center, the Uffculme Clinic, housed in the former Cadbury Mansion in Birmingham, in a manner which provided a prototype of his idea of a comprehensive psychiatric care facility. He tried to develop the same model when he moved to the United States. At the same time he also emphasized the use of mental health principles in community planning. This found expression for the first time in 1966, in a comprehensive plan submitted to the Secretary of Health of Maryland, on the application of behavioral sciences to the planning of neighborhoods. The concept of a "healing community," he formulated in this document won him a citation from the Governor of the State.

To meet the needs of "behavioral medicine" Elkes' first wife, Charmian embarked upon a training program for "mature woman." The "Phipps Ladies," as the trainees became known, were rigorously selected for their stability, maturity, empathy, and interpersonal skills.

When an opportunity arose for the planning of a completely new city, Columbia, Maryland, by the Rouse Company, Elkes was instrumental in designing and creating a prepaid, low-fee mental health service, functioning alongside the major primary care specialties – medicine, pediatrics, and obstetrics and gynecology. (See more details in Part Nine, Chapters

28 and 29). While serving on the advisory council for the planning of the new city, he developed, in collaboration with colleagues, a survey of human resources for the community.

In the same vein, at the University of Louisville, Elkes created the "Wellness Forum," a community resource dedicated to educating the corporate sector, the professions, and the public in matters of "health maintenance," "health enhancement," and "self care." It was a consortium, sponsored by the county medical society, the university, the chamber of commerce, and other civic organizations, to promote the concepts of preventive health care, and long term health research in the community. As the honorary president of the forum, and a member of the health advisory council of the State, Elkes was actively engaged in furthering the cause of a State funded center for health promotion and disease prevention in Kentucky during the 1980s.

III.5 Humanizing medical education: the behavioral sciences in the service of medicine

All through his professional life Elkes has had an abiding interest in what is conventionally referred to as the "mind/body connection," and in the emerging concepts of psychosomatic medicine. He acted on his convictions by reading widely in the field and getting personal exposure to the phenomena of yoga, relaxation, meditation, and imagery. While engaged in his studies in physical chemistry, he was impressed by the restorative powers of these techniques, and incorporated some very elementary exercises in his daily life during the stressful years of the second World War.

Elkes has also been interested in Hans Selye's concept of "stress" since the time of its inception in the late 1930s. He knew Selye, and assisted him in founding both, his International and American Stress Institute. He was founding president of the latter.

Elkes was trying to incorporate some concepts and techniques of stress management into the practice of his clinics, and the education of his students, in Birmingham; however, the first real opportunity to do so presented itself at Johns Hopkins, where he succeeded in introducing an "introductory course in behavioral sciences" for medical students. The core message of the course was to connect the behavioral sciences to medicine as a whole, i.e., not merely to psychiatry, and provide each student an opportunity to meet him/herself, and use his/her own "body/mind" thoughtfully in daily living. (See more details in Part Seven, Chapter 19). The course was built around theories of Human Development, Human Learning, Human Communication, and the operation of the "Social Field." A common thread running through the course was "behavioral biology," and some emerging concepts of regional chemical regulation (and self regulation) of the brain. The course was one of the first attempts to make sense of the biological origins and correlates of symbolic life, and to convey to the student a deep respect for personal awareness, self observation, and the realities of "psychobiology."

Elkes' experience at Hopkins made him aware of the great stresses undergone by students in the course of their training, and when the opportunity at the University of Louisville arose, he created in collaboration with Leah Dickstein a "Health Awareness Program" for incoming medical students. The objective of the program was the correction of the lack of training in preventive medicine, and of the inattention-by-default to the personal wellbeing of students in medical institutions. The program was based on the assumption that "other-care" is best begun with "self-care;" and that "awareness of self and others" is at the very heart of humane medical practice; and on the belief that if awareness is coupled with training in simple life skills and lifestyle principles – all based on common sense; it may go some way to help future physicians cultivate the same skills in their patients.

The "connection course" was another elective he introduced. It was a collaborative effort between the Division of Attitudinal and Behavioral Medicine and the Department of Family Practice at the University of Louisville. The purpose of the course was to focus attention on the reality of mind/body interaction in the practice of medicine. The course was centered on chronic illness, and involved visits to patients' homes.

Elkes succeeded also in introducing a Program in the arts in medicine. He observed that arts can reach areas of emotional life inaccessible to traditional approaches; recognised that they can move beneath and beyond words; and believed that art therapies, at their best, are deeply restorative and healing. The implementation of this program was part of his overall effort to humanize medical education. His aim was to bring about a meeting of two cultures – the culture of the arts and of the medical sciences. (See more details in Part Twelve.)

Finally, before leaving almost six decades of professional activities, Elkes developed a proposal for the creation of a center for comprehensive medicine and health enhancement which, by widening the concept of health to include mental, social and spiritual well-being, would create a climate that could play a significant part in changing the prevailing culture of medical institutions.

IV. IMPACT THROUGH TRAINING OF PROFESSIONALS

The impact of Elkes' professional activities on the development of neuropsychopharmacology through training of professionals is unparalleled. The list of the people who passed through his laboratories reads like a Who's Who of American Psychopharmacology (4). At the University of Birmingham he drew together a cohort of researchers, including Philip Bradley, Brian Key, Michael Chance, Charmian Elkes, and Willy Mayer-Gross, with seminal contributions to the establishment of the field. At the NIMH in Washington he started with a secretary (Anne Gibson) and by the time he left for Johns Hopkins he had a large staff of prominent researchers and clinicians including Floyd Bloom, Max Hamilton, Eliot Hearst, Anthony Hordern, John Lofft, Richard Michael, Shepherd Kellam, G.C. Salmoiraghi, Steven Szara, Neil Waldrop, Hans Weil-Malherbe, Harold Weiner, and many others (9). And while he was chairman at Johns Hopkins, Solomon Snyder began with his pathbreaking neurochemical studies while still a resident in psychiatry, Joe Brady built primate-laboratories for his far-reaching program in behavioral biology, Ross Baldessarini began with his career in clinical psychopharmacology, and "Uhli" Uhlenhuth, Lino Covi, and Len Derogatis developed their rating scales and engaged in important outpatient studies.

During his working years Elkes has contributed to the development of some 35 to 40 investigators who have assumed prominent, and in some instances leading positions. The span of activities of these investigators has been wide, ranging from cellular biology (Floyd Bloom and Solomon Snyder), clinical psychiatry and psychology (Freyhan, Kellam and Weingartner), clinical psychopharmacology (Baldessarini and Van Kammen), to the study of the states of consciousness (Stanislav Grof). Among Elkes' former associates there are two past presidents of the prestigious Society of Neuroscience (Bloom and Snyder), three deans of medical schools (De Vaul, Freeman and Knorr), and some fourteen chairman and/or institute and program directors, including the chairman of psychiatry at Harvard (Coyle), and the director of Research of the Mayo Clinic at Jacksonville (Richelson).

V. THE CONTENT OF THIS BOOK

This book reflects an attitude to Psychopharmacology. Its content is not restricted to a collection of Joel Elkes' papers in neuropsychopharmacology, but includes also his contributions to other areas in the behavioral sciences and some of his personal reflections.

Joel Elkes connects. His interests range wide – from the molecular building blocks of the brain to social behavior. In each area his inquisitive spirit poses questions; questions which he continues to ask even if answers are not readily forthcoming.

It is the intention of this editor to present Joel Elkes, the man. It took long arguments into the night to convince him to allow the inclusion of non-technical material, and his Art. For that reason, the material is, at times, repetitious, and references are missing. However, all relevant references are comprised in the papers quoted.

REFERENCES

1. De Montigny, C (1998) The CINP-Pfizer Pioneer in Neuropsychopharmacology Award. CINP Newsletter, Fall: 3-4
2. Elkes J (1952) Discussion. In JM Tanner (ed.) Prospects in Psychiatric Research (pp. 126-135). Oxford, Blackwell Publications
3. Elkes J (1966) Introduction to Section IV Psychopharmacology. In M Rinkel (ed.) Biological Treatment of Mental Illness (pp. 437-439). New York, L.C. Page & Co., Division of Farrar, Straus and Giroux
4. Healy D (1998) Pioneers in Psychopharmacology. International Journal of Neuropsychopharmacology 1: 191-194
5. Ban TA (1999) Interview with Joel Elkes. (Unpublished)
6. Elkes J, Frazer AC, Stewart HC (1939) The composition of particles seen in normal human blood under ground illumination. J Physiol (London) 95: 68
7. Elkes J (1989) Dr. Elkhanan Elkes of the Kovno Ghetto. A Son's Holocaust Memoir. Brewster (Mass.), The Paraclete Press
8. World Health Organization (1958) Ataractic and Hallucinogenic Drugs in Psychiatry. WHO Technical Report No. 152. Geneva, WHO
9. Elkes J (1970) Psychopharmacology: On beginning of a new science. In FJ Ayd, B Blackwell (eds.) Discoveries in Biological Psychiatry (pp. 30-52). Philadelphia/Toronto, J.B. Lippincott Company
10. Elkes J, Finean JB (1953) X-ray diffraction studies on the effect of temperature on the structure of myelin on the sciatic nerve of the frog. Experimental Cell Research 4: 69-81
11. Elkes J, Finean JB (1953) Effects of solvents on the structure of myelin in the sciatic nerve of the frog. Experimental Cell Research 4: 82-95
12. Elkes J (1955) The Department of Experimental Psychiatry. The University of Birmingham Gazette, 11 March
13. Elkes J, Todrick A (1955) On the development of the cholinesterases in the rat brain. In H Waelsch (ed.) Biochemistry of the Developing Nervous System. New York, Academic Press
14. Elkes J, Eayrs JT, Todrick A (1955) On the effect and the lack of effect of some drugs on postnatal development in the rat. In Waelsch (ed.) Biochemistry of the Developing Nervous System. New York, Academic Press
15. Bradley PB, Elkes J (1957) The effects of some drugs on the electrical activity of the brain. Brain 80: 77-117
16. Elkes J, Elkes C, Bradley PB (1954) The effects of some drugs on the electrical activity of the brain and behaviour. J. Ment. Sci 100: 125-128
17. Elkes J, Elkes C (1954) The effect of chlorpromazine on the behaviour of chronically overactive psychotic patients. British Medical Journal II: 560-576

Thomas A. Ban
Editor

INTRODUCTION

I am honored to be part of this work and to have the opportunity to express my sincere appreciation for the marvelous series of inspirational achievements that characterize the careers of Joel Elkes. My first meeting with him arose unexpectedly when I was invited to NIH to compete for a two year opportunity to be a Research Associate. A not-to-be denied side benefit of that job was that it came with a commission in the US Public Health Service and the ability to satisfy my Medical Selective Service obligation while learning how to do research.

Being called for interviews was already a sign that some of the studies I had done as a student were seen as suggesting potential, and I was very optimistic. However, when I got my interview schedule, prominently absent was the one person, my MD Thesis Advisor, Gordon Schoepfle, who, I felt, was most likely to take me. Fortunately for me, Robert Berliner then Director of Intramural Research, suggested I might want to take a taxi ride over to St. Elizabeth's Hospital where the NIMH had only recently installed a new enterprise called the Clinical Neuropharmacology Research Center (CNRC) in the infamous Wiiliam A. White Building (where prefrontal lobotomies were once performed). I did, and it changed the course of my future life.

The CNRC was organized with the main offices on the 5th floor and all the laboratories 6 levels below in the basement. G. C. (Nino) Salmoiraghi, who eventually was to be my friend, mentor, and training boss, was busily engaged in making intracellular recordings from neurons in the cat medulla and determining the effects of nearby intra-arterially injected cholinergic drugs on their firing rate. Around his laboratories were a biochemistry laboratory (headed by Hans Weil-Malherbe) trying to understand how the brain reacted to elevations in plasma ammonia in hepatic coma, a psychopharmacology laboratory (headed by Steve Szara) trying to determine how different hallucinogens worked, and a behavioral unit (headed by Elliot Hearst). The three occupied floors in between had become active research wards.

The reason for this mixed environment became clear when I was taken back to the top floor to meet Joel Elkes. When I sat beside his large desk to lay out my reprints and some recent data, Joel was busily engaged in cleaning and refilling what I thought must be the smallest pipe in the world. His excitement for my student's thesis work soon made me feel the trip to St. Elizabeths was going to be a wise decision. It turned out that Joel was well steeped in "axonology" although from a structural viewpoint rather than from an electrophysiological one. His interest had been to apply physical imaging methods like X-ray diffraction to try to define the physicochemical nature of myelin long before the structure was defined chemically or by electron microscopy. He thought that my data, which dealt with dynamic changes in ion potential and the actions of drugs on these processes, could be usefully carried into the central nervous system. He explained the theories that he and Seymour Key were promulgating of "regional neurochemistry", and that the things that mattered in the brain were lost when it was homogenized, and could only be understood in terms of what went on in discrete functional regions.

Joel has frequently stated that his and Kety's goals in setting up the CNRC were to try to integrate all those skills and research disciplines into the brain of individual researchers. In that way, he hoped that future scientists with this style of analysis would think not in terms of only biochemistry, or electrophysiology, or anatomy or behavior. Instead they could become "trans-disciplinarians" who would understand the value of their work for those other fields of investigation.

Needless to say, I left there pretty excited about what I might be able to learn, and was elated (and relieved) a few days later when I was notified that I would be accepted as a Research Associate in Nino Salmoiraghi's Section on Neurophysiology, beginning in July 1962.

During my first two years there, I recall most vividly Joel's lightening-like forays through the basement laboratories, usually with a guest scientist in tow, showing off what wonderful things we were all learning. My two very productive years there included a great deal of modern neuropharmacology learned at the elbow of Mimo Costa who spent more than half of his time helping Salmoiraghi and I characterize responses as real by using drugs known to block each of their receptors. Time went by quickly.

It never really occurred to me then just how significant that two year post in the basement of St. Elizabeths turned out to be. For one thing, the sheer transparency of the multidisciplinary attack on the brain's secrets was never really questioned. However, the scale of interaction was very macro. My desire to understand where, at the synaptic level, these neurotransmitters were located (so as to be better able to know where to point the pipettes) led me to abandon internal medicine for histochemistry the year after the Swedes invented fluorescence histochemistry. When I came back a third time in 1968, Joel had begun his era at Hopkins; NIMH had become its own Bureau, and the St. Elizabeths operations were now a major Division of the NIMH Intramural Program, which Nino headed. Our Laboratory of Neuropharmacology was treated to be inherently interdisciplinary and none of us has really ever questioned the world in which we were allowed to see this future.

One of the highlights of renewing friendships with Joel frequently over the next several years has been how many mutual activities and colleagues we continue to share, from ACNP to Jonas Salk, from neuroscience to psychopharmacology, from training to educating, and always he has inspired me with his eloquence, his creativity, and his undying curiosity. This collected volume of selected examples will certainly be an inspiration to all those who know and love this remarkable person.

Floyd E. Bloom

INTRODUCTION

The papers reprinted in this volume represent a selection of the publications of Joel Elkes, who is one of the founders of Psychopharmacology. They fall, roughly, into two main groups which can be related to the two principal periods of his career, that spent in the U.K. and latterly in the United States. The message, however, is the same throughout, as the reader will discover.

Joel Elkes was born in Koenigsberg, East Prussia. His father, a distinguished physician in Lithuania, who served in the Russian army in the First World war, died in Dachau concentration camp, while his mother, Miriam survived the holocaust and moved to Israel after the Second World war. Joel was educated in Lithuania and Switzerland. He came to England in 1931 and studied medicine at St. Mary's Hospital, London. He moved to Birmingham in 1941 to join his friend, Alastair Frazer, in the Department of Pharmacology.

I first met Joel in the summer 1949. I had recently graduated and was looking for interesting work, preferably with a research element, when I heard that someone in the Pharmacology Department at Birmingham University was looking for a research student. A visit to Birmingham led to the offer of a post which I accepted and, after attending a short course in electroencephalography at the Burden Neurological Institute in Bristol, I moved to Birmingham and started work. These were exciting times. I soon discovered that Joel's interests extended into a number of basic disciplines in the neurosciences, as well as my own area of electrophysiology and neuropharmacology. In the early 1950s, new drugs acting on the brain were being discovered and we received one of the first samples of chlorpromazine (Largactil) for both experimental and clinical investigations.

In 1950, Joel was awarded a Fulbright Fellowship to study in the United States. On his return to Birmingham in 1951 the university created a new department of Experimental Psychiatry for him, including experimental animal laboratories and a strong clinical section comprising an outpatient clinic, a day hospital and a forty-bed unit, together with ancillary services. I was invited to join this new department and to take charge of the experimental laboratories.

Everything seemed to be going well and generous funding was being provided by sources on both sides of the Atlantic when, in 1957, Joel decided to accept an offer to head a new Clinical Neuropharmacology Research Center at St. Elizabeth's Hospital in Washington. While it cannot be denied that Joel's sudden departure was severe blow to those of us who remained in Birmingham, we survived and ultimately two departments (pharmacology and psychiatry) emerged.

Between 1963 and 1975, Joel was professor of Psychiatry and Behavioral Sciences at the John Hopkins University, Baltimore. When he retired he moved to McMaster University in Canada where he helped to create a psychopharmacology programme. Subsequently he moved to Louisville where with his wife J. Rhodes he founded the Genesis Centre for the management of chronic illness. He is currently a Fellow of the Fetzer Institute, Kalamazoo.

Joel Elkes has received many awards and honours. He is a Life Fellow of the American Psychiatric Association and of the American College of Neuropsychopharmacology. He is also a Fellow of the American Academy of Arts and Sciences. He is a Founding Fellow and Senior Scholar-in-Residence of the Fetzer Institute. Although not present at the Founding Meeting of the International Collegium of Neuro-Psychopharmacology in 1957, his help and guidance in its birth was considerable and in 1998 he was awarded the Pioneer Award.

Joel Elkes' many former students and associates, some of whom now occupy senior positions will, I feel sure, wish him and this book every success.

Philip B. Bradley

Part One

OVERVIEWS

PAPERS

1. J. Elkes: *Towards footings of a science: Personal beginnings in psychopharmacology in the forties and fifties.*
   Reprinted with the kind permission of the Collegium Internationale Neuro-Psychopharmacologicum from T.A. Ban, D. Healy, E. Shorter (eds.) *The Rise of Psychopharmacology and The Story of CINP* (pp. 15-25). Budapest, Animula, 1998
2. J. Elkes: *The Department of Experimental Psychiatry.*
   Reprinted with the kind permission of The University of Birmingham from the *University of Birmingham Gazette,* 11th March, 1955
3. J. Elkes: *Psychopharmacology: Finding one's way.*
   Based on invited lecture delivered at the Annual Meeting of the American College of Neuropsychopharmacology.
   Reprinted with the kind permission of Elsevier Science from *Neuropsychopharmacology* 12: 93-111, 1995
4. J. Elkes: *The American College of Neuropsychopharmacology: A note on its history and hopes for the future.*
   Reprinted with the kind permission of The American College of Neuropsychopharmacology from the *ACNP Bulletin* 1: 2-3, 1962

CONTEXT

The program on "Drugs and the Mind" developed in the Department of Pharmacology, University of Birmingham (England) between 1947 and 1951, i.e., before the advent of the major tranquilizers. It received recognition by the University as an independent Department – the Department of Experimental Psychiatry – in 1951. This was the first Department of its kind in the world.

Areas in neurochemistry, electrophysiology, animal behavior, and the clinical experiment and clinical trial were all represented in the small group in Birmingham. Slowly, these areas emerged as the footings of a new science, which, at that time had no name.

The first two papers outline the genesis of the program in Birmingham, and the development of laboratory studies and clinical facilities. Paper 1 (1996) gives a retrospective overview. Paper 2 (1955) was written for a general audience.

Paper 3 (1995), an invited address to the American College of Neuropsychopharmcology in 1994, records the above and later developments as they shaped in the United States at the National Institute of Mental Health/St. Elizabeths Center and at Johns Hopkins University. It also refers to national (US) and international responses, as the work proceeded.

Paper 4 (1962) summarizes Elkes' address at the end of his tenure as first President of the American College of Neuropsychopharmacology. The reader may wish to note the concluding comments in the last two paragraphs.

PAPER 1

TOWARDS FOOTINGS OF SCIENCE: PERSONAL BEGINNINGS IN PSYCHOPHARMACOLOGY IN THE FORTIES AND FIFTIES

Joel Elkes

Reprinted with the kind permission of the Collegium Internationale Neuro-Psychopharmacologicum from T.A. Ban, D. Healy, E. Shorter (eds.) *The Rise of Psychopharmacology and The Story of CINP* (pp. 15-25). Budapest, Animula, 1998

A PROGRAM ON "DRUGS AND THE MIND" – EXPERIMENTAL PSYCHIATRY IN BIRMINGHAM, ENGLAND

The inverted telescope of recollection is apt to diminish and obscure persons and events. However, in this instance, they remain clear, distinct, and warming to recall. I have referred to them more extensively in a recent invited address (1). It also carries a fuller bibliography.

The dialectic between Psychiatry and Molecules began quite early in my life. As a medical student at St. Mary's Hospital, London, in the thirties, I was deeply attracted to psychiatry. However, the excellent lectures and demonstrations in the local mental hospital left me bewildered, curious and hungry, and groping for a physiology and chemistry which at the time did not exist. Immunology was very strong at St. Mary's (where, some ten years later, Fleming discovered penicillin). So, one read wildly in immunology, particularly on Paul Ehrlich's ideas about cell surfaces, receptor configuration, specificity, side-chains ("Seitenketten") and the like. Soon, the lipoprotein structure of cell membranes became a consuming interest. I spent two gorgeous summers in the Department of Colloid Science at Cambridge under Sir Eric Rideal, spreading monomolecular films and reading on crystallography. Getting into microstructures (membranes, organelles) became a persistent visual game. I did not know it then, but I was heading into pharmacology.

The opportunity came in 1941, when I accompanied my erstwhile chief and friend Alastair Frazer to Birmingham to help him found what, in retrospect, was to become a major department of pharmacology. Psychiatry was always beckoning in the background: but in those days, there were few bridges leading from cell biology to psychiatry, and it was not easy to convince university authorities that "Mental Disease Research" (as it was called) was a worthwhile enterprise. The leading laboratories were small, not very well equipped, and usually functioned outside universities, being mostly supported by local hospital boards. Yet, in retrospect, I was most fortunate. In Birmingham, I found acceptance of my interest in the chemistry of the brain and, more importantly, while teaching conventional pharmacology I was allowed to stray. My colleagues and I strayed into the study of the cholinesterases, and the very powerful and specific anticholinesterases. We began mapping the distribution of these enzymes in the brain noting their unevenness in the hope of finding a clue to the action of hypnotics. I was also fortunate in another respect. Tracking back to my days in physical chemistry, Bryan Finean (as my first PhD student) engaged in X-ray diffraction studies of living myelin, demonstrating clearly its ordered lamellar, paracrystalline structure (2). After two years of work in this field I found myself anchored. Neurochemistry extended its powerful pull, with psychiatry moving ever closer. At about this time (1945), another pivotal event took place. A small unit of "Mental Disease Research," loosely administered from the Dean's Office, became available. It fell under the aegis of the Department of Pharmacology, through the retirement of its director, Dr. A. Pickworth. I was put in charge of two rooms in the medical school. There was also some seed money. An enormous step in my life had been taken; I knew I was in biological psychiatry for good.

I began to read avidly, to train myself by seeing patients in the local mental hospital (the Winson Green Mental Hospital), and to familiarize myself with the drug treatments then available. The old reliable triad – bromine, chloral hydrate, and the barbiturates – was ever present, and the anti-epileptic drugs were coming into their own at the periphery. There was, of course, also insulin coma and ECT. Vast questions beckoned everywhere: I felt like a naturalist advancing into a strange continent. Deeply moved by what I saw and heard in the ward, I found myself discussing my bewilderment with Charmian, my late first wife, who was in general practice at the time. We talked into the night, pulled by the same curiosity. One day, after a meeting in London, we came upon reports on the effects of drugs on catatonic schizophrenic stupor. The syndrome was not uncommon in our mental hospital, and we were struck by the combination of mask-like rigidity, withdrawal, and cyanosis of the limbs. Quietly, Charmian suggested that we plan a study.

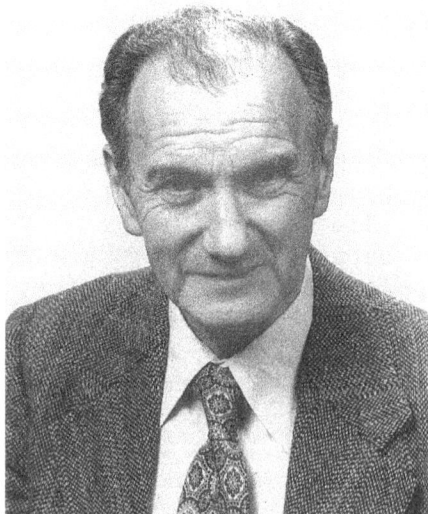

Joel Elkes

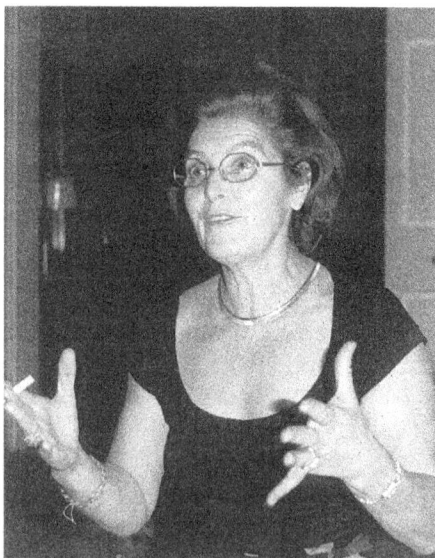

Charmian Elkes

When we proposed this to Dr. J.J. O'Reilly, superintendent at Winson Green Mental Hospital (The Birmingham City Mental Hospital – now All Saints Hospital), he readily agreed and remained our supporter and friend in years to come.

Dr. O'Reilly put a small research room at our disposal and allowed us to choose patients, using our criteria; he also gave us nursing help. We used homemade gadgetry to measure "muscle tone" (i.e., rigidity) and foot temperature by thermocouple, and we also developed our own rating scales to measure change. The study taught us the enormous value of working in a real mental hospital setting. Sodium amytal, administered in full hypnotic doses intravenously, led to a paradoxical awakening of patients from catatonic stupor. a relaxation of muscle tone, and a rise in foot temperature. The effect of amphetamine was equally paradoxical. It led to the deepening of the stupor, an increase in muscle rigidity, and a deepening cyanosis. We also tried mephenesin, which had been shown by Frank Berger to be a powerful spinal internuncial neuron blocking agent and, through his prescient insights, later led to meprobamate and the whole family of anxiolytics. When tested in catatonic schizophrenic stupor, mephenesin produced marked muscle relaxation. There was, however, little effect on psychomotor response or peripheral temperature. The ability of patients to draw – for ten minutes, without prompting – while under the influence of drugs proved particularly interesting. Amytal markedly increased this ability, and amphetamine inhibited it. The experiments which we reported later (3) thus suggested *selectivity* in the action of drugs on catatonic stupor and raised the question of the relation of hyperarousal to catatonic withdrawal and, possibly, schizophrenia. Most important, however, these experiments established – at a tangible and a conceptual level – the need of working in parallel. The laboratory and the ward became ends of a continuum of related activities. I began to think of this continuum as *experimental psychiatry.*

At that time, then, there were two anchoring points for our work: neurochemistry, at the bench level, and human behaviour, as influenced by drugs. There was nothing in between, no indicator that could relate the effects of drugs on the brain to behaviour. I began to hunt again. The EEG was at that time coming into its own. Hill and Pond were publishing on the dysrhythmias, and Grey Walter and Gastaut were, in their own idiom, trying to relate functional states in man to EEG activity. And across the water there beckoned the great papers of Herbert Jasper and Wilder Penfield. I plumbed for the effect of drugs on, the electrical activity of the brain in the conscious animal. There were very few data available in those days – except, a little later, those of Abraham Wikler and of James Toman's review (4). I obviously could not do it alone, and again, I was in the market for an associate.

I cannot recall now who told Philip Bradley about me or me about Philip Bradley, but I remember clearly his coming to my office and telling me of his experience and his interests. He had been trained in zoology and had carried out microelectrode studies in insects. He seemed interested in the problem, and a salary was available. So, after some consultation with Dr. Grey Walter, arrangements were made for him to spend some time with Walter to learn EEG techniques

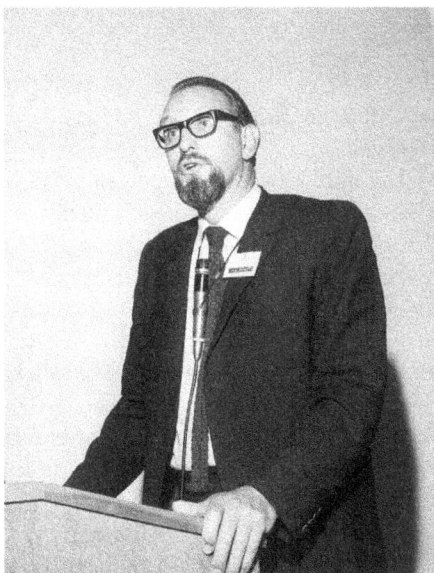

Philip B. Bradley

and then set up his own laboratory in the second of the two rooms of "Mental Diseases Research." This was duly done, and in 1949, Philip was working alongside us, developing his pioneering technique for recording electrical activity in conscious cats, a procedure that in those days (the days of sulfonamides – *not* penicillin) was quite a trick. The work proceeded well, and quickly established reference points for a pharmacology of the brain, inasmuch as it relates to behaviour. I still treasure a copy of Philip's thesis completed in October 1952 (5). It was a joy to see the clear and unambiguous effects of physostigmine, atropine, hyoscyamine, and amphetamine (and later, LSD-25) on the electrical activity of the brain in relation to behaviour. It was also particularly satisfying to find how these drugs grouped themselves in terms of their dependence on midbrain structures, and how information arriving at that time from Morruzzi and Magoun's (6) studies could be related to our own findings. There gradually emerged (and this was my own view) a concept of the presence of *families* of compounds that had arisen in the brain, in the course of chemical evolution. These compounds seemed chemically related to powerful neurohumoral transmitters familiar to us at the periphery. Three types of receptors, centering around members of the cholinester, the catecholamine, and later the indole family, were proposed (7, 8). Implicit in this concept of families of compounds was the notion of small regional *chemical fields* and of the interaction between molecules governing the gating, storage, and flow of information in self-exciting neural loops.

As we wrote at the time (9):

> It is likely that neurons possessing slight but definite difference in enzyme constitution may be unevenly distributed in topographically close, or widely separated areas in the central nervous system: these differences probably extend to the finest level of histological organization... It would perhaps be permissible to speak of the operation of chemical fields in these regions. The agents in question may be either identical with or, more likely, derived from neuro-effector substances familiar to us at the periphery. Their number is probably small, but their influence upon integrative action of higher nervous activity may be profound. The basic states of consciousness may well be determined by variations in the local concentration of these agents.

It gives me special satisfaction to reflect on Philip Bradley's subsequent illustrious career and the influence he has exerted on the course of Neuropsychopharmacology in Europe and the world.

The third area to occupy us in those years concerned hallucinogenic drugs, which, from time to time, had been noted in literature. We began to read about them and formed a small discussion group to explore the possible relation of endogenously-produced hallucinogenic metabolites to schizophrenia. Hofmann's historic report to Stoll was written on April 22, 1943, and Stoll's paper on LSD-25 appeared in 1947 (10). We were immediately struck by the very low dose level, suggesting a specificity of very high order. Our own work in cats and a small number of human volunteers (of whom I was the first), using a single small dose (half a microgram per kilo) led us to conclude, later, that LSD-25 was acting on a serotonin-mediated receptor, peculiarly related to the afferent system (possibly the medial collaterals) (8) and exerting a selective inhibitory role on the organisation of sensory information and the serial organisation of information in time.

Thus, by about 1949-1950, three elements were in place in our small unit in Birmingham.

There was a representation of neurochemistry; a laboratory for the study of electrical activity of the brain in the conscious animal, and there was Charmian's clinical investigation in the mental hospital. A *continuum* was in place. In our presentations and applications for funding, we referred to our program as a program of "Drugs and the Mind."

It is only fair to say that not everybody was friendly to our approach. The pharmacologists (with a few distinguished exceptions) regarded us as "odd men out" and we were strangers to the psychiatrists. But there was also solid support at the core. My chief, Alastair Frazer, was a staunch friend and supported us through thick and thin. I suspect too, that he was a little proud to have our unit emerge in a large department preoccupied with lipid transport and fat absorption. And our Dean, Professor Leonard (later Sir Leonard) Parsons, gave us, at all times, the feeling that he truly understood what we were about. Sir Leonard was succeeded as Dean by Professor Arthur (later Sir Arthur) Thomson. When, on one particular occasion. I mentioned to him the need for more clinical facilities, he readily agreed. The Queen Elizabeth Hospital built us a small research wing adjoining the Medical School. But, more significantly, the Superintendent of the Mental Hospital, J.J. O'Reilly, put at our disposal an entire clinic, which had been used to house cases of chronic schizophrenia and organic psychoses. The house had at one time been the magnificent mansion of the Cadbury chocolate family. Over a period of nine months, it was steadily emptied (a result of deliberate policy of Dr. O'Reilly's); and sometime in 1952, we moved into a beautiful, well-equipped facility – standing among old trees with a rose garden at the back – and comprising forty-four beds. a day hospital, an out-patient clinic, and even an ethology laboratory, in which Michael Chance could carry out his pioneer studies on the effect of social setting on drug activity! When we were visited by the Rockefeller Foundation and the Medical Research Council (who supported us munificently), we could present a continuum extending from laboratories to clinic, and from the Medical School to the purview of the Regional Hospital Board.

In 1951, while in the United States on a Fulbright Fellowship to study psychiatry, I received a telegram informing me that I had been appointed the Head of a newly created Department of Experimental Psychiatry in the University of Birmingham. I returned humbled, thrilled, and bewildered by this extraordinary opportunity. A dream had come true.

We did not have to wait long for another major event. Sometime in late 1952, or early 1953, there walked into my office Dr. W. R. Thrower, Medical Director of Messrs. May and Baker. Dr. Thrower told me that May and Baker had acquired the British rights for chlorpromazine and presented me with Delay and Deniker's reports (11). They had a supply and could make up the necessary tablets. Would we care to perform a blind-controlled trial? Being very impressed by Delay and Deniker's pathbreaking studies, I said we certainly would and suggested that we would do so at the Winson Green Mental Hospital. Again, I asked Charmian, whether she would be interested. She was, and it was she who assumed full responsibility for the management of what was to prove, I think, a rather important step in clinical psychopharmacology. For, as I think back on it, all the difficulties, all the opportunities, all the unpredictable aspects of conducting a trial in a mental hospital were to show up clearly in that early trial: the preparation of the ward, the training of the personnel, the gullibility of us all (the so-called "halo" effect), the importance of nursing attendants, relatives, and patients themselves as informants; the use of rating scales and the calibration of such scales – all these elements came into their own, once Charmian (and to a lesser extent I) were faced with the realities of working in a "chronic" mental hospital ward. I still remember the morning when we all trooped into the boardroom of the hospital, spread the data on the large oak table, and broke the code after the ratings and side effects had been tabulated. The trial involved 27 patients chosen for gross agitation, overactivity, and psychotic behaviour: 11 were affective, 13 schizophrenic, and 3 senile. The design was blind and self-controlled, the drug and placebo being alternated three times at roughly six-week intervals. The dose was relatively low (250 to 300 mg per day). We kept the criterion of improvement conservative, which was reflected in our discussion. Yet there was no doubt of the results: 7 patients showed marked improvement; 11 slight improvement; there was no effect in 9 patients. Side effects were observed in 10 patients. Our short paper (12), which conclusively proved the value of chlorpromazine and was the subject of an editorial in *The British Medical Journal*, was a blind self-controlled trial. But it was more, for it was a statement of the opportunities offered by a mental hospital for work of this kind, the difficulties one was likely to encounter, and the rules that one had to observe to obtain results. As we wrote (12):

> The research instrument in a trial of this sort being a group of people, and its conduct being inseparable from the individual use of words, we were impressed by the necessity for a 'blind' and self-controlled design and independent multiple documentation. For that reason the day and night nursing staff became indispensable and valued members of the observer team. We were warmed and encouraged by the energy and care with which they did what was requested of them, provided this was clearly and simply set out at the beginning. A chronic 'back' ward thus became a rather interesting place to work in. There may well be a case for training senior nursing staff in elementary research method and in medical documentation. This would make for increased interest, increased attention to, and respect for detail, and the availability of a fund of information, all too often lost because it has not been asked for.

GROPING TOWARDS FOOTINGS OF A SCIENCE

By the mid-fifties, the good boot of empiricism had propelled our field mightily forward. New drugs were beckoning on the horizon and facts were hunting for an explanation. Yet the *science* of it all was sparse, a mere silhouette. New methods, new facts, new connections were needed to generate new hypotheses, to fill in details, and to give the field coherence and structure.

As we were working away in Birmingham, it became apparent to me that we were dealing with a science of a very peculiar kind. It was not a discipline in a traditional sense, but an *inter*science par excellence. It depended on the free flow of information between disparate fields; transdisciplinary communications were at the heart of progress. To be sure, the component fields were developing at different rates: but they induced questions between domains, which proved provocative and catalytic.

The five areas which seemed important to us at the time were *functional neuroanatomy* (as exemplified by the work of Magoun, McLean, Nauta, Jung, and Olds); *neurochemistry,* particularly *regional neurochemistry* of the brain; *electrophysiology* of the brain, particularly in the conscious animal; *animal behaviour* studies; *human subject studies* and the refinement of the *clinical trial.* These seemed to be footings on which the new science could stand and grow. I have expanded on these concepts in an older review (13). Nowadays, of course, we could add molecular biology and genetics.

Equally important, as one thought of it, seemed the creation of environments, which would facilitate such interdisciplinary conversation. This was not always easy, but possible, as I found out in later ventures at the NIMH and at Johns Hopkins.

INTO A WIDER FIELD: CONTACTS, MEETINGS, AND SYMPOSIA

It is hard to recapture the sheer elan and energy, which developed in us all in those early fifties and the contacts which generated spontaneously as we went on in our work. The little handwritten blue airletters carried prepublication news, and were eagerly awaited. I vividly remember Hy Denber's first visit to us, soon after the publication of our chlorpromazine paper, and our discussion on dosage levels. There was an exciting correspondence with Nate Kline, whom I had first met in 1950, concerning reserpine. Later the Killams came, and a life-long friendship ensued, and Jim Hance, who had worked for Phil Bradley and subsequently went to work with the Killams. Warren McCullough and Pitts visited us and fascinated our group with their mathematical models of self-regulation. Tinbergen (since a Nobel laureate) spoke on ethology at the Uffculme Clinic soon after it opened. and Leonard Cook. a most welcome visitor from Smith, Kline and French (SKF), shared with us some of the new and exciting techniques in the emerging field of behavioural pharmacology that he was developing. There were contacts with Ed Fellows, of SKF, who had introduced "Dexamyl," and David Rioch and Joseph Brady of the Walter Reed; later we contacted Jim Olds. Most importantly, the Macy Foundation began to organize its excellent Macy conferences on neuropharmacology, which brought us all together regularly. Also, in 1953, Hudson Hoagland organized an important interdisciplinary symposium at the Batelle Institute, at which we began. for the first time, to talk about the importance of social setting in relation to drug effects. This was called "sociopharmacology," a strange new concept to the orthodox pharmacologist. I had started to commute to the States regularly, visiting colleagues and comparing notes as the field was shaping. One such visit was of particular consequence: I believe it took place in 1952 or early 1953. A number of us met to discuss the need for an international symposium in neurochemistry, the first of its kind. Included were Seymour Kety, by that time Director of the Intramural Program for the NIMH; Heinrich Waelsch, Professor of Neurochemistry at Columbia; Jordi Folch-Pi, Director of the McLean Hospital Laboratories at Harvard; and Lou Flexner, Chairman of Anatomy at Pennsylvania. Also, I got in touch with Derek Richter and with Geoffrey Harris, who later was to emerge as a father of modern neuroendocrinology. As the theme of this symposium, we chose the "Biochemistry of the Developing Nervous System." As a place to hold it, we chose Magdalen College, Oxford. I was charged with being the Organizing Secretary, and I could not have done so without the devoted help of my British colleagues. The Symposium took place in the summer of 1954: sixty-nine colleagues from nine countries participated. It may very well be that at this Symposium the term "Neurochemistry" was used officially for the first time. As Heinrich Waelsch and I put it in our introduction to the Proceedings (14):

> … We agreed, also, that from the start it would be well to consider the brain as a biological entity in all its complexity of morphology and function, rather than as a homogenate, or an engineering problem.

Three subsequent symposia reflected the momentum that was developing at this historic first meeting. The second on "The Metabolism of the Nervous System" was held in Aarhus, Denmark in 1956. The Proceedings were edited by D. Richter. The third on "The Chemical Pathology of the Nervous System" followed in Strasbourg, France, in 1958. The Proceedings were edited by Jordi Folch-Pi. The Fourth International Symposium centered on "Regional

Neurochemistry." It was held in Varenna, Italy, in 1960. Seymour Kety and I edited the Proceedings.

Again, it is hard to convey the productivity that attended these meetings, as they steadily shaped some basic concepts in our field. Bit by bit, the footings of our new science were being put into place. Neurochemistry, and particularly the regional neurochemistry of the brain, was being related to electrophysiology; electrophysiology was being related to the emerging reward systems of Jim Olds, Joe Brady and Peter Dews. Behaviour analysis techniques were applied to the study of the effects of drugs on behaviour, and there was steady refinement of the clinical trial. In a word, things began to *connect.* In 1956, under the joint chairmanship of Jonathan Cole and Ralph Gerard, a milestone conference in psychopharmacology was held under the aegis of the National Research Council, the National Academy of Science, and the American Psychiatric Association (15), during which year also, Cole's Psychopharmacology Service Center was created – a step of enormous consequence for the future development of the field all over the world.

In 1957, the World Health Organization invited me to convene a small study group on the subject of "Ataractic and Hallucinogenic Drugs in Psychiatry." The following participated:

Ludwig von Bertalanffy, USA (Systems Theory)
U. S. von Euler, Sweden (Pharmacology
E. Jacobsen, Denmark (Pharmacology)
Morton Kramer. USA (Epidemiology)
T. A. Lambo, Nigeria (Transcultural Psychiatry)
E. Lindemann, USA (Psychiatry)
P. Pichot, France (Psychiatry)
D. McK. Rioch, USA (Neurosciences)
R. A. Sandison, England (Psychiatry)
P. B. Schneider, Switzerland (Clinical Pharmacology)
J. Elkes, England (Rapporteur)

I wrote the report (16), which, incidentally, carried Eric Jacobsen's pioneer classification of the main drugs according to their pharmacological properties. In the meantime, the scientific command of the U.S. Air Force, through its principal representative in Europe, Colonel James Henry, had catalyzed meetings, at which the international implications of brain research became steadily more apparent. After preliminary meetings in 1958 and 1959, a number of us met at UNESCO House in 1960 to draft the Statutes and Bylaws of IBRO... the International Brain Research Organization. The disciplines of neuroanatomy, neurochemistry, neuroendocrinology, neuropharmacology, neurophysiology, behavioural sciences, neurocommunication, and biophysics were represented. Dr. Daniel Bovet and I represented Neuropharmacology in the first Central Council of IBRO. Our emerging field had now a major international presence.

TOWARDS THE CINP, THE ROME CONGRESS, THE NIMH, AND HOPKINS

In the Spring of 1955 or 1956 – I cannot remember which – Professor Ernst Rothlin and Mrs. Rothlin paid us a leisurely three-day visit in Birmingham. During our conversations, in which Charmian, Philip Bradley, William Mayer-Gross, and I participated, two broad ideas kept surfacing. One was the need for an international forum to discuss and serve the advances in our field. The other, the need for an international journal. I do not rightly recall whether the Latin name of *Collegium* was used in our discussion, but the need for an organization certainly kept recurring.

As for the journal, preliminary work had already been done. Willie Mayer-Gross had been in touch with R. Jung of Munich. Springer, the publishers had been approached and appeared interested. Further discussions involved Jean Delay, P. Deniker, P. Pichot of Paris, and most importantly, Abe Wikler of Lexington. It took quite a number of telephone calls and letters to persuade Abe to assume the co-editorship of this new journal. I served on the editorial board and still recall the excitement when the first slim yellow issue of *Psychopharmacologia* landed on my desk.

Perhaps this is also the place to emphasize the prescient vision of psychopharmacology that Abe Wikler had developed at the time. He saw, long before most of us the true dimensions of the field, defining it beautifully in his book on the *Relation of Psychiatry to Pharmacology,* (17) now out of print. It set a standard of rigour and excellence – a standard he set for *Psychopharmacologia*, which continued as a model for years to come. Our contacts with the Rothlins and the Sandoz Group remained very much alive.

In 1957 at the invitation of Seymour Kety and Robert Cohen, I moved to the United States to establish the Clinical Neuropharmacology Research Center at St. Elizabeth Hospital, where Nino Salmoiraghi, Steve Szara, Hans Weil-Malherbe, Fritz Freyhan, and Floyd Bloom, joined us in rapid succession. Max Hamilton was our first visiting scholar. After I left (in 1963). Nino Salmoiraghi assumed the directorship. He was followed by Floyd Bloom and later by Richard Wyatt, the present incumbent.

Philip Bradley remained in contact with European colleagues. As he, Deniker, and Radouco-Thomas reported (18): At a meeting on psychotropic drugs in 1957 in Milan, "a small group of interested people representing pharmacology, psychiatry, psychology, and so on, held informal discussions and decided that regular opportunities should be provided for workers in the various fields of research and clinical investigation, to meet and discuss their common problems." The idea was taken further at the Second International Psychiatric Congress in Zurich in September of the same year (I could not attend, having just moved to Washington). It was at this Congress that our new *Collegium* was formally inaugurated, and it was Professor Trabucchi's invitation which led to our first Congress in Rome in 1958.

I attended the Congress, co-chairing the third Symposium and reading a paper on the "Relation of Drug Induced Mental Changes to Schizophrenia" (18) at the fourth. Across a span of nearly fifty years, one cannot help but be encouraged and thrilled by the vision of the organizers and the sheer span, grasp and inclusiveness of the program. For at what earlier international forum had the four footings of our science – neurochemistry, electrophysiology, animal behaviour, and the refinement of the clinical trial – been so skilfully juxtaposed? Where had one encountered papers on the measurement of subtleties of subjective experience in drug-induced states and discussed rating scales for subjective experience and objective behaviour? Or had been considered, in context, the huge policy implications of the psychoactive drugs for the mentally ill? I feel that by the end of the Congress, the silhouette had filled out and sharpened, presenting a new landscape in clear light. Biochemistry, physiology, psychology, and behaviour were looking each other in the face in a new kind of recognition. We had a map. It is exciting to recall this historic encounter.

As for my own paper (19), I could only submit an abstract – having been preoccupied with our newly formed group in Washington. I presented an expanded version of the same ideas at the Third International Neurochemical Symposium in Strasbourg during the same year. In this paper (20) I examined schizophrenia as a possible disorder of information processing by the brain, drew attention to the possible place of subcortical structures (putamen, caudate, globus pallidus and hippocampus) in the processing and misprocessing of such information, and considered the role of amines, particularly serotonin, norepinephrine, and dopamine in such misprocessing.

In 1963, I was invited to assume the chair at Johns Hopkins and the directorship of the Henry Phipps Psychiatric Clinic. But this "epistle" is already far too long, and I must defer details of this most fruitful and meaningful period to another occasion. Let me simply say that at Hopkins we went on doing "more of the same." Sol Snyder began his pathbreaking neurochemical studies while still a resident and now heads up the superb Department of Neuroscience at Hopkins. Joe Brady built primate laboratories for his far-reaching program in behavioural biology. Joe Coyle advanced developmental neurobiology in a way which inspired many residents to follow in his footsteps; he is now chief of Psychiatry at Harvard. Ross Baldessarini is director of the Mailman Laboratories at Harvard. "Uhli" Uhlenhuth, Lino Covi and Len Derogatis developed their rating scales and engaged in important outpatient studies. Uhli was also president of the ACNP at its twenty-fifth anniversary. Last but not least, reaching back to joint times at the NIMH, Floyd Bloom is now editor-in-chief of Science. There are many, many others one wishes to mention, but 'tis time to stop.

CLOSING

In 1961 the newly constituted American College of Neuropsychopharmacology did me the immense honour of electing me as their first president. Looking back on my year of service, I said (21):

> It is not uncommon for any one of us to be told that Psychopharmacology is not a science. and that it would do well to emulate the precision of older and more established disciplines. Such statements betray a lack of understanding for the special demands made by Psychopharmacology upon the fields, which compound it. For my own part, I draw comfort and. firm conviction from the history of our subject and the history of our group. For I know of no other branch of science which, like a good plough on a spring day, has tilled as many areas in Neurobiology. To have, in a mere decade, questioned the concepts of synaptic transmission in the central nervous system: to have emphasized compartmentalization and regionalization of chemical process in the unit cell and in the brain: to have given us tools for the study of chemical basis of learning and temporary connection formation; to have resuscitated that oldest of old remedies, the placebo response. for careful scrutiny; to have provided potential methods for the study of language in relation to the functional state of the brain: and to have encouraged the Biochemist, Physiologist, Psychologist, Clinician, Mathematician, and Communication Engineer to join forces at bench level, is no mean achievement for a young science. That a chemical text should carry the imprint of experience, and partake in its growth, in no way invalidates the study of symbols, and the rules among symbols, which keep us going, changing, evolving, and human. Thus, though moving cautiously, Psychopharmacology is still protesting; yet, in so doing, it is, for the first time, compelling the physical and chemical sciences to look behaviour in the face, and thus enriching both these sciences and behaviour. If there be discomfiture in this encounter, it is hardly surprising; for it is in this discomfiture that there may well lie the germ of a new science.

In our branch of science, it would seem we are as attracted to soma as to symbol; we are as interested in overt behaviour as we are aware of the subtleties of subjective experience.

There is no conflict here between understanding the way things are and the way people are, between the pursuit of science and the giving of service. So we must go on along lines we began: talk to each other, and keep talking. Psychopharmacology could prove a template for a truly comprehensive psychiatry of the future. We must train colleagues who do good science and. above all, who also listen: For, like it or not, our humanity will never leave us in our molecular search.

REFERENCES

1. Elkes, J. (1995) Psychopharmacology: Finding one's way. Neuropsychopharmacology 12: 93-111.
2. Elkes, J. and Finean, J. (1953) X-ray diffraction studies on the effects of temperature in the structure of myelin in the sciatic nerve of the frog. Exp. Cell Res 4: 69.
3. Elkes, J. (1957) Some effects of psychotomimetic drugs in animals and man. In Neuropharmacology: Transactions of the Third Conference, New York Josiah Macy Jr. Foundation 11: 205-294.
4. Toman, J. and Davis, J. P. (1949) The effects of drugs upon the electrical activity of the brain. Pharmacological Reviews 1: 425.
5. Bradley, P. B. (1952) Observations of the Effects of Drugs in the Electrical Activity of the Brain, Doctoral thesis. University of Birmingham, England.
6. Morruzi, G. and Magoun, H.W. (1949) Brain-stem reticular formation and activation of the EEG. Electroencephalography Clinical Neurophysiology 1: 455.
7. Bradley, P.B. and Elkes, J. (1953) The effects of atropine. Hyoscyamine, physostigmine and neostigmine on the electrecal activity of the brain of the conscious cat. J. Physiol. (London) l20: 14.
8. Elkes, J. (l958) Drug effects in relation to receptor specificity within the brain: some evidence and provision formulation. In G. Wostenholme (ed.) CIBA Foundation Symposium in Neurological Basis of Behaviour (pp. 303-332) London: Churchill.
9. Bradley, P.B., and Elkes, J. (1957). The effects of some drugs in the electrical activity of the brain. Brain 80: 113-114.
10. Stoll, A. (1947) Lysergs"ure-Diaethylamid – ein Phantasicum aus der Mutterkorngruppe. Schweiz Arch. Neurol. Neurochirurg Psychiat 60: 279-323.
11. Delay, J., and Deniker, P. (1953) Les neuroplegiques en therapie psychiatrique. Therapie 8: 347-364.
12. Elkes, J. and Elkes, C. (1954) Effects of chlorpromazine on the behaviour of chronically overactive psychotic patients. British Medical Journal. 2: 560.
13. Elkes, J. (1955) The Department of Experimental Psychiatry. University of Birmingham Gazette. March 11.
14. Waelsch, H. (ed.) (1955) Biochemistry of the developing nervous system: Proceedings of the First International Symposium in Neurochemistry (p. 5) New York: Academic Press.
15. Cole, J., and Gerard, R. W. (eds.) (1957) Psychopharmacology: Problems in Evaluation. Washington, D.C.: National Academy of Science and National Research Council.
16. Elkes. J. (Rapporteur) (1958). Atatactic and hallucinogenic drugs in psychiatry. WHO Tech. Rep. Series. 152. Geneva: World Health Organization
17. Wikler. A. (1957). The Relation of Psychiatry to Pharmacology. Baltimore: Williams and Wilkins.
18. Bradley. P. B., Deniker P. and Radouco-Thomas. C. (eds.) (1959) Neuropsychopharmacology, I. Pcoceedings of the First Meeting of the Collegium Internationale Neuro-Psychopharmacologicum. Rome, September 1958. (pp. vii-viii). Amsterdam. Elsevier.
19. Elkes, J. (1959) On the relation of drug-induced mental changes to the schizophrenias. In: P.B. Bradley, P. Deniker. and C. Radouco-Thomas (eds.) Neuro-Psychopharmacologium, 1. Proceedings ot the First Meeting of the Collegium Internationale Neuro-Psychopharmacologium, Rome, September 1958. (p. 166). Amsterdam, Elsevier.
20. Elkes, J. (1961) Schizophrenic disorder in relation to levels of neural organization: the need for some conceptual points of reference. In: M. Folch-Pi (ed.) The Chemical Pathology of the Nervous System (pp. 648-645). London: Pergamon Press.
21. Elkes, J. (1963). The American College of Neuropsychopharmacology: A note in its history and hopes for the future. American College of Neuropsychopharmacology Bulletin, 1: 2-3.

PAPER 2

THE DEPARTMENT OF EXPERIMENTAL PSYCHIATRY
Joel Elkes

Reprinted with the kind permission of The University of Birmingham from the
University of Birmingham Gazette, 11th March, 1955

The Department of Experimental Psychiatry was founded in 1951. Its aim is the application of scientific and experimental method to problems of clinical psychiatry.

The extent of the problem of mental ill-health is not generally realised. Thus, according to recent official returns, nearly half the total hospital beds in the country are occupied by the mentally ill. Accurate figures for attendances at overcrowded and understaffed psychiatric out-patient clinics are lacking, as are figures for the incidence of the milder forms of mental disorder in general practice. There is, however, general agreement that the proportion is high.

Psychiatry is a clinical subject, and can be nothing else. It deals with phenomena, such as disturbances of awareness, thought, emotion, communication, personal and social adjustment, which are uniquely human, and which can be reproduced in the animal experiment only in the most rudimentary and questionable way. However useful the animal experiment may be in advancing basic knowledge, research in psychiatry implies investigation in the ward, the outpatient department and quite possibly, the surgery (office) of the suitably trained and interested general practitioner. The aim of the Department is therefore twofold. On the one hand it is to advance knowledge in the laboratory, particularly in relation to the physiology and chemistry of the brain; on the other, to apply such knowledge as exists already in the most efficient and economical way. The first calls for "basic science" laboratories, now situated in the Medical School; the second, for clinical investigation and research units, such as are about to be provided through the generosity of the United Birmingham Hospitals and the Birmingham Regional Hospital Board.

The laboratory work of the Department rests on the assumption that the various manifestations of gross mental disorder and milder dysfunction have their counterpart in a disturbed physiology of the brain, and that the study of the chemistry, the cellular constitution, and the electrical activity of the brain may contribute to an understanding of its function as the highest integrating organ. In this context the selective effect of some drugs on mental function is of particular interest: an interest enhanced by the knowledge of the low order of dose (in some instances 20 millionths of a gram) in which these drugs are effective. This, if nothing else, points to specificity of interaction at an enzymological level.

The first problem to be attacked some time ago, however, was the submicroscopic constitution of a number of structural components of neural tissue. Nervous tissue is particularly rich in certain fatty compounds, the ubiquitous distribution of which indicated an important, though still ill-understood, function. These fatty bodies (the so-called neurolipids) are built into the membrane covering the individual nerve cell. Equally, most nerve fibres are encased in a thick fatty sheath of peculiar resilience. This sheath (the "myelin sheath") is wrapped round the nerve fibre somewhat in the manner of the layers of a leek. These regular layers have been found to be liquid crystals. In conjunction with the Department of Pharmacology, the detailed crystalline structure of these highly organised elements is being investigated by combination of X-ray diffraction and microchemical techniques. The dimensions of the individual units have been established, and the role of water, of certain fatty bodies, and of a number of key polar groups (as if were the nuts and bolts of the unit) have been determined. The effect of some solvents, such as chloroform and ether (well-known anaesthetics), upon the structure of these crystal) has also been studied. And, since the myelin sheath is affected in conditions known as demyelinating diseases, notably disseminated sclerosis, a field of study is opening up in this area also.

The second problem to be investigated was the distribution of some enzymes and enzyme systems in various areas of the brain. The enzymes are the naturally occuring catalysts which govern the rate of certain chemical reactions known to occur in the brain. It is becoming quite apparent that some areas of the brain are richer in certain enzymes than others. Moreover, if, for example, the brains of fishes, birds and higher mammals are compared, phylogenetic as well as ontogenetic differences can be established. These differences extend to a much finer level of organisation than hitherto supposed. For example, a layered structure such as the cortex of the brain, shows slight but quite definite differences in the chemical constitution according to the layer of cells which one is investigating. Chemically the brain is thus an *in*homogeneous organ. Certain enzymes appear characteristic for certain types of cells. A particular type of cell may be scattered at random throughout a region, or be condensed into sheets, clusters or bundles in geographically close or widely separated areas. The susceptibility of a particular region to a particular drug will thus depend on its dominant cell population. Basic information of the geography and, if one may be permitted to use the term, the chemical geology of the brain thus becomes a prerequisite if one is to take the study of drugs from a descriptive and empirical level to a fuller understanding.

Yet another method of study is available in the use of the inhibitors of the enzyme systems studied. These drugs, some of which are effective in a concentration of one in a hundred million, inhibit chemical processes discriminately and specifically. Their effect on overall behaviour and learning in animals, on growth and maturation, and on the emergence of certain automatic behaviour patterns during development is being studied in conjunction with the Department of Anatomy.

A further method of investigation is the recording of the electrical activity of the brain. This activity indirectly reflects chemical events. Recording can be carried out unobtrusively in the conscious animal, or in man, and the effect of some drugs on the electrical activity in relation to behaviour can then be studied. The electrical patterns shown by the quiescent, relaxed and contented animal are quite different from those seen in the alerted animal or in the animal, which is emotionally disturbed. It can be shown that whereas some drugs alter behaviour and electrical activity in a corresponding way, other drugs, while profoundly affecting the electrical activity of the brain, do not exert a comparable effect on behaviour. Furthermore, it appears from related chemical studies that the former group of compounds acts on receptors situated in the so-called upper brain stem, a developmentally old part of the brain buried deep at its base. It may be that threshold amounts of well-defined naturally occuring chemical substances at this area govern the basic states of consciousness such as sleep, wakefulness and attention: and, quite possibly, the storage of information known as memory.

As pointed out above, such animal experiments can only be in the nature of preliminary steps when viewed against the perspective of clinical psychiatry. Here clinical investigation, experiment and trial are the final and, indeed, the only arbiters. Present clinical studies in the Department centre on the mode of action of drugs on mental function. Relevant here are, first, the very specific psychological effect of some drugs in the normal; and secondly, the effects of some drugs in the mentally ill.

The so-called hallucinogenic drugs which include among others the alkaloid mescaline and the very powerful diethylamide of lysergic acid (LSD-25) produce disturbances of awareness, perception, imagery, feeling, movement and overall behaviour which have been compared with an acute schizophrenic episode. The work of the Department now includes a programme for the development of antagonists to these compounds. There are strong indications that both mescaline and LSD-25 may interfere with the chemical turnover of a naturally occurring substance in this brain. Through the ready co-operation of chemical industry, both in this country and the United States, compounds are being prepared which might, at least theoretically, be expected to compete with the "hallucinogens" for these very receptors. It will then be also a somewhat natural step to look into the intermediate metabolism of these drugs in schizophrenic patients.

Experiments over the past three years have shown striking and often paradoxical differences between the responses of psychotic patients and normal subjects to some common drugs. Thus, for example, a sedative (a barbiturate) given in doses sufficient to induce sound sleep in the normal will "wake" a schizophrenic patient from extreme catatonic withdrawal; and a stimulant (amphetamine, Benzedrine), which normally produces talkativeness and elation, will deepen stupor in such patients. These changes in accessibility (which are well known) are accompanied by profound changes in the reactivity of the autonomic nervous system. Similarly, other drugs, while reducing subjective anxiety, may exert little effect on skeletal musculature. Both clinical and laboratory experiments thus confirm the existence of elective chemical affinities within the nervous system.

This is borne out further by the recent introduction of a new family of compounds, which exert a peculiar calming effect in the agitated, hallucinated and overactive patient. When put the controlled "blind" trial in which active and identical inactive placebo tablets are alternated in the same patient unknown to observers over many weeks these drugs have proved of definite, though limited, value in mental hospital practice. Patients thus treated, though still hallucinated, become quieter, less tense, and less disturbed by their hallucinations, more responsive to their family and friends. They also put on weight in a striking fashion. It is quite likely that this group of drugs (which originated in France) is but the forerunner, and that more powerful and more specific agents will follow.

The above remarks refer to investigations into the metabolic background of mental disorder, which can be carried out in the laboratory and in the mental hospital. There is, however, a growing recognition of the role of psychiatry outside the mental hospital, particularly in relation to the general hospital and in relation to prevention, and the need for intermediate early treatment facilities. Through the generous help of the Board of Governors of the United Birmingham Hospitals, a research block for the Department is now being erected on the Queen Elizabeth Hospital site. This block will include biochemical, pharmacological and hormone assay laboratories and a small suite of clinical investigation rooms. Work here will centre on problems applicable to the clinical material seen in a general hospital, and will be related, wherever possible, to the work of the other Professorial Units in the Clinical Research Block.

Here, too, there will be scope for investigating (in biochemical and neurohumoral terms) the reactions of the normal; this should provide a much-needed baseline for related clinical studies.

Another project is the establishment of a centre for research into Early Treatment Method at Uffculme Hospital, Moseley. This has received the full and generous support of the Birmingham Regional Hospital Board. The prime object of this centre will be to further, develop and test procedures designed to keep patients *out* of mental hospitals, and to assist in the rehabilitation of the mentally ill. If successful, it may go some way towards bridging the gap between the psychiatric outpatient clinic and the admission ward of a mental hospital. A reasonable turnover at such a centre should result in a saving of mental hospital beds.

At this Early Treatment Hospital it is proposed to develop outpatient, day hospital, and inpatient facilities in that order. The day hospital is a relatively new development and particularly relevant. Its aim would be to provide full therapeutic, social, occupational, and recreational and club facilities during the day, while at the same time enabling the patient to return home at night. Family and patient could thus be guided in a slow process of mutual readjustment. Severe cases could be admitted as in-patients, go through a stage of day attendance, and finally be discharged as outpatients. Minor problems would be treated at an outpatient clinic as hitherto.

Our present state of knowledge in psychiatry does not justify extravagant claims on behalf of any particular therapeutic technique. In the research centres which are envisaged it is absolutely necessary to have full access to any methods that are available. It goes without saying that mental illness is a disorder of the whole person and, as often as not, presents an admixture of genetic, social, psychological and physiological factors. An attempt should be made to separate these factors wherever possible. The principal advantage of long-term research of this kind would be that, often unknown to the patient, information concerning these various aspects could be systematically collected, sifted and assessed in relation to the breakdown and to subsequent recovery. Quantitative information, based on record systems which it is hoped will be developed in conjunction with the Department of Medical Statistics, could thus be slowly gathered, and expanded and supported by larger-scale surveys of the general population in the region. The two centres would thus serve as mutually complementary laboratories for wider scale studies of mental health in the community. Furthermore, they would form a useful nucleus for the training of medical and non-medical psychiatric personnel, and for conveying to the general practitioner the psychiatric implications of the problem with which he is called to deal. Links with the public health services could further strengthen these trends.

The opportunities in Birmingham are indeed great.

PAPER 3

PSYCHOPHARMACOLOGY: FINDING ONE'S WAY

Joel Elkes

Reprinted with the kind permission of Elsevier Science from
Neuropsychopharmacology 12: 93-111, 1995

ABSTRACT

The paper recalls the experiences of the author over the past forty-eight years in a field which later became known as psychopharmacology. The author began in physical chemistry and traditional pharmacology. His interest in the nervous system stemmed from X-ray diffraction studies on the structure of living myelin, and led, by way of studies on the distribution of cholinesterases and the effects of atropine, to the study of the effects of drugs on the electrical activity of the brain in the conscious animal. At the clinical level it included studies of the effects of drugs on catatonic schizophrenic stupor. These studies took place before the discovery of chlorpromazine. They led to the creation, in 1951, of the Department of Experimental Psychiatry in Birmingham, England, the first department of its kind in the world. The department included neurochemical, electrophysiological, and animal behavior laboratories and a strong clinical facility (the Uffculme Clinic). The first blind trial of chlorpromazine was carried out in that department in 1953 and 1954. The existence of families of neuroregulatory compounds, having uneven distribution in the brain, and exerting regional chemical field effects in relation to function was postulated on the basis of experimental and clinical findings. The work of colleagues and participants in the various studies is gratefully acknowledged in the text. In 1954 the author served as convening executive secretary of the first International Symposium on Neurochemistry at Oxford, England, the first meeting of its kind. He came to the United States in 1957 and founded, and served as first director of, the new Clinical Neuropharmacology Research Center, now the Center for Neuroscience at St. Elizabeth's Hospital, Washington, DC. He directed this program from 1957 to 1963. Subsequent activities at Johns Hopkins, the World Health Organization, and the International Brain Research Organization (IBRO) are recalled. In 1961 he was elected first president of the American College of Neuropsychopharmacology. In looking back, he notes the sparse and personal nature of the field in the late 1940s and early 1950s, its explosive growth in the wake of the major clinical discoveries, and above all, the emergence of a new science through the interaction of neurochemistry, electrophysiology, studies of animal behavior, and the refinement of the clinical trial. He regards the emergence of concepts of regional chemistry of the brain as particularly significant, and feels that psychopharmacology is ideally positioned to act as an intermediary between classical pharmacology and quantum biology. The transdisciplinary nature of psychopharmacology provides a template for a comprehensive psychiatry of the future – a discipline which is now positioned to lead. He also feels that future discoveries in psychopharmacology will pose a most poignant ethical dilemma for medicine, and argues for a timely readying for these responsibilities.

I am much honored to be part of this illustrious series. In their distinguished contributions that preceded my own, Drs. Frank Ayd (1991) and Heinz Lehmann (1991) have given us – each in their own idiom – a fine account of how our field and our college came to be. So when Dr. Oakley Ray intimated that I was to follow them, I asked him – a little hesitatingly – what I should talk about. "Your times, and how you found your way," said he. By the time I left his office, I had my title: "Finding One's Way" is what this talk is about; though, on reflection, "Trial and Error" might have been even more appropriate.

Personal beginnings are hard to trace; they appear most clearly in retrospect. My entry into psychopharmacology was far from direct. It happened in the mid-forties through a fortunate play of synchronicities. Let me explain.

Physics and the mind have been with me since my youth, but physics came first. At high school, I had three heroes: Einstein, Ehrlich, and Goethe. I spent my first prize monies on accounts of the new physics. To this day, I recall the awe with which I viewed cloud chamber photographs that rendered visible the mysterious geometry of particle paths in collision. As a novice (I had no mathematical training beyond calculus) I could not go beyond first principles. And yet, as I read myself into the field (French 1979) and as I tried to grasp the curious transforms, jumps, symmetries, and asymmetries operating in particle physics, I kept on imagining the life of the mind as a molecular process, linking it in some way to particle physics. It was, of course, a fatuous exercise; yet, it gave me strange satisfaction to engage in such molecular games. Much, much later, I came upon Pauling's concepts of the "hydrogen bond" (Pauling 1945). I still recall the thrill of the first reading, like discovering a new and profound piece of music.

Quite early, thus, I began to think of molecules visually; and when my father, a prominent physician, directed me to Paul Ehrlich's writings (Himmelweit 1956), that interest quickened apace. His concept of receptors, accompanied by his famous "lock and key" diagram, implied stereochemical "fit." Ehrlich wrote on the elective affinities of dyes for tissues and bacteria; he had a consuming curiosity about the molecular basis of immunological memory. He also envisioned the fashioning (in our day we would say, "engineering") of drugs that would selectively attack themselves to specific receptors. Tissues could learn, and rational chemotherapy, to him, was an elaborate imitation of nature.

Why Goethe? I cannot truly account for Goethe's lifelong influence on me, except to say that, with Thomas Jefferson, he represents to me the most comprehensive and comprehending of men. The Germans refer to such people as "eine Natur," a magnificent phenomenon of nature. There is also another term "Naturforscher" – a searcher of nature. Goethe's life was a continuous conversation between the Without and Within (Nevinson 1931). He cultivated an inner awareness that was never allowed to interfere with the affairs of the world. (He was statesman, counselor, war correspondent.) Long before Freud, he befriended his unconscious; and from that teeming laboratory, sent his images out into the world. Man, to him, was a piece of nature that he tried to map and comprehend. There was another dialectic. Alongside poetry, there was science, and even the titles of some of his novels, such as "Elective Affinities," reflect this dialectic. His studies in physics (color theory and crystals), botany, and paleontology were fed by the same joyous energy that permeates his conversations and correspondence. Many of his conclusions were wrong. Yet one continues to marvel at his leaps, and his insights. Goethe was a seeker and a seer. Long before concepts of homeostasis and biofeedback, information flow and self regulation, he was a systems man to his marrow. I believe he would have been very intrigued by psychopharmacology.

These three patron saints were at my side as I entered the portals of St. Mary's Hospital Medical School, University of London, where, in retrospect, I was extraordinarily fortunate. I was taught bacteriology by Alexander Fleming (penicillin) and medicine by Charles Wilson (later Lord Moran, Churchill's physician). Sir Almroth Wright, the great immunologist, gave a few select tutorials. Most importantly, I was appointed Student Demonstrator in Physiology by my erstwhile beloved chief, Alastair Frazer. My co-demonstrator was Geoffrey Harris (who later mapped the hypothalamic-pituitary axis and became one of the fathers of modern neuroendocrinology.) Martin Roth (later Sir Martin, Founding President of the Royal College of Psychiatry) was a fellow student. Early (and as part of my duties) I read Sir Charles Sherrington's Integrative Action (1911) and to this day feel the impact of Sherrington's concepts of integration as the ordered, reciprocal play of selective excitation and inhibition. Later, I attended, by invitation (and hiding safely in the dark of a back seat), a meeting of the august British Physiological Society, at which Dr. Adrian (later Lord Adrian) demonstrated the firing of neurons. The loudspeaker crackled as he touched a cat's single vibrissa; it remained silent as he touched another. These two events – the reading of Sherrington, and witnessing an emergent neurophysiology – firmly implanted themselves in my mind, and made me determined to get into the nervous system, come what may. Much later, I read a quotation from Sherrington (1941) that proved prophetic:

> The body of a worm and the face of a man alike have to the taken as chemical responses. The alchemist dreamed of old that it might be so. The dream, however, supposed a magic chemistry. There they were wrong. The chemistry is plain everyday chemistry. But it is complex. Further, the chemical brew in preparation for it time has been stirring unceasingly throughout some millions of years in the service of a final cause. The brew is a selected brew.

I had to await my turn to get within reach of the "brew." My chief, Alastair Frazer, proposed that I put my interest in physical chemistry to use. His field was not the nervous system, but fat absorption, and he suggested that I work on the structure of the surface coating of the chylomicron, a physiologically present fatty particle that floods the circulation from the thoracic duct after a fatty meal. The envelope was a lipoprotein, and carried a pH-sensitive ionic charge. I developed microelectrophoretic cell and various flocculation techniques as means of characterizing the nature of this lipoprotein coating (Elkes et al. 1939).

I suppose what intrigued me then (and still intrigues me) was inferring the properties of a macromolecular structure from physicochemical measurements, building up a. mental picture of the basis of collateral evidence. This wish to visualize, to have a map, often a wrong map, has stayed with me all my life. Playing with macromolecular configurations, fitting models together, became quite a hobby with me and my friends. In any event, with chylomicron, and with its lipoprotein envelope, my quest into the interface between physical chemistry and biology began. I started to read widely, pulled, I supposed, by a wish to penetrate the fundamental building blocks of life; I also ventured into surface chemistry, and the spreading and study of the monomolecular films. It was, of course, the pursuit of an illusion; but even then, the sense of pattern, of configuration, and the effects of subtle variations of an arrangement and charge distribution on a molecule's physicochemical properties became a game that whiled away some idle hours in medical school.

In 1941, Alastair Frazer invited me to join him in starting a Department of Pharmacology in Birmingham, England. Birmingham, even then, had the makings of the great university that it has since become. For one thing, it had a splendid campus, all compact. Within five minutes' walk of the medical school there were the basic science departments : there were giants in physics (Peierls and Oliphant), chemistry (Haworth), statistics (Hogben), genetics (Medawar), and anatomy, and science policy (Zuckerman). Conversation at lunch was propitious and soon turned to the structure of biological membranes and, of course, to lipoproteins. The structure of liquid crystals – the nature of forces, polar, nonpolar and steric – the bonding that made for their ordered cohesion, continued to excite. I found myself visualizing the architecture of membranes, streaming through special pores like a sodium ion, negotiating various channels and portals, with chains collapsing spring-like as these tiny compartments opened and closed. And then, one day I realized that the nervous system was full of lipoproteins, and that myelin was a highly ordered lipoprotein liquid crystal structure.

I came upon the papers of Francis Schmitt (1935, 1941), who was then at St. Louis. I wrote to him and got back a handsome collection of reprints describing his work on the structure of the myelin sheath. I was fascinated by his diagrams. Here was a highly ordered, aesthetically beautiful arrangement, which fit the facts and which made it possible to envision how bimolecular leaflets were built into a highly specialized structure. Myelin, I thought, could provide a model for understanding the structure of a membrane that was ion sensitive and electrochemically responsive. My friend Alastair Frazer concurred, but I found it hard to convince others. However, one fine thing happened: Bryan Finean walked into my laboratory as my first Ph.D. student.

Bryan Finean had got his degree in chemistry doing crystallography of the traditional kind. Looking at the Schmitt diagrams, we posed an obvious question. Schmitt had worked on dried nerve. Could low-angle x-ray diffraction be made to work on a nerve that was irrigated and alive? It did not take long for Bryan to design a cell that would allow us to irrigate the nerve, test its viability, expose a segment of it to changes in moisture, and to solvents (such as alcohol or ether), while at the same time obtaining low-angle x-ray diffraction patterns. Within three months or so, we were looking at the first x-ray diffraction photograph of living sciatic nerve; I still remember the thrill of seeing that film. To me there was also a profound personal and psychological element in this engagement. I was moving from somebody else's field, fat absorption, and entering the field that mysteriously pulled me, the nervous system, albeit by creeping up the myelin sheath!

Our studies gave us a picture, a sort of basic scaffolding, into which specialized receptors could fit. Cholesterol and phospholipids were accommodated in these diagrams. We also examined the effects of temperature, moisture, alcohol, and ether on myelin structure (Elkes and Finean 1949, 1953a,b). Gradually, in a small circle of physical chemists, and what was then the nucleus of molecular biology in Britain, we made some headway. However, when we demonstrated our findings to the Physiological or the Pharmacological Society, we got very peculiar looks. People were very sceptical of the model value of the myelin for the study of the structure of biological membranes, and only a few stopped by our demonstration stalls. It is significant who they were: Lord Adrian, Sir Henry Dale, J. H. Gaddum, and Alan Hodgkin. They were interested. So was Astbury, father of "biomolecular structure," and Bernal, a great crystallographer and physicist. As Bryan Finean's work was recognized, as he went to MIT, to Caracas, to Stockholm, as he published his monographs, including one with Engstrom (Engstrom and Finean 1958, Finean 1961) his views gathered strength. Today, he is a recognized and respected authority in his field, and I am glad for him, and a little proud at having had something to do with his success.

For me, there was also a much more personal satisfaction. I was in the nervous system, yet, as it is apparent, still edging safely at the periphery, a long way from behavior, and the mode of action of psychoactive drugs. However, once again, lucky chance cleared the way.

PHARMACOLOGY AND EXPERIMENTAL PSYCHIATRY
IN BIRMINGHAM, ENGLAND

There was in Birmingham, in the laboratory immediately below the Department of Pharmacology, a small subdepartment of two rooms administered from the Dean's office, called "Mental Diseases Research." In charge of it was a gifted neuropathologist, Dr. F.A. Pickworth, who held the view that mental disease was a capillary disease, and that all disorders were reflected in an abnormal cerebral vascular bed (Pickworth 1941). He had developed beautiful benzidine staining techniques for demonstrating the small cerebral vessels, and the laboratory was filled with innumerable slices and slides of the brain in all manner of pathological states, stained by his methods. This treasury represented Dr. Pickworth's life work.

Dr. Pickworth retired, and again serendipity took me by the hand. For the laboratory reverted to the Department of Pharmacology, and I became administratively responsible for its program. Our Department of Pharmacology was growing by leaps and bounds. When we arrived in Birmingham in 1942, there were two people; when I left, in 1950, there were 42 in the department. I was getting my taste for administration and helping people to perform. While Bryan Finean and I were busy with our studies, another event took place. The war had ended. Our military intelligence had given us insights into the secret German chemical warfare work, and particularly the anticholinesterases and their tremendous specificity for certain enzymes in the brain. We were asked to work with the anticholinesterases: DFP, TEPP, and the like. We started mapping the cholinesterases in various areas of the brain; inhibiting the "true" and "pseudo" enzymes from birth; observing the effect of such inhibition on the emergence of various inborn reflexes (Elkes, Eayrs and Todrick 1955). It was a long, long way from fat absorption, and some way from lipoproteins. But, at long last, it was the brain, it was drugs; and I was even beginning to "smell" that mysterious entity called behavior. In those days, there were few texts on neurochemistry. There was Irvine Page's seminal book (1937); there were Quastel's papers (Michaelis and Quastel 1941); there were Harold Himwich's (Himwich et al. 1940), and Derek Richter's early contributions (1940); and there was, of course, always Thudichum (1884). I also started reading Masserman (1946) and McDougall (1935), in the hope of linking chemistry to behavior. And then there appeared, in 1948, Feldberg and Vogt's classical paper in the *Journal of Physiology* (1948) questioning the universal role of acetylcholine in the central nervous system.

In retrospect, it becomes apparent to me that I was once again approaching my central interest, gingerly and carefully, as if I were defusing a bomb. For it is plain that what attracted me to research in psychiatry was an urge to leave the bench and get to people; and what made me circumambulate this purpose was my feeling of safety with things. Somehow, mental disease research, or "experimental psychiatry" (as I was beginning to call it in my mind), presented a sort of compromise. It led inevitably to human work, but it did so by way of experiment and control. This double bookkeeping worked for a time, for an astonishingly long time; it took a further five years to break through the barrier.

As we were feeling our way through the distribution of the cholinesterases, I began to read on the psychoactive drugs. The first required dissection in the cold room and mapping of the enzymes in various parts of the brain by a succession of extraction elution, incubation and bioassay, a tedious approach to regional neurochemistry: the second involved human studies. Kluver's papers on mescaline (1942) proved an illumination. Here was an extraordinary range of observations, with profound implications for a chemical pathophysiology of the psychoses.

By accident, too, I came across descriptions of the somatic and psychologic accompaniments of catatonic stupor, and saw some patients exhibiting this syndrome in the local mental hospital. At that time, Jean Delay came over to London (this was before the discovery of chlorpromazine). It was his first contact across the Channel since the war, and he told us of his experiments of the effects of amytal in catatonic stupor. (I was not aware of Lindemann's work [Lindemann and Malamud 1934] at that time.) Shorvon was developing his ether abreactive techniques (Sargant and Shorvon 1945). It was not long before we decided to embark on a study of the effects of drugs on catatonic stupor and began to look for clinical material. I obtained a small grant for this work from the hospital research fund and advertised for a research associate. No response was forthcoming, but one evening, when I was despondently telling Charmian, my former wife (who was in general practice at the time), about the lack of appeal for a job of this kind, another of those taps of fate took place. For quietly she asked me whether I had thought of her in this context. I said that I honestly hadn't and was delighted at her interest. She weighed things very carefully, finally deciding that she would give the job a try.

We began to work at the Winson Green Mental Hospital (The Birmingham City Mental Hospital, now All Saints Hospital), whose superintendent, J.J. O'Reilly, proved a real friend. He put a small research room at our disposal and allowed us to choose patients using our criteria; he also gave us nursing help. Thus, our catatonia study developed. We used homemade gadgetry to measure muscle "tone" and foot temperature and developed our own rating scales to measure change. The study taught us the enormous value of working in a realistic mental hospital setting. We communicated the results first to the Pharmacological Society of Great Britain, and then, some years later, to psychiatric groups (Elkes 1957). They created a good deal of attention. Amytal, administered in full hypnotic doses intravenously, led to a paradoxical awakening of patients in catatonic stupor, a relaxation of muscle tone, and rise in foot temperature. The effect of amphetamine was equally paradoxical. It led to a deepening of the stupor, increase in muscle rigidity, and deepening cyanosis. We also tried mephenesin, which had been shown by Frank Berger (Berger and Bradley 1946) to be a powerful spinal internuncial neuron blocking agent, and through his prescient insights, later led to meprobamate, and a whole family of anxiolytics. When tested in catatonic schizophrenic stupor, mephenesin produced marked muscle relaxation. There was, however, little effect on psychomotor response or peripheral temperature. We also studied the ability of patients to draw – for ten minutes, without prompting – while under the influence of drugs. Amytal markedly increased this ability, and amphetamine inhibited it. The experiments thus suggested *selectivity* in the action of drugs on catatonic stupor, and raised the question of the relation of hyperarousal to catatonic withdrawal. Most important, however, these experiments established – at a tangible, as well as a conceptual level – the need of working in parallel. The laboratory and the ward became ends of a *continuum* of related activities.

It was then, I suppose, that I decided that experimental psychiatry was clinical, or that it was nothing. Let it draw on the bench sciences, let it look for neural correlates of behavior in the animal model, let it delve deeply into processes governing the chemically mediated organ of information that we carry in our skull; but unless this yield from the bench is clearly and continuously related to the uniquely human events that are the business of psychiatry and of neuropsychology, the implications of such knowledge must, of necessity, remain conjectural. All this is pretty obvious nowadays. In those days, however, in a Department of Pharmacology in Birmingham, it became part of a plan. I felt instinctively that the drugs we were working with, and drugs still to come, could be tools of great precision and power, depending (if one was lucky) on one or two overriding properties. It is this kind of precision pharmacology of the central nervous system that made me hopeful, and made me take up my stance in the face of raised eyebrows, which I encountered not only in the Physiological Society but also in psychiatric circles, where I was regarded as a maverick, newcomer, and a curiosity.

At that time, then, there were two anchoring points for our work in the mental disease field: neurochemistry, at the bench level, and human behavior, as influenced by drugs. There was nothing in between, no indicator that could relate the effects of drugs on the brain in the conscious animal to behavior, nor any correlation between behavior and chemistry of the brain. I began to hunt again. The EEG was at that time coming into its own. Hill and Pond (Hill 1944; Hill and Pond 1952) were publishing on the dysrhythmias, and Grey Walter (Walter and Walter 1949) and Gastaut (1950) were, in their own idiom, trying to relate functional states in man to EEG activity. And across the water there beckoned the great papers of Herbert Jasper (1949) and Wilder Penfield (1947). I plumbed for the effect of drugs on the electrical activity of the brain in the conscious animal. There were very few data available in those days except, a little later, those of Abraham Wikler (1952) and James Toman's review (Toman and Davis 1949). I obviously could not do it alone, and again I was in the market for an associate.

I cannot recall now who told Philip Bradley about me or me about Philip Bradley, but I remember clearly his coming to my office and telling me of his experience and his interests. He had been trained in zoology and had carried out microelectrode studies in insects. He seemed interested in the problem, and a salary was available. So, after some consultation with Dr. Grey Walter, arrangements were made for him to spend some time with Grey Walter, to learn EEG techniques and then set up his own laboratory in the second of the two rooms of "Mental Diseases Research." This was duly done; and in 1949, Philip was working alongside, developing his pioneering technique for recording the electrical activity in the conscious animal (Bradley 1953), a procedure that in those days (the days of sulfonamide – *not* penicillin), was quite a trick. The work proceeded well and quickly established reference points for a pharmacology of the brain, inasmuch as it relates to behavior. I still treasure a copy of Philip's thesis completed in October 1952 (Bradley 1952). (Figures 1-5). It was a joy to see the clear and unambiguous effects of physostigmine, atropine, hyoscyamine, and amphetamine (and later, LSD-25) on the electrical activity of the brain in relation to behavior (Bradley and Elkes 1953, 1957). It was also particularly satisfying to find how these drugs grouped themselves in terms of their dependence on midbrain structures, and how information arriving at that time from Moruzzi and Magoun's studies (1949) could be related to our own findings. There gradually emerged (and this was my own view) a concept of the presence of *families* of compounds that had arisen in the brain, in the course of chemical evolution, and that were chemically related to powerful neurohumoral, transmitters familiar to us at the periphery (Elkes 1953, 1958, 1961). Three types of receptors, centering around members of the cholinester, the catecholamine and, later, the indole family, were proposed. Implicit in this concept of families of compounds was the concept of small, local, regional *chemical fields;* and of the *inter*action and interdependence between molecules governing and modulating the gating, storage, and flow in self-exciting neural loops. Reciprocal inhibition was regarded as the agent of structure in the central nervous system. I have modified these ideas somewhat since, and expressed them in various papers (Elkes 1953, 1958, 1961, 1966, 1967), but the concept of families of compounds, derived and evolved from respective common chemical root, governing the physiology of the brain (and, by implication, the chemistry of awareness, perception, affect, and memory) was a steady part of my thinking as we worked away in Birmingham; and to the best of my knowl-

Fig. 2. Plug carried by cat in harness, back view: protective flap open Reproduced by kind permission of P.B. Bradley from his thesis, 1952.

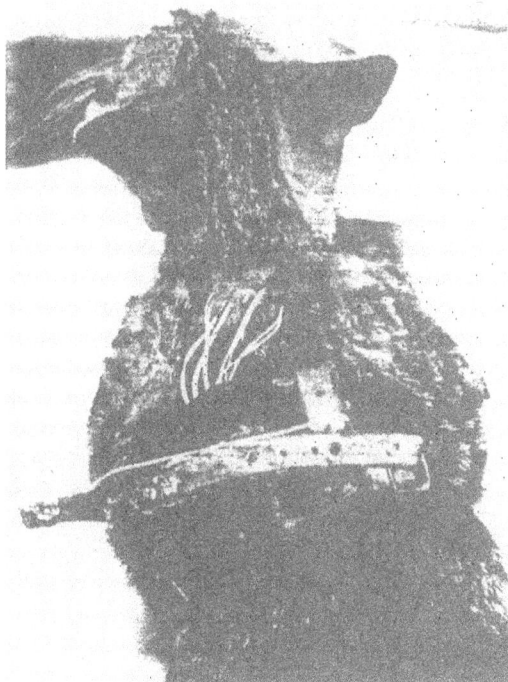

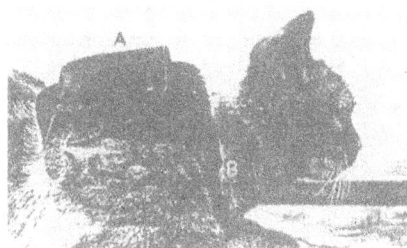

Fig. 1. Leads of implanted electrodes emerging through skin leading to plug held in special harness Reproduced by kind permission of P.B. Bradley from his thesis, 1952.

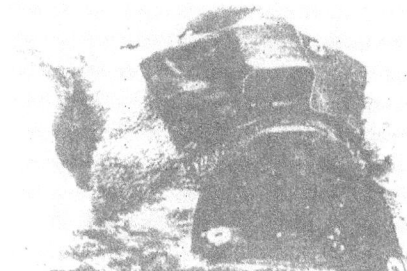

Fig. 3. Plug carried by cat in harness, side view. A, protective flap, closed when in use; B, cross straps with press studs that can be released for periodic inspection of the skin. Reproduced by kind permission of P. Bradley from his thesis, 1952.

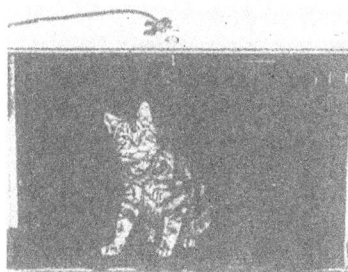

Fig. 4. Observation chamber, front open, cat "plugged in". The lead moves freely on bicycle hub bearings. The rim of the stroboscope lamp can be seen on left. Reproduced by kind permission of P.B. Bradley from his thesis, 1952.

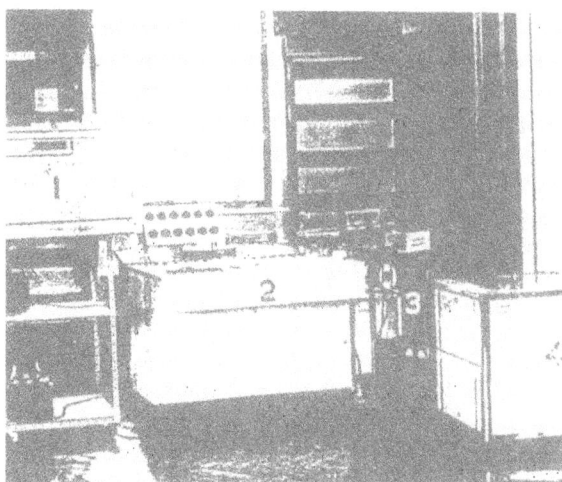

Fig. 5. Arrangement for recording the effects of drugs on the electrical activity of the brain in the conscious cat (Birmingham, England, 1948 onward): (1) constant environment chamber (underneath: stroboscope unit, and accumulators for D.C. supplies); (2) six channel electroencephotograph with electrode selector mounted on top; (3) rack carrying trigger unit for stroboscope control and test equipment; (4) wave analyzer. Reproduced by kind permission of P.B. Bradley from his thesis, 1952

edge, represents an early formulation of these ideas. It gives me special satisfaction to reflect on Philip Bradley's subsequent illustrious career and the influence he has exerted on the course of neuropsychopharmacology in Europe and the world. He has now retired from the chairmanship of pharmacology in Birmingham.

As we wrote at the time (Bradley and Elkes 1957, pp. 113-114):

> Perhaps rather than thinking in unitary terms, it may at this stage, be advisable to think in terms of the possible selection by chemical evolution of small families of closely related compounds, which by mutual interplay would govern the phenomena of excitation and inhibition in the central nervous system. Acetylcholine, nor-adrenaline and 5-hydroxy-tryptamine may be parent molecules of this kind; but one has only to compare the effects of acetylcholine with succinylcholine, or nor-adrenaline with its methylated congener to realize how profound the effects of even slight changes of molecular configuration can be. The astonishing use which chemical evolution has made of the steroids is but another example of the same economy. It is likely that neurons possessing slight but definite differences in enzyme constitution may be differentially susceptible to neurohumoral agents. Such neurons may be unevenly distributed in topographically close, or widely separated areas in the central nervous system; these differences probably extending to the finest level of histological organization. Phylogenetically older parts, and perhaps, more particularly, the midline regions and the periventricular nuclei may, in terms of cell population and chemical constitution be significantly different from parts characteristic of later development... It would perhaps be permissible to speak of the operation of chemical fields in these regions, which would depend on the rate of liberation, diffusion and destruction of locally-produced neurohumoral agents. The agents in question may be either identical with or, more likely, derived from neuro-effector substances familiar to us at the periphery. Their number is probably small, but their influence upon integrative action of higher nervous activity may be profound. The basic states of consciousness may well be determined by variations in the local concentration of these agents.

Bradley and I reported on the effects of amphetamine and LSD-25 at the January 1953 meeting of the Physiological Society (Bradley and Elkes 1953), and at the April 1953 meeting, Gaddum reported his now classic observation of the antagonism of LSD-25 and serotonin (1953). All our experimental facts became relevant in proposing later that the LSD-sensitive receptor might be peculiarly related to the afferent system (possibly to the medial afferent collaterals) and exercise a selective inhibitory role in the organization of sensory information (Elkes 1958), a proposal not out of keeping with Aghajanian's more recent findings on the effects of LSD-on the Raphe' nuclei (1970). Thus, in Birmingham we were developing a small experimental and clinical base for the study of the effects of drugs on brain and behavior. As mentioned earlier, we were impressed by the paradoxical effects of amytal, amphetamine, and mephenesin in catatonic schizophrenic stupor. We were also taken with the findings of Hill and Pond (Hill 1944, Hill and Pond 1952) and others suggesting temporal lobe dysfunction in aggressive antisocial states and possibly in schizophrenia. We were wondering whether the so-called antiepileptic drugs had a place in the treatment of these disorders. However, we did not know what awaited us. For one day there walked into my office Dr. W.R. Thrower, Clinical Director of Messrs. May and Baker. He said it was not a routine visit. He showed me, in English translation, the findings of Delay and Deniker concerning chlorpromazine (1953), findings that have been so admirably reviewed by Dr. Frank Ayd (1991). Dr. Thrower told me that May and Baker had acquired the British rights for chlorpromazine. They had a supply and could make up the necessary tablets. Would we care to perform a blind-controlled trial? Being very impressed by Delay and Deniker's reports, I said we certainly would and suggested that we could so at Winson Green Mental Hospital. I asked Charmian whether she would be interested. She was, and it was she who assumed full responsibility for the management of what was to prove, I think, a rather important step in clinical psychopharmacology. For, as I think back on it, all the difficulties, all the opportunities, all the unpredictable qualities of conducting a trial in a mental hospital were to show up clearly, and to be dealt with clearly, in that early trial: the preparation of the ward, the training of personnel, the gullibility of us all (the so-called "halo" effect), the importance of nursing attendants, relatives, and patients themselves as informants; the use of rating scales and the calibration of such scales – all these elements came into their own, once Charmian (and to a lesser extent I) were faced with the realities of working in a "chronic" mental hospital ward. I still remember the morning when we all trooped into the board room of the hospital, spread the data on the large oak table, and broke the code after the ratings and side effects had been tabulated. The trial involved 27 patients chosen for gross agitation, overactivity, and psychotic behavior: 11 were affective, 13 schizophrenic, and 3 senile. The design was blind and self-controlled, the drug and placebo being alternated 3 times at approximately six-week intervals. The dose was relatively low (250 to 300 mg per day). We kept a criteria of improvement conservative, which was reflected in our discussion. Yet there was no doubt of the results: 7 patients showed marked improvement; 11 slight improvement; there was no effect in 9 patients. Side effects were observed in 10 patients. Our short paper, which conclusively proved the value of chlorpromazine (Elkes and Elkes 1954), and was the subject of an editorial in *The British Medical Journal,* was a blind self-controlled trial. But it was more; for it was a statement of the opportunities offered by a mental hospital for work of this kind, the difficulties one was likely to encounter, and the rules that one had to observe to obtain results. As we wrote (Elkes and Elkes 1954, p. 573):

> Perhaps we may be allowed to draw attention to one last point – namely, the lessons we feel we have learned from the trial itself. The research instrument in a trial of this sort being a group of people, and its conduct being inseparable from the individual use of words, we were impressed by the necessity for a "blind" and self-controlled design and independent multiple documentation. Furthermore, we were equally impressed by the false picture apt to be conveyed if undue reliance was placed on interview alone, as conducted in the clinic room. The patients behavior in the ward was apt to be very different. For that reason the day and night nursing staff became indispensable and valued members of the observers' team. We were warmed and encouraged by the energy and care with which they did what was requested of them, provided this was clearly and simply set out at the beginning. A chronic "back" ward thus became a rather interesting place to work in. There may well be a case for training senior nursing staff in elementary research method and in medical documentation. This would make for increased interest, increased attention to, and respect for detail, and the availability of a fund of information, all too often lost because it has not been asked for.

The trial took place in a department, which by that time (1951) I had been invited to found. My dean, Sir Leonard Parsons, gave me the courage to begin, and his successor, Sir Arthur Thomson, continued with steadfast support. We called the new department, the Department of Experimental Psychiatry. I believe it was the first department of its kind anywhere. I chose the name deliberately to emphasize the research objectives of our enterprise. As indicated, the laboratory facilities were already available and had grown out of our previous work. But, as mentioned earlier, psychiatry, even experimental psychiatry, is clinical or it is nothing. Thus, quite early, we decided on the need for a clinical arm. The neurophysiology and neuro-chemistry laboratories were situated in the school of medicine and in a small new building provided by the Hospital Board (we were already working at the City Mental Hospital). What was needed was an Early Treatment Center, comprising inpatient and outpatient facilities. Again, we were fortunate. Through Dr. J.J. O'Reilly intervention, a mansion that had been previously the home of the Cadbury Chocolate Family became available. The name of the house was "Uffculme" and the name of our Clinic thus became the "Uffculme Clinic." Standing in its own lovely grounds, it comprised 42 beds, a day hospital, and an outpatient clinic. William Mayer-Gross joined us as Principal Clinical Associate in 1954, and John Harrington became Director of the Clinic in 1957. There were also biochemical laboratories, and an Ethology Laboratory to accommodate the work of Dr. M.R.A. Chance, I believe the first animal ethology laboratory in a psychiatric clinic.

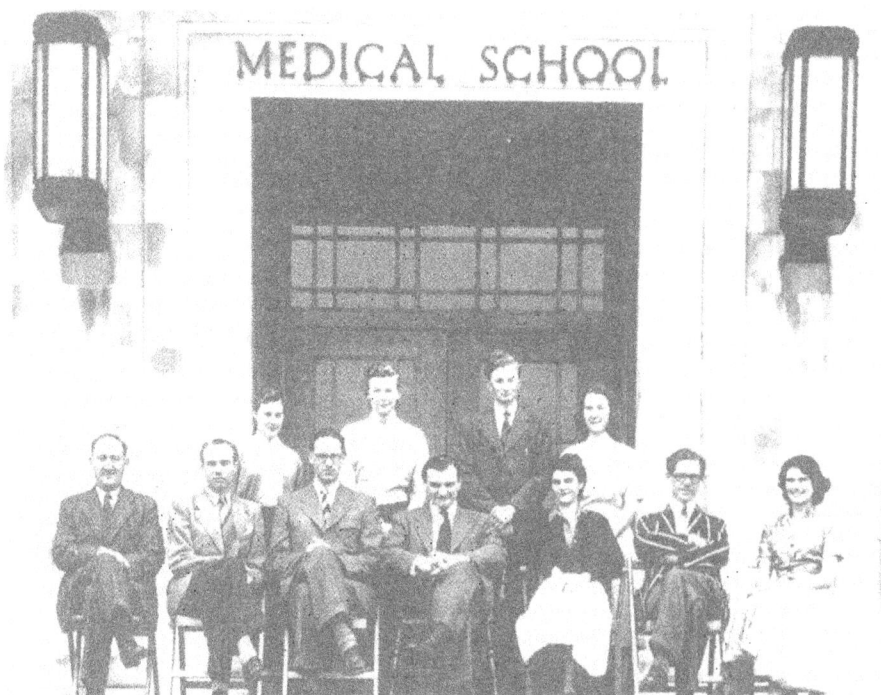

Fig. 6. The Department of Experimental Psychiatry, University of Birmingham, Birmingham, England, 1953. Front row: (from left) A. Todrick, M. Piercy, P.B. Bradley, J. Elkes, C. Elkes, A. Baker, and L. Allan; back row: (technical colleagues) second from left, B. Bayliss; third from left, E. Bailey

We developed and maintained many productive and encouraging contacts. I still remember vividly Hy Denber's first visit to us soon after the publication of our chlorpromazine paper and our discussion on dosage levels. We had used 250 mg with marked effects; across the water dosages had been much higher. There was exciting correspondence between Nate Kline (whom I had first met in 1950) and ourselves concerning reserpine. The Killams came, and a lifelong friendship ensued; and Jim Hance, who had worked with Phil Bradley, subsequently went to work with the Killams. Warren McCulloch and Pitts visited and fascinated our group by their mathematical models of self-regulation. Tinbergen (since, a Nobel Laureate) spoke at the Uffculme Clinic on ethology, and Leonard Cook, a most welcome visitor from S.K.F., shared with us some of the new and exciting techniques in the emerging field of behavioral neuropharmacology that he was developing. There were contacts with Ed Fellows (who had introduced "dexamyl"), with David Rioch and Joseph Brady at the Walter Reed, and later with Jim Olds. It was a tribute to the foresight of the Macy Foundation that they organized the splendid Macy Conferences on Neuropharmacology that brought us all together regularly.

In 1953, Hudson Hoagland organized an important interdisciplinary symposium at the Battelle Institute, at which we began to talk of social setting in relation to drug effects – sociopharmacology – a new and strange concept to the orthodox pharmacologist. The Rothlins spent three days as our guests in Birmingham, at which time, with Willy Mayer Gross and Philip Bradley, we began to talk about the need for a new journal, and possibly an international college. We were glad to learn that Springer, the publishers, were interested. Further discussions involved R. Jung (of Munich), J. Delay, P. Deniker, and P. Pichot (of Paris) and most importantly, Abraham Wikler (of Lexington). Perhaps this is the point to emphasize the prescient vision of psychopharmacology that Abe Wikler had developed at the time. His work on dependence and addiction was a model of rigor and clarity; from the vantage point of someone working both at the bench and in the clinic, he saw, long before most of us, the true dimensions of our field. He defined this beautifully in his book, *The relation of Psychiatry to Pharmacology* (1957), now out of print. We were glad that we managed to persuade him to assume the coeditorship of *Psychopharmacologia.* I still remember the excitement when the first, slim, yellow-cover issue of *Psychopharmacologia* landed on my desk.

After my departure for the United States in 1957, our department was divided into a Department of Experimental Neuropharmacology, under Professor Philip Bradley, and a Clinical Department of Psychiatry, under Professor William (now Sir William) Trethowan, later Dean of the Medical Faculty. I am glad to say that until recently Uffculme Clinic was functioning very well as a postgraduate teaching center of the Birmingham Regional Hospital. Now there stands, on university grounds, the brand new Queen Elizabeth Psychiatric Hospital, the inauguration ceremonies of which I had the immense pleasure of attending last year.

NEUROPHARMACOLOGY AND PSYCHOPHARMACOLOGY IN WASHINGTON, D.C., AND AT JOHNS HOPKINS, BALTIMORE

As I mentioned earlier, I had spent a year (1950 to 1951) in the United States, having had the good fortune, through the offices of Ted Wallace of S.K.F., to be awarded the first Smith, Kline, and French Traveling Fellowship in England, and to get a Fulbright Award. I had a stimulating time at the late Samuel Wortis' Institute at New York University, also visiting Fritz Redlich's Institute at Yale, and also worked very productively at the Pratt (New England) Diagnostic Center at Boston with John Nemiah, later Editor-in-Chief of the *American Journal of Psychiatry*, who taught me much. Once again, the mental hospital exerted its pull. When I met with Dr. Redlich, I asked him whether it would not be advisable for me to get to know an American state hospital at first hand. It was duly arranged that I should spend five months at Norwich State Hospital, Connecticut. This was done through the courtesy of the late Dr. Kettle, Superintendent of the Hospital, a wonderful person to work with, and for. At that time, too, we discussed the question of building a research center at Norwich State Hospital, and some 10 years later that I got a joyous letter from Dr. Kettle that he had obtained funds to create such a Center, which now is the Abraham Ribicoff Center for Mental Health Research at Norwich State Hospital.

It is during that time too, that I met Danny Freedman for the first time. To this day, I remember his comment at a seminar I gave concerning the possible relation of upper brain stem chemistry to schizophrenia. We saw alike and continued our exchanges later, distance notwithstanding. However, one of the most decisive meetings of my life was still to come. Before returning from the United States to England, I asked my friends at S.K.F. to arrange a visit with Seymour Kety, whose fundamental work on cerebral circulation I had admired from a distance for some years. This was duly done and one morning in the summer of 1951, I was in his laboratory at the University of Pennsylvania. We started talking and went on talking through a four-hour lunch. Seymour told me that he had just been appointed Scientific Director of the Intramural Program at NIMH, and I shared with Seymour that I was going back to England to occupy the newly created Chair of Experimental Psychiatry in the University of Birmingham. We talked of the possibilities of biological research in psychiatry and the exciting methods for in vivo work in man, which were just emerging. On a more personal level, a link was forged that day that has remained one of the most precious constants of my life.

Indeed, it is strange to reflect how constant are such constants. For when, in 1957, I received an invitation from Drs. Robert Cohen and Seymour Kety to create the Clinical Neuropharmacology Research Center at NIMH, we all felt that biological research would gain by being in a realistic mental hospital setting. The hospital under consideration was St. Elizabeth's in Washington, DC. Dr. Winfred Overholser, the superintendent, was duly approached and was very receptive. With Robert Felix's strong and continuous support, and with the exceptional understanding and enthusiasm of Drs. Bob Cohen and Seymour Kety, we established the Center at the William A. White building of the hospital. I will not hide the fact that it was hard going at first. We started, in 1957, with a secretary (Mrs. Anne Gibson) and myself in a large, dark, "Continued Care" building accommodating

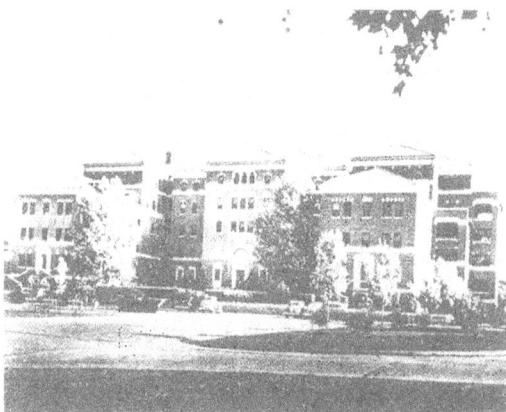

Fig. 7. The William A. White Building, St. Elizabeths Hospital, Washington, D.C. Site of the first Clinical Neuropharmacology Research Center, NIMH, founded in 1957. Now site of The Neuroscience Center, NIMH.

some 300 patients. However, time, energy, persistence, and support prevailed, and it became a research institute within two years. Again, the plan was the same: laboratories below, clinic above, and patients all around. The facilities grew and grew. Colleagues joined: Drs. Floyd Bloom, R. Byck, Richard Chase, R. Gjessing, R. Gumnit, Max Hamilton, Eliot Hearst, Tony Hordern, Shepherd Kellam, Don Lipsitt, John Lofft, Richard Michael, Herbert Posner, G.C. Salmoiraghi, S. Szara, R. von Baumgarten, Neil Waldrop, Hans Weil-Malherbe, Harold Weiner, Paul Wender, R. Whalen, and many others. In 1961, Fritz Freyhan arrived as the Center's Director of Clinical Studies.

Again, some of the same themes (in variation) reappeared, though I cannot mention them all: microelectrophysiology, which, in Nino Salmoiragh s hands mapped the pharmacology of respiratory neurons (1962) and later with Floyd Bloom, became a pioneering technique for the study of the pharmacology of individual neurons in the central nervous system (Salmoiraghi and Bloom 1964); amine metabolism, under H. Weil-Malherbe (Weil-Malherbe et al. 1962), which also initiated a collaboration with J. Axelrod (Axelrod et al. 1959), the metabolism of psychodysleptic tryptamine derivates, under Szara (Szara et al. 1962); animal behavioral studies, combining Skinnerian avoidance training with metabolic experiments under Eliot Hearst (Szara and Hearst 1962); the effect of locally and isotopically labeled implanted hormones on behavior, under Richard Michael (1961); human behavior analysis studies under Harold Weiner (1962); the methodology of clinical drug trials under Hordern and Lofft (Hordern et al. 1963), the quantification of social interaction in a psychiatric ward under Shepherd Kellam (1961); Max Hamilton, a visiting Fellow gave seminars on the methodology of Clinical Research, and the conceptualization of comprehensive mental health care in a given community by Fritz Freyhan (Freyhan and Mayo 1963); and studies on dependency, depression, and hospitalization by Don Lipsitt (1962). Later, with the help of the late Dr. Winfred Overholser, the Behavioral and Clinical Studies Center of St. Elizabeth's was created as a complementary entity, under the direction of Dr. Neil Waldrop.

Over the last two decades, the program – later the Division of Special Mental Health Programs of the National Institute of Mental Health – assumed dynamic leadership under Dr. G.C. Salmoiraghi and later, under Drs. Floyd Bloom and Ermino Costa, who, in their subsequent, remarkable careers, have made deep and lasting contributions to the neurosciences and psychopharmacology. The leadership of the program then passed into the very capable hands of Dr. Richard Wyatt, its well-known contributions continuing to this day.

In 1963, I was invited to assume the chairmanship of the Department of Psychiatry at Johns Hopkins, vacated the previous year by my friend, Seymour Kety. Here again, fate was kind. The University provided us with some new laboratories, and the old Phipps Clinic, still standing since Adolf Meyer opened it in 1913, provided room for some 80 patients and an outpatient clinic. I count myself most fortunate in the colleagues who were with us, in the residency and fellowship programs, and in major staff positions: Drs. Ross Baldessarini, Joseph Brady, Lino Covi, Joe Coyle, Len Derogatis, Louis Faillace, Jerome Frank, Arthur Freeman, Richard Hall, Nelson Hendler, John Money, Dennis Murphy, Candace Pert, Elliott Richelson, Solomon Snyder, Nahum Spinner, Joseph Stephens, Eberhard Uhlenhuth, Daniel van Kammen, Bill Webb, Herbert Weingartner, among others.

Three major developments began to take shape in my time: Dr. Solomon Snyder established his group in neuropharmacology, from a laboratory initially jointly supported by our department and the Department of Pharmacology. Dr. Paul Talalay, Chairman of Pharmacology and a true friend, showed a rare understanding for the emerging new field of psychopharmacology. It is a matter of deep joy and satisfaction to have watched Dr. Snyder's group grow to the world leadership position that it now occupies. He now holds the post of Distinguished Service Professor at Johns Hopkins and is head of the Department of Neurosciences, created for him in the university.

Dr. Joseph Brady, who joined us from Walter Reed, brought us another important component. As a clinical psychologist with a Skinnerian background, he developed behavior analysis and operant conditioning as a major research approach to the study of the effect of drugs on behavior. Bringing his great originality and boldness of approach into the clinical arena, he rapidly created at Johns Hopkins, the Division of Behavioral Biology and Behavioral Medicine, foreseeing clearly the shape of things to come. At the same time, Drs. Eberhard

Uhlenhuth, Lino Covi, and later, Len Derogatis established much of the technology for quantitative trials in an outpatient setting. We also revived an old interest in the use of diphenylhydantoin in anxiety and depression (Dr. J. Stephens); and maintained contact with Drs. Al Kurland's and Stanislaw Grof's group at the Maryland State Psychiatric Institute. It is good to know that research activities now continue vigorously in the new Adolf Meyer building under Dr. Paul McHugh, and it warms the heart that we celebrated the 25th anniversary of our College under the leadership of "Uhli" Uhlenhuth, and that Joe Coyle is now leading psychiatry at Harvard.

FOOTINGS OF A NEW SCIENCE: NEUROCHEMISTRY, ELECTROPHYSIOLOGY, ANIMAL BEHAVIOR AND THE CLINICAL TRIAL

Looking back, with large national and international organizations in psychopharmacology spanning the globe, and vast industrial undertakings engaged in research, development, and manufacture, it is a little hard to visualize the sparse and intimate nature of our field some 40 years ago. As I said earlier, neurochemistry as we know, didn't really exist. And when I began, acetylcholine was still regarded as the principal chemical mediator in the central nervous system. Regional "elective affinities" of drugs for receptors remained in Henry Maudsley's memorable phrase, still to be "shadowed out" in the brain (Maudsley 1882), and Paul Ehrlich's "receptors" still an analogy. I remember sitting in Heinrich Waelsch's study overlooking the Hudson in August 1951, just before returning to England to take up my newly-created post. "What is experimental psychiatry?" asked Heinrich Waelsch, giving me that whimsical penetrating look of his. The newly named professor did not rightly know. "I suppose," I said, hesitatingly, "it is the application of experimental research method to clinical psychiatry; I suppose, in my own case, it is the application of chemistry to an analysis and understanding of behavior. I will tell you when I have done it for a while."

Photo of letter written by Heinrich Waelsch, Professor of Neurochemistry, Columbia University, to Joel Elkes on the occasion of his 50th birthday (11/12/63). It reads: "I am afraid that you will have to lift yourself into the second half of your century without my midwifery but with my best wishes. I can probably guess what goes on in your mind at this occasion. Some satisfaction with what has been accomplished, some surprise that it has been done and most of all a feeling of great urgency that much is still to do, and will probably stay undone. But it is just this what keeps us alive, and the arteries relatively elastic. I cannot help but taking stock at this occasion of our joint efforts. We probably have not done too badly as things go, but we have educated ourselves more in the process than others."

Later, back in England, I got in touch with Drs. Derek Richter and Geoffrey Harris; Heinrich Waelsch met with Drs. Seymour Kety, Jordi Folch-Pi, and Louis Flexner. Our joint hope, which we had shared at a previous small meeting, was to organize an International Neurochemical Symposium, the first of its kind. As the theme of the symposium, we significantly chose "The Biochemistry of the Developing Nervous System." As a place to hold it, we chose Magdalen College, Oxford. I was charged with being organizing Secretary, but could not have done it without the devoted help of my British colleagues. Sixty-nine colleagues from nine countries participated. It was a fine symposium. It may be that it was at this symposium that the term "neurochemistry" was used officially for the first time. The spirit of the meeting is conveyed in an extract from the Preface that Heinrich Waelsch and I wrote for the *Proceedings* (Waelsch and Heinrich 1955, p. 5):

> We agreed, also, that from the start it would be well to consider the brain as a biological entity in all its complexity of morphology and function, rather than as a homogenate, or an engineering problem. For that reason, we felt that the most useful contribution of a symposium of this kind would be an attempt to reintegrate biochemical process with structure and function, particularly with respect to the chemical topography of the brain, which, to us, seemed of greatest moment in an understanding of function. The program thus not only represents the framework of a conference, but also expresses an attitude; and of necessity includes discussion of structural, genetic, and pathological aspects, as well as subject matter that in the more limited sense may be termed "neurochemical." We feel that this approach may be helpful in slowly building the foundations for a rational therapy of disorders of the nervous system.

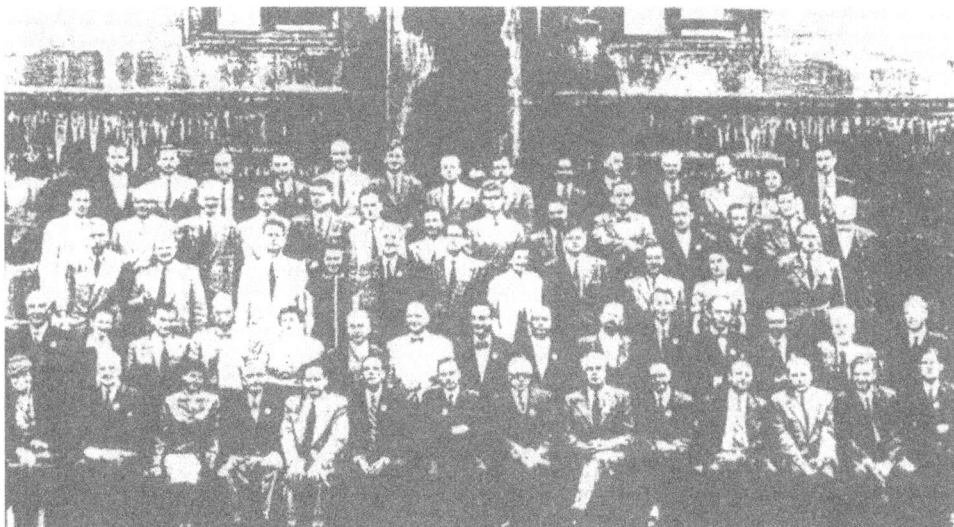

The First International Neurochemical Symposium held at Magdalen College, Oxford, 1954.

Three subsequent symposia reflected the momentum that was developing at this historic first meeting. The second on "The Metabolism of the Nervous System" was held in Aarhus, Denmark in 1956. The *Proceedings* were edited by D. Richter (1957). The third on "The Chemical Pathology of the Nervous System" followed in Strasbourg, France in 1958. The *Proceedings* were edited by Jordi Folch-Pi (1961). The Fourth International Symposium centered on "Regional Neurochemistry." It was held in Varenna, Italy in 1960. Seymour Kety and I edited the *Proceedings* (1961).

It is impossible to convey the excitement and productivity that attended these meetings as they steadily shaped some basic concepts in our field. I can only mention a very few examples, perforce omitting others of equal merit, referring the reader to the respective *Proceedings*.

There were, for example, the remarkable studies of the chemistry of single neurons using X-ray microphotometry by Holger Hyden (1955) and the chemical micromethods of Oliver Lowry, making possible the mapping the layer-by-layer of enzyme distribution in the retina and Ammon's horn (1955); quantitative cytochemical studies by Al Pope (1955); the early work on the distribution of cholinesterase by Koelle (1961); descriptions of the biochemical specificities of neurons by R.W. Sperry (1955); the classical cerebral circulation studies by Seymour Kety (1957) and Lou Sokoloff (1961); studies on the metabolic responses to electric stimulation by Paul Greengard and H. McIlwain (1955); and the whole concept of metabolic pools by H. Waelsch (1961).

There came, in quick succession, the classical reviews of the place and regional distribution of acetylcholine by Feldberg (1957), norepinephrine by von Euler (1957) and Marthe Vogt (1957); serotonin by Udenfriend, Bogdanski and Weissbach (1957) covering the early work of Gaddum (1953), Wooley and Shaw (1954), and Brodie, Pletscher, and Shore (1955), in the history of this key mediator in the brain; of gamma amino butyric acid by Roberts (1961). An excellent early review on noncholinergic transmission (including Substance P, vasodilator substances, ATP, and histamine) was given by J. Crossland (1957). Most importantly, there was also the early presentation of the occurrence and effect of the nerve growth factor by Rita Levi Montalcini and P.U. Angeletti (1961). It is said that the highest compliment to a piece of work is its acceptance by the public to the point of anonymity of its authors. The names I mentioned are not exactly household words in psychopharmacology today; yet we owe some fundamental concepts of our science to them.

Similarly, in electrophysiology the early work on the sequential iontophoretic application of drugs and metabolites to single cells that started with the muscle end plate (Fatt 1954) and extended into the work of Curtis (1961) and into the classical studies of Salmoiraghi and Bloom (1964), leading later to study of susceptibility to neurotransmitters in individual cells in mixed populations. These approaches complemented studies on the pharmacology of the reticular formation by the Killams (1956) and Bradley (1957), the effects of drugs on the electrical activity of the brain in the conscious animal mentioned above (Bradley and Elkes 1957), studies that quickly led to an analysis of the electrophysiological effects of chlorpromazine (Bradley and Hance 1956).

Imagine, however, the excitement when these findings were put into the context of the effect of drugs on self-stimulation of the Reward systems in the hands of James Olds (1958) and the application of the Skinnearian approach to an analysis on the effects of drugs on behavior by Brady (1956) and Sidman (1956), and Dews (1955), the development soon thereafter of cognate approaches in the hands of many others too numerous to mention. In a word, as meetings proceeded, things began to *connect:* neurochemistry connected to electrophysiology, and electrophysiology to behavior: and animal behavior to the clinical trial. The difficulties in evaluation were faced early and honestly (Cole and Gerard 1959 see below). Suddenly, an array of evaluation techniques was available. Industrial psychopharmacology took note and very rapidly moved our field mightily into the marketplace. Yet, our small group continued to do science by correspondence; I still remember the illegible notes, often on blue airmail letters (no fax in those days!), which brought the latest news. Those were heady days, to be sure. The process felt in some way like the collective painting of a mural; it all looked a bit weird at first, but month by month, and certainly year by year, it was beginning to make increasing sense: some pieces remained blurred, but others looked quite beautiful.

THE EMERGENCE OF ORGANIZATIONS

In the meantime, other important events were stirring. The Macy Symposia on Neuropharmacology, initiated by Dr. Harold Abramson in 1954, brought a number of us together (1954) and in 1956, under the joint chairmanship of Drs. Jonathan Cole and Ralph Gerard, a milestone Conference on Psychopharmacology was held under the aegis of the National Research Council, the National Academy of Sciences, and the American Psychiatric Association (1959), during which year also Dr. Cole's Psychopharmacology Service Center was created, a step of enormous consequence for the future development of the field all over the world.

In 1957, the World Health Organization invited me to serve as consultant and convened a small study group on the subject of Ataractic and Hallucinogenic Drugs in Psychiatry. The following participated: Ludwig von Bertalanffy, USA (Systems Theory), U.S. von Euler, Sweden (Pharmacology), E. Jacobsen, Denmark (Pharmacology), Morton Kramer, USA (Epidemiology), T.A. Lambo, Nigeria (Transcultural Psychiatry), E. Lindemann, USA (Psychiatry), P. Pichot, France (Psychology), D. McK. Rioch, USA (Neurosciences), R.A. Sandison, England (Psychia-

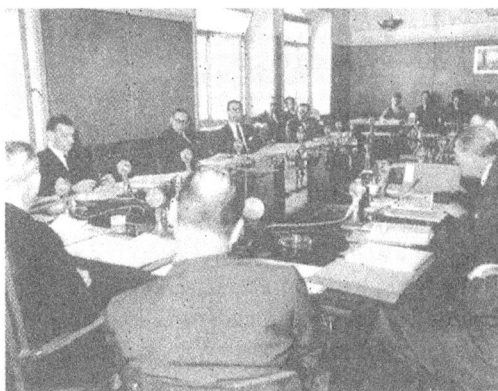

Meeting of the First World Health Organization Study Group on Ataractic and Hallucinogenic Agents, Geneva, 1957. In photo second from left: J. Elkes (USA, Chair); third from left: P.B. Schneider (Switzerland); fourth from left: M. Kramer (USA); and middle right, in profile: E. Jacobsen (Denmark).

WORLD HEALTH ORGANIZATION

TECHNICAL REPORT SERIES

No. 152

ATARACTIC AND HALLUCINOGENIC DRUGS IN PSYCHIATRY

Report of a Study Group

This report contains the collective views of an international group of experts and does not necessarily represent the decisions or the stated policy of the World Health Organization.

WORLD HEALTH ORGANIZATION
PALAIS DES NATIONS
GENEVA

1958

The title page of World Health Organization first Technical Report on psychoactive drugs (1958). Joel Elkes wrote this report.

try), P.B. Schneider, Switzerland (Clinical Pharmacology), J. Elkes, England (Rapporteur).

I wrote the report (1958) which, incidentally, carried Eric Jacobsen's pioneer classification of the main drugs according to their pharmacological properties. In the meantime, the Scientific Command of the U.S. Air Force, through its principal representative in Europe, Col. James Henry, had catalyzed important work in the neurological sciences in a number of European laboratories. Through these meetings, the international implications of brain research became steadily more apparent. After preliminary meetings in 1958, 1959, and 1960, a number of us met in UNESCO House in 1960 to draft the statutes and bylaws of IBRO, the International Brain Research Organization. The disciplines of neuroanatomy, neurochemistry, neuroendocrinology, neuropharmacology, neurophysiology, behavioral sciences, neurocommunication, and biophysics were represented. Dr. Daniel Bovet and I represented neuropharmacology on the First Central Council of IBRO.

At about the same time, national groups in psychopharmacology began to form, at first loosely and informally, and later in more definitive ways. That most important international body, the Collegium Internationale Neuro-Psychopharmacologicum was born in 1956, and, as mentioned earlier – reflecting Drs. E. Rothlin's and Abraham Wikler's energy and devotion – our own journal of *Psychopharmacologia*, representing our new science, saw the light of day in 1959, and has continued as a yardstick of excellence since. In 1970, I had the great pleasure of founding the Israel Center for Psychobiology, a national center comprising representation from five universities and two research institutes. Psychopharmacology was richly represented in its work. Drs. A. Carmon and M. Abeles succeeded me as Directors; and Dr. H. Belmaker, distinguished psychopharmacologist has led the field in Israel since its inception. The Center is now known as the Israel National Institute for Psychobiology. I was also honored later, to be elected a Charter Fellow of the Canadian College of Neuropsychopharmacology.

CLOSING

There are many other memories that flood the mind, but clearly these reminiscences have gone on much too long, and I must come to a close. When, through the initiatives of Drs. Ted Rothman, Paul Hoch, Jonathan Cole and some of us, as I have recorded elsewhere (1963), the American College of Neuropsychopharmacology was constituted in Washington in 1960, and did me the immense honor of electing me its first President, I could not help remembering that this had happened only 15 years after I played with macromolecular models and the x-ray diffraction of myelin in my laboratory in Birmingham, and only 10 years after we had created a Department of Experimental Psychiatry in Birmingham. I could not help reflecting on the unique power of our field to act not only as a catalyst, but as a binder; a catalyst bringing into being whole new areas of science, but also as a binder and a relater of these sciences to each other. For we had not only to create fields of investigation and measuring devices in many disciplines, but also a degree of understanding and interaction between disciplines which is very rare. As I said at the time (1963):

> It is nut uncommon for any one of us to be told that Psychopharmacology is not a science, and that it would do well to emulate the precision of older and more established disciplines. Such statements betray a lack of understanding for the special demands made by Psychopharmacology upon the fields which compound it. Fur my own part, I draw comfort and firm conviction from the history of our subject and the history of our group. For I know of

no other branch of science which, like a good plough on a spring day has tilled as many areas in Neurobiology. To have, in a mere decade, questioned the concepts of synaptic transmission in the central nervous system; to have emphasized compartmentalization and regionalization of chemical process in the unit cell and in the brain; to have given us tools for the study of chemical basis of learning and temporary connection formation; to have emphasized the dependence of pharmacological response on its situational and social setting; to have compelled a hard look at the semantics of psychiatric diagnosis, description and communication; to have resuscitated that oldest of old remedies, the placebo response, for careful scrutiny; to have provided potential methods for the study of language in relation to the functional state of the brain; and to have encouraged the Biochemist, Physiolo-

American College of Neuropsychopharmacology

FIRST ANNUAL MEETING

January 24 - 27th, 1963

PROGRAM

THE WOODNER HOTEL

3636 Sixteenth Street, Northwest

Washington 10, D. C.

1962   OFFICERS   1963

President — Joel Elkes, M.D.
President - Elect — Paul H. Hoch, M.D.
Vice - President — Klaus R. Unna, M.D.
Secretary - Treasurer — Theodore Rothman, M.D.
Assistant Secretary - Treasurer — Milton Greenblatt, M.D.

COUNCIL

Frank J. Ayd, Jr., M.D.   Bernard B. Brodie, Ph.D.
Jonathan O. Cole, M.D.   Heinz E. Lehmann, M.D.
James E. P. Toman, Ph.D.   Joseph Zubin, Ph.D.

PROGRAM AND SCIENTIFIC COMMUNICATIONS COMMITTEE

Jonathan O. Cole, M.D., Chairman
Bernard B. Brodie, Ph.D.   Conan Kornetsky, Ph.D.
Seymour S. Kety, M.D.   Milton Greenblatt, M.D.
Keith F. Killam, Ph.D.

Pages from the program of the First Annual Meeting of the American College of Neuropsycho-pharmacology.

gist, Psychologist, Clinician, the Mathematician and Communication Engineer to join forces at bench level, is no mean achievement for a young science. That a chemical text should carry the imprint of experience, and partake in its growth, in no way invalidates study of symbols, and the rules among symbols, which keep us going, changing, evolving and human. Thus, though moving cautiously, psychopharmacology is still protesting; yet, in so doing, it is, fur the first time, compelling the physical and chemical sciences to look behaviour in the face, and thus enriching both these sciences and behavior. If there be discomfiture in this encounter, it is hardly surprising; for it is in this discomfiture that there may well lie the germ of a new science.

In our branch of science, it would seem we are as attracted to soma as to symbol; we are as interested in overt behavior as we are aware of the subtleties of subjective experience. There is here no conflict between understanding the way things are and the way people are, between the pursuit of science and the giving of service.

As new borderlands beckon, and as our science moves into fresh terrain, the chemical languages in which the nervous system, the endocrine system, and the immune system converse are becoming increasingly known. They are very precise. Receptors of common lineage suggest a remarkable economy in chemical evolution. Like a modern Rosetta Stone, psychopharmacology holds the key to much that is puzzling today. We must deepen our discourse with psychoimmunology, for we have much to offer to each other; and in a wider perspective, we may yet prove powerful brokers between quantum physics and the neurosciences. Concepts of electromagnetic fields (Adey 1988) may be needed to supplement our present concepts of chemical messaging: Who knows? The brain may emerge as a unique amplifier of very fast quantal events. As I delve into modern physics (Dyson 1988), I continue to be reminded of the physics I read in my youth. When, in years to come, the chemical code is more fully read, new understanding will continue to astonish. There will be new approaches to healing, new hopes for many; and with it an ethical dilemma remorseless in its recurrent dialectic.

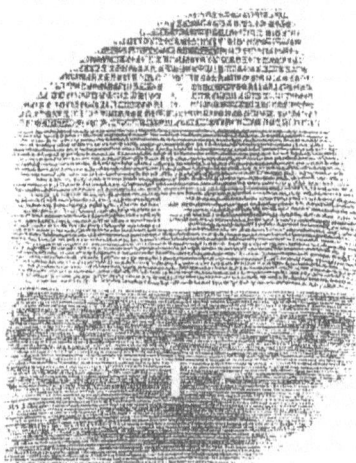

Like the Rosetta Stone, Psychopharmacology provides a key to three languages: the nervous system (N); the endocrine system (E); and the immune system (I).

Today, street drugs are a tragedy, and smart drugs still a joke: But when our college meets a quarter of century hence, huge new questions will loom, and will not go away. Let us, therefore, while there is still time, develop structures to guard us from the consequences of our own curiosity, and – dare I say it? – our own ambitions. I remember discussing such matters with Leo Szilard to whose seminal insights we owe the very origins of the atomic bomb. We met shortly before he died. You may recall that very early in the game, he and his colleagues created the "Bulletin of the Atomic Scientists." On the face sheet there was displayed a clock, the position of its hands reflecting the political stability of our world. At the time of the Cuban missile crisis, they read a few seconds to twelve; they may have shifted to a more reassuring position since. Perhaps we should think of our own bulletin, in which we could speak of our hopes, achievements, and fears to society. There is no greater safeguard against the consequences of our inventiveness than an informed public. As for our clock, and the ticking of what my wife, Josephine, calls the "Brain Bomb," I do not know what time the hands would show this fine morning in December 1992; but I suspect it may be later than we think.

ACKNOWLEDGMENTS
The author wishes to express his sincere thanks to Professor P.B. Bradley, Professor Emeritus, University of Birmingham, England, for his kind permission to reproduce photographs from his thesis; to Dr. Frank J. Ayd for his permission to draw on an earlier paper given by the author at a meeting convened by Dr. Ayd in 1970 [Discoveries in Biological Psychiatry, F.J. Ayd and Barry Blackwell (editors) Lippincott, 1970]. He deeply appreciates the hospitality given him by the Fetzer Institute, Kalamazoo, Michigan, during the preparation of this article, and the expert technical assistance of Ms. Carolyn Dailey, Administrative Assistant at the Institute

REFERENCES
Adey WR (1988): Physiological signalling across cell membranes and cooperative influences of extremely low frequency electromagnetic fields. In Frohlich, H (ed), Biological Coherence and Response to External Stimuli. Springer-Verlag, pp 148-170
Abramson HA (ed) (1954): Neuropharmacology. New York, Josiah Macy Jr. Foundation
Aghajanian GK (1970): Effects of LSD-on raphe nuclei neurons. Neurosciences Res Program Bull 8:40-54
Axelrod J, Weil Malherbe H, Tomchik R (1959): The physiological disposition of H(3) epinephrine and its metabolite metanephrine. J Pharmocol Exptl Therapeutics 127:251-256
Ayd FJ (1991): The early history of modern psychopharmacology. Neuropsychopharmacology 5; 71-85
Berger FM, Bradley W (1946): The pharmacological properties of χ:β dihydroxy-γ-(2-methylphenoxy)-propane (Myanesin). Brit J Pharmacol 1:265
Bradley PB (1952): Observations of the Effects of Drugs on The Electrical Activity of the Brain. Thesis, submitted as a candidate to qualify for the degree of Philosophae Doctor, University of Birmingham, England
Bradley PB (1953): A technique for recording the electrical activity of the brain in the conscious animal. Electroenceph Clin Neurophysiol 5:451
Bradley PB (1957): Microelectrode approach to the neuropharmacology of the reticular formation. In Garratini S, Ghetti V (eds), Psychotropic Drugs. Amsterdam, Elsevier, p 201
Bradley PB, Elkes J (1953): The effect of atrophine, hyoscyamine physostigmine and neostigmine on the electrical activity of the brain of the conscious cat. J. Physiol (London) 120:14
Bradley PB, Elkes J (1957): The effects of some drugs on the electrical activity of the brain. Brain 80:77-117
Bradley PB, Elkes J (1953): The effect of amphetamine and d-lysergic acid diethylamide (LSD-25) on the electrical activity of the brain of the cunscious cat. J Physiol (London) 120:13
Bradley PB, Hance AJ (1956): The effects of chlorpromazine and methopromazine of the electrical activity of the brain in the cat. EEG Clin Neurophysiol 6:191-215
Brady JV (1956): Assessment of drug effects on emotional behavior. Science 123:1033
Brodie BB, Pletscher A, Shore PA (1955): Evidence that Serotonin Has a Role in Brain Function. Science 122:968
Cole J, Gerard RW (eds) (1959): Psychopharmacology: Problems in Evaluation. Washington, DC, National Academy of Science and National Research Council
Crossland J (1957): The problem of non-cholinergic transmission in the central nervous system. In Richter D (ed), The Metabolism of the Nervous System, Oxford, Pergamon, pp 523-541
Curtis DR (1961): The effects of drugs and amino acids upon neurons. In Kety 55, Elkes J, (eds), Regional Neurochemistry, Oxford, Pergamon, pp 403-422
Delay J, Deniker P (1953): Les neuroplegiques en therapeutique psychiatrique. Therapie 8:347
Dews PB (1955): Studies on behavior. I. Differential sensitivity to pentobarbital of pecking performance in pigeons depending on schedule of reward. J Pharmacol Exp Therap 113:393
Dyson F (1988): Infinite in all directions: The Gifford Lectures. New York, Harper and Row
Elkes J (rapporteur) (1958): Ataractic and Hallucinogenic Drugs in Psychiatry. WHO Tech Rep Series, 152. Geneva, World Health Organization
Elkes J (1963): The American College of Neuropsychopharmacology: A note on its history and hopes for the future. Amer College Neuropsychopharmacology Bulletin 1:2-3
Elkes J (1957): Some effects of psychotomimetic drugs on the experimental animal and in man. In Neuropharmacology, Transactions of the Third Conference, New York, Josiah Macy, Jr. Foundation, pp 205-294
Elkes J (1953): In Tanner, JM (ed), Prospects in Psychiatric Research. Oxford (England), Blackwell, p 126
Elkes J. (1958): Drug effects in relation to receptor specificity within the brain: Some evidence and provisional formulation. In Wostenholme, G (ed), Ciba Foundation Symposium on the Neurological Basis of Behavior. London, Churchill, pp 303-332
Elkes J. (1961): Drugs influencing affect and behavior: Possible neural correlates in relation to mode of action. In Simon A (ed), The Physiolvgy of Emotions. Springfield (IL), Thomas, p 95
Elkes J (1966): Psychoactive drugs: Some problems and approaches. In Solomon P (ed), Psychiatric Drugs. New York, Grune, pp 4-21

Elkes J. (1967): Behavioral pharmacology in relation to psychiatry. In Gruhle HW, Jung R, Mayer-Gross W, and Muller M (eds), Psychiatrie der Gegenwart, Berlin, Springer, pp 931-1038

Elkes J., Eayrs JT, Todrick A (1955): On the effect and the lack of effect of some drugs on postnatal development in the rat. In Waelsch H (ed), Biochemistry of the Developing Nervous System, New York, Academic, p 409

Elkes J, Elkes C (1954): Effects of chlorpromazine on the behaviour of chronically overactive psychotic patients. Brit Med J 2:560

Elkes J, Elkes C, Bradley PB (1954): The effect of some drugs on the electrical activity of the brain and on behavior. J Ment Sci 100:125

Elkes J, Finean JB (1949): The effect of drying upon the structure of myelin in the sciatic nerve of the frog. In Discussion of the Faraday Society (Lipoproteins), London, p 134

Elkes J, Finean JB (1953): X-ray diffraction studies on the effects of temperature on the structure of myelin in the sciatic nerve of the frog. Exp Cell Res 4:69

Elkes J, Finean JB (1953): Effects of solvents on the structure of myelin in the sciatic nerve of the frog. Exp Cell Res 4:82

Elkes J, Frazer AC, Stewart HC (1939): The composition of particles seen in normal human blood under dark ground illumination. J Physiol 95:68

Elkes J, Todrick A (1955): On the development of the cholinesterases in the rat brain. In Waelsch H (ed), Biochemistry of the Developing Nervous System. New York, Acad Press, p 309

Engstrom A, Finean JB (1958): Biological Ultrastructure. New York, Academic Press

Fatt P (1954): Biophysics of junetional transmission. Physiol Rev 34:674

Feldberg W (1957): Acetylcholine. In Richter, D (ed), The Metabolism of the Nervous System, Oxford, Pergamon, 493-510

Feldberg W, Vogt M (1948): Acetylcholine synthesis in different regions of central nervous system. J Physiol (London) 107: 372

Finean JB (1961): Chemical Ultrastructure in Living Tissues. Springfield (IL), Thomas

Folch-Pi J (ed) (1961): The Chemical Pathology of the Nervous System, Proceedings of the Third International Symposium in Neurochemistry. Oxford, Pergamon

French AP (ed) (1979): Einstein: A centenary volume. Cambridge (MA), Harvard University Press

Freyhan F, Mayo JA (1963): Concept of a model psychiatric clinic. Amer J Psychiat 120:222

Gaddum JH (1953): Antagonism between lysergic acid diethylamide and 5-hydroxytryptamine. J Physiol (London) 121:15

Gastaut H (1950): Combined photic and metrazol activation of the brain. Electroenceph Clin Neurophysiol 2:263

Greengard P, Mcllwain H (1955): Metabolic response to electrical pulses in mammalian cerebral cortex during development. In Waelsch, H (ed), The Biochemistry of the Developing Nervous System, New York, Academic, pp 251-260

Himmelwait F (ed) (1956): The Collected Papers of Paul Ehrlich. London/New York, Pergamon

Himwich HE, Bowman KM, Fazekas JF, Goldfarb W (1940): Temperature and brain metabolism. Amer J Med Sci 200:347

Hill D (1944): Cerebral dysrhythmia: Its significance in aggressive behavior. Proc Roy Soc Med 37:317

Hill D, Pond DA (1952): Reftections of one hundred capital cases submitted to electroencephalography. J Ment Sci 98:23

Hordern A, Hamilton M, Waldrop FN, Lofft JC (1963): A controlled trial on the value of prochlorperazine and trifluoperazine and intensive group treatment. Brit] Psychiat 109:510-522

Hyden H (1955): The chemistrv of single neurons; A study with new methods. In Waelsch H (ed), Biochemistry of the Developing Nervous System. New York, Academic, pp 359-371

Jasper H (1949): Symposium: Thalamocortical relationships; diffuse projection systems: Integrative action of thalamic reticular system. Electroenceph Clin Neurvphysiol 1:406

Kellam SG (1961): A method for assessing social contact: Its application during a rehabilitation program on a psychiatric ward. J Nerv Ment Dis 132:277

Kety S, Elkes J (eds) (1961): Regional Neurochemistry, Proceedings of the Fourth International Symposium in Neurochemistry. Oxford, Pergamon

Kety SS (1957): General metabolism of the brain in vivo. In Richter D (ed), The Metabolism of the Nervous System, Oxford, Pergamon, pp 221-237

Killam KF, Killam EK (1956): A comparison of the effects of reserpine and chlorpromazine to those of barbiturates on central afferent systems in the cat. J Pharmacol Exp Ther 116:35

Kluver H (1942): Mechanisms of hallucinations. In MeNemar Q, Merrill MA (eds), Studies in Personality. New York, McGraw-Hill, p 175

Koelle GB (1961): Evidence for differences in primary functions of acetylcholinesterase at different synapses and neuroeffector junctions. In Kety S, Elkes J (eds), Regional Neurochemistry. Oxford, Pergamon, pp 312-323

Lehmann H (1991): "Before they called it psychopharmacology" – invited ACNP lecture, presented at 30th Annual Meeting of the American College of Neuropsychopharmacology, San Juan, Puerto Rico, December 10th

Levi-Montalcini R, Angeletti PU (1961): Biological properties of a nerve growth promoting protein and its antiserum. In Kety SS, Elkes J (eds), Regional Neurochemistry, Oxford, Pergamon, pp 363-377

Lindemann E, Malamud W (1934). Experimental analysis of the psychopathological effects of intoxicating drugs. Amer J Psychiat 13:853

Lipsitt DR (1962): Dependency, depression, and hospitalization: Towards an understanding of a conspiracy. Psychiat. Quarterly 30537-554

Lowry OH (1955): A study of the nervous system with quantitative histochemical methods. In Waelsch H (ed), The Biochemistry of the Developing Nervous System, New York, Academic, pp 350-357

Masserman JH (1946): An analysis of the intluence of alcohol on experimental neuroses in cats. Psychosom Med 8:36

Maudsley H (1882): The Physiology and Pathology of the Mind, Third Edition, Part 2. New York, Appleton, p 195

McDougall W (1935): The Frontiers of Psychology. Cambridge (England), Cambridge University Press

Michael RP (1961): An investigation of the sensitivity of circumscribed neurological areas to hormonal stimulation by means of the application of oestrogens directly to the brain of the cat. In Kety S, Elkes J (eds), Regional Neurochemistry. Oxford (England), Pergamon, p 465

Michaelis M, Quastel JH (1941): Site of action of narcotics in respiratory processes. Biochem J 35:518.

Moruzzi C, Magoun HW (1949): Brainstem reticular formation and activation of the EEG. Electroenceph Clin Neurophysiol 1:455

Nevinson HW (1931): Goethe: Man and Poet: Written for the Centenary of Goethe's Death. London (England), Nisbet

Olds J (1958): Selective effects of drives and drugs in "reward" systems of the brain. In Wostenholme G (ed), Ciba Symposium on Neurological Basis of Behavior. London, Churchill, p 124

Page IH (1937): Chemistry of the Brain. Springfield (IL), Thomas

Pauling L (1945): The Nature of the Chemical Bond and the Structure of Molecules and Crystals: An Introduction to Modern Structural Chemistry. Ithaca (NY), Cornell Universitv

Penfield W (1947): Ferrier lecture: Some observations on the cerebral cortex of man. Proc Roy Soc Med 134:329

Pickworth FA (1941): Occurrence and significance of small vascular lesions in brain. J Men Sc 87:50-76

Pope A (1955): The relationship of neurochemistry to the microscopic anatomy of the nervous system. In Waelsch H (ed), Biochemistry of the Developing Nervous System, New York, Academic, pp 341-349

Richter D (1940): Inactivation of adrenaline in vivo in man. J Physiol (London) 98:361

Richter D (ed) (1957): The Metabolism of the Nervous System, Proceedings of the Second International Symposium in Neurochemistry. Oxford, Pergamon

Roberts E (1961): Metabolism of gamma amino butyric acid in various areas of the brain. In Kety SS, Elkes J (eds), Regional Neurochemistry, Oxford, Pergamon, pp 324-339

Salmoiraghi GC (1962): Pharmacology of Respiratory Neurons, Proceedings of First International Pharmacology Meetings. Oxford, Pergamon, pp 217-229

Salmoiraghi GC, Bloom FE (1964): Pharmacology of individual neurons. Science 144:493

Sargant W, Shorvon HJ (1945): Acute war neuroses. Arch Neurol (Chicago) 54:231

Schmitt FO (1935): X-ray diffraction studies on nerve. Radiology 25 :131

Schmitt FO (1941): X-ray diffraction studies on structure of nerve myelin sheath. J Cell Physiol 18:31

Sherrington CS (1911): The Integrative Action of the Nervous System. New Haven, Yale University Press

Sherrington CS (1941): Man on His Nature. Cambridge (England), Cambridge University Press, p 104

Sidman M (1956): Drug behavior interaction. Ann NY Acad Sc 65:282

Sokoloff L (1961): Local cerebral circulation at rest and during altered cerebral activity induced by anaesthesia or visual stimulation. In Kety S, Elkes J (eds), Regional Neurochemistry, Oxford, Pergamon, pp 107-117

Sperry RW (1955): Problems in the biochemical specification of neurons. In Waelsch H (ed), The Biochemistry of the Developing Nervous System, Oxford, Pergamon, pp 75-84

Szara S, Hearst E (1962): The 6-hydroxylation of tryptamine derivatives: A way of producing psychoactive metabolites. Ann NY Acad Sci 96:134

Szara S, Hearst E, Putney F (1962): Metabolism and behavioral action of psychotropic tryptamine homologues. Int J Neuropharmacol 1:111

Thudichum JWL (1884): A Treatise on the Chemical Constitution of the Brain. London, Balliere

Toman J, Davis JP (1949): The effects of drugs upon the electrical activity of the brain. Pharmacol Rev 1:425

Udenfriend S, Bogdanski DF, Weissbach H (1957): Biochemistry and metabolism of serotonin as it relates to the nervous system. In Richter D (ed), The Metabolism of the Nervous System, Pergamon, pp 567-577

Vogt M (1957): Distribution of adrenaline and noradrenaline in the central nervous system and its modification by drugs. In Richter D (ed), The Metabolism of the Nervous System, Pergamon, pp 553-565

Von Euler US (1957): Noradrenaline. In Richter D (ed), The Metabolism of the Nervous System, Pergamon, 543-552

Waelsch H (ed) (1955): Biochemistry of the Developing Nervous System, Proceedings of the First International Symposium in Neurochemistry. New York, Academic, p 5

Waelsch H (1961): Compartmentalized biosynthetic reactions in the central nervous system. In Kety SS, Elkes J. (eds), Regional Neurochemistry, Oxford, Pergamon, pp 57-64

Walter VJ, Walter WG (1949): The central effects of rhythmic sensory stimulation. Electroenceph Clin Neurophysiol 1:57

Weil Malherbe H, Smith ERB (1962): Metabolites of catecholamines in urine and tissues. J. Neuropsychiatry, 113-117

Weiner H (1962): Some effects of response cost upon human operant behavior. J Exp Anal Behav 5:201

Wikler A (1952): Pharmacologic dissociation of behavior and EEG "sleep patterns" in dogs; morphine, n-allyl-normorphine and atropine. Proc Soc Exp Biol Med, 79:261

Wikler A (1957): The Relation of Psychiatry to Pharmacology. Baltimore, Williams and Wilkins

Wooley DW, Shaw E (1954): A Biochemical and Pharmacological Suggestion about Certain Mental Disorders. Proc Nat Acad Sciences 40:228

PAPER 4

THE AMERICAN COLLEGE OF NEUROPSYCHOPHARMACOLOGY: A NOTE ON ITS HISTORY, AND HOPES FOR THE FUTURE

Joel Elkes

Reprinted with the kind permission of The American College of Neuropsychopharmacology from the *ACNP Bulletin* 1: 2-3, 1962

It is both timely and pleasant to recall, on the occasion of the first issue of the Bulletin, the events which led to the establishment of our young organization.

On November 12-13, 1960, a Conference for the Advancement of Neuropsychopharmacology was held at the Barbizon-Plaza Hotel, New York City, organized by the convening Secretary, Dr. Theodore Rothman, under the Chairmanship of Dr. Paul Hoch. The main purpose of the Conference was to stimulate critical discussion and suggest proposals for the advancement of Neuropsychopharmacology.

There were twenty participants, and above twenty guests present at this Conference. The program was introduced by Dr. Rothman. The present situation in Neuropsychopharmacology and Psychiatry was discussed by Dr. Paul Hoch and Dr. Heinz Lehmann. Proposals were made to improve the evaluation of the psychoactive agents, and the dissemination of accurate information to investigators. These discussions were led by Dr. Paul Feldman and Dr. Jonathan Cole. Dr. Bernard Brodie opened a session dedicated to an evaluation of the present state of neuropsychopharmacological research; his paper was discussed by Dr. Abram Hoffer. Dr. Eugene M. Chaffey and Dr. Joseph M. Tobin spoke on the need of collaborative multidisciplinary research. Recommendations were made by Conference participants, and were summarized by Dr. Arnold Scheibel and Dr. James T. Ferguson. The most important of these was a recommendation for the creation of a Committee to organize an American College of Neuropsychopharmacology. Dr. Theodore Rothman was elected Chairman of this Organizing Committee; other members were Dr. Frank J. Ayd, Dr. Bernard B. Brodic, Dr. Jonathan O. Cole, Dr. Paul Feldman and Dr. Paul H. Hoch.

Dr. Rothman and the Organizing Committee met numerous times during the following months and spent many hours investigating, inquiring, studying and readying plans for an organizational meeting of interested individuals drawn from Neuropsychopharmacology and its allied fields, with the set purpose of creating a permanent Society for the Advancement of Neuropsychopharmacology. A draft of a Constitution and By-Laws was formulated, and steps taken to form a non-profit, scientific research corporation in the State of Maryland, to be known as the American College of Neuropsychopharmacology. These preparations led ultimately to the First Organizational Meeting of the American College of Neuropsychopharmacology, which was held in Washington, D. C., on October 7-8, 1961.

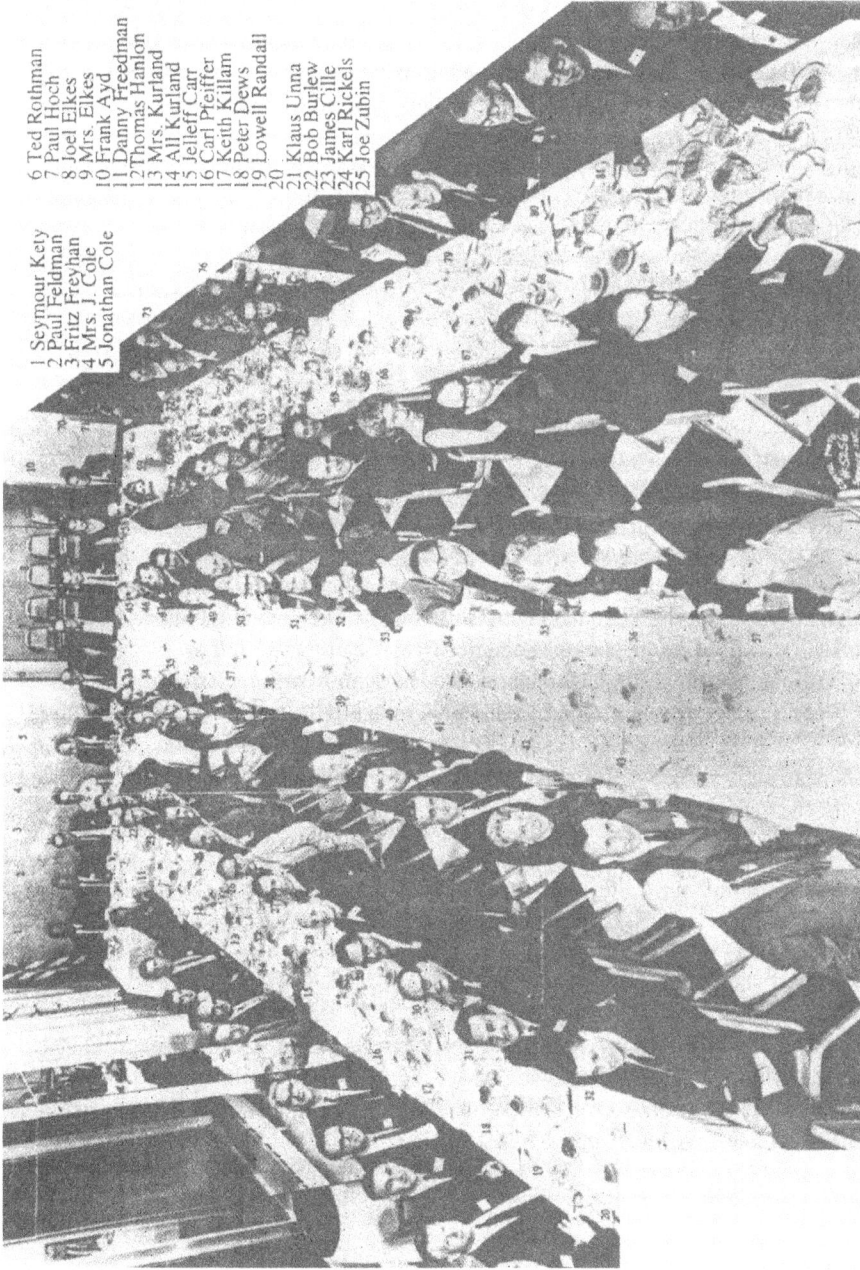

1 Seymour Kety
2 Paul Feldman
3 Fritz Freyhan
4 Mrs. J. Cole
5 Jonathan Cole

6 Ted Rothman
7 Paul Hoch
8 Joel Elkes
9 Mrs. Elkes
10 Frank Ayd
11 Danny Freedman
12 Thomas Hamlon
13 Mrs. Kurland
14 All Kurland
15 Jelleff Carr
16 Carl Pfeiffer
17 Keith Killam
18 Peter Dews
19 Lowell Randall
20
21 Klaus Unna
22 Bob Burlew
23 James Cille
24 Karl Rickels
25 Joe Zubin

26 Sy Fisher
27 Murray Jarvik
28 Sam Irvin
29 Ernest Sigg
30 Lincoln Clark
31 Al DiMascio
32 Bud Veech
33 Erminio Costa
34 Mrs. Costa
35 Guy Everett
36 Alex Karczmar
37 Sid Malitz
38 Stan Lesse
39 Mervin Clark
40 Len Cook
41 Conan Kornetsky
42 Lorraine Bouthilet
43 Charles Shagass
44 Dick Wittenborn
45 Max Rinkel
46 Jim Toman
47 Hussain Azima
48 Mrs. Winkelman
49 Bill Winkelman
50 Burt Schiele
51 Elsie Kris
52 Doug Goldman
53 Max Fink
54 Gerry Klerman
56 Sherman Ross
57 Mrs. Ross
58 Herb Freed
59 Mrs. Freed
60 Max Reiss
61 Mrs. Reiss
62 John Pearse
63 Al Freedman
64 Mrs. Hines
65 Lein Hines
66
67 Werner Koella
68 John Burns
69 Abe Wikler
70
71
72 Rita Ayd
73 N.D.C. Lewis
74 Henry Brill
75 Barbara Fish
76 Heinz Lehmann
77 Arnold Friedhoff
78 Eugene Roberts
79 Paul Greengard
80 Henry Beecher
81 Jean Bennett

American College of Neuropsychopharmacology, First Organizational Meeting Dinner, Washington, October 8, 1961

This meeting was chaired by Dr. Theodore Rothman. Dr. Jonathan O. Cole spoke briefly on the needs for an American College and Dr. Paul H. Hoch discussed the proposals and objectives for the College. The ninety participating members present at the meeting recommended that a multi-disciplinary group of one hundred and twenty-three be accorded temporary Charter Fellowship. A Credentials Committee was formed to study all temporary fellowships and report to the members at the next Annual Meeting of the ACNP.

During the course of the meeting, I moderated a symposium on the contributions of the Basic Sciences to Neuropsychopharmacology; Dr. Fritz Freyhan moderated a symposium on the contributions of the clinician to the Science of Neuropsychopharmacology; and Dr. Jonathan O. Cole spoke on the current program of the Psychopharmacology Servier Center, NIMH.

The participating members represented twenty-two states and two Canadian provinces; they approved a Constitution and By-Laws for the College. All disciplines immediately concerned with Neuropsychopharmacology, including Pharmacology, Psychiatry, Psychology, Neurophysiology and Biochemistry, were represented at the meeting.

It was during this meeting, also, that the Assembly elected the following officers; President-Elect, Dr. Paul H. Hoch; Vice-President, Dr. Klaus R. Unna; Secretary-Treasurer, Dr. Theodore Rothman; Assistant Secretary-Treasurer, Dr. Milton Greenblatt; and did me the great honor of electing me First President. Council members elected were: Drs. Frank J. Ayd, Bernard B. Brodic, Jonathan O. Cole, Heinz E. Lehman, James E. P. Toman, and Joseph Zubin.

In keeping with its mandate from this first organizational meeting, Council proceeded to structure the work of the College by way of its various committees. These committees comprised the Nominating Committee (Chairman, Dr. M. Rinkel); Credentials Committee (Chairman, Dr. Fritz A. Freyhan); Program and Scientific Communications Committee (Chairman, Dr. Jonathan O. Cole); Finance and Budget Committee (Chairman, Dr. Paul H. Hoch); Publications Committee (Chairman, Dr. Theodore Rothman). Other committees concerned themselves with matters pertaining to Liaison with Government Agencies and Industry (Chairman, Dr. Henry Brill); Liaison with Learned Societies (Chairman, Dr. Ralph W. Gerard); Ethical Matters (Chairman, Dr. Nolan D. Lewis); and Education and Training (Chairman, Dr. Klaus R. Unna). The reports of the Committees will be included in the next issue of the Bulletin.

However, as with all committees, their work can but reflect the work of the membership at large. Ours is an active association; and it was indeed warming to me to receive, during the early days of the College, such ready response to my suggestion that we form Study Groups within the College. The small size of our College is our ally in this venture. Members know one another well, thus providing a ready opportunity to clarify some controversial issues through frank debate in small groups. It was suggested that Study Groups address themselves to an examination of topics which were either vague or controversial, or of special relevance to the practical pursuit of some areas of investigation; and that they do so over a period of time to ensure a definitive summary of the state of a given field. The topics chosen initially were:

Individual Variation in the Metabolism of Psychoactive Drugs (Co-Chairman: Drs. B.B. Brodie and Albert Kurland)

Analysis of the Effect of Drugs on the Electrical Activity of the Brain (Co-Chairman: Drs. James E.P. Toman and Max Fink)

Individual Animal Differences in Drug Responses; Determining Factors (Co-Chairman: Drs. Samuel Irwin and Conan Kornetsky)

Social Factors and Individual Expectation in Relation to Drug Responses in Man (Co-Chairman: Drs. Milton Greenblatt and Seymour Fisher)

Advantages and Limitations of the Controlled Clinical Trial in Psychopharmacological Investigation (Co-Chairman: Drs. Jonathan Cole and Heinz Lehmann)

The Effects of Drugs on Communication Processes in Man with Special Reference to Problems of Verbal Behavior (Co-Chairman: Drs. Joseph Zubin and Louis Gottschalk)

Pharmacology of Memory and of Learning (Co-Chairman: Drs. Murray E. Jarvik and Sherman Ross)

Toxicity of Psychoactive Drugs (Chairman: Dr. Klaus Unna)

Members were invited to express preferences for one or another of the Study Groups. The groups having been once constituted, met at the call of their co-chairman and gave lively consideration to their topics for a whole day at the First Annual Meeting of the College, on Friday, January 25th. It is anticipated that, with the help of a generous grant from the National Institute of Mental Health, this work will now continue for the next two years.

Council also considered a further suggestion; namely, the institution, at an appropriate time in the future, of practical Courses and Workshops in various aspects of Psychopharmacology This suggestion stemmed from the conviction that the Science of Psychopharmacology can only be as good as its methods; and that it was appropriate for the College to face the responsibility of providing training opportunities in the various techniques currently used in the field, and to make available to members (and possibly, to others) the reservoir of skills comprised within the College. It is quite conceivable that such Practice Training Workshops may lead to the development of training manuals in various areas, resulting, over the years, in a series of authoritative, up-to-date Teaching Texts in Research Methods in Psychopharmacology. These could range from Neurobiological to Behavioral Techniques and comprise both Experimental and Clinical aspects.

In looking back over its short history from that early meeting at the Barbizon-Plaza to the present day, it is hard not to be encouraged by the vigor and variety of programs developing within our small association. It is not uncommon for anyone of us to be told that Psychopharmacology is not a science, and that it would do well to emulate the precision of older and more established disciplines. Such statements betray a lack of understanding for the special demands made by Psychopharmacology upon the fields which compound it. For I know of no other branch of science which like a good plough on a spring day, has tilled as many areas as Neurobiology. To have, in a mere decade, questioned the concept of synaptic transmission in the central nervous system; to have emphasized compartmentalisation and regionalization of chemical process in the unit cell, and in the brain; to have focussed on the interaction of hormone and chemical process within the brain; to have given us tools for the study of the chemical basis of learning and temporary connection formation; to have emphasized the dependence of pharmacological response on its situational and social setting; to have compelled a hard look at the semantics of psychiatric diagnosis, description and communication; to have resuscitated that oldest of old remedies, the placebo response, for careful scrutiny; to have provided potential methods for the study of language in relation to the functional state of the brain; and to have encouraged the Biochemist, Physiologist, Psychologist, Clinician and the Mathematician and Communication Engineer to join forces at bench level, is no mean achievement for a young science. That a chemical text should carry the imprint of experience, and partake in its growth, in no way invalidates study of the symbols, and the rules among symbols, which keep us going, changing, evolving, and human.

Thus, though moving cautiously from set habit to positive scepticism, Psychopharmacology is still protesting; yet, in so doing it is, for the first time, compelling the physical and chemical sciences to look behavior in the face, and thus enriching both. If there be discomfiture in this encounter, it is hardly surprising; for it is in this discomfiture that there may well lie the germ of a new science.

Part Two

EARLY PAPERS:
PHYSICAL CHEMISTRY
AND X-RAY DIFFRACTION

PAPERS

5. J. Elkes, A.C. Frazer, J.H. Schulman and H.C. Stewart: *Reversible adsorption of proteins at the oil/water interface. I. Preferential adsorption of proteins at charged oil/water interfaces.*
Reprinted with the kind permission of The Royal Society from the *Proceedings of the Royal Society* (London) B184 (996): 102-115, 1944

6. J. Elkes and J.B. Finean: *X-ray diffraction studies on the effect of temperature on the structure of myelin in the sciatic nerve of the frog.*
Reprinted with the kind permission of Academic Press from *Experimental Cell Research* 4: 69-81, 1953

7. J. Elkes and J.B. Finean: *Effects of solvents on the structure of myelin in the sciatic nerve of the frog.*
Reprinted with the kind permission of Academic Press from *Experimental Cell Research* 4: 82-95, 1953

CONTEXT

Joel Elkes has had an abiding interest in the structure of cell surfaces and lipid/protein interaction in biological membranes. He started by studying the properties of lipid and lipoprotein monomolecular films, using a Langmuir trough. This work continued in the study of the preferential adsorption of proteins at charged oil/water interfaces using detergent stabilized emulsions as a marker system. (Paper 5 – 1944). The system allowed for inference concerning the formation of firmly gelled monolayers of protein at the oil/water interface.

This interest in the structure of layered lipoproteins in biological sytems continued in studies of the liquid crystal structure of myelin – a lipoprotein of ubiquitous distribution, but of uncertain function in the nervous sytem.

Papers 6 and 7 (1953) report on the work done jointly with J.B. Finean, a crystallographer and first Ph. D. student of Elkes. They describe x-ray diffraction studies of living myelin using an irrigated frog sciatic nerve preparation. The dimensions of the basic crystal micelle of myelin were determined and the effects of temperature, drying, and of solvents – alcohol and ether – on nerve conductivity and crystal structure were studied in parallel. Reversible and irreversible changes were noted, and correlated with clear changes in the crystal structure, as reflected in x-ray diffraction patterns.

PAPER 5

REVERSIBLE ADSORPTION OF PROTEINS AT THE OIL/WATER INTERFACE
I. Preferential adsorption of proteins at charged oil/water interfaces

J.J. Elkes[*], A.C. Frazer[*], J.H. Schulman, H.C. Stewart[*]

Pharmacology Department, University of Birmingham;
Colloid Science Department, Cambridge; and Physiology Department,
St. Mary's Hospital Medical School, London

Reprinted with the kind permission of The Royal Society from the
Proceedings of the Royal Society (London) B184 (996): pp 102-115, 1944

The behaviour of positively and negatively charged oil-in-water emulsions, stabilized with hexadecyl trimethyl ammonium bromide and sodium hexadecyl sulphate respectively in the presence of protein solutions has been studied.

Under certain conditions proteins will adsorb to a charged oil/water interface. When finely dispersed oil-in-water emulsion was used to a provide this oil/water interface, adsorption of protein resulted in flocculation of the oil droplets.

Flocculation of emulsion on the addition of protein is pH conditioned and occurred on the acid side of the isoelectric point of the protein with negatively charged and on the alkaline side with positively charged oil globules. No flocculation occurred on the alkaline side of the isoelectric point with a negative emulsion or the acid side with a positive emulsion.

The amount of protein required to cause maximum clarification of the subnatant fluid corresponded with that needed to give a firmly gelled protein monolayer at the interface, namely, 2.5 mg of protein/sq.m. of interfacial area. With that amount of protein the flocculated oil globules remained discrete and no coalescence or liberation of free oil occurred. If only 1 mg of protein/sq.m of interfacial area was added, flocculation was followed by rapid coalescence of oil globules and liberation of free oil. If smaller amounts still were used, no greater amounts than 2.5 mg/sq.m of interfacial area, up to ten times the monolayer concentration was adsorbed to the interface.

Sodium chloride affected the flocculation range, and instead of the clear-cut change-over between the positive and negative interfaces at the isoelectric point of the protein, overlapping occurred. 5% sodium chloride shifted the flocculation point about 1 unit of pH. The addition of sodium chloride also altered the point of maximum clarification. Thus with haemoglobin the maximum clarification point was shifted from 2.5 to 1.7 mg/sq.m of interfacial area by the addition of 1% sodium chloride.

The adsorption of protein on to charged oil/water interfaces was reversible. This was best demonstrated with haemoglobin. Thus, haemoglobin was adsorbed at pH 5.0 to a negative emulsion – the red floccules were washed and transferred to a buffer at pH10. The haemoglobin thus released and the emulsion was redispersed.

The effect of adsorption and desorption on the structure of the protein molecule has been studied with haemoglobin. By solubility and colour tests it was shown that the haemoglobin molecule was changed to parahaematin by adsorption and subsequent desorption from a charged oil/water interface.

---

[*] Sir Halley Stewart Research Fellows

Molecular weight and shape determinations were carried out on the desorbed protein.

Two proteins have been separated by this adsorption mechanism. This was demonstrated on a mixture of albumin and haemoglobin.

Some applications of the flocculation technique are indicated and the significance of the phenomena described are discussed.

Recent work on the significance of emulsification of fat in intestinal absorption (Frazer 1943, Frazer, Schulman & Stewart 1944), the structure of the chylomicron in the blood (Elkes, Frazer & Stewart 1939), and the reversible detoxification of snake venom and bacterial toxins by oil-in-water emulsions (Frazer & Walsh 1934, 1939; Frazer & Stewart 1940) has encouraged a quantitative approach to the study of the charged oil/water interface in relation to proteins by the use of surface physicochemical methods.

The behaviour of protein molecules when they are brought into relation with an air/water or oil/water interface has been extensively studied. The protein molecule has three main possible configurations dependent upon its position in the water phase before or after adsorption or when it is fixed at the interface. The effects of these changes in structure on the biological activity of the protein molecule is, of importance. If the oil/water interface is in the form of a finely dispersed oil-in-water emulsion, the adsorption of the protein to this interface results in changes in dispersion and stability of the emulsion. Changes of this nature in the particulate fat in the body may have biological significance. The object of this paper is to put forward evidence of the pH conditioning and the reversible nature of adsorption at the charged oil/water interface in oil-in-water emulsions. Evidence of structural changes in the haemoglobin molecule after adsorption is given and the preferential adsorption one protein from a mixture of two proteins is described. The possible significance of these observations is discussed.

TECHNIQUE

1. Emulsions and interfaces

The emulsions and throughout the experiments described were 5% olive oil or paraffin emulsions, except where otherwise stated. 0.2% of stabilizer was used in these emulsions, and they were prepared using the apparatus described by Frazer & Walsh (1933). The particle size was of the order of 0.5μ which gives an oil/water interfacial area of approximately 0.6 sq.m/c.c. of emulsion.

The stabilizer used to give a negatively charged interface was sodium hexadecyl sulphate, and hexadecyl trimethyl ammonium bromide was used to give a positively charged interface. The 0.2% concentration of stabilizer was chosen since most of the agent would thus be at the interface and not in the continuous phase. It further ensures a saturated interfacial film of the stabilizer.

2. Protein solutions

Solutions of the serum proteins were prepared by fractional ammonium sulphate precipitation and dialysis against distilled water; 0.6% NaCl was used for γ globulin. The albumin fraction was recrystallized by the method of Adair & Robinson (1930). The oxyhaemoglobin was prepared by lysis of washed cells with distilled water, centrifugation and subsequent dialysis against distilled water. A small number of experiments have been made using carboxy-haemoglobin. The concentration of the protein solutions was determined by Adair's refractometric method and by micro Kjeldahl. The haemoglobin concentration was determined by colorimetry and protein estimation. The structure of the molecule was studied by spectroscopy determination of osmotic tests as described in the text.

The serum proteins used for most experiments were from the horse, and the fractions were derived from Burrougs and Wellcome's no. 3 horse serum. A small number of experiments were conducted with human protein fractions. The haemoglobin used was from human red cells and a series has also been studied using sheep haemoglobin.

3. Buffer solutions

The buffer range studied was pH 3.5-10.0. The buffers used had the following composition, and were all adjusted to a contrentation sufficient to buffer against strong protein solutions. The pH of all buffers and mixtures was checked by glass electrode measurements:

Range pH 3.5–4.8, Sörensen's citrate/HCl.
Range pH 4.8–.5, Sörensen's citrate/NaOH
Range pH 5.8–8.6, dihydrogen phosphate/NaOH
Range pH 8.0–10.0, Boric acid/NaOH
These buffers were compiled from the formulae given by Clark (1928).

Di- and triphosphates in acid solution were avoided in the buffer range, since the polyvalent anions would discharge the positive interface formed by hexadecyl trimethyl ammonium bromide and break these emulsions.

4. Flocculation method and criteria

The buffer and protein solutions were mixed, and to this was immediately added the emulsion. After mixture, the tubes were kept at room temperature and examined macroscopically with the hand lens and microscopically with dark-ground illumination. Observations were repeated every hour for 3 hr. and finally after 24 hr., which allowed for maximum clarification in flocculated specimens. The following phenomena were observed:

(a) *No change:* the whole tube appeared as a homogenous milky fluid. Under dark-ground the particles were seen to be single and discrete and in violent Brownian movement.

(b) *Flocculation:* the particles aggregated in clumps and these could be seen macroscopically like pepper grains on the side of the tube if it was tilted. Later these clumps "lifted" and formed a thick white layer with no free oil at the top of the tube while the subnatant fluid clarified and became water clear. Under dark-ground these particles were seen in clumps but the individual particle size did not change. There was no Brownian movement (figure 2B).

(c) *Breaking of the emulsion:* the particles ran together and formed a cream on the top of fluid. Gradually free oil was seen on the side of the tube and finally a layer of free oil separated at the top. Under dark-ground and an increase in rise of the oil particles could be seen. There was no Brownian movement. With coloured proteins such as haemoglobin a further aid to interpretation was afforded by the transference of the pigment with the protein from the continuos phase to the interference or vice versa.

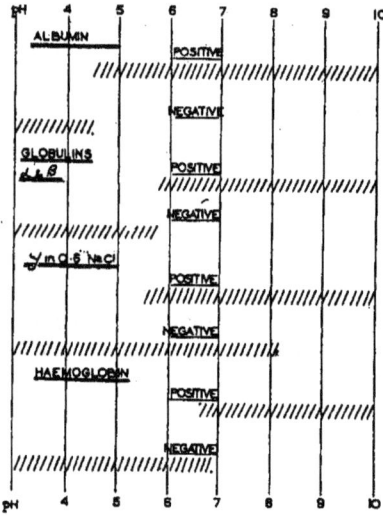

Fig. 1. Flocculation reactions of proteins with positively and negatively charged oil-in-water emulsions. Cross-hatching indicates the flocculation range in each case.

EXPERIMENTAL RESULTS

1. Flocculation over the pH range 4.0-10.0 with positively and negatively charged interfaces

Each series was put up using equal quantities of buffer and protein solution; to this mixture a further aliquot of emulsion was added. The changes in the dispersion of the emulsion were noted and in flocculated tubes maximum clarification of the subnatant fluid was obtained in 24 hr. The changes appeared immediately and became more pronounced overnight. The results of these experiments with albumin α, β, and γ globulin and haemoglobin are shown in figure 1 and figure 3A, B. Probable isoelectric points for the proteins are respectively pH 4.65, 5.2, 6.4 and 6.9 as determined by other methods (Svedberg & Pedersen 1940). The isoelectric points determined by this method show identical figures for serum albumin and haemoglobin, but are somewhat higher for the globulins, being 5.8 and 6.8 respectively. It can be seen that flocculation occurred with each protein on the acid side of its isoelectric point if a negatively charged interface was used, and on the alkaline side with a positively charged interface. No change was found on the alkaline and acid sides of the isoelectric point with negatively and positively charged surface respectively within the stability ranges of these proteins.

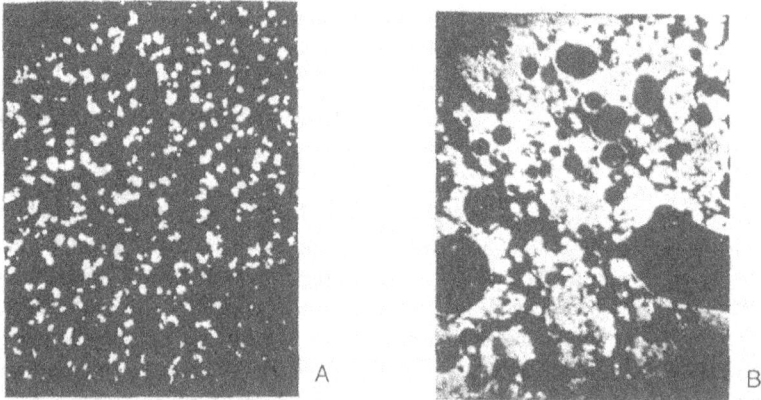

Fig. 2. Untouched micro-photographs to show the difference between flocculation and breaking of emulsion. The photographs were taken of specimens under dark-ground illumination using 1/6 in objective and 8 eyepiece (mag. 96), 2 min. exposure. The emulsion before flocculation showed a mass of free particles in violent Brownian movement. The individual particles were only just visible under this magnification. A. Flocculation. Particles in clumps; no Brownian movement; no free oil liberated. B. Breaking. Particles in clumps: no Brownian movement; large masses of free oil separating out.

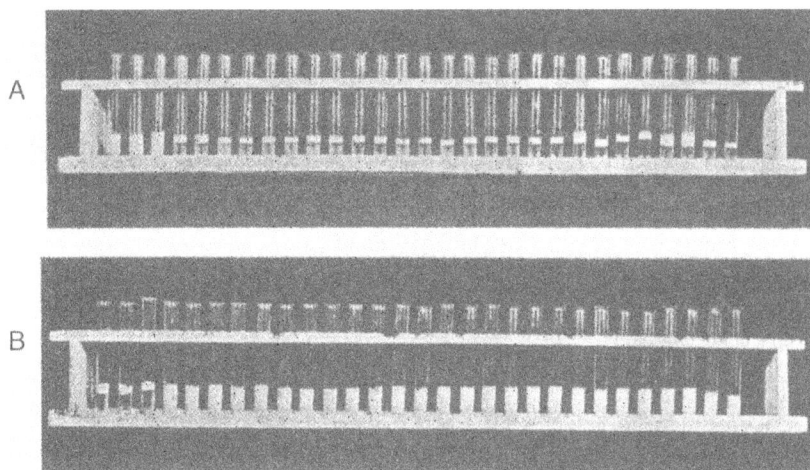

Fig. 3. Untouched photograph of characteristic flocculation range experiment. Both series of tubes contain equal amounts of protein solution and emulsion with buffer added, so that the resultant pH ranges from 4 on the left of the rack to 10 on the right-hand side. In series A a positively charged emulsion was used, and in series B a negatively charged emulsion. It will be seen that flocculation occurs on the alkaline side of the isoelectric point in A and to the acid side in B.

2. The effect of protein concentration and interfacial area on the flocculation phenomenon

Numerous series of mixtures were studied with variable protein content and constant interfacial area and using constant protein with varying emulsion concentration.

(a) Point of maximum clarification threshold (table 1)

The point of maximum clarification of the subnatant fluid was found to be when 2.5 mg of protein was added per sq.m of interfacial area. Identical results we obtained with both negative and positive interfaces at appropriate pH levels to give flocculation and also in experiments in which the protein was kept constant and the interfacial area was varied. At threshold or greater concentration of protein there was no breaking of the emulsion.

TABLE 1

Determination of point of maximum clarification. pH.5.0 Variable protein: constant interfacial area. Protein: human haemoglobin. Interface: 50% paraffin-in-water emulsion stabilized with 2% sodium hexadecyl sulphate. In each tube 1 c.c. of dilute protein solution +0.1 c.c. of emulsion. Flocculation occur throughout											
tube	1	2	3	4	5	6	7	8	9	10	11	12
Hb conc	$\frac{1}{100}$	$\frac{1}{200}$	$\frac{1}{300}$	$\frac{1}{400}$	$\frac{1}{500}$	$\frac{1}{600}$	$\frac{1}{700}$	$\frac{1}{800}$	$\frac{1}{900}$	$\frac{1}{1000}$	$\frac{1}{1500}$	$\frac{1}{2000}$
Subnatant fluid	increasing depth of red colour due to free Hb					clear, no free Hb		increasing turbidity due to free emulsion				
If 1% sodium chloride added to each tube												
		increasing depth of red colour due to free Hb						clear, no free Hb		increasing turbidity due to free emulsion		

(b) Subthreshold concentrations (table 2 and figure 4)

When a subthreshold concentration was added, two effects were seen. With grossly sub-threshold amounts no visual effect was obtained. With a just-subthreshold level of about 1 mg/sq.m interfacial area, the emulsion broke and free oil accumulated at the surface. The normal emulsion was resistant to this same pH. The breaking can be accelerated if the flocculated emulsion particles are resuspended in fresh buffer at the same pH.

TABLE 2

Flocculation at threshold level.
Constant protein,, variable interfacial area. pH 4.6.
Protein: sheep's haemoglobin
Interface: 5% olive oil emulsion,, stabilized with 0.2% sodium hexadecyl sulphate.
0.9 c.c. of a 1/15,000 haemoglobin solution in each tube.
Emulsion diluted progressively as indicated,, and 0.1 c.c. of dilutions added to corresponding tubes.
Flocculation occurs throughout

tube	1	2	3	4	5
dilution of emulsion	1/1	1/2	1/4	1/8	1/16
emulsion	++	none	none	none	none
free oil	many free	no free	no free	no free	no free
subnatant fluid	emulsion particles	emulsion particles	emulsion particles	emulsion particles	emulsion particles

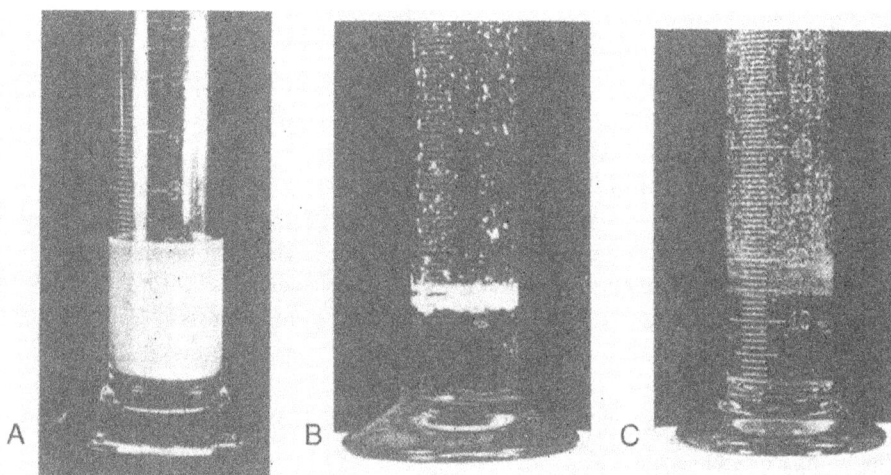

Fig. 4. Untouched photograph of three mixtures of protein and emulsion with variable protein content. A. Emulsion to which a grossly subthreshold amount of protein has been added. There is no flocculation visible macroscopically. B. Emulsion to a which a protein contrentation of about 1 mg/sq.m of interfacial area has been added. There is no flocculation visible macroscopically. B. Emulsion to a which a protein contrentation of about 1 mg/sq.m of interfacial area has been added. Flocculation and coalescence of the fat globules has occurred. Free oil can be seen on the surface. C. Emulsion to a which 2.5 mg/sq.m of interfacial area of protein has been added. Flocculation has occurred and the flocculated oil globules have remained discreet. No free oil can be seen in this specimen.

(c) Super-threshold concentrations

Using haemoglobin, the effect of super-threshold concentrations was studied:

(i) When a constant amount of emulsion was added to varying concentrations of haemoglobin only a threshold or possibly a double threshold concentration allowed of complete clearing of haemoglobin from the subnatant fluid. Owing to the decrease in the interfacial area by flocculation, greater amounts of haemoglobin were not adsorbed.

(ii) When a 5% emulsion was added to a strong haemoglobin solution (2%)'adsorption of greater amounts of haemoglobin up to approximately 20 mg/sq.m of interfacial area occurred. This might be due to the greater area available before flocculation could be effective.

3. Effect of sodium chloride concentration

Two effects have been observed:

(a) Increasing concentration of NaCl displaced the flocculation range towards the alkaline side with a negative interface and to the acid side with a positive interface causing an overlap of the two flocculation ranges. This phenomenon can be easily demonstrated with albumin or γ globulin, but only slight overlapping occurs with α and β globulins. A gradation of overlapping is obtained with increasing concentration of sodium chloride from 1 to 5%. The maximum overlapping obtained with 5% sodium chloride is 1 unit of pH.

(b) When sodium chloride was added to the variable protein concentration series (table 1) a lowering of the clarification threshold concentration of protein was demonstrated. Thus in the absence of sodium chloride, the clarification threshold occurred with the haemoglobin concentration of 2.5 mg/sq.m of interfacial area, while in the presence of 1% sodium chloride, the threshold was found to be 1.7 mg of protein per sq.m of interfacial area.

4. Desorption of protein from the interface

This has been studied with haemoglobin since observation was facilitated by the pigment. The haemoglobin was adsorbed to a negatively charged interface at a pH of 5.0. The resultant red floccules were washed thoroughly in buffer solution at pH 5.0. They were then transferred into a buffer solution at pH 10.0. Redispersion of the emulsion occurred and the fluid became red. This was centrifuged at 10,000 r.p.m. and the emulsion formed a whitish layer at the top, while the deep red pigment was seen in clear solution below. Adsorption and subsequent desorption readily occurred when concentrated solutions were used. If a threshold concentration of protein was used, desorption only occurred after repeated washing and centrifuging in an alkaline buffer, the emulsion breaking towards the end of the experiment. Since breaking also occurred in control emulsions repeatedly centrifuged without protein at pH 10, it was concluded that the stabilizing soap film was removed by this procedure. The desorbed pigmented material has been studied in order to determine what changes, if any, have occurred in the molecular structure as a result of adsorption to and desorption from the oil/water interface. The results of these investigations are shown in table 3. The sedimentation diagram obtained from the ultracentrifuge is shown in figure 5. The conclusion arrived at from these investigations was that human and sheep haemoglobin was changed by adsorption into pure soluble parahaematin (Keilin 1926).

TABLE 3. Effect of reversible adsorption on the haemoglobin molecule*

	before adsorption	after adsorption
pigment colour	red	red
spectral bands	two well-marked bands at 578 and 540	three very faint bands,, one in red and two in green part of spectrum
effect of reduction: colour	purple	reddish brown
spectral bands	one broad band at 565	two marked bands at 558 and 520
eefect of addition of 1.5 M phosphate buffer at pH 6.8	pigment freely soluble	pigment precipitated
effect of heating	no change	red changes to brown
effect of subsequent cooling	no change	brown changes to red
effect of pH change 8-12	no change	reversible red to brown
† sedimentation constant $S_{20}^{0} \times 10^{13}$	4.48	3.9
† molecular shape or hydration f/f_o (in ultracentrifuge)	1.16	1.33
molecular weight by osmotic pressure	68000	68000
conclusion	pigment: oxyhaemoglobin	pigment: parahaematin

* Blank results with the stabilizing agents without the oil were carried out and gave no significant results at the concentrations used.
† See figure 5 on ultracentrifuge results.

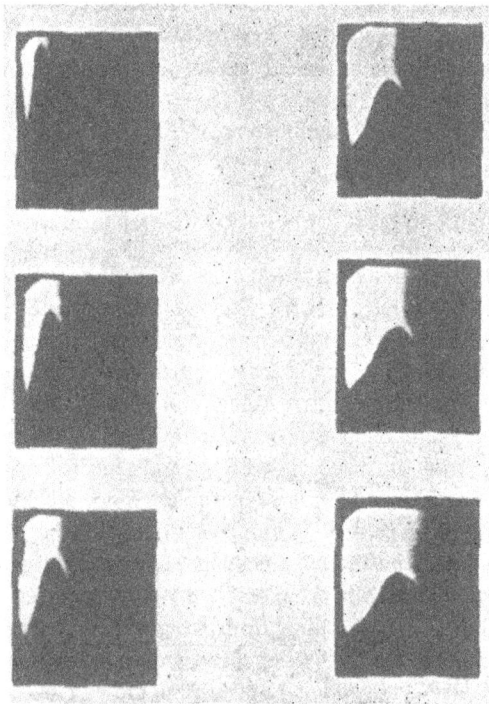

Fig. 5. A solution of desorbed haemoglobin removed from a negative emulsion at pH 10 and ultracentrifuged. It was adsorbed at pH 5.0. Six "Schlieren" photographs are given in course of the centrifuging:

$$S_{20}^{0} x 10^{13} \quad f/f_0$$

Haemoglobin	4.48	1.16
Desorbed Hgb (parahematin)	3.9	1.33

Phosphate buffer at pH = 8.6

$$\eta_{o\varepsilon\lambda} = \frac{\eta_{buffer}}{\eta_{buffer}} = 1.020 \pm (0.005)$$

Concentration of protein = 0.50 g./100 c.c.
   Rev./sec. = 1266
   Centrifugal field = 182.000 g.

In addition to the peak which gives a measure of dc, dx at different positions of the cell, owing to the colour of the protein the depth of the shading in the background makes possible an estimate of protein contrentation.

5. Preferential adsorption of protein from a mixture of two proteins

A mixture of haemoglobin and albumin was placed in a buffer solution at pH 5.5. Flocculation occurred and the floccules were red in colour; the subnatant fluid was decolorized. When these floccules were removed by centrifugation and further emulsion was added to the subnatant fluid no fresh flocculation occurred, but if the pH of the subnatant fluid was changed to 4.6, white flocculation readily occurred owing to adsorption of the albumin. The proteins can be readily desorbed from the oil/water interface by transference into an alkaline buffer.

DISCUSSION

It has been shown that the results of a study of molecular interactions at an air/water interface can be directly applied to phenomena occurring at an oil/water interface, or at an emulsion particle interface (Schulman & Cockbain 1940). Nearly all proteins spread, or can be made to spread, by suitable dispersion in solutions of alcohols and salts, at the air/water interface and better at the oil/water interface in the form of a monolayer over a large range of pH in the underlying solution. This process entails a radical alteration in the structure of the protein molecule, which has been considered by many workers in this field to be an irreversible change (Langmuir & Waugh 1940, Langmuir & Schaefer 1939). The experimental results show that adsorbed proteins can readily be made to go back into solution again, although the structure of the adsorbed protein in the various cases quoted has still to be established. The protein molecule has three main configurations. The structure of the regenerated protein in relation to the other two forms, and the biological activity of a protein molecule in these three configurations are of considerable interest.

Form I. Before adsorption
There is evidence from ultracentrifuge studies that the protein molecule in solution is globular or nearly globular in form, with the ionized carboxyl and amine groups at the end of short hydrocarbon chains orientated into the aqueous solution, and the associating non-polar side chains orientated towards the centre of the large molecule. The charge and isoelectric points of the protein molecule are directly related to the ratio of the positive NH_3 and negative COO ionic groups at the end of their side chains.

Thus on the acid side of this isoelectric point, suppression of the ionization of the carboxyl ion takes place and the protein molecule behaves as a positively charged colloid. Conversely on the alkaline side the protein behaves as a negatively charged colloid.

Form II. Adsorbed protein
When a protein molecule of the above description comes into contact with an oil/water or air/water interface, the non-polar portions of the molecule will be separated from the polar and ionic groups owing to the strong asymmetric field at the interface. Thus, the molecule with other unrolled molecules, forms a triplex monolayer. The non-polar side chains will be pulled towards the oil phase or air, and the side chains with the ionic or polar groups towards the water phase, leaving the ketoamido backbone in between. The protein molecules will adlineate to one another according to the stresses placed on the valence linkages by this separation of the non-polar portions (due to the asymmetric field at the interface) and the intramolecular association of these groups (Schulman & Cockbain 1939).

The approach of a protein molecule to a charged oil/water interface is more specific than at the uncharged oil/water interface. At the air/water interface where the surface is covered by a monolayer which does not interact with an injected protein solution, no change as measured by surface potentials, surface pressure, surface viscosity, or rigidity takes place. Examples are: serum proteins injected under lecithin (Hughes 1935) or long-chain ester films (Schulman, unpublished). If the proteins can associate with the film-forming molecules, penetration of the interfacial films takes place with radical changes in the above-mentioned film properties (Schulman, unpublished).

It is a known fact that if protein is adsorbed from a solution to the interface of either oil/water or air/water, the adsorbed film can become thicker than that of a monolayer obtained by the surface-spreading technique. The structure of the proteins in these thick layers is of great interest. Whether these thick layers are unrolled proteins in a laminated monolayer form, or due to adsorption in a globular form, or primarily a monolayer followed by a globular adsorption, will be discussed later (Danielli & Davson 1943).

Form III. Desorbed protein

If surface pressure is exerted on an interfacial protein film, besides increase in surface concentration two things may occur; the molecule may be forced back into solution again, or it may become so involved with its neighbouring molecules that the interfacial film collapses forming pleats and rolls. These pleats and rolls, having a hydrophilic core with the non-polar side chains on the outside can be spun off the surface as threads which do not spread again on the aqueous solution Schulman & Cockbain 1939). The ease with which a protein molecule can be pushed back into solution again is dependent on its size and on the lipoid content of a mixed film. Thus, it has been shown that, in a 20% cholesterol mixed protein film the protein molecule can be readily forced back into solution again without the film crumpling (Schulman & Rideal 1937). Desorption of a protein molecule from a charged oil/water interface can be brought about in a much more convenient way than at the air water or uncharged oil/water interface. This is achieved by simply suppressing the ionization of the associating group of opposite sign and the bringing into action the repulsive forces between ions of like sign. Another method is to break the emulsion by removal of or interference with, the stabilizing agent. The structure of the desorbed protein has been investigated by determination of its molecular weight, shape (sedimentation constant), and, if pigmented, by its absorption spectrum and, if biologically active, by comparable biological tests with the unadsorbed protein.

It will be seen from the experimental results that these general principles of the behavior of protein molecules at an oil/water interface can be applied to the study of the reactions which occur when protein solutions are mixed with finely dispersed oil-in-water emulsions. If an emulsion is used in which the oil particles are stabilized with a soap so that the oil globule carries either a positive or a negative charge. Adsorption of the protein to the interface is indicated by flocculation of the emulsion particles. This flocculation is due to the reduction of the surface charge on the oil particle. Brownian movement ceases and repellent forces between individual particles no longer exist. The oil particles will, however, remain as separate and discrete globules provided that there is a sufficiently large concentration of protein present.

A number of factors affecting the adsorption of protein, consequent flocculation and the stability of the flocculated particles have been studied from the experimental results. The most important factors can be seen to be: The reaction of the continuous phase, the relative concentrations of protein to interfacial area, the nature of the stabilizing agent and the presence of electrolytes, and the molecular weight of the protein.

Effect of reaction of continuos phase

If protein solutions are taken at concentrations above 2 mg/sq.m of emulsion interface over the whole range of pH from 4 to 10 for negatively and positively charged emulsions, adsorption, as signified by flocculation of the emulsions, occurs at pH levels below the isoelectric point for negative interfaces, and above this point for positive interfaces. No flocculation occurs above the isoelectric point of the proteins for negative interfaces or below for positive interfaces.

For serum proteins with a molecular weight up to approximately 70,000, the change-over from adsorption to no adsorption over a pH range is very sharp. With high molecular weight proteins such as γ globulin there is an overlap. This might be due to the size of molecule giving it extra Van der Waals associating forces as compared with a smaller molecule; this would enable it to adsorb against a small surface charge. The overlap with γ globulin is about 1.5 pH units on either side of its isoelectric point of pH 6.8. It will be seen that serum albumin in distilled water gives a sharp change-over at the isoelectric point of pH 4.65. The addition of electrolyte to the albumin creates a flocculation overlap at the isoelectric point similar to that seen with γ globulin 0.6% of NaCl solution. A pH shift of 1 on either side of the isoelectric point is obtained with a 5% concentration of sodium chloride. This may be due to the effect of electrolyte reducing the potential and thus extending the flocculation range.

The effect of protein concentration

The initial flocculation of the emulsion occurs at a protein concentration of approximately 1 mg/sq.m of oil/water interface. This concentration is that at which a protein film forms a coherent monolayer at the air/water interface. Alexander & Teorell (1939) show from surface studies of proteins at the uncharged oil water interface that the oil can expand the protein monolayer uniformly beyond the point of a coherent monolayer which would be formed at an air/water interface These expanded protein films are fluid but the gelation point remains the same at air/water and oil/water interfaces. The flocculated emulsion with this low protein concentration breaks up into large oil droplets (figure 4), and it is significant that the protein monolayers at low surface pressures are fluid and possess low viscosity as compared with a protein film at its equilibrium spreading pressure where it is a strong gel. Thus the oil droplets have become discharged by adsorption of the protein monolayer, but the protein coat around the droplets at this surface concentration is too fragile to stop the discharged oil droplets from coalescing. At a protein concentration of 2.5 mg/sq.m of interface a firmly gelled monolayer is formed. The emulsion is flocculated in large clumps, each droplet remaining discrete, no free oil being visible and the subnatant solution becoming completely clear of the emulsion droplets which float to the top of the solution as a white layer. If emulsion is mixed with a protein concentration series, this clear tube with stable flocculated emulsion droplets rapidly becomes apparent. This concentration is approximately 0.15% of protein per 1 c.c. of 5% emulsion with 0.6 sq.m of interface. This gives a figure of 2.5 mg of protein/sq.m which agrees well with that obtained for a strongly gelled protein monolayer compressed to its equilibrium spreading or collapse pressure (Schulman & Cockbain 1939).

Further, an adsorption of protein in globular form can here be ruled out since the smallest globular unit would have a diameter of 55Å which is five and a half times greater in thickness than that obtained for the monolayer at 1 mg/sq.m and some two or three times thicker than the strong gelled monolayers giving maximum clarification of the emulsion. The emulsion particles have a mean diameter of 0.5μ and one rarely obtains any particles in the emulsions used above 1μ.

It can be shown that an emulsion will go on adsorbing protein beyond the monolayer concentration in a manner similar to the adsorption of the strong and thick gel films obtained from a floating protein solution at the air/water and oil/water interface. This can be demonstrated more readily with pigmented proteins. Thus, the concentration of haemoglobin which can be removed by an emulsion to give a colourless solution is of the order of 10 monolayers in thickness. This can only be obtained by the use of a strong protein solution, i.e. 2%. The structure of these films of adsorbed protein is at present not quite clear. Whether they are laminated monolayers comparable to soap films or adsorbed globular proteins must be established by work on biologically active proteins. The first view would appear more in line with the available facts since adsorbed haemoglobin comes off as parahaematin, showing that a change has occurred in the protein molecule which would be unlikely if it had been adsorbed in its globular form. This denaturation may, however, only occur with proteins which posses large oil soluble pigmented prosthetic groups. These might irreversibly distort the protein portion of the molecule by their separation at the oil/water interface.

Desorption of protein, from charged oil/water interface

The experimental results described show that a protein molecule can only approach a charged oil/water interface when the charges of the two colloids are of the opposite sign, and that the protein molecule occupies the same area at the interface as a protein molecule in the form of a monolayer at the uncharged oil/water interface. If a protein such as haemoglobin is adsorbed at pH 5.0 on a negative emulsion or at pH 8.5 on a positive interface, and the pH of the solution is now changed so that the sign of the two colloids is the same, repulsion takes place between the adsorbed protein layer and the adsorbed emulsion stabilizing agent (i.e. at pH 10 and 4.6 respectively). With the pigmented haemoglobin the desorption of the protein back into solution again can be readily observed. The flocculated emulsion, which was red in the case of haemoglobin, becomes white again and redisperses to form a fine emulsion. The solution which was originally red becomes decolorized when the emulsion is added under adsorption conditions and the emulsion becomes red. This agglutinated emulsion can be washed with the appropriate buffer solution and then centrifuged. When it is placed in a buffer solution of the opposite reaction, repulsion occurs between the ions of the stabilizing soap film and the ionized groups of the protein molecules in the mixed lipoprotein monolayer at the emulsion interface. Under these conditions the protein molecule redisperses into solution again, and, in the case of the pigmented proteins, colours the solution. That this interfacial film is a mixed monolayer can be seen from penetration experiment at the air/water interface by injecting protein solutions under monolayers of ionizing compounds (Schulman, unpublished). Work with the ultracentrifuge suggests that the molecular weight and shape of the desorbed protein, parahaematin, represents a modified haemoglobin in which the position of the pigmented prosthetic groups and its attached groups have changed. This might be due to the reorientation of the porphyrin group on adsorption at the oil/water interface, so that on desorption it associates non-specifically with the protein molecule. From the osmotic pressures and membrane potentials as measured by G.S. Adair, the evidence shows that the charge but not the molecular weight has changed from that of the original haemoglobin.

Preferential adsorption, of proteins from mixed solutions

From a study of figure 1 it can be seen that at pH 5.5 on a negative emulsion, haemoglobin will be adsorbed, but serum albumin will not. In a mixed protein solution at pH 5.5, haemoglobin should therefore be adsorbed leaving albumin behind in the solution. This occurs readily; the emulsion at this pH agglutinates into red floccules. When this flocculated red emulsion is centrifuged off and fresh emulsion is added, it remains suspended. But this emulsion gives a white flocculation if the pH of the solution is now moved to pH 4.6 showing that the albumin has now become adsorbed.

These adsorbed proteins on the two emulsion fractions can now be desorbed by placing them in an alkaline solution of pH 10. Thus it can be established that protein can be preferentially adsorbed out of mixed solutions as a function of their isoelectric points, the sign of the charge on the oil/water interface, and the pH of the solution and can readily be desorbed. Adsorption and desorption with large foreign prosthetic groups results in some change in molecular structure (table 3) but it is possible that other protein molecules may be adsorbed and desorbed without any change in structure.

Work on possible charges in biological activity of ferments adsorbed in the form of monolayers and multilayers at solid interfaces has been carried out by Langmuir and his co-workers. This work has been discussed and enlarged upon by Lawrence Miall, Needham & Shih-Chang Shen (1944).

The standardized flocculation technique can be used for the study of certain properties of proteins or for the separation of some protein mixtures. It is also being used for the measurement of interfacial area in emulsions and for the determination of film structure at the oil/water interface. This method is being employed in the study of fat particles during and after absorption from the intestine, and in the investigation of the factors concerned in the stability of particulate fat in the blood. The whole of this work is being continued and extended in order to determine the possible changes in the relationships between proteins and interfaces in vitro and in vivo. Such changes undoubtedly occur in immunological and other reactions and it is hoped that the study of the simple system described in this paper may of assistance in the elucidation of more complex biological phenomena of a similar type.

We are indebted to Professor H. R. Dean for much help and encouragement in the initial experiments. We should like to thank Dr G. S. Adair, F.R.S., for assistance with the experiments on haemoglobin, Dr P. Johnson who carried out the centrifuge experiments on the haemoglobin fractions, W. J. Pardoe for assistance in the preparation of figure 1 and photographs, and Professor E. K. Rideal, F.R.S., for much helpful criticism and advice. We are also indebted to the Sir Halley Stewart. Trust for financial assistance in carrying out this work. Thanks are due to Mrs G. S. Adair for giving us fractions of the serum proteins.

REFERENCES

Adair, G.S. & Robinson, J. 1930. Biochem. J. 24, 993.
Alexander, A. E. & Teorell, T. 1939. Trans. Faraday 5oc. 35, 727.
Clark 1928 The determination of the hydrogen ions. Bailliece, Tindal and Cox.
Danielli, J. F. & Davson, H. 1943. Permeability of natural membranes. Cambridge.

Elkes, J. J., Frazer, A. C. & Stewart H. C. 1939. J. Physi.ol. 95, 68.

Frazer, A. C. 1943. J. Phyziol. 102, 306.

Frazer, A. C., Schulman, J, H. & Stewart, H. C. 1940. J. Physiol.103, 306. ,

Frazer, A. C. & Stewart, H. C. 1940. Brit. J. Exp. Path. 21, 361.

Frazer, A. C. & Walsh, V. G. 1933. J. Physiol. 78, 467.

Frazer, A. C. & Walsh, V. C. 1934. Brit. Industr. J. 424.

Frazer, A. C. & Walsh, V. G. 1939. J. Pharmacol. 67, 476.

Hughes, A. H. 1935. Biochem. J. 29, 430, 437.

Keilin, D. 1926. Proc. Roy. Soc. B, 100, 187.

Langmuir, I. & Schaefer V. J. 1939. Chem. Rev. 24, 181.

Langmuir, I. & Waugh, D. F. 1940. J. Amer. Chem. Soc. 62, 2771.

Lawrence, A. S. C., Miall, M., Needham, J. & Shen, S.-C. 1944, J. Gen. Physiol. 27, 233.

Schulman, J. H. & Cockbain, E. G. 1939. Trans. Faraday Soc. 35, 1266.

Schulman, J. H. & Cockbain, E. G. 1940. Trans. Faraday Soc. 36. 651.

Schulman, J. H. & Rideal, E. K. 1937. Proc. Roy. Soc. B,122, 29.

Svedberg, T. & Pedersen, K. O. 1940. The Ultracentrifuge. Oxford Univ. Press.

PAPER 6

X-RAY DIFFRACTION STUDIES ON THE EFFECT OF TEMPERATURE ON THE STRUCTURE OF MYELIN IN THE SCIATIC NERVE OF THE FROG

J.J. Elkes and J.B. Finean

Department of Pharmacology, University of Birmingham; and
Davy Faraday Laboratory
The Royal Institution, London, England

Reprinted with the kind permission of Academic Press from
Experimental Cell Research 4: 69-81, 1953

Observation the X-ray diffraction pattern of irrigated frog sciatic nerve, and a study of the effect of drying upon this pattern, have been reported (8, 4, 5). Present experiments are concerned with some effects of temperature on whole nerve, and on total nerve lipids.

EXPERIMENTAL

Materials. Frog sciatic nerve was used throughout. Total nerve lipid extract was obtained by refluxing the tissue with alcohol followed by ether, and evaporating the pooled extract to dryness at reduced pressure.

Source of radiation, and diffraction cameras. These have been previously described (4, 5) In all exposures made at long specimen-to-film distances, hydrogen was used to reduce air scatter (5).

Observation cells. Three cells were employed. The first of these (Fig. 1) was used to cover a range of temperature from 20°C to –90°C. The freshly dissected sciatic nerve preparation, with spinal column attached, was mounted in the irrigation chamber, through which frog Ringer solution was circulated continuously. The nerve, which had been ligatured at its point of entry into the gastrocnemius muscle, was passed through an aperture in the bottom of the irrigation chamber, and was allowed to hang freely inside the brass cylinder. A small weight (0.6 g) attached to the nerve served to steady it during the experiment. The cylinder was fitted with cellophane windows for passage of X-rays. The system was cooled by liquid air which was introduced into the bottom of the cylinder through a side tube at a controlled rate. As the liquid air evaporated, it produced a stream of cold air which served to cool the specimen before escaping through an aperture at the top of the cell. A heating coil around the brass cylinder was used to keep the cellophane windows free from frost at temperatures down to about –5°C. Frosting at lower temperatures was prevented by directing a jet of air against the windows. The temperature was measured by means of a thermocouple hooked around the nerve at the point of incidence of the X-ray beam.

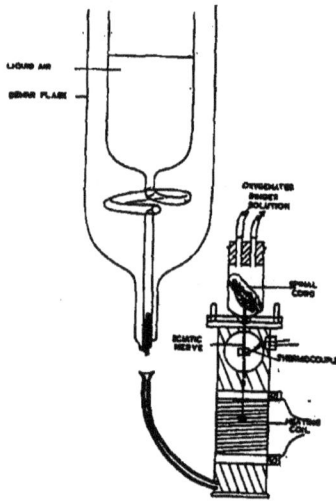

Fig. 1. Diagram of low temperature cell
(cooled by liquid air).

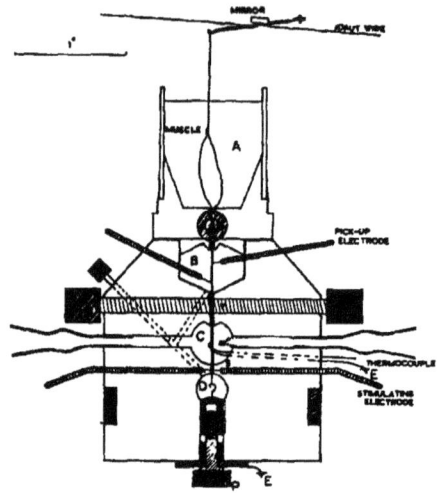

Fig. 2. Diagram of irrigation

In some experiments, short segments of fresh nerve, ligatured at each end, were attached to a metal frame, and a stream of liquid air directed against them. Cooling to –180°C was thus quickly achieved, and the diffraction pattern was recorded at this temperature.

The second cell (Fig. 2) used over a range of + 80°C to –40°C, was a modification of one previously described (5), and made provision for the simultaneous recording of the X-ray diffraction patterns and nerve conductivity. A sciatic nerve with the gastrocnemius muscle attached was used in these experiments. The muscle was mounted in the manner indicated in Fig. 2, and the muscle response recorded by means of an optical lever. A stream of air (which had been pre-cooled by passing through a copper coil immersed either in a solid CO_2 alcohol mixture or in liquid air) was blown into compartment C, and cooled the nerve segment in this compartment. The temperature of the specimen was controlled by the rate of air flow, regulated by a needle valve. A thin-walled glass or cellulose acetate capillary tube was slipped over the segment of nerve in compartment C to prevent drying. When a glass tube was used, a short segment of nerve at the bottom of the compartment was left unprotected so that direct contact with the thermocouple could be made. An interval of 5 to 10 minutes was allowed for equilibration of temperature. As most of the segment of nerve in compartment C was exposed to the X-ray beam, temperature readings at the bottom of the cell could be taken as representing mean values within the limits of the experiment. In experiments in which nerve conductivity was studied simultaneously, however, this arrangement left some doubt as to the exact temperature at which changes of activity took place; a large (4 mm) segment of nerve was affected by the temperature changes, and the variation of the temperature along the specimen was not known. This difficulty was to some extent obviated by using cellulose acetate capillary tube, and by inserting the thermocouple through a hole in the side of the tube. The specimen was then heated or cooled by a fine jet of air which impinged on the tube at the same height as, but opposite to the thermocouple. In this way only a small section of the nerve was affected, and the temperature was measured at that point. The X-ray diffraction patterns were not recorded in these experiments.

To study ranges above room temperature, warm air was blown into compartment C. In this cell, temperatures could be maintained to within $\pm^1/_2°C$ for periods of up to two hours.

A third cell served to cover a range up to 300°C. This consisted of a brass block, electricaly heated, in which the temperature was controlled through an electric contact thermometer which was in thermal contact with the brass block. The specimen was placed in a compartment in the block, and a thermocouple touching the specimen served to record the temperature. The exposed surfaces of the cell were insulated with a layer of asbestos. Temperatures could be maintained to within a degree for periods up to three hours. It was not found necessary to provide windows for the specimen compartment.

METHODS

Experiments with fresh nerve were carried out over a range of temperatures from +80°C to –90°C. In many experiments, series of exposures were made using the same specimen, the temperature being raised or lowered between exposures. Between temperatures of +8°C and –5°C, and 58°C and 63°C, the diffraction patterns were examined at intervals of $^1/_2°C$ to 1°C; other ranges were covered at intervals varying from 2°C to 5°C.

The effects of speed of cooling, and of freezing a second time after thawing, were also examined. In studying the diffraction patterns obtained after thawing, the length of time during which the nerve-had remained frozen, and the temperature at which it was maintained, were taken into consideration.

In all experiments, the specimens were finally dried to constant weight, and the diffraction patterns compared with that of normal dried nerve.

The effects of temperature on the diffraction pattern of normal dried nerve, nerve dried after freezing and thawing, and total lipid extract of nerve, were also studied. A temperature range of –20°C to +200°C was covered, the region between –20°C and +60°C at intervals of 5°C to 10°C, and higher regions at intervals of 20°C to 30°C. The diffraction patterns of lipid-in-water emulsions were examined at temperatures of –20°C to 100°C, with particular reference to +2°C to –2°C.

RESULTS

In the figures which follow, most of the dimensions given for diffraction spacing represent mean values derived from a number of experiments carried out under slightly varying conditions. The maximum variations observed in these experiments are stated.

Some diffraction bands, particularly the very weak ones, were not observed in a sufficient number of patterns for satisfactory mean values to be obtained. In such cases only approximate spacing are given.

a) Fresh nerve. Cooling. 85 exposures were made at temperatures below 20°C. Of these, 50 were taken between +8°C and –5°C. In all exposures, the X-ray beam was perpendicular to the fibre direction. Fig. 3 summarizes the findings, and typical diffraction patterns are shown in Fig. 4. There were no variations in diffraction pattern which could be attributed to the rate of cooling, the pattern depending solely on the actual temperature at the time of exposure.

The first changes in the nerve pattern were observed near the freezing point of Ringer solution, as indicated by the appearance of an ice diffraction pattern in the short spacing photographs. At this point (i.e. between 0°C and –2°C) the normal fresh nerve pattern was replaced

Spacings

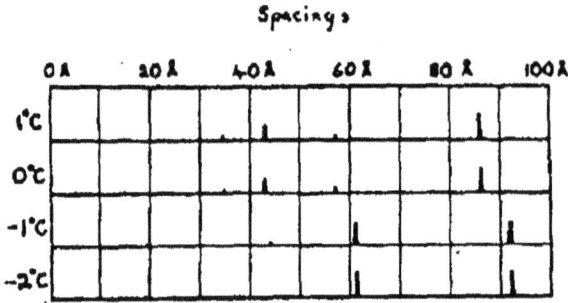

Fig. 3. Summary of changes in diffraction pattern observed over the temperature range +1°C to –2°C.

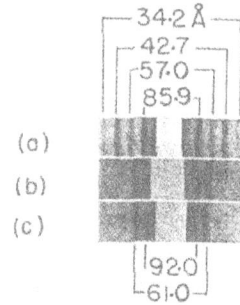

Fig. 4. Examples of diffraction patterns observed during cooling: (a) at 20°C; (b) at –40°C.

by one showing intense diffraction bands at 61.0±1.5Å and 92.0±2.5Å (Fig. 4b). Some patterns showed an additional faint band at about 46Å. The 15.0±0.2Å of fresh nerve disappeared on freezing, and was replaced by a band at 19.65±0.5Å which showed less equatorial orientation. The 4.7±0.1Å band was difficult to examine because of interference by diffraction's from ice and from the cellophane window, but it did not appear to have undergone any marked change. As the temperature was lowered further (to –90°C) there was a steady decrease in intensity of the 92.0±2.5Å band in relation to the one seen at 61.0±1.5Å. At –180°C, the diffraction pattern consisted of a broad, diffuse band at about 63Å, and a very faint band at about 90Å.

Thawing and drying. In eight experiments the fresh nerve specimen was frozen for 15 minutes (i.e. the time usually required for recording the diffraction pattern), allowed to thaw, and then immersed in Ringer solution for at least thirty minutes. Material treated in this way showed two well defined diffraction bands at 97.4±6.0Å and 47.8±3.0Å. The variation of spacings in these patterns was greater than the estimated maximum experimental error, and appeared to be related to the duration of freezing, and the temperature maintained during this period. In general, it seemed that the longer the period of freezing and the lower the temperature, the higher the spacing seen on thawing and immersing in Ringer solution. Further faint bands were observed at about 15Å and 20Å, and occasionally at about 40Å. In some experiments in which the flow of Ringer solution down the speciman was very slow, the first pattern to be recorded after thawing resembled of fresh nerve. However, after further treatment with Ringer solution, the pattern changed to the one just described.

When dried, all specimens gave a pattern which consisted of an intense band at 42.8±1.0Å, and weaker bands at 59.6±1.5Å and 92.4±3.5Å (Fig. 5d). In addition, some patterns showed a very faint band at about 34Å. The relative intensities of the 92.4±3.5Å, and 59.6±1.5Å bands appeared to vary according to the conditions of the experiment. The longer the duration of freezing, and the lower the temperature maintained, the weaker the 92.4±3.5Å band.

Freeze-drying. Freeze-dried nerve furnished diffraction patterns similar to those obtained from normal dried nerve material (Fig. 5c).

Refreezing. In some of the experiments, the specimen was allowed to thaw for a few minutes, and then frozen again. In such cases, there was a further decrease in intensity of the 92.0±2.5Å band relative to the one at 61.0±1.5Å. Repeated freezing and thawing resulted in

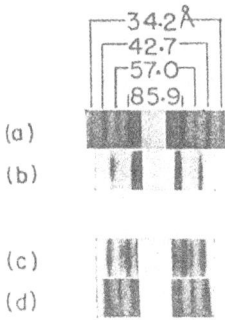

Fig. 5. Effects of thawing and drying on the diffraction pattern of fresh nerve. (a) Fresh nerve pattern; (b) Pattern after freezing and thawing. (c) Normal dried nerve pattern. (d) Pattern of nerve, dried after freezing and thawing.

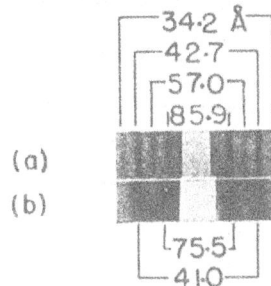

Fig. 6. Effect of heating on the diffraction pattern of fresh nerve. (a) At 20°C. (b) At 62°C

the almost complete disappearance of the 92.0±2.5Å band. The intensity of the 92.4±3.5Å band in the pattern of the dried specimen showed a corresponding decrease.

Heating. 15 exposures were made between 40°C and 70°C, 11 of these being taken between 50°C and 60°C. The normal fresh nerve pattern persisted up to about 55°C but above this temperature the bands began to decrease in intensity and to become diffuse. Between 58°C and 61°C there was a definite change in diffraction pattern. The new pattern (Fig. 6b) consisted of a moderately intense but somewhat diffuse band at 75.5±4.0Å, and a very broad and weak band at 41.0±1.2Å. At higher temperatures the general intensity of this pattern decreased.

Cooling (following initial heating) and drying. When the specimen was cooled to room temperature after initial heating to 65°C for 15 minutes, the 75.5±4.0Å band showed an increase in dimension and definition, whilst the diffuse band at 41.0±1.2Å showed a decrease in intensity, and was eventually replaced by a sharp band at about 54Å. In six experiments the nerve was heated in the irrigation cell, removed after cooling, and left in Ringer solution at 20°C for an hour. Specimens thus treated gave diffraction patterns which showed well-defined and intense bands at about 96Å and 48Å (Fig. 7) the former being the more intense. In some cases, very faint bands could also be seen at about 59Å and 35Å.

In other experiments, lengths of nerve, ligatured at either end, were heated in Ringer solution, and then left to cool before the diffraction patterns were examined. When the bath of Ringer solution was maintained at a temperature of 60°C for ten minutes, and then allowed to cool slowly, the final diffraction pattern was similar to that obtained in the previous experiment. In all, seven such specimens were examined. When subsequently dried, each gave a diffraction pattern which showed a moderately intense band 44.6±1.5Å, a less intense band either at about 56.7Å or at about 60Å, and a higher spacing which varied considerably both in magnitude (80 to 105Å), and intensity. These variations again appeared to bear some relation to the extent of previous heating and immersion in Ringer solution.

Effect of temperature on impulse conduction. This was found to vary a good deal, and to depend upon the rate of change of temperature, as well the actual temperature level. Thus, on cooling rapidly, conduction was blocked at temperatures as high as 6 or 8°C, though on lowering the temperate slowly, conduction could often be maintained until just above the freezing point of Ringer solution. No muscle response was ever observed after ice had formed in the specimen (as detected by the ice diffraction pattern in the short spacing photograph).

In cases where blocking was seen at temperatures above the freezing point, activity was usually restored almost instantaneously when cooling was discontinued. One freezing had taken place, however, no recovery was seen upon thawing.

Somewhat similar results were observed on heating. Blocking was seen at temperatures as low as 35°C, though recovery could usually be brought about by cooling. At higher temperatures, recovery was delayed, though it must be stressed that in our experiments, no consistent blocking temperature could be determined. The findings are in general agreement with those of previous workers (1, 2, 3, 6, 7, 9).

b) Dried nerve and dried lipid extract. Three series of experiments, involving a total of 30 exposures were carried out on dried nerve. Å similar number of observations was made on total lipid extract.

The changes in diffraction pattern with temperature of normal dried nerve and dry total lipid extract showed marked similarities. The 73.5±1.5Å and 143±3.0Å bands of the dried nerve pattern appeared to be relatively unaffected over the whole range of temperatures cov-

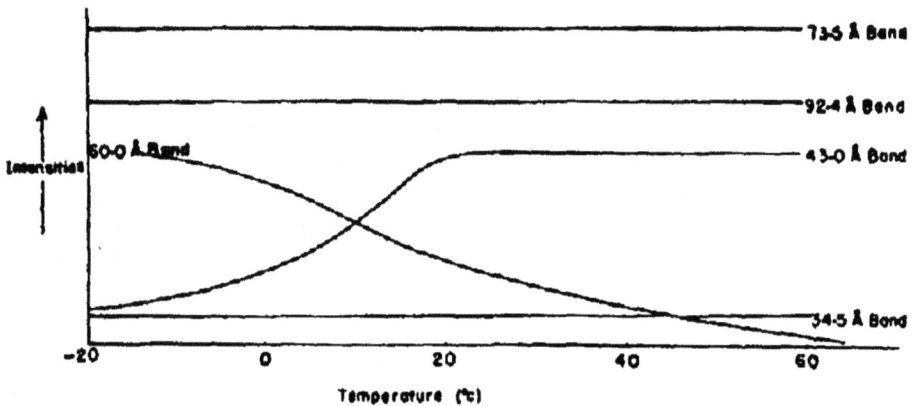

Fig. 7. Diagrammatic representation of the variations of intensities with temperature of diffraction bands in the patterns of normal dried nerve, total lipid extract, and nerve, dried after initial freezing and thawing.

ered (Fig. 207). The 34.5±1.0Å band, which was observed in both dried nerve and lipid extract patterns, showed little change below a temperature of 150°C to 170°C. At this temperature the band became diffuse and weak. Because of their relative stability these three bands at 73.5±1.5Å, 143±3.0Å and 34.5±1.0Å, formed useful standards for comparison. Marked variations in intensities where encountered in the 43.0±1.0Å and 60.0±1.0Å bands. Here again there was good agreement between dried nerve and total lipid extract. The approximate changes in intensities of the diffraction bands from dried nerve, total lipid extract, and nerve dried after initial freezing and thawing are summarised in Fig. 7. Temperatures were maintained only whilst the X-ray diffraction pattern was being recorded (usually about 15 mins.). Diffraction patterns of dried nerve and total lipid extract at various temperatures are shown in Fig. 8.

Fig. 8. Examples of diffraction patterns obtained from normal dried nerve and total lipid extract of nerve at different temperatures.

At 20°C, the 43.0±1.0Å band was much more intense than the 60.0±1.0Å band, but on cooling, the intensity of the former decreased while that of the latter increased. Eventually the 60.0±1.0Å band became the more intense of the two. The intensity of the 43.0±1.0Å band appeared to be at a maximum at about 20°C, and remained relatively unchanged up to about 150°C. At this temperature the band became diffuse and weak. The intensity of the 60.0±1.0Å band decreased with rise in temperature, and the band was not seen at temperatures above 60°C to 70°C.

All spacings showed a gradual contraction as the temperature was raised from 20°C to 150°C. The effect was most marked in the case of the 43.0±1.0Å spacing which was reduced to about 39Å before the band finally became diffuse at about 150°C.

The effects of temperature on the pattern of nerve dried after initial freezing and thawing (Fig. 5d) were very similar to those observed in normal dried nerve and total lipid extract. The 92.4±3.5Å spacing was not reduced by more than 1 to 2Å on heating to about 200°C.

c) Lipid emulsion. Total lipid extract was emulsified with an equal amount of Ringer solution. The diffraction pattern of the freshly prepared emulsion was always diffuse, but the definition of the bands improved when the preparation was allowed to stand for a day or two. At a temperature of 20°C, the diffraction patterns showed a fairly intense band which varied from 75Å to 95Å in different preparations. In addition, there was a less intense band at about half of this dimension. On cooling the emulsion, the only marked change in diffraction pattern was observed at the freezing point. Here, the pattern changed abruptly to one which showed only a broad and intense band at 61.9±2.0Å (Fig. 9). The value of this spacing appeared to be independent of the initial spacings of the emulsion at room temperature.

On heating the emulsion, there appeared to be a gradual contraction of spacings (to the extent of about 10Å at 100°C). At this temperature, the stronger band was seen to be split into two distinct spacings; one approximately equal to that observed at room temperature and the other corresponding to the spacings noted in the pattern of the frozen emulsion. Both bands were quite sharp, and the changes were reversible.

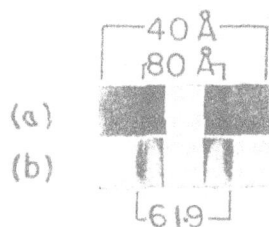

Fig. 9. Effect of freezing on the diffraction pattern of a 50% emulsion of total lipid extract in Ringer solution.
(a) At 20°C. (b) At –5°C.

DISCUSSION

The diffraction patterns of fresh nerve, normal dried nerve and of nerve studied during intermediate stages of drying, have been previously discussed (8, 4, 5). The conclusions will be used in a consideration of the above results. When fresh nerve was cooled in Ringer solution, the most marked change in diffraction pattern was observed in the region of the freezing point (about $-1°C$). Owing to slight fluctuations of temperature within the irrigation cell, and possible temperature variations over the comparatively large segment of nerve examined, it was impossible to establish whether or not these changes in diffraction pattern took place abruptly at the freezing point. The experiments showed that between $0°C$ and $-2°C$ the normal fresh nerve pattern was replaced by a pattern characterised by well-defined diffraction bands at 19.65 ± 0.5Å, 61.0 ± 1.5Å, and 92.0 ± 2.5Å.

In interpreting the diffraction pattern of frozen nerve, two possibilities must be borne in mind. The diffraction bands may all be related to a single fundamental structural unit, or they may be derived from several different systems existing as separate phases.

The three main spacings could be identified with second, third and ninth orders of a hypothetical fundamental unit of about 180Å. This might mean that the changes observed on freezing reflect an expansion of the 171Å unit (proposed in the interpretation of the fresh nerve pattern; 8, 4, 5) to about 180Å. Such expansion may be due to the conversion of water into ice. If the expansion is not restricted in any direction, and there is water throughout the length of the 171Å unit of fresh nerve, the increase in length on freezing would be about 3 per cent or 5 to 6Å. With expansion restricted in a direction at right angles to the long axis of the unit (e.g. by van der Waals cohesive forces between hydrocarbon chains), the increase in the length of the unit due to freezing might be considerably more than 3 per cent. If the patterns of normal and frozen nerve are to be related in this way, the explanation for the marked differences in relative intensities of orders may lie in a possible rearrangement of diffracting material within the unit, which could be brought about by an uneven expansion of the structure, changing the positions of diffracting groups relative to the length of the unit.

A comparison of the diffraction pattern of frozen nerve and that observed on freezing a 50 per cent lipid-in-Ringer emulsion suggests an alternative explanation of the changes in diffraction pattern which accompany the freezing of fresh nerve. The frozen emulsion gives a diffraction pattern which shows only one intense band at 61.9 ± 2.0Å, whereas frozen nerve shows a 61.0 ± 1.5Å band and an additional intense band at 92.0 ± 2.5Å. The 61.0 ± 1.5Å band of frozen nerve may reflect the existence of a free component of similar constitution to that of the total lipid extract, but additional band at 92.0 ± 2.5Å would indicate that myelin contains structure which is not reproduced in the lipid extract.

A similar conclusion is reached when the diffraction pattern of normal dried nerve and that of dried total lipid extract are compared (Fig. 10). The three lower spacings (34.5 ± 1.0Å, 43.0 ± 1.0Å, and 60.0 ± 1.0Å) of dried nerve are reproduced by the total lipid extract, but not the 73.5 ± 1.5Å and 143 ± 3.0Å bands. The stability of the latter spacings at (73.5 ± 1.5Å and 143 ± 3.0Å) distinguishes them from the shorter lipid spacings. They are, however, affected by lipid solvents. It is possible that these longer spacings reflect a complex or complexes which involve lipid material, either alone or in combination with some non-lipid component, and that such complexes are broken down during extraction with lipid solvents.

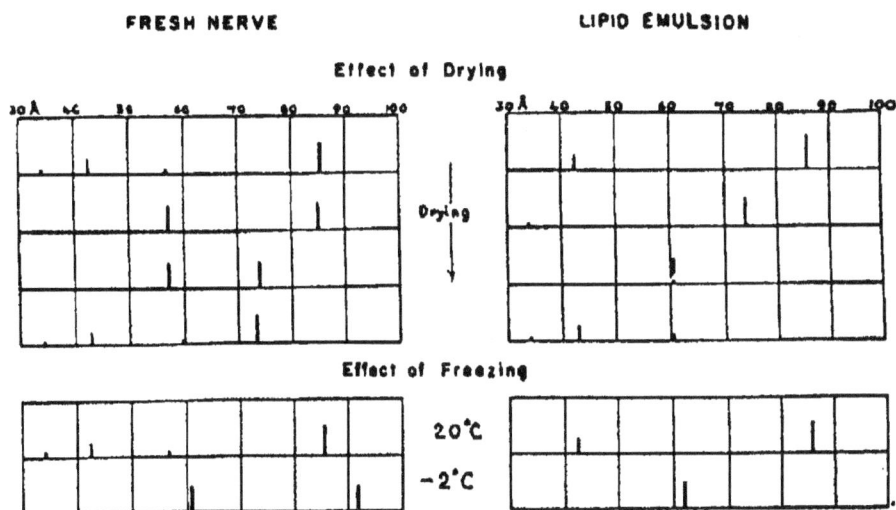

FRESH NERVE　　　　　　　　LIPID EMULSION

Effect of Drying

Effect of Freezing

Fig. 10. Diagram comparing the effects of drying and of freezing on the diffraction patterns of fresh nerve and a 50 per cent emulsion of total lipid extract in Ringer solution.

There is a marked similarity between the diffraction pattern observed at the end of stage I of the drying of fresh nerve (5), and that of frozen nerve. In both cases the pattern appears to indicate the separation of a labile lipid component from the complex. However, the changes in diffraction pattern observed during the first stages of drying are reversible, whereas those associated with freezing are not. In this connection, it is perhaps significant that freeze-dried preparations give a diffraction pattern which is identical with that of normal dried nerve, whereas a frozen nerve which is allowed to thaw before drying gives a diffraction pattern which differs from that of normal dried nerve in that it shows a band at 92.4 ± 3.5Å rather than at 73.5 ± 1.5Å. There is a corresponding difference between the higher spacings (i.e. in the region of 140 to 160Å). It is thus possible that a significant change in structure takes place on thawing.

The fact that the pattern changes accompanying the freezing of an emulsion of total lipid extract are reversible, suggests that it is the complex component (not reproduced in the total lipid extract) rather than the labile lipids of myelin which is affected irreversibly by freezing and thawing.

The temperature changes in the diffraction pattern may be due to a change in a protein component, or a lipid component, or both. The presence of a protein component in nerve myelin has been suggested (8, 4, 5), but there is no positive X-ray diffraction evidence for its existence. Any diffraction from a small quantity of protein in myelin would probably be masked by diffraction from the larger amounts of protein in other components (e.g. axon, neurilemma, connective tissue). Nevertheless, it is of interest that the irreversible changes in diffraction pattern of myelin come within the range of protein denaturation. The changes in organisation of lipid might be expected to be reversible. Investigations of the nerve lipids are being continued.

SUMMARY

1. The effects of temperature on the X-ray diffraction patterns of fresh nerve, normal dried nerve, total lipid extract, and emulsified total nerve lipids, have been studied.

2. Maximal changes in diffraction pattern of fresh nerve were noted between 0°C and −2°C, and between 58°C and 61°C. The patterns of dried nerve and total lipid extract showed wide variations in the relative intensities of the 43.0±1.0Å, and 60.0±1.0Å bands. Except for a slight decrease in spacings, the other bands remained relatively unaffected over most of the range covered (−20°C to 200°C). Total nerve lipids emulsified in Ringer solution, showed a marked change in diffraction pattern at the freezing point.

3. A comparison of the changes in diffraction patterns of fresh nerve and emulsified total lipid extract, and those of dried nerve and dried total lipid extract, suggests the presence in myelin of a lipid or lipoprotein complex not present in total nerve lipid extract. The changes in the structure of this complex with temperature appear irreversible. The irreversible changes occur within the range of protein denaturation.

We wish to thank Professor E. K. Rideal, F.R.S., and the Managers of the Royal Institution for facilities provided to us at the Davy Faraday Laboratory of the Royal Institution; Professor A. C. Frazer for his interest and encouragement; Mr. J. Teale for helpful discussion; Mr. H. Smith for valuable technical assistance; and the Medical Research Council and Sir Halley Stewart Trust for financial support.

REFERENCES

1. Boyd, T. E., and Ets, H. N., Amer. J. Physiol., 107, 76 (1934)
2. Bremer, F., and Titeca, J. Compt. Rend. Soc. Biol., 118, 371 (1935)
3. Denny-Brown, D., Adams, R. D., Brenner, C., and Doherty, M. M., J. Neuropathol. Exptl. Neurol., 4, 305 (1945).
4. Elkes, J., and Finean, J. B., Recent Advances in Surface Chemistry. Butterworth, London, p. 289, 1949.
5. Discussions of the Faraday Society, No. 6 (Lipoproteins) p. 134 (1949)
6. Hannon, I. F. and Boyd, T. E., Amer. J. Physiol., 114, 85 (1935.
7. Hodgkin, A. L. J. Physiol., 90 183 (1937)
8. Schmitt, F. O., Bear R. S., and Palmer, K. J., J. Cellular Comp. Physiol., 18, 31 (1941)
9. Schmitt, F. O., and Fourt, L., Amer. J. Physiol., 115, 564 (1936)

PAPER 7

EFFECTS OF SOLVENTS ON THE STRUCTURE OF MYELIN IN THE SCIATIC NERVE OF THE FROG

J. Elkes and J.B. Finean

Department of Pharmacology, University of Birmingham,
and Davy Faraday Laboratory
The Royal Institution, London, England

Reprinted with the kind permission of Academic Press
from *Experimental Cell Research* 4:82-95, 1953

The effects of drying, and of temperature changes on the structure of myelin in the sciatic nerve of the frog have been previously reported (2, 3). The purpose of this communication is to present some data on the effects of lipid solvents on the structure of myelin as studied in X-ray diffraction.

EXPERIMENTAL

Materials. Frog sciatic nerve was used in all experiments.

Apparatus. The source of X-rays, diffraction cameras, and observation cells have been described (1-3).

Methods. 1. *Exposure to solvent vapours.* Fresh nerve was mounted in the irrigation cell (2, 3) and slow stream of air, bubbling through alcohol, ether or acetone, was passed into chamber C (2, 3). A series of diffraction patterns was recorded during this treatment. Immediately after recording the last diffraction pattern, the specimen was either dried by blowing a stream of air into the chamber, or re-wetted with Ringer solution. Action potentials were recorded during these experiments.

2. *Exposure to Ringer solution containing lipid solvents.* Fresh nerve was placed in Ringer solution, to which varying proportions of alcohol or acetone had been added. The diffraction patterns were obtained after varying periods, the specimens being bathed in the solvent-Ringer mixture during exposures. Specimens were dried at various stages of treatment, and the diffraction patterns of the dried material compared with those of normal dried nerve.

3. *Exposure to pure solvents.* (a) Extraction of lipid from both fresh and dried nerve was carried out at low temperature, reduced pressure, or under normal atmospheric conditions. The diffraction patterns, both of the residual tissue, and of dried lipid extract, were recorded.

(b) The effects of refluxing solvents over dried nerve were studied in a special distillation cell (2). The solvents used were alcohol, acetone, and ether.

RESULTS

In the figures which follow, most of the dimensions given for diffraction spacings represent mean values derived from a number of experiments. The maximum variation observed in these experiments is stated. In cases where the number of observations made was insufficient only the approximate values of the spacings are given.

1. *Solvent vapours.* Ten series of experiments (each involving four to ten exposures) were carried out using alcohol, four series using acetone, and five using ether.

When a slow stream of air was bubbled through alcohol and passed into chamber C of the irrigation cell, the action potentials of the fresh nerve were blocked within a few minutes, and a series of changes in diffraction pattern was observed. A summary of these changes is given in Fig. 1. and examples of the diffraction patterns in Fig. 2.

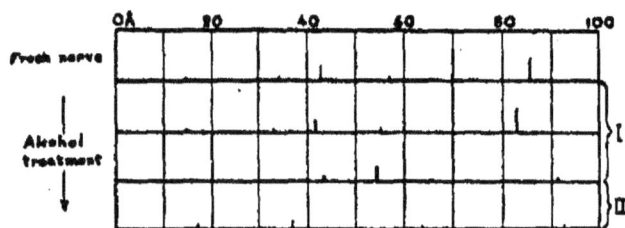

Fig. 1. Summary of changes in diffraction pattern observed during treatment of fresh nerve with alcohol vapour.

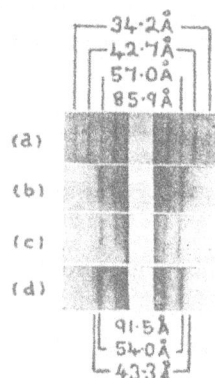

Fig. 2. Examples of diffraction patterns obtained during treatment of fresh nerve with alcohol vapour. (a) Fresh nerve pattern. (b), (c) and (d) Patterns obtained during treatment with alcohol vapour.

The changes in diffraction pattern can be conveniently described as occurring in two stages, During stage I, all the spacings of the normal fresh nerve pattern showed a slight contraction, and at the same time the intensity of the band at $57.0 \pm 1,5$Å (seen in fresh nerve pattern) began to increase. This increase in intensity, together with a further reduction in spacing, continued after the other spacings had reached a minimun and had started to increase again. In four experiments minimum spacings of 41.5 ± 0.3Å and $82.7 \pm 0,6$Å were recorded, but by the time the intermediate band (initially at 57.0 ± 1.5Å) had reached its maximum intensity, the main spacings of the pattern were 43.3 ± 1.0Å, 54.0 ± 1.7Å and 91.5 ± 4.0Å. Some patterns showed additional faint bands at about 35Å and 17Å. Spacings above 100Å were not recorded.

In stage II, the pattern appeared to change rather abruptly to one which showed a fairly sharp and intense band at 37.0 ± 1.0Å, and fainter bands at 63.4 ± 1.5Å and 17.0 ± 0.1Å band was greater than in stage I. These spacings were calculated from nine diffraction patterns, and in every case the nerve specimen appeared to be quite soft and moist after the exposure. When treatment with alcohol vapour was discontinued after stage I, and the specimen well irrigated with Ringer solution, the diffraction pattern changed to one which resembled fresh nerve pattern, but showed an appreciable general increase in spacing (e.g. from 85.9 ± 1.5Å to about 98Å, with corresponding increases in other spacings). This treatment with Ringer solution did not restore the activity of the nerve. When the alcohol treatment was continued to the end of stage II, and the specimen then well-irrigated with Ringer solution, the diffraction pattern obtained showed two well-defined bands of moderate intensities at about 110Å and 55Å. The first of these bands was the stronger. In addition, some patterns showed faint bands at about 70Å and 40Å.

In six experiments, treatment with alcohol was continued into stage II and dry air was then blown into the cell in order to drive off the solvent. After a few hours the diffraction patterns were examined. All patterns showed a sharp and intense band at 47.2 ± 1.0Å, and a very faint band at 90 to 100Å. Three of the patterns showed a band at 57.6 ± 1.1Å which was of a similar intensity to the 47.2 ± 1.0Å band, whilst in the other three a less intense band at 61.5 ± 0.5Å replaced the band at 57.6 ± 1.1. The more intense patterns also showed weak bands at 35.7 ± 1.2Å, and at about 17Å.

If the alcohol-treated specimen were treated with Ringer solution before drying, the relative intensity of the band at 90 to 100Å was markedly increased.

When the above experiments were repeated using acetone instead of alcohol, changes in diffraction pattern were observed which were very similar to those seen in stage I of the alcohol treatment (Fig. 3). At this stage, the patterns showed an intense band at 52.2 ± 0.7Å, a less intense band at 43.2 ± 1.8Å, and a faint band at about 90Å (Fig. 3b). On further treatment with acetone vapour, the diffraction pattern changed to one showing a relatively strong band at about 42Å, and weak bands at about 62Å and 82Å (Fig. 3c). On drying, the pattern underwent further slight changes, the lower spacing increasing to 45.4 ± 1.0Å, and the relative intensities of the diffraction bands undergoing some readjustments (Fig. 4). When the acetone treated specimen was re-wetted with Ringer solution, the pattern changed to one showing two well-defined bands at about 48 and 95Å (Fig. 5.). Specimens treated with Ringer solution before drying gave a pattern very similar in appearance to that obtained from specimens which had been dried immediately after the acetone vapour treatment.

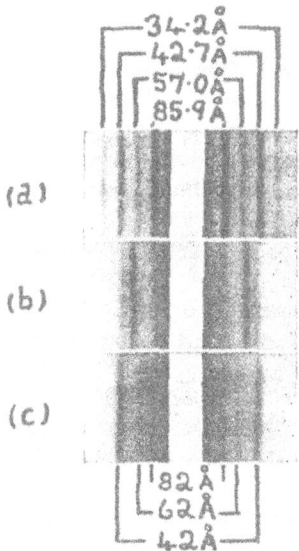

Fig. 4. X-ray diffraction pattern obtained after treatment of fresh nerve with acetone vapour and subsequent drying.

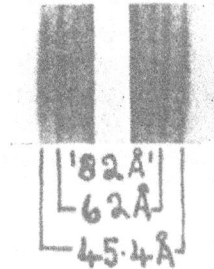

Fig. 5. X-ray diffraction pattern obtained after treatment of fresh nerve with acetone vapour and subsequent treatment with Ringer solution.

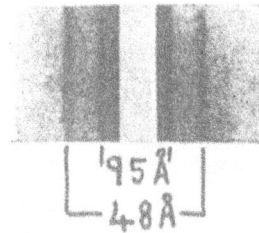

Fig. 3. Examples of the diffraction patterns obtained during the treatment of fresh nerve acetone vapour. (a) Fresh nerve pattern. (b) and (c). Patterns obtained during treatment with acetone vapour.

A slow stream of air passing through ether and into the cell had no immediate effect on the diffraction pattern of fresh, Ringer-irrigated nerve or on the action potentials. A rapid stream of ether vapour appeared to dry the specimen, the changes in diffraction pattern following a similar sequence to that of normal drying (2).

2. *Ringer solution containing lipid solvents.* Twelve experiments, involving a total of fifty exposures, were

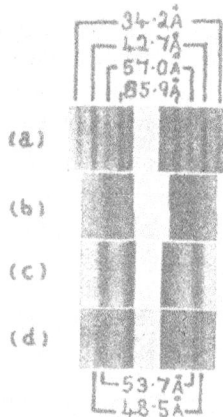

Fig. 6. Examples of diffraction patterns obtained during treatment of fresh nerve with varying proportions of alcohol and Ringer solution. (a) Fresh nerve pattern. (b) Fresh nerve after immersion for 12 hours in a 1:1 alcohol-in-Ringer solution. (c) Fresh nerve after ixnmersion for 24 hours in a 2:1 alcohol-in-Ringer solution. (d) Fresh nerve after about 24 hours in a 3:1 alcohol-in-Ringer solution.

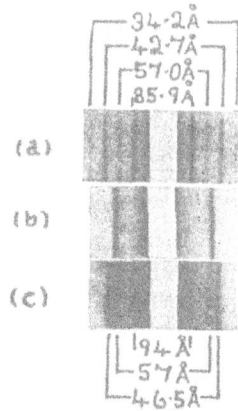

Fig. 7. Examples of diffraction patterns obtained during treatment of fresh nerve with varying proportions of acetone and Ringer solution. (a) Fresh uerve pattern. (b) Fresh nerve after immersion for 4 hours in a 3:1 acetone-in-Ringer solution. (c) Fresh nerve after 4 hours to pure acetone.

carried out with varying concentrations of ethyl alcohol in Ringer solution. Six series of experiments were carried out using acetone in Ringer.

When fresh nerve was immersed in a medium consisting of one part of ethyl alcohol and three parts Ringer solution, the intensity of the 57.0 ± 1.5Å band of the fresh nerve pattern increased relative to the other bands, until, after about twenty hours, it was of the same order as that of the next lower spacing (corresponding to the 42.7 ± 1.0Å spacing in the fresh nerve pattern). This change was accompanied by a slight general increase in spacings.

In a mixture containing a 1:2 proportion of alcohol and Ringer solution, this general increase in spacings became more marked, and the intensity of the band seen originally at 57.1 ± 1.0Å in fresh nerve now became comparable with that of the higher spacing (85.9 ± 1.5Å in the fresh nerve pattern).

In a 1:1 alcohol-Ringer mixture the fresh nerve pattern was eventually replaced by a pattern which showed an intense band at about 54Å, and very faint bands at about 110Å and 43Å (Fig.ÿ206b).

In solutions containing greater proportions of alcohol, the faint hands were no longer observed, and the intense band was replaced hy to well-defined and equally intense diffractions at 48.5 ± 0.5Å and 53.7 ± 0.6Å (Fig. 6c and d). In absolute alcohol the diffraction pattern showed only a very faint band at about 42Å.

When similar experiments were carried out with acetone in Ringer solution, the initial changes in diffraction pattern were very much like those observed with alcohol-Ringer mixtures. After four or five hours in a 3:1 mixture of acetone and Ringer solution, the diffraction pattern showed an intense band at about 53Å and a faint one at about 10Å (Fig. 7b). In pure acetone the pattern showed an intense band at about 46.5Å, and progressively weaker ones at about 57Å and 94Å (Fig. 7c).

Specimens immersed for twenty-four hours in a mixture containing 1:2 or 1:3 proportions of alcohol (or acetone) and Ringer solution and subsequently dried, gave a diffraction pattern which showed bands at approximately 34.5Å, 43.0Å, 60.0Å, 80.0Å and 160.0Å (Fig. 8). A similar pattern could be obtained by treatment with solutions containing greater proportions of solvent for short periods of time. In this pattern the three lower spacings coincided with those found in normal dried nerve, but in the solvent-treated specimen the 60Å band appeared relatively much more intense than in the normal. Also, the relative intensities of the 80 and 160Å bands appeared to differ appreciably from those of the corresponding 73.5±1.5Å and 143.5± 3.0Å bands in the normal dried nerve pattern. When the treatment with low proportions of solvent in Ringer solution was carried out at low temperatures (0 to 3®MDSU⁻oC), the dried specimen gave a pattern which was identical with that of normal dried nerve.

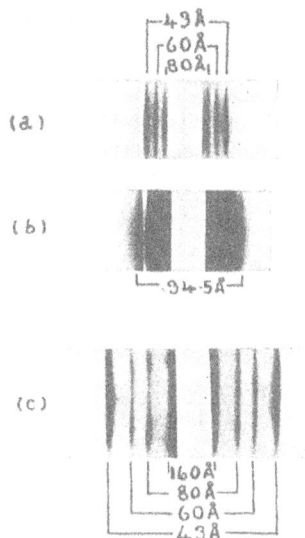

Fig. 8. X-ray diffraction pattern obtained after immersion of fresh nerve for 24 hours in a 1:3 acetone-in-Ringer solution, and subsequent drying to constant weight. In (a) and (b) the centre of the film has been masked with a thin sheet of aluminium foil to reduce halation from higher spacings.

The diffraction patterns obtained from nerve specimens which had been treated with Ringer solution containing the higher proportions of solvent for periods up to twenty-four hours and dried subsequently, showed further increases in the higher spacings (i.e. above 70Å) and corresponding decreases in intensities. With alcohol, these bands eventually became too weak to be detected. In some of these patterns spacings of the orders of 46 to 48Å and 53 to 55Å were often found to replace the more usual ones of 43.5±1.0Å and 56.5±1.0Å or 60.0±1.0Å. These spacings could be reduced to the normal values (as in dried nerve) by re-immersing the specimens in Ringer solution and then re-drying. This treatment did not reduce the higher spacings (i.e. those above 70Å), but it was often observed to increase their intensities.

3. *Pure solvents.* When alcohol was refluxed over normal dried nerve, the bands of the dried nerve pattern became progressively more faint and diffuse, eventually there remained only a faint general scatter from 40Å to 60Å. When refluxing was discontinued, the first definite diffraction band to reappear was at about 37 to 38Å. This was initially rather diffuse, but the definition gradually improved as the intensity increased. At the same time the spacing increased to about 44Å (Fig. 9). Before these changes were completed, a further diffraction band had appeared at about 58Å, and this too became sharper, the spacing increasing steadily to about 62Å. When the specimen was dried to constant weight, the long spacing diffraction pattern (Fig. 10a) showed intense diffractions at 43.6±1.2Å and 62.6±1.4Å, and well defined, but faint ones at 34.8±1.0Å and at about 17.2Å, but this could be reduced to the more usual value by immersing the specimen in Ringer solution for about thirty minutes and then re-drying. As compared with the pattern of normal dried nerve, there appeared to be appreciable increases in the intensities of the bands at 62Å, 35Å, and 17Å, relative to the one at 43Å.

Spacings above 70Å were no longer observed. When alcohol was once more refluxed over the specimen, the diffraction bands again became faint and diffuse, the 43.6±1.2Å and

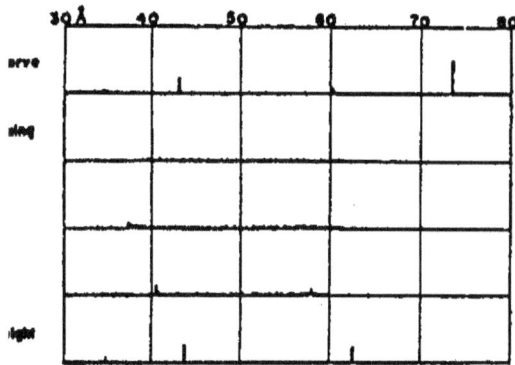

Fig. 9. Summary of changes in diffraction patterns observed during cooling following a 20 minute period of refluxing with alcohol.

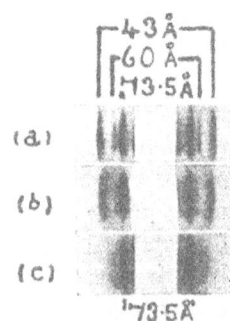

Fig. 10. Effect of alcohol on the X-ray diffraction pattern of dried nerve. (a) Pattern obtained after refluxing with alcohol for 5 minutes, and subsequent drying. (b) Slow refluxing repeated after treatment as in (a). Pattern obtained during the first 15 minutes of refluxing.

62.6±1.4Å bands being affected before the ones at 34.8±1.0Å and 17.2Å (Fig. 10b). Continued refluxing resulted in a gradual decrease in intensity of all the diffraction bands in the pattern of the dried specimen. Again it was observed that in cases where a faint diffraction band persisted in the region of 90 to 100Å, its intensity could be increased by immersing the specimen in Ringer solution, and then re-drying. After prolonged refluxing with alcohol (i.e. when the higher spacings could no longer be detected in the diffraction of the dried specimen), this treatment had no effect.

Refluxing acetone over dried nerve resulted in the complete disappearance of the 60Å band (Fig. 11b). The 34.5±0.5Å band appeared to be relatively unaffected, the 43.5±1.0Å and 73.5±1.5Å spacings being reduced by about 3Å during refluxing, but returning to their normal values when refluxing was discontinued. Refluxing was maintained for two hours without appreciably affecting the definition of these spacings. The 60.0±1.0Å band reappeared on cooling.

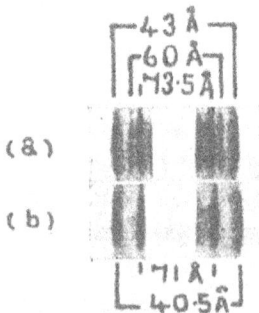

Fig. 11. Effect of acetone on the X-ray diffraction pattern of dried nerve. (a) Normal dried nerve pattern. (b) Pattern obtained during the refluxing of acetone over the specimen. The exposure (of 15 min. duration) was started after 5 min. of preliminary refluxing.

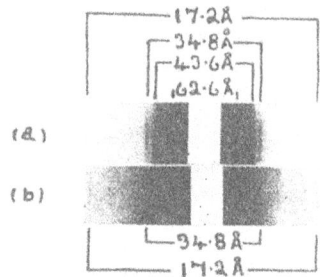

Fig. 12. Effect of ether on the X-ray diffraction pattern of dried nerve. (a) Normal dried nerve pattern. (b) Pattern obtained after suspending dried nerve over ether in the distillation cell for 12 hours. (b) Pattern obtained during refluxing. Exposure (of 15 min. duration) started after 5 min. of preliminary refluxing.

When dried nerve was suspended in the distillation cell over ether, the intensity of the 60.0±1.0Å band was observed to decrease even before distillation commenced. On refluxing, the 60.0±1.0Å band disappeared completely, and after about thirty minutes, the 43.5±1.0Å band became faint and diffuse (Fig. 12c). The 73.5±1.5Å band was unaffected by ether in these experiments. When refluxing was discontinued, the definition of the 43.5±1.0Å band improved again, and the intensity increased. The 60.0±1.0Å band did not reappear until the specimen had been taken out of the cell, and left in air for an hour. Continued refluxing resulted in the complete disappearance of the 34.5±0.5Å band from the pattern of dried specimen, and a marked increase in the intensity of the band at 43.5±1.0Å.

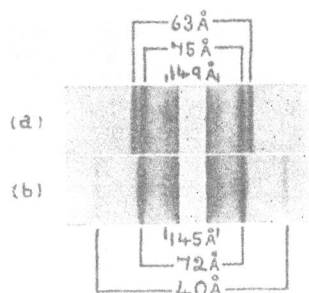

Fig. 13. (a) X-ray diffraction pattern obtained after refluxing dried nerve with ether for 24 hours, and subsequent drying. (b) Specimen as in (a), when heated to 100°C.

The treatment with ether was repeated under carefully controlled conditions in a separate distillation apparatus. The temperature of the solvent in contact with the specimen was kept at 12°C. From time to time the distillation apparatus was opened up, and a segment of nerve removed. This was dried, and the X-ray diffraction pattern recorded. After about twenty-four hours' refluxing, the pattern consisted of two sharp and intense bands at about 75.5Å and 60Å, and a fainter band at about 148Å (Fig. 13a). Continued treatment under these conditions did not appear to effect any further changes. The effect of heating on the pattern obtained after treating with ether for twenty-four hours is shown in Fig. 13. The band at about 63Å was replaced by a less intense diffraction at about 40Å, but the higher spacings remained unaffected. This effect was completely reversible.

A number of experiments were carried out in which nerve was partially extracted, and the diffraction patterns of both the residual dry tissue and the dried lipid extract were examined. The extraction was subsequently completed, and the diffraction pattern of this second lipid extract was also studied. The amount of lipid extracted, and the proportions of cholesterol and phospholipid in each specimen were determined. A summary of the findings is given in Fig. 14. At room temperature and reduced pressure, acetone and ether appeared to extract lipids in proportions corresponding approximately to the relative intensities of the diffraction bands in the dried nerve pattern. At low temperature (i.e. below 3°C), acetone and ether extracted cholesterol preferentially. Alcohol would extract practically all the lipid, but when diffraction patterns (of a dried specimen) were recorded after only part of the lipid had been removed, the 60.0±1.0Å band was much more intense than in the pattern of normal dried nerve.

In the experiments in which fresh nerve was treated with solvent vapours and dried nerve with refluxing solvents, interference from the diffraction of the cellophane (or polythene) windows of the observation cells made an interpretation of the short spacing patterns impracticable.

When small amounts of solvent were added to the Ringer solution in which fresh nerve was immersed, the short spacing ring (4.7Å) showed no appreciable change. When high proportions of solvent (more than 50 per cent) were used, a sharp diffraction ring at 4.2Å was superimposed on the diffuse 4.7Å ring. When such specimens were subsequently dried, the sharp 4.1Å ring became much more marked.

LIPID (as % of total lipid)	CHOLESTEROL (as % of total cholesterol)	PHOSPHOLIPID (as % of total phospholipid)		30 40 50 60 70 80 90 100
ACETONE EXTRACTION *(refluxing at reduced pressure)*				
49.2	100	31.6	Acetone extract	
			Residual tissue	
50.8	0	68.4	Extract of residual tissue	
ETHER EXTRACTION *(refluxing at reduced pressure)*				
14.4	9.8	13.1	Ether extract	
			Residual tissue	
85.6	90.2	86.9	Extract of residual tissue	
ACETONE EXTRACTION *(at 0-3°c)*				
11.1	31.9	0	Acetone extract	
			Residual tissue	
88.9	68.1	100	Extract of residual tissue	
ETHER EXTRACTION *(at 0-3°c)*				
16.4	31.3	11.7	Ether extract	
83.6	68.7	88.3	Extract of residual tissue	

Normal dried nerve

Total lipid extract

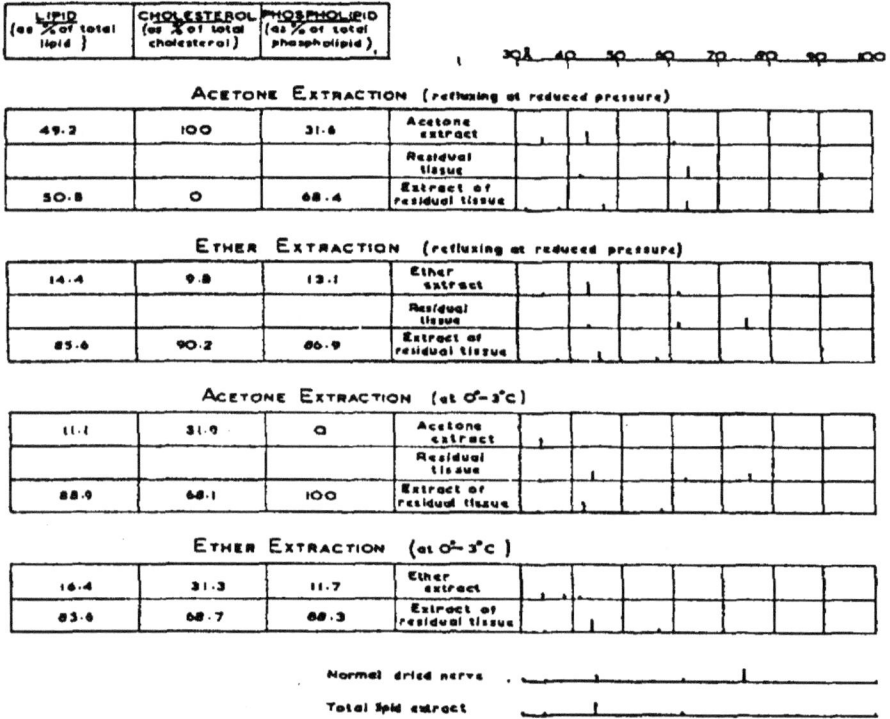

Fig. 14. Summary of the effects of partial lipid extraction on the X-ray diffraction pattern of nerve.

DISCUSSION

The diffraction patterns of fresh nerve, normal dried nerve, and total lipid extract of nerve, and the effect of drying and temperature on such patterns, have been discussed elsewhere (1, 2, 3, 4). These finding indicated the existence in myelin of a highly ordered lipid-lipoprotein unit. Present results are in keeping with this hypotheses.

Small amounts of alcohol and acetone vapours have an almost immediate effect on action potentials and the diffraction patterns of irrigated fresh nerve, whilst ether has no such immediate effect. This is presumably due to the complete miscibility of water with acetone and alcohol but not with ether.

The initial effect of alcohol is probably one of dehydration. This effect is reflected in the initial shrinkage of all spacings, and in the increase in intensity of the diffraction band corresponding to the 57 ± 1.5Å band in the fresh nerve pattern, a change very similar to those seen in the initial stages of normal drying. These changes may be due to either an extensive rearrangement of the diffracting groups in the original unit, or to the break-up of the unit. The apparently independent variation both in position and intensity of some of the diffraction bands during exposure to alcohol, suggests the separation of two or more independent components during some stages of the treatment. Previous data (2, 4) suggested the existence in dried nerve of separate lipid phases and a residual lipoprotein. A similar separation of lipid phases may be brought about by treatment with solvents. However, the effect of alcohol appears to go further in its modification of structure than does normal drying. Even at the end of stage I, the alcohol-treated specimen shows a diffraction band at 91.5±4.0Å, which when the specimen is dried gives rise to a faint band at 90 to 100Å (as compared with the much more intense band at 73.5±1.5Å found in normal dried nerve). The total effect of stage I of treatment of fresh nerve with alcohol vapour appears to be a dehydration, accompanied by a greater modification of the residual lipoprotein complex (as indicated by the higher spacings) than is brought about by normal drying. Further modifications of this complex probably occurs in stage II. The diffraction patterns during this stage show some resemblance to those obtained from dried specimens which have been refluxed with alcohol, and examined whilst some of the alcohol remained in the structure. Thus it is quite possible that stage II of the alcohol vapour treatment reflects a penetration, and partial solvation, of some of the lipid components.

When alcohol was added to the Ringer solution and allowed to act on fresh nerve, the sequence of changes observed resembled that seen when alcohol vapour was used. In absolute alcohol, however, the nerve specimen showed only one diffraction band at about 42Å. This probably indicates a more extensive penetration, or a more complete solvation than is possible using alcohol vapour. Moreover the low intensity of the bands above 70Å appears to indicate a still further modification of the lipoprotein complex.

The increase in intensity of the 90 to 100Å band in specimens previously exposed to absolute alcohol and then treated with Ringer solution and dried subsequently, probably reflects a recrystallisation of the residual lipoprotein complex. When such treatment has resulted in the complete disappearance of the higher spacings, treatment with Ringer solution has no appreciable effect.

The gradual decrease in intensity of the bands below 70Å after refluxing and drying, probably reflects the extraction of lipid components.

The changes brought about by acetone are similar to those observed during the first stages of alcohol treatment. However, its effect on the spacings above 90Å is not so marked. After stage I, an intense band appears at about 42Å, just as in the later stages of normal drying. It would therefore appear that acetone vapour simply brings about a dehydration without any indication of penetration into the free lipid components (as represented by the 42 and 62Å bands). However, when nerve was treated with liquid acetone, the diffraction pattern showed a band at about 90Å which decreased to about 82Å when the acetone was evaporated. Acetone thus apparently will penetrate the lipoprotein complex at least when it is applied to fresh nerve and modify the spacing of the complex, which in normal dried nerve has the value of 73.5±1.5Å.

The changes brought about by refluxing acetone over dried nerve could probably be explained in terms, of temperature effects alone. Previous experiments on the effects of temperature on the diffraction pattern of dried nerve have shown that all spacings show a contraction with rise in temperature above 20°C, and that the intensity of the 60.0±1.0Å band falls rapidly when the specimen is heated.

Refluxing ether over dried nerve does not involve any appreciable increase in temperature. Thus the effects observed on the 43.0±1.0 and 60.0±1.0Å bands must be due to penetration of the ether into these particular components. In the limited time in which the ether was refluxed over the dried nerve, there was no change in the complex spacing (73.4±1.5Å). Even on prolonged treatment with ether (100 hrs), the bands at 73.5±1.5Å and 143.5±3.0Å in the dried nerve pattern were relatively unaffected. However, the 60.0±1.0Å band became much more intense than in the normal dried nerve pattern and the 43.5±1.0Å band disappeared entirely. This change is similar to the one observed when dried nerve was cooled to about –20°C, and which may be due to the existence of two polymorphic forms of a lipid component, the one showing a predominant band at about 40Å, and the other at about 60Å. The effect of ether might thus be interpreted as a transition from the 40Å form to the 60Å form. The 63Å band was replaced by one at about 40Å on heating the ether-treated specimen to about 100°C, but on cooling the process was completely reversed. If the initial effect of ether had been merely to recrystallise the lipid component, one would have expected the effect to disappear after subsequent heating and cooling, and the resulting pattern to resemble that of normal dried nerve. The fact that this is not the case suggests that ether may actually change the composition of the lipid component.

The bands occasionally observed at 53 to 55Å and 46 to 48Å in the patterns of specimens which had been treated with solvents before drying, probably indicate further polymorphic forms of the main 40 to 60Å lipid component.

Possible polymorphic transitions may also in part, explain some of the changes observed during partial extraction of nerve by lipid solvents. In many of the patterns of residual tissue, the relative intensity of the 60.0±1.0Å band is unusually high, and though preferential extraction may be part of the explanation (particularly in the case of the early disappearance of diffraction band at 34.5±1.0Å) the principal effect on the 60.0±1.0Å and 34,5±1,0Å spacings is a shift in emphasis between them. Another possibility could be a partial break down of the lipoprotein complex, with consequent liberation of lipid components, and affecting the relative intensities of the bands below 70Å (the free lipid bands). Thus, in partial extraction of nerve, three factors may be involved: the preferential extraction of lipid, a polymorphic transition from one lipid form to another, and a liberation of fresh lipid from a lipoprotein complex.

SUMMARY

1. The effects of ethyl alcohol, ether and acetone on the X-ray diffraction patterns of fresh nerve and dried nerve have been studied.

2. Ethyl alcohol and acetone vapours produced rapid changes in the diffraction pattern of fresh nerve. Ether vapour relatively little effect. The effects of mixtures containing varying proportions of alcohol or acetone in Ringer solution were similar to those of the solvent vapours. Ethyl alcohol, acetone, and ether, all readily affected the spacings below 70Å in the dried nerve pattern. The spacings above 70Å were much more susceptible to alcohol treatment than in ether and acetone.

3. The results are in keeping with the existence in myelin of a highly-ordered lipid–lipoprotein unit.

We wish to thank Professor E.K. Rideal, F.R.S. and the Managers of the Royal Institution for facilities provided to us at the Davy Faraday Laboratory of the Royal Institution, London; Professor A.C. Frazer for his encouragement and interest in this work; Dr. H.G. Sammons for the lipid estimations; Dr. J. Teale for much helpful discussion; Mr. H. Smith for valuable technical assistance; and the Medical Research Council and Sir Halley Stewart Trust for financial support.

REFERENCES

1. Elkes,J., Finean, J.B., Recent Advances in Surface Chemistry, London, p. 289. (1959)
2. Discussions of the Faraday Society, No. 6. (Lipoproteins) p. 134. (1949)
3. Exptl. Cell Res. 4, 09, (1953)
4. Schmitt, F.O., Bear, R.S., Palmer, K.J., J. Cellular comp. Physiol., 18, 21 (1941)

Part Three

ELECTROPHYSIOLOGICAL STUDIES IN BIRMINGHAM AND AN EARLY CLINICAL TRIAL

PAPERS

8. J. Elkes: *Discussion: Prospects in Psychiatric Research.*
   Reprinted with the kind permission of Blackwell Science Ltd. from J.M. Tanner (ed.) *Prospects in Psychiatric Research* (pp. 126-135). Oxford, Blackwell Scientific Publications, 1952

9. J. Elkes, C. Elkes and P.B. Bradley: *The effect of some drugs on the electrical activity of the brain and behaviour.*
   Reprinted with the kind permission of The British Journal of Psychiatry from the Journal of Mental Science 100: 125-128, 1954

10. P.B. Bradley and J. Elkes: *The effects of some drugs on the electrical activity of the brain.*
    Reprinted with the kind permission of the Oxford University Press from Brain 80: 77-117, 1957

11. J. Elkes: *Drug effects in relation to receptor specificity within the brain: Some evidence and provisional formulation.*
    Reprinted with the kind permission of John Wiley & Sons from Ciba Foundation Symposium on the Neurological Basis of Behavior (pp. 303-332). London, Butterworth, 1958

12. J. Elkes and C. Elkes: *Effect of chlorpromazine on the behaviour of chronically overactive psychotic patients.*
    Reprinted with the kind permission of the BMJ Publishing Group from the British Medical Journal II: 560-576, 1954

ARGUMENT

Papers 8 (1952) and 9 (1954) are early summary reports on the work proceeding in Birmingham in the late forties and early fifties. As noted, the Department of Experimental Psychiatry was founded in 1951. Paper 8 was an invited contribution to the first conference on "Prospects in Psychiatric Research," convened in 1952 and sponsored by the newly founded Mental Health Research Fund. Paper 9 was an invited paper delivered at the Annual Meeeting of the Royal Medico-Psychological Association held in July 1953.

Paper 8 outlines some ideas on the "use of pharmacology in the study of mental organisation." It takes up some neurochemical issues and the possible use of neurotransmitters familiar at the periphery as reference points for the study of central events. It defines (see p. 118) some "simple desiderata" which one would like to see fulfilled by a substance claiming to act as a neurotransmitter in the central nervous system, (i.e., presence; presence of specific enzymes for synthesis and breakdown; observable effects of specific blockade; effects of application of substance in question by systemic or local route). These desiderata are only partly met by several putative agents. It outlines the idea of families of neuroregulatory compounds, possibly evolved as variants of original parent molecules associated with different neurone populations, which vary in density and distribution according to region, or even in the same region. "A particular type of neurone may be scattered at random throughout a region, or condensed into sheets, clusters and bundles in topographically close or widely separated areas. The pharmacological susceptibilities of a region will be those of its dominant cell population" (see p. 119) and of related cell populations influencing it from nearby or afar. The paper also emphasizes the importance of *interaction* and balance between cell populations carrying different receptors – a theme which draws on the demonstrated facilitatory (permissive) or inhibitory interaction between neurotransmitters at peripheral sites. Paper 8 gives names, but no references. The names are well-known and references are to be found scattered throughout this book.

These papers also summarize studies, then in active progress, on the effects of drugs on the electrical activity of the brain in the animal proceeding in the laboratory of P.B. Bradley; and Charmian Elkes' studies on the effects of drugs in catatonic schizophrenic stupor.

In short, the papers provide a conceptual outline of the work within the Birmingham department, as it was evolving at the time.

Papers 10 (1957) and 11 (1958) report in more detail on studies on the effects of drugs on the electrical activity of the brain, and on behavior. Previous short communications on the same topic are referenced in the paper. Paper 11 (1958) takes the discussion further, and also includes reference to other model systems, e.g., the peristaltic reflex.

The discussion sections of these papers in essence introduce some – at the time novel – concepts of the existence in the brain of distinct families of neuroregulatory compounds ("neurotransmitters") related to chmically distinct neurone populations carrying specific receptors. It is argued that these populations, derived from peripheral autonomic nets, may have differentially "colonised" the brain during evolution, making for chemical inhomogeneity at the finest level of histological organization, as well as for sharp chemical differences in some nodal areas, particularly in the evolutionarily older parts of the brain. The three types of neurone population, related respectively to acetylcholine, norepinephrine and serotonin are regarded as mere forerunners for cell populations related to other, akin, neurotransmitters.

The possible operation of chemical fields (shifts in local "titre") in some nodal areas is seen as influencing the activity of larger neurone pools at a distance. These concepts are seen as potentially helpful in understanding the effects of drugs, such as chlorpromazine. Rather than emphasizing a single, highly specific overriding effect (like the anticholinesterases), it is suggested that these drugs may possibly affect the stochastic *balance*, and interplay between different neurone populations, condensed in some areas and also widely distributed in others and mediated by related transmitters of different kinds. The basic states of appetitive behavior and of consciousness may very well be determined by subtle chemical shifts in regionally organised cell mosaics. Chemically mediated discriminate inhibition is regarded as the agent of structure in the central nervous system.

Paper 12 (1954) is a report of a blind-controlled trial of chlorpromazine, carried out by Charmian Elkes in collaboration with Joel Elkes. It records the effects of chlorpromazine in twenty seven overactive psychiatric patients. The results of the trial – which was initially approached with a great deal of skepticism – proved reasonably convincing. Seven patients who showed definite improvement on chlorpromazine, relapsed strikingly on placebo. The paper also draws attention to "the lessons the investigators have learned from the trial itself." It acknowledges gratefully the "energy and care" which the nursing personnel brought to the conduct of the trial; and enters a plea for setting up clinical research units in chronic wards of mental hospital, and "the training of senior nursing staff in research methods and medical documentation."

PAPER 8

DISCUSSION: PROSPECTS IN PSYCHIATRIC RESEARCH

Joel Elkes

Reprinted with the kind permission of Blackwell Science Ltd. from J.M. Tanner (ed.)
Prospects in Psychiatric Research (pp. 126-135). Oxford, Blackwell Scientific Publications, 1952

The use of pharmacology in the study of mental organisation is inseparable from its use in the broader field of neurophysiology, and its contribution to psychiatry will be measured by its contribution to an understanding of the brain as an integrating, feeling and computing organ. The vast cell population and the continuous activity of the central nervous system militate against a convenient study of the relation of the part to the whole. Nevertheless, an ever-growing body of knowledge is rapidly leading to a much clearer understanding of the physiological basis of perception (Adrian 1948, 1952, Walter 1950) and to the recognition of some, as yet qualitative and approximate, relationships between cells and groups of cells within the central nervous system (Dempsey & Morison 1942, Jasper 1949, Magoun 1950). It is here, in the modification of individual cell function, and in the relationship between cells, that pharmacological tools may find their application. Their discriminate use in systems of varying complexity may be helpful in an understanding of the organisation of these systems.

It may be useful to think in terms of some broad and common theoretical pathways by which chemical agents may exert their effect on the central nervous system. They may, for example, act by modifying the energy metabolism of the cell along some selective Lines, or alternatively, by altering the ionic or humoral environment of neurones either generally, or at some specific sites. The distinction between the power-economy of the cell, the integrity and function of its membrane, and the possible local elaboration of highly specific humoral agents, is a distinction which is conveniently made in the mind; it is quite unlikely to be made in the cell, where the several processes overlap, and are mutually complementary and interdependent. Thus energy metabolism is almost certainly related to membrane integrity, and, as is well known, membrane permeability, can be profoundly altered by specific neurohumoral agents, e. g. acetylcholine. The uses of these arbitrary distinctions lie principally in defining approach, and field of work. There would appear to be some disproportion of data at present available in these three areas. For example, a great deal is known of the intermediate energy metabolism of brain tissue (Himwich 1951), yet the evidence of the precise effects of chemical agents upon its various stages remains incomplete. Similarly, our recent understanding of conditions obtaining at the neurone membrane (Hodgkin 1950, Keynes 1951) poses many a pressing pharmacological problem. The position of potential humoral synaptic transmitters in the central nervous system is peculiar. Abundant data are available on neurohumoral transmission at such peripheral sites as autonomic ganglia, secretory cells, and smooth and skeletal muscle; the mode of action of various drugs at these sites has been extensively studied. Yet the relevance or otherwise of these findings to the central nervous system can only be determined in the light of further information obtained from, and within the central nervous system itself. Such information is now gradually coming forward.

There are certain simple desiderata which one would like to see fulfilled by a substance claiming a transmitter role in the central nervous system. Four of these come to mind. Firstly, the substance should be present in the central nervous system; it should also vary in quantity with the functional state, and should be identifiable by sensitive, reliable and unequivocal tests. Secondly, there should be enzymes present, responsible both for the synthesis and the breakdown of the substance in question. Thirdly, the blocking of these enzymes by specific inhibitors should result in effects related to either lack or accumulation of the hypothetical transmitter. Fourthly, the application of the substance to the central nervous system by either local or systemic routes should have demonstrable effects on the function of the tissue.

It is perhaps natural that the attempted identification of central neurohumoral mediators should have begun with acetylcholine. With certain important reservations, this substance appears to satisfy the above criteria. It is present in the central nervous system, and, as has been shown by Richter and Crossland (1949), can vary in concentration with the functional state of the animal. Thus, it is high in anaesthesia and in sleep, and diminished in excitement. Again, enzyme systems both for synthesis and breakdown have been identified; these are cholineacetylase, and the so-called specific and non-specific ("true" and "pseudo") cholinesterases. In their important studies, Feldberg and Vogt (1948), and, later, Feldberg, Harris and Lin (1951) have demonstrated a curiously uneven distribution of acetylcholine synthesising power throughout the central nervous system. Thus, for example, the anterior roots are rich in the enzyme, though the pyramidal tracts are poor, and whereas the enzyme is low in the sensory roots, it is abundant in the gracile and cuneate nuclei. This at least suggests the possible existence of cholinergic as well as non-cholinergic neurones within the central nervous system. A universal transmitter role for acetylcholine would thus seem unlikely (Feldberg 1950) although there can be no doubt of its activity at some neurones.

This activity is borne out by a third group of data concerning the central effects of cholinesterase inhibitors which appear to be attributable to the accumulation of acetylcholine at some central synapses. The number of such inhibitors is steadily increasing, their specificity for the enzyme receptors is high, and their effective concentration correspondingly low (in some instances as low as one in ten billion). They can be reversible in their attachment to the enzyme (for example Physostigmine or Neostigmine), irreversible (DFP; Adrian, Feldberg & Kilby 1947, Rowntree, Nevin & Wilson 1950) or partly reversible (TEPP; Hobbiger 1951); they can have a predilection for the "true" cholinesterase (e. g. Nu 1950; Hawkins & Mendel 1949) or, the non-specific pseudo cholinesterase (e. g. TOCP; Earl and Thompson 1952). It is important, incidentally, to distinguish between these two enzymes. Most emphasis has hitherto been laid on the "true" cholinesterase of the brain. There is little doubt, however, from our own work and work in other laboratories (Burgen & Chipman 1951), of the existence of the non-specific "pseudo" enzyme in some areas of the central nervous system. Just what roles it, and its unknown substrate play in function, further specific inhibition studies may be expected to show.

The fourth line of evidence concerns the effects of local application of acetylcholine to the central nervous system, or its administration by a selected vascular route. This approach has a long and varied history; and the evidence has been admirably summarised in a recent review (Feldberg 1950). Added acetylcholine can undoubtedly exert *some* influence on function in the central nervous system. But, again, one is impressed by the weight of negative evidence, suggesting that substances other than acetylcholine, of equally wide or wider distribution, may play a complementary part.

One's mind, of course, turns to *nor*adrenaline and adrenaline. It is of great interest that noradrenaline has recently been identified in the hypothalamus and the medial thalamic nuclei of the cat (Vogt 1952), though we know, as yet, nothing of its synthesis, its role, or its possible breakdown by amine oxidase (Burn 1952) in these regions. Similarly the central effects of inhibitors of amine oxidase such as ephedrine (Gaddum & Kwiatkowski 1938) require much fuller study. Again, the extremely interesting work on the effects of addition of adrenaline to perfusates of the superior cervical ganglion (Bülbring 1944) or the spinal cord (Bülbring & Burn 1941), suggesting an interplay between acetylcholine and adrenaline, invites similar experiments at higher levels of the central nervous system. There are also curious structural affinities between nor-adrenaline, adrenaline, ephedrine, amphetamine, methylamphetamine and mescaline; and our most powerful "phantasticum", lysergic acid diethylamide (LSD-25; Stoll 1947), acting in doses of 30 to 50 micrograms by mouth in man, is a synthetic ergot derivative, ergot being a parent substance of some adrenaline-blocking agents. There is thus no lack of suggestive evidence. Nevertheless, care has to be exercised if one is to avoid a facile carrying-over of interpretation from one system to another, and it is wise to stick to some of the desiderata mentioned earlier. In the case of *nor*adrenaline they remain unfulfilled, and only further experiment will determine its role, or the possible role of the vasodilator substance of nervous origin recently studied by Holton and Holton (1952).

One cannot help wondering whether one would not be nearer the truth if, instead of thinking in purely unitary terms, one began to think in terms of groups or families of compounds, possibly evolved as variants of original parent substances. There may be esters other than acetylcholine and amines other than *nor*-adrenaline or adrenaline taking part in a continuous turnover, regulated by the activity of corresponding enzymes. The balance may be delicate, and the effects of slight changes in molecular configuration of a substance profound. One need not go further than the steroids to seek an analogy of a family of compounds, or the effects of "local hormones" (Burn 1950) on function to see just how fine the balance between chemically mediated excitation and inhibition can be.

Basic information on the enzyme constitution of neurones thus becomes one pre-requisite before we can hope to take the study of the action of drugs on the central nervous system from a descriptive and empirical level towards a more precise understanding. Certain enzymes may be characteristic of certain types of neurones or glia, and magnitude of number of elements in the central nervous system need not necessarily reflect multitude and variation in kind. It is, in fact, not unlikely that the nervous system may be built on a relatively simple plan, and that variation and distribution of a limited number of types may make for apparent complexity. Thus a particular type of neurone may be scattered at random throughout a region, or be condensed into sheets, clusters or bundles in topographically close or in widely separated areas. The pharmacological susceptibilities of a region will be those of its dominant cell population, and of cells "impinging" (Feldberg 1950) upon it from nearby, or from afar. To talk of "levels" of action, as for example of predominant cortical, thalamic, hypothalamic effects, although in some instances perhaps empirically true, is apt to be misleading. Delicate shifts of balance between various cell groups would seem more likely.

There are certain advantages in assuming the existence of neurohumoral substances in the central nervous system. These lie in the fact that a good deal is known of the action of some chemical mediators at peripheral sites, and that the properties of some drugs can be partly or mainly ascribed to highly specific effects on the metabolism and effectiveness of local transmitters at these sites. The action of the anticholinesterase substances has already been mentioned. Drugs antagonising the peripheral effects of acetylcholine, adrenaline and histamine furnish further examples. Thus atropine blocks acetylcholine at autonomic nerve endings, and the curariform agents block transmission at the motor end plate; Dibenamine (Nickerson 1949) antagonises the peripheral effects of adrenaline, and the antihistamines the local effects of histamine. It is perhaps of interest that atropine (and, to a lesser extent, some of the antihistamine compounds) exert a protective effect against DFP and TEPP poisoning, and that in the case of atropine vis- -vis TEPP the evidence strongly suggests a central effect (Douglas & Matthews 1952). The ill-defined nature of the central effects of such compounds need not deter one from closer scrutiny for their merit may not so much lie in these actions, as in the possession of an overriding property which, by slow trial and error, may lead to a better understanding of these central effects and the enhancement of similar effects by possible analogues. The possession of a few pharmacological precision tools may thus be helpful in interpreting the less definite, composite, statistical states so common in the central nervous system, and also aid an understanding of the mode of action of other drugs whose properties are less apparent. Cross-relationships between actions are constantly coming to light. The recent development of drugs used in the treatment of Parkinsonism from some antihistamine compounds (Bovet, Durel & Longo 1950) furnishes but one example of this trend.

It is with such chemical and physicochemical considerations in mind that one should also re-examine the central relaxing substances (e. g. mephenesin; Henneman, Kaplan & Unna 1949) the barbiturates, analgesics and anticonvulsants. Similarly the central effects of the ganglion-blocking agents (Paton & Zaimis 1951) and their analogues are only slightly known, and may be full of interest.

The above drugs, though exerting some central effects, are hardly characterised by selective effects on higher mental function. It is to these latter substances that the attention of the psychiatrist inevitably turns. The origin and properties of such agents is varied, and the mere mention of alcohol, some of the volatile anaesthetics, the barbiturates, morphia, cocaine, cannabis, amphetamine, mescaline and, lately, the very powerful diethylamide of lysergic acid (LSD-25), will indicate the scope of the problem. The florid symptoms produced by some members of this group (particularly the so-called "phantastica", e. g. mescaline, cannabis, cocaine and LSD-25), despite the remarkable penetration and insight of some workers, have not always encouraged a careful and quantitative approach. The symptoms are well known, and need not detain us: disturbances in sensory perception, body image, time sense, affect, and in some instances autonomic and motor function, set in a state of consciousness which, though fluctuating, allows detailed self-observation; the lack of gross disturbances of speech despite interference with the normal imagery of language – all these sufficiently resemble some symptoms of the major psychoses to challenge further use of such drugs in a study of higher mental organisation. It is, however, well to remember the limitations of such an approach as well as its conceivable promise. To argue from the results of intoxication experiments to the aetiology of mental disorder is totally unjustified by the available facts.

It clearly reflects our present state of ignorance that we know almost as little of the mode of action of these phantastica as, for example, of the analgesics. Knowledge usually depends on method, and here at least, there is some promise of progress in the foreseeable future.

What are these methods? The relevance of the purely biochemical approach has already been stressed and, no doubt, will be stressed elsewhere during this meeting. The enzyme constitution of heterogeneous cell and fibre populations may slowly yield to microchemical and histochemical techniques. Possible effects of drugs on enzyme systems may be assessed just as directly from small tissue samples (Holter & Linderstr"m-Lang 1951) or tissue culture (Abood, Cavanaugh, Tschirgi & Gerard 1951), as indirectly from the accumulation of one or other of the metabolites in tissue fluids. The use of radioactive tracer techniques, especially if coupled with methods recently developed for studying cerebral circulation (Schmidt 1950) will no doubt make their contribution to the basic biochemical data.

But the fact that interneuronal events are temporally related makes a fuller understanding of these time-relationships indispensable, and it is here that the rapid recording methods of the electrophysiologist become invaluable in a study of drug action. Microelectrode techniques (Brock, Coombs and Eccles 1951), recording from single or a limited number of neurones can be used alongside electroencephalographic methods furnishing data on the overall electrical activity of large cell populations. In animals, cortical and stereotactically placed sub-cortical electrodes may be employed, either in acute experiments, or permanently implanted for work with the conscious, unrestrained preparation. Dr. P.B. Bradley in our laboratory has recently developed such a technique. Up to ten electrodes can be implanted into the skull of a cat, the leads being brought out through the skin of the shoulder area and attached to a miniature multiple socket, carried by the animal in a small harness. It is thus possible to plug in directly into the various cortical and subcortical leads. With suitable precautions sepsis in these chronic preparations can be avoided, and animals have been kept in good condition for periods up to one year, though, more usually, they are killed after three months to check electrode placement. Observations in the conscious animal are usually carried out in a constant-environment chamber, which makes possible simultaneous recording of behaviour and electrical activity. The effect of sensory, (for example rhythmic photic), stimulation can also be studied. Drugs can be applied singly or in combination, and the vitiating effect of anaesthetics is completely avoided. The information thus obtained is, of course, complementary to that yielded by acute experiments, where chemical agents may be applied to the brain by the systemic or carotid routes, or by direct local microinjection into selected areas. Interruption of pathways, and destruction of isolated cell groups are further procedures designed to reduce the number of variables in such studies.

Animal behaviour offers another large and useful field, and the effects of chemical agents on basic activities such as sleep, food, and sexual habit, on the processes of discrimination and learning, on conflict and conditioned behaviour (Masserman 1943) invite further detailed study. Here again a combination of experimentally produced anatomical and biochemical lesions may be helpful, and parallel studies on the electrical activity of the brain in such experimentally induced behaviour disorders, or the effects of electrical stimulation upon them, may add further information.

Whatever data animal experiments may yield, however, must be regarded as only preparatory, and complementary to data obtained in man, where subjective sensations communicated by means of speech add a fund of information inaccessible in the animal experiment. Two groups of observations are relevant here. The first concerns the effects of some drugs on mental function in normal subjects; the second the modification of abnormal mental function in patients by pharmacological means. The gross effects of the "phantastica" on normal volunteers are well known, and well documented (see Mayer-Gross 1951). Although there is little doubt that some effects are peculiar to some drugs, the final picture of intoxication depends upon the personality of the subject. I do not know that one need always go to full intoxication in such pharmacodynamic studies. It may perhaps be equally useful to work with the early symptoms and to see whether they can be enhanced or arrested by some controlled chemical or physical means. We have recently begun to record in some detail the illusions (of colour, pattern and movement) induced by rhythmic photic stimulation by white light at frequencies from 4 to 24 cycles per second, and the possible effects of some drugs upon them. Subjective sensations at each frequency are sound-recorded, transcribed, and the transcript analysed subsequently for relevant elements. Our experience with this method is as yet very limited, and because of its time-consuming nature, it may be a long time before sufficient data are ready for review and assessment. Nevertheless, even at this stage, one cannot help noticing the curious resemblance between the coloured, fine, ordered geometrical patterns reported as visual hallucinations in mescal intoxication, and the patterns induced by some frequencies of photic stimulation in normal subjects in the absence of any medication. Both phenomena may perhaps represent a shift in the time base, (that is in the "beat" of some elements of the visual pathway), the shift being induced, in one instance, by rhythmic stimulation of the visual fields, and in the other by some selective interference with a cycle of chemical events in certain neurones. Whether such changes are related to recent evidence concerning a triple pathway along the visual system (Clark 1941, Chang 1951) only future experiment can tell.

The second group of data concerns the effects of some drugs on mental and somatic function in clinical material. The amytal interview, the ether abreaction, the effect of dextro-amphetamine on mood and appetite are simple and well-known examples of such effects. The remarkable increase in accessibility brought about by small doses of intravenous sodium amytal in long-standing cases of catatonic stupor forms a useful starting point for pharmacological investigations of this kind. Dr. Charmian Elkes in our laboratory has recently had occasion to compare the effects of intravenously administered sodium amytal, amphetamine, and mephenesin in nine cases of catatonic stupor, who were selected according to a number of criteria out of an original group of 23 patients. Amytal increased accessibility, as shown both in terms of verbal productivity and of drawing; there seemed to be a better correlation between this increase of accessibility and foot temperature than between accessibility and muscle tone (as measured in the flexors of the elbow by a simple weighting device). Optimum psychomotor effect was only rarely accompanied by muscular relaxation. Amphetamine decreased accessibility, a finding unlike its more common effects in control material. Mephenesin regularly reduced muscle tone (i. e. the weighting figures) without appreciably altering either accessibility or foot temperature.

What developments such transient effects of drugs on normal and abnormal mental function foreshadow, it is difficult to say at this stage; but no one will question the challenge implicit in such simple facts. The critical study of familiar chemical agents, and of deliberately fashioned analogues, (used either singly, or in combination, so as to emphasise or attenuate some particular property) offers an inviting field to physiologist, psychologist and physician alike. Problems of perception, of affect, and of the cognitive, adaptive, and integrative functions commonly comprised by the term "ego" may perhaps be aided by the study of the effects of such agents. As yet we know little of the chemical basis of learning, remembering and forgetting; and it is not unlikely that both electroconvulsive therapy and leucotomy will in time yield to more discriminate chemical means. Drugs have begun to find their use in diagnosis and therapy, but their real value will keep step with their use as research tools. Our understanding of their action will depend on our understanding of the coding and cipher employed by the brain in the elaboration and storage of its patterns, and yet such understanding may be enhanced and supported by the very agents we employ. Perhaps time may turn out to be the denominator shared by brain patterns and the physicochemical activities of its constituent neurones.

Certainly for the present the gaps far exceed the body of knowledge. Looking at this field, one is rather reminded of Cézanne's later paintings, where, shining through surfaces of subtle and delicate colour, there are large areas of bare canvas. He is reputed to have said that he left them bare because he was not certain. Yet they form part of the picture. It is as good to wonder as to explain.

PAPER 9

THE EFFECT OF SOME DRUGS ON THE ELECTRICAL ACTIVITY OF THE BRAIN AND BEHAVIOUR[*]

J. Elkes, C. Elkes and P. B. Bradley

Department of Experimental Psychiatry,
University of Birmingham and Winson Green Hospital, Birmingham

Reprinted with the kind permission of The British Journal of Psychiatry
from the Journal of Mental Science 100: 125-128, 1954

Peripheral neuro-effector sites within and outside the autonomic nervous system form useful reference points for the study of the central effects of some agents. Nevertheless, ready analogies between peripheral neurohumoral mediation, and central synaptic transmission may be grossly misleading, and reliance must solely be placed on data derived from within the central nervous system itself.

A number of drugs known to have both peripheral an central actions (atropine, *d*- and *l*-amphetamine and *d*-lysergic acid diethylamide) were studied in terms of their effects on behaviour, and on the electrical activity of the brain in the experimental animal; observations on some effects of *d*-lysergic acid diethylamide on catatonic stupor were also made.

Conscious, unrestrained cats, carrying multiple, permanently implanted cortical and stereotactically placed subcortical electrodes were used for the animal experiments (1). Simultaneous observation on behaviour and electrical activity were made possible by the use of a constant environment chamber. Acute preparations subjected to high spinal or midbrain sections (the so-called *encéphale* and *cerveau isolé*) (2), and preparations anaesthetized with pentobarbitone, furnished complementary information.

In the conscious animal, large doses of atropine (1–2 mgm./kgm. i.p.) produces large-amplitude, slow waves, interspersed by bursts of fast activity. These patterns bore some resemblance to those characteristic of sleep. They did, however, differ from the latter in their failure to show a cortical alerting response to sensory stimuli, although the animals could, in fact, be roused. *l*-Hyoscyamine induced effects similar to those seen with atropine: the dose, however, was lower (1–2 mgm./kgm. i.p.). *d*-Hyoscyamine was ineffective, even in high doses. Physostigmine (0.5–1.0 mgm./kgm. i.p.) abolished the slow activity induced by atropine and *l*-hyoscyamine, the resultant low-amplitude, fast activity resembling the normal alert pattern. Such activity was also produced by physostigmine alone. This activity, however, was not necessarily accompanied by a corresponding change in behaviour. Neostigmine left the

---

[*] An abstract of a paper read at the Annual Meeting of the Medico-Psychological Association held at Barnwood House, Gloucester, on 10 July, 1953.

electrical activity of the brain unaffected, even in doses which produced marked peripheral parasympathomimetic effects.

D- and *l*-Amphetamine in full doses (3–5 mgm./kgm. by mouth) produced rhythmic fast (15–30 cycles per second) activity in all regions. This was accompanied by a corresponding change in behaviour, the animal regularly becoming more attentive and excitable. The cortical response to rhythmic photic stimulation recorded over the visual area was increased in amplitude at all frequencies between 2 and 25 cycles per second. *d*-lysergic acid diethylamid (15–25 microgm./kgm. by mouth) exerted effects somewhat similar to those of amphetamine on both electrical activity and behaviour. There was, however, no change in the reponse to photic stimulation.

In preparations anaesthetized with pentobarbitone (30 mgm./kgm. i.p.) the characteristic waxing and waning activity (the so-called barbitone "spindling") was changed by both physostigmine (0.5–1.0 mgm./kgm. i.v.) and D.F.P. (administered i.v. in divided doses up to a total of 3–4 mgm./kgm.); the spindle bursts were abolished, and replaced by continuous rhythmic activity at 4–4 cycles per second. Atropine sulphate abolished this continuous activity, and restored spindle bursts. Mid-brain section either reduced or abolished the D.F.P.-induced rhythmic activity. Amphetamine had little effect on the electrical activity of a barbiturate anaesthetized animal as recorded at the cortical level. There was, however, some increase in the response to photic stimulation when recorded at the level of the lateral geniculate body. Large doses of *d*-lysergic acid diethylamide (50–100 microgm./kgm. i.p.) completely abolished the electrical activity characteristic of moderate barbiturate anaesthesia, the anaesthesia continued apparently unaffected.

The characteristic waxing and waning activity seen in the corticogram of the brain sectioned *in situ* at the level of the first cervical vertebra, or superior colliculus (2) was abolished by physostigmine and restored by atropine. In such experiments, simultaneous recordings of blood pressure and electrico-cortical activity showed the cortical activity to be unrelated to the transient changes in blood pressure produced by thes drugs. The intermittent electro-cortical activity of the *encéphale isolé* was abolished by amphetamine (in doses of 1.5–3.0 mgm./kgm. i.v.). This activity was, however, restored by section at mid-brain level in the same preparation, and remained unaffected by the administration of further doses of amphetamine. *d*-lysergic acid diethylamide (in doses of up to 100 microgm./kgm. i.p.) had no effect on the electrical activity of either of these acute preparations.

The effects of amphetamine and *d*-lysergic acid diethylamide on the corticogram thus differ from those of atropine, *l*-hyoscyamine and physostigmine in their apparent dependence upon mesencephalic or spinal connections. Again, there is better correlation between electrical activity and behaviour in the case of amphetamine and *d*-lysergic acid diethylamide, than there is with atropine, *l*-hyoscyamine and physostigmine. Magoun (3) has drawn attention to the existence in the upper brain stem of reticular activating system, concerned with arousal by sensory stimuli. Amphetamine is structurally related to tyramine, *nor*-adrenaline, adrenaline and not unrelated to mescaline; *d*-lysergic acid diethylamide is related to other adrenaline blocking agents of the ergot group. It is perhaps of interest that *nor*-adrenaline (4) and 5-hydroxytryptamine (5) have been recently identified in some areas of the brain, and that *d*-lysergic acid diethylamide has been found to antagonize 5-hydroxytryptamine (6). Possible effects of these drugs on the general and local cerebral circulation, and on intermediate metabolism (7) must, however, be very clearly borne in mind.

The symptoms of *d*-lysergic acid diethylamide (LSD-25) intoxication were studied in 12 male and 3 female volunteers. The drug was administered in doses of 15 to 100 microgm. by mouth, and particular attention was paid to the effects of rhytmic photic stimulation (at 4 to 24 cycles per second) on the symptoms of intoxication. Subjective sensations, including the peculiar illusions of form, colour and movement experienced under these conditions, were sound recorded for each frequency, both before and after the administration of the drug. The sound-record was transcribed, and the transcript subsequently analysed independently for relevant elements. EEG records were also taken.

The symptoms described by Stoll (8) were confirmed. Depersonalization, heightened awareness and fluctuating incongruous affect were the common symptoms. Visual symptoms were seen in 8 subjects, and 7 experienced distortion of body image. Mild dysarthria was seen 11, and thought-blocking in 6 subjects. Rhytmic photic stimulation enhanced the symptoms in 12 out of 15 subjects; in 3 out of these 12, symptoms were brought out where no symptoms of any kind had been experienced before. An uncommunicative, trance-like state during photic stimulation following LSD-25 was experienced by six subjects, and in three there was a slight, transient, but quite definite alteration in muscle tone, not unlike that seen in catatonia. This persisted for up to 20 minutes after photic stimulation had ceased. EEG records were taken in 13 subjects. In terms of resting record, 2 of the subjects belonged to the micro-alpha, 5 to the responsive alpha, and 6 to the persistent alpha group (9). Following LSD-25 the micro-alpha subjects showed little change in their resting record. One responsive subject showed micro-alpha activity, and four others became more responsive. Of the 6 persistent alpha subjects, 5 became completely responsive, and one remained persistent.

The effects of amytal (120–240 mgm. i.v.), amphetamine (7–15 mgm. i.v.), mephenesin (750–1000 mgm., administered as a 5 per cent solution in saline) and *d*-lysergic acid diethylamide (60–100 microgm. by mouth) were compared in 9 cases of catatonic stupor. The mental response was assessed in terms of verbal productivity and of drawing. The somatic changes recorded included blood pressure, pulse rate, foot temperature (recorded by multiple thermocouple), muscle tone (as measured in the flexors of the elbow by a simple weighting device) and sweat secretion. The well known effect of amytal on accessibility showed itself as an increase of both verbal productivity, and of drawing. There was better correlation between this change, and a rise in foot temperature, than between accessibility and muscle tone. An optimum mental response was only rarely accompanied by full muscular relaxation. Amphetamine decreased accessibility (10), a finding unlike its more common effects in normal subjects Mephenesin regularly reduced muscle tone without changing either accessibility or foot temperature. LSD-25 produced a response peculiar to itself, and unlike that seen either with amytal or amphetamine. This was characterized by unmotivated laughter and crying, bizzare uncontrolled behaviour, and an apparent activation of hallucinatory and delusional material. There was a blunting of the amytal response with repeated administration. Premedication with neostigmine (0.5–0.75 mgm. s.c.) or physostigmine (1.0 mgm. s.c.) did not modify the amytal response.

The above phenomena suggest the existence of elective affinities within the central nervous system. It is possible thet chemical evolution has, at certain stages, accompanied phylogenetic evolution and, in the central nervous system, made use of selected variants of substances familiar to us as powerful neuro-humoral transmitters at the periphery. There may be subtle and definite chemical differences between phylogenetically older and newer parts of the brain; and even if such differences be confined to a few nodal points, a delicate shift in balance at these points could have profound effects on the function of the brain as a whole. Clear cut "levels" of action are perhaps less likely than changes in the temporal relation between the activities of unevenly distributed cell groups.

The above material was communicated to the Physiological Society at its meetings of January 16th (11, 12), and June 5th (13, 14), 1953. We wish to express our thanks to the Superintendent of Winson Green Hospital, Dr. J.J. O'Reilly, for the facilities so generously put at our disposal at the hospital.

REFERENCES

1. Bradley, P.B., and Elkes, J., EEG Clin. Neurophysiol., 1953, 5, 451.
2. Bremer, F., L'activité électrique de l'écorce cérébrale, 1938, 46 pp. Hermann: Paris.
3. Magoun, H.W., Res. Publ. Ass. Nerv. Ment. Dis. 1952. 30. 480.
4. Vogt, M., Communication to the British Pharmacological Society, 5 January, 1952.
5. Amin, A.H., Crawford, T.B.B., and Gaddum, J.H. Communication to the British Pharmacological Society, 7 July, 1952.
6. Gaddum, J.H., J. Psychol., 1953, 121, 15 P.
7. Mayer-Gross, W., McAdam, W., and Walker, J.W., Nature, 1951, 168, 827.
8. Stoll, W.A., Schweiz. Arch. Neurol. Psych. 1947. 60, 279.
9. Golla, F., Hutton, E.L., and Walter, W.G., J. Ment. Sci., 1943. 89, 216-223.
10. Delay, J., Proc. R. Soc. Med., 1949, 42. 491.
11. Bradley, P.B., and Elkes, J., J. Physiol., 1953, 120. 13.
12. Bradley, P.B., and Elkes, J., Ibid., 1953, 120. 14.
13. Bradley, P.B., Elkes, C., and Elkes, J., Ibid., 1953. 121. 50.
14. Bradley, P.B., Cerquiglini, S., and Elkes J., Ibid., 1953. 121. 51.

PAPER 10

THE EFFECTS OF SOME DRUGS ON THE ELECTRICAL ACTIVITY OF THE BRAIN

P.B. Bradley and J. Elkes

Department of Experimental Psychiatry,
University of Birmingham

Reprinted with the kind permission of the Oxford University Press from Brain 80: 77-117, 1957

INTRODUCTION

There is no lack of data on the effect of drugs on the electrical activity of the brain. Ever since Berger (1933) observed the effects of barbiturates on the human alpha rhythm numerous studies have attempted to describe and interpret the effects of drugs on the electrical activity of cortical and subcortical areas (Adrian and Matthews 1934, Gibbs, Gibbs and Lennox 1937; Grinker and Serota 1938 and Gerard and Libet 1940). The effect on the activity of isolated units has also been studied (Amassian 1952). In so far as they concern the so-called autonomic drugs, which form the burden of this paper, particular attention has centred on the possible role of acetylcholine as a central neurohumoral transmitter. Sympathomimetic and other noncholinergic agents have received relatively little attention, though, with the recent advent of drugs exerting peculiar effects on mental function, some shift of interest is now apparent. The field has been reviewed by Toman and Davis (1949).

The drugs in question have been applied by various routes. Thus Bonnet and Bremer (1931) and Bremer and Chatonnet (1949) injected acetylcholine and physostigmine into the carotid artery in unanaesthetized preparations (*encéphale isolé*). They found that acetylcholine, in quantities of less than 0,5 μg. caused a reduction in voltage and rise in the electrocortical activity. Physostigmine and neostigmine given intra-arterially in doses of 0.1-0.5 mg/kg produced similar effects to those of acetylcholine, but these were longer lasting. All these effects could be abolished (or blocked) by intravenous atropine in doses of 0.5 mg/kg. Hampson et al. (1950) administered di-isopropylfluorophosphate (DFP) in graded doses by the intracarotid route. They observed the emergence of seizure patterns characterized by high amplitude waves which could be related to a decrease in the cholinesterase activity of cortical tissue.

Topical application to the exposed cerebral cortex of anaesthetized animals has provided another route, the electrical activity being recorded either from the area to which the drug had been applied, or adjacent areas. Miller, Stavraky and Woonton (1940), obtained spike discharges, and also motor effects, when they applied a 1 per cent solution of acetylcholine to an area of exposed cortex previously treated with 1 per cent neostigmine. They also found that atropinization blocked these effects. Chatfield and Dempsey (1942) obtained similar effects with 1 per cent acetylcholine following 1 per cent neostigmine, and found that alone, acetylcholine exerted no effect. They also noted that atropine (1 mg./kg., intravenously) did not abolish the spike discharge. Brenner and Merritt (1942) obtained localized discharges with acetylcholine alone, but used higher concentrations (2.5 to 10 per cent). They observed that neostigmine enhanced the responses and lowered the threshold to acetylcholine. Intravenous atropine (1 mg./kg.) did not antagonize these effects.

Forster (1945) injected acetylcholine intracisternally in cats in doses of 10 to 25 mg and obtained depression of electrical acclivity, followed by high voltage discharges. Similar effects were obtained by Forster and McCarter (1945) with 5 to 25 per cent solutions of acetylcholine applied to the exposed cortex, and Forster, Borkowski and McCarter (1946) found that the depression of activity preceding the spike discharge was not related to the systemic effects, and could be obtained with solutions of acetylcholine which were too weak to produce a discharge. This initial depression of activity was also observed by Beckett and Gellhorn (1948) and Hyde, Beckett and Gellhorn (1949) who were able to show that high voltage discharges from the cortex could be obtained with a variety of agents having little in common. These included mescaline, streptomycin and acid fuchsin, as well as established convulsants such as metrazol and picrotoxin. More recently, depression of electrical activity on local application of acetylcholine (in 2 to 20 per cent solutions) was observed by Essig, Adkins and Barnard (1953). This was occasionally followed by paroxysmal spikes. Cooke and Sherwood (1954) obtained an increase in spindle activity in *encéphale isolé* preparations after intraventricular injections of 10 to 20 μg. of acetylcholine. This was depressed by atropine.

Similar patterns of activity to those seen with intra-cisternal or topical application of the drugs in question have been obtained by way of the intravenous route. Thus DFP, when administered in doses of 1 to 2 mg./kg. produced *grand mal* patterns (Freedman et al. 1949) and this effect could be abolished by intravenous atropine in doses of 2 to 4 mg./kg. Funderburk and Case (1951) found that atropine when administered alone in doses of 0.4 to 1.2 mg./kg. intravenously, produced sleep patterns in the EEG of curarized cats. They also note that whereas atropine increased the spiking due to the topical application of curare and penicillin, it decreased or abolished that due to acetylcholine. Wikler (1952) recorded the electrical activity of the brain in unanaesthetized dogs, and observed that although the administration of atropine was followed by excitement, the EEG showed "sleep patterns." A similar dissociation between behaviour and electrical activity using atropine, was observed independently by Bradley and Elkes (1953b) in the conscious cat.

All workers draw attention to the similarity between the high voltage discharges obtained with acetylcholine and epileptic seizure records, and there have been numerous suggestions (Tower and Elliott 1952) that acetylcholine may play an important part in the mechanism of epileptic seizures. On the other hand, it is well known that high voltage discharges can be obtained by applying a variety of agents to the cortex (Hyde, Beckett and Gellhorn 1949, Funderburk and Case 1951).

Relatively little attention has been paid to the effects of sympathomimetic agents on the electrical activity of the brain. Toman and Davis (1949) found no change in the EEG of animals treated with amphetamine. Changes in the EEG have been observed in the conscious cat following the administration of *r-*, *d-* and *l-*amphetamine (Bradley and Elkes 1953a) and in the dog following *d-*amphetamine (Schallek and Walz 1953). In all these experiments the changes in the EEG paralleled the effects on behaviour. The effects of adrenaline on the EEG and its possible significance in the mechanism of arousal, has recently been studied by Bonvallet,

Dell and Hiebel (1954), who recorded the effects of this drug in acute preparations sectioned at various levels of the brain stem. The effect of *d*-lysergic acid diethylamide (LSD-25) on the electrocorticogram in rabbits has been studied by Delay et al. (1952) and in the conscious cat by Bradley and Elkes (1953b).

Many of the reports on the effects of drugs on the electrical activity of the brain are contradictory. They are, in the main, based on experiments carried out in anaesthetized preparations, or in acute preparations immobilized by spinal section, or by curare. Behaviour could not readily be studied in these experiments. Since, however, some drugs do affect behaviour, and the relation between electrical activity and behaviour seemed particularly important, some time was devoted to the development of a technique for the recording of electrical activity simultaneously with behaviour in the conscious, unrestrained and unanaesthetized animal (Bradley and Elkes 1953c). An additional advantage of this technique was that it enabled the operator to become familiar with the normal behaviour and EEG patterns of each animal. Slight effects produced by drugs could thus be more easily detected, and the differences between individual animals be given their due weight.

In addition to the chronic unrestrained preparations, acute preparations were also used. These were the so-called *encéphale* and *cerveau isolé* (Bremer 1935, 1936), where both systemic blood pressure and heart rate could be recorded simultaneously with the electrical activity. In addition, drugs could be injected both by the intracarotid and intravenous route, and the effects of the planes of section on the responses observed.

The aim of the study was an attempt to answer the following questions:
(a) What is the effect of the drugs studied on the electrical activity of the brain and on behaviour in the normal conscious animal?
(b) Is there any correlation or lack of correlation between electrical activity and behaviour with any of these drugs?
(c) Is their any interaction between the drugs used?
(d) Can any clues as to their mode of action be derived from these experiments?

The preliminary results of the experiments which follow have been communicated to the Physiological Society (Bradley and Elkes 1953a,b) and the 3rd International EEG Congress (Bradley 1953).

METHODS

Fifty-four cats and six monkeys were used in the study. Most of the experiments were carried out in the conscious animal using chronic cat preparations with implanted electrodes. The operative technique has already been described (Bradley and Elkes 1953c). In a few cases a cannula for the intraventricular injection of drugs (Feldberg and Sherwood 1953) as well as electrodes were implanted. In all, fourteen chronic preparations were used, and experiments were carried out over a period of approximately six months before killing the animals and checking the electrode placement. For the simultaneous observation of behavior, a specially constructed chamber (Bradley and Elkes 1953c) was used. An occasional film record was also made.

For acute experiments, the Bremer preparations (the so-called *encéphale isolé* and *cerveau isolé*) were used almost exclusively. These were prepared under ether anaesthesia combined with local infiltration of procaine. A tracheal cannula was introduced, and wherever necessary, the carotid or femoral artery and the femoral vein were cannulated.

To prepare the *encephalé isolé*, the neck muscles were dissected away from the occipital region of the skull, the occipital joint exposed and the dura incised between the foramen magnum and the first cervical vertebra. The spinal cord was then transected through this aperture by means of a blunt leucotome, whilst full anaesthesia was maintained. Artificial respiration was then applied. Cortical recording electrodes were inserted through burr holes in the skull to record various regions of the cortex, and an earthing electrode inserted into the bone overlying the frontal sinus. The electrodes were of the same type as those used in chronic preparations. When all operative procedures had been completed, the administration of ether was discontinued and artificial respiration alone maintained. At least one hour was allowed to elapse before the experiment was commenced. This ensured an adequate wearing off of the anaesthetic. At the end of each experiment the brain was dissected out and fixed in formol saline to confirm the electrode positions and to check the completeness of the spinal section.

In some early experiments the *cerveau isolé* was prepared from the *encephalé isolé*; in others the mid-brain section was made in the intact animal. This was done in two ways. In some cases, a leucotome was inserted on either side of the mid-line through holes just anterior to the supra-occipital ridge, and slid down over the edge of the tentorium until it reached the base of the skull. In more recent experiments, a new method of making the lesion was tried, and found to be more successful. Here a fronto-parietal bone flap was turned, exposing almost the whole of one cerebral hemisphere. The dura was then incised and the occipital lobe gently pulled forward to give a clear view of the superior colliculus. The lesion was then made at the inter-collicular level, using suction. A fine glass pipette was employed and the negative pressure kept to a minimum. The tissue was removed very gently, and the lesion gradually extended to the opposite side to give a complete transaction of the mid-brain. Local bleeding or oedema was controlled by means of small pledgets of gelatine sponge. The occipital lobe was then allowed to fall back into place, the bone flap replaced and held in position by one or two sutures in the temporalis muscle. Recordings of electrical activity were taken from the opposite, undisturbed hemisphere. In all cases the brain was fixed in formol saline at the end of the experiment, and the position and extent of the lesion checked subsequently.

Five experiments were carried out under barbitone anaesthesia where the effects of barbiturates in combination with other drugs were being studied.

Recordings of blood pressure in the acute experiments from either the carotid or femoral arteries were made either on a kymograph, or using an electronic manometer which recorded the blood pressure on the same trace as the electrical activity.

In all experiments recordings of electrical activity were made with bipolar electrode connections. A Mitchell 6-channel Electroencephalograph in conjunction with an Ediswan Low Frequency Wave Analyser was used in early experiments. Later, 4-channel Ediswan Portable Recording Equipment was used.

TABLE 1

Drugs	Preparations
Physostigmine sulphate	Conscious animal
Physostigmine salicylate	
Neostigmine methylsulphate	
Di-isopropylfluorophosphate	Encéphale isolé
Atropine sulphate	
d-hyoscyamine sulphate	
l-hyoscyamine sulphate	Cerveau isolé
r-amphetamine sulphate	
d-amphetamine sulphate	
l-amphetamine sulphate	Anaesthetized animal
Mescaline sulphate	
d-lysergic acid diethylamide	

A list of drugs, together with the types of preparation, is given in Table 1. In most cases, the solutions were freshly made up in normal saline, or sterile distilled water. In a few cases dispensed solutions were used. In experiments in the conscious animal, drugs were given mostly by the intraperitoneal route, but in some experiments they were given orally, intramuscularly or subcutaneously, and in others by intraventricular injection. In acute experiments, drugs were administered either by way of a cannula in the femoral vein, or by intracarotid injection.

RESULTS

I. THE ELECTRICAL ACTIVITY OF THE BRAIN OF THE NORMAL CONSCIOUS CAT

The spontaneous resting acclivity of the unrestrained conscious cat has been described by a number of authors (Rheinberger and Jasper 1937, Bradley 1952, Hess, Koella and Akert 1953) and their findings are in very close agreement. Our own observations may be summarized as follows:

(a) In the waking, fully alert state, with the animal showing maximum awareness of the environment and spontaneous movement, the amplitude of the electrical activity was at a minimum. No dominant rhythm could be detected and components were present at many frequencies. These usually ranged between 15 to 20 c/s and 25 to 30 c/s (Hess et al. have observed frequencies up to 40 c/s). The appearance of the record was flat and desynchronized (Fig. 1A). This type of record characterized the alert state in all our animals, and appeared in all regions from which recordings were taken. It was referred to as the "alert" or "activation" pattern.

(b) In the resting or relaxed state, in which the animal was often seen sitting or lying down with its eyes open or closed and obviously not markedly interested in its environment, bursts of rhythmic activity et a frequency of 5 to 8 c/s were noted (Fig. 1B). These had an amplitude of up to 200 μV, but were not uniformly distributed over the whole of the cortex. They appeared more in the cortical areas which were not primary sensory or motor areas and in the medial nuclei of the thalamus rather than the lateral nuclei. In some animals these bursts were often preceded and followed by shorter bursts at frequencies between 12 and 16 c/s.

(c) The third stage corresponded to drowsiness or light sleep. In this state the electrical activity consisted of slow waves at 1 to 3 c/s with an amplitude of up to 500 μV., together with bursts of spindle activity at 12 to 15 c/s (Fig. 1C). This activity appeared in all the regions from which recordings were taken.

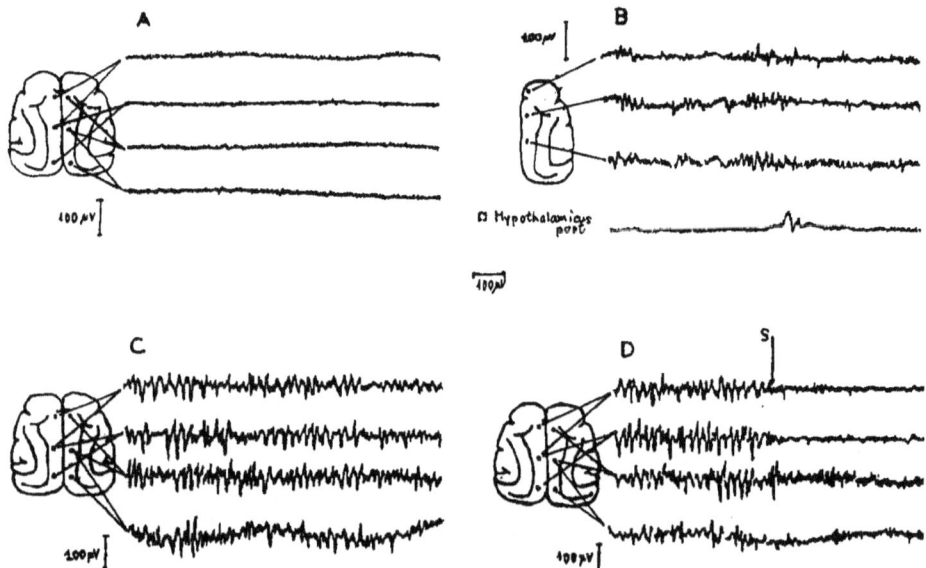

Fig. 1. Typical records of the electrical activity of a normal conscious cat in different behavioral states. A: fully alert; B: quiet; C: drowsy; D: arousal from the drowsy state through a sensory stimulus (noise) at "S."

In either the resting or drowsy state an arousal response could be obtained if a suitable sensory stimulus was applied. This could be either tactile or auditory, the latter usually being more convenient, and, irrespective of the previous state. of the animal, the activation pattern was immediate, produced, the behaviour changing correspondingly (Fig. 1D). In no case did we fail to obtain this response in the normal animal; it was regularly tested for in every experiment before any of the drugs were administered.

Although the patterns described above were those seen normally in most of the chronic preparations, and no other type of pattern was encountered, there were individual variations in certain cases. These however, always followed the observed behaviour. For example, in one animal which was very restless and never really settled down in the constant environment chamber (although it was put in at weekly intervals over a period of months), the activity characteristic of the drowsy state never fully developed. Equally, the animal was never seen to be drowsy or sleeping under experimental conditions. On the other hand some animals settled down very quickly, and after two or three periods of acclimatisation would go to sleep almost at once. Here only a transient response to the arousal stimulus was usually seen. This was characterized behaviourally by merely lifting the head and opening the eyes.

There were also variations between experiments with the same animal on different occasions. Some animals were more restless on some occasions than others but always showed the type of electrical pattern that one would expect from the observed behaviour. We never noticed any change in the behaviour of these animals as a result of previous experiments. They remained perfectly friendly and even affectionate, and never resisted being manually restrained for injections.

These observations serve to emphasize the importance of observing behaviour simultaneously with electrical activity; of observing each animal over long periods so that the operator could become thoroughly familiar with the normal individual pattern of each animal; and of providing a relatively constant environment so that, as far as possible, the only variable operating during the experiment was the pharmacological agent under study.

II. THE EFFECTS OF PARASYMPATHOMIMETIC AND PARASYMPATHOLYTIC SUBSTANCES ON ELECTRICAL ACTIVITY, AND ON BEHAVIOUR

(a) In the Conscious Animal

(i) *Physostigmine.* This drug was given alone or preceding other drugs in twelve experiments in the conscious chronic preparation and produced consistent changes in the electrical activity of the brain. Within five to ten minutes after the administration of the drug, the electrical activity from all regions consisted of flat low amplitude potentials similar to those seen in the normal alert animal (Fig. 2B). However, the behaviour of the animals was unchanged and they remained quiet or even apparently sleeping, whilst the electrical activity was of a type seen in the normal animal only in the waking state. The dose required to produce these effects varied between 0.2 to 1.0 mg/kg for the salicylate, which was used in five of these experiments; and between 0.05 and 0.1 mg/kg for the sulphate, the drug in all cases being given intraperitoneally. No peripheral effects were obtained with these doses, but with larger doses salivation incontinence and respiratory embarrassment were observed and the animals became more alert in their behaviour as a result of these effects. Smaller doses than those given above produced a less marked change in electrical activity.

Recovery of the normal electrical pattern was usually complete in two or three hours but the effects could be abolished earlier by the administration of atropine (Fig. 2C) or *l*-hyoscyamine.

There was no noticeable change in the response to rhythmic photic stimulation after these doses of physostigmine.

(ii) *Neostigmine.* This was given in two experiments, in the form of the methyl sulphate, in doses of 0.2 and 0.4 mg./kg., intraperitoneally. With the smaller dose, no change in the electrical activity was observed and with the larger dose marked peripheral effects were seen. These included excessive salivation, incontinence, muscular fasciculation and respiratory embarrassment; the effects on the electrical activity were those which would be expected from such a disturbance of behaviour. When the animal was quiet, the electrical activity was unchanged.

(iii) *Di-isopropylfluorophosphate (DFP).* This drug has been used in only two experiments in the conscious animal owing to its long-lasting effects. In each case the experiment was pre-terminal and the animals were pre-medicated with atropine (1.0 mg/kg). The respective doses of DFP were 3.0 and 6.5 mg/kg in the two experiments.

With the smaller dose, (3.0 mg/kg) no change in the electrical activity was seen. The larger dose caused (6.5 mg/kg) an increase in the amount of fast activity in the record, and bursts of activity at 20 to 30 c/s (with an amplitude of about 100 μV.) were observed. The behaviour changes were very slight. The rate of respiration increased slightly (from 35 to 46 per minute with 3.0 mg/kg) and some unsteadiness of gait was noted. Both animals were less active and did not move unless they were disturbed. No change in the response to rhythmic photic stimulation was observed.

(iv) *Atropine.* This drug was given alone, or preceding other drugs in 22 experiments in the conscious animal. In 18 of these it was given by intraperitoneal injection, in doses of 1.0 to 3.0 mg/kg of the sulphate. Doses of less than 1.0 mg/kg had no effect on

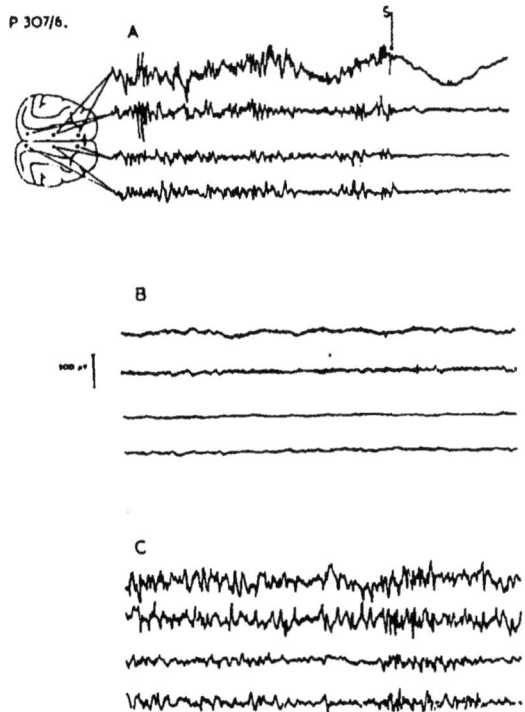

Fig. 2. Records from an experiment of a chronic preparation in which physostigmine was given first, followed by atropine. A: control record of the conscious animal showing an arousal response; B: ten minutes after an intraperitoneal injection of 0.08 mg/kg of physostigmine sulphate; C: twenty minutes after the subsequent injection of 3.0 mg/kg of atropine sulphate (intraperitoneally).

electrical activity but caused dilation of the pupils. Larger doses (2.0 to 3.0 mg/kg) caused a marked change in the electrical activity in all cases. Some 15 to 20 minutes after the adminis-

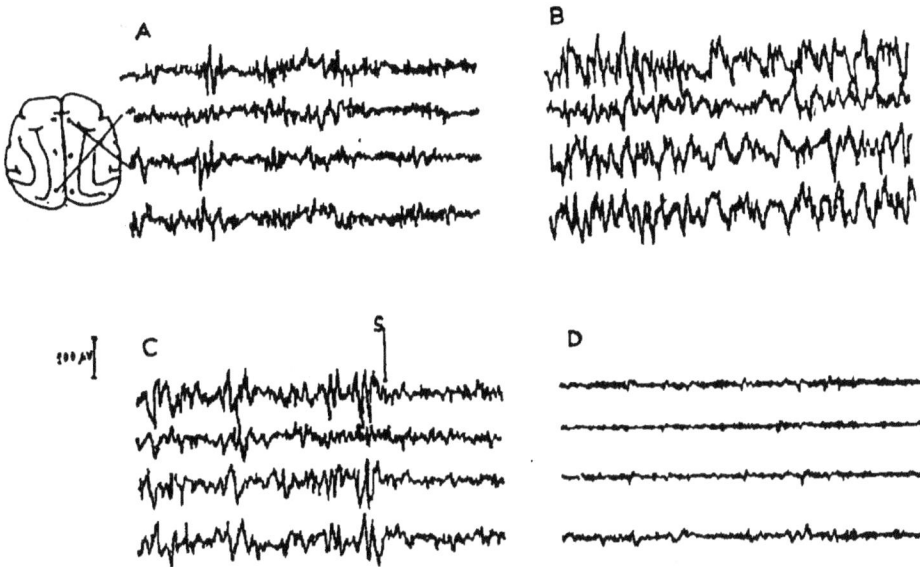

Fig. 3. Records from an experiment in which atropine was given to the conscious animal and followed by physostigmine in divided doses. A: control record; B: twenty minutes after an intraperitoneal injection of 2.0 mg/kg of atropine sulphate; C: ten minutes after the subsequent injection of 0.5 mg/kg of physostigmine sulphate (intraperitoneally) showing the return of the arousal response; D: fifteen minutes after a total of 0.9 mg/kg of physostigmine had been given.

tration of the drug large amplitude slow waves appeared in all regions of the cortex and in the leads from the thalamus, hypothalamus and caudate nucleus (Fig. 2C and 3B). This activity was very similar to the activity seen in the drowsy or sleeping state, but the amplitude was sometimes larger. There were also bursts of spindle activity at 12 to 15 c/s in most cases, similar to those seen in the drowsy animal. In all these experiments, although large amplitude slow waves dominated the electrical recordings, sleep or drowsiness were never observed and the animals remained fully awake. In some cases slight excitement was noted after the drug had been given. The application of an arousal stimulus (e. g. a noise) which would normally alert the animal and produced a corresponding change in electrical activity, evoked the normal behaviour response (i.c. alerting) but produced no change in the electrical patterns. Thus the slow waves persisted irrespective of the behaviour of the animal.

When doses of between 1.0 and 1.5 mg/kg were used the slow activity appeared in bursts and was less persistent. With these lower doses it could still be blocked by sensory stimuli. No change was observed in the response to rhythmic photic stimulation after atropine sulphate, and the response recorded from the visual cortex was often seen superimposed on the slow activity. This effect was never observed when the slow activity of the drowsy state was present in the normal animal. Under such conditions the response to photic stimulation was very much reduced or lost.

In four experiments atropine sulphate was injected into the lateral ventricle in the conscious animal by means of an implanted cannula. The doses used were between 200 and 500 µg., and the behavioural effects observed were similar to those described by Feldberg and Sherwood

EXP. 307/5   A

500 μV

1 sec   B

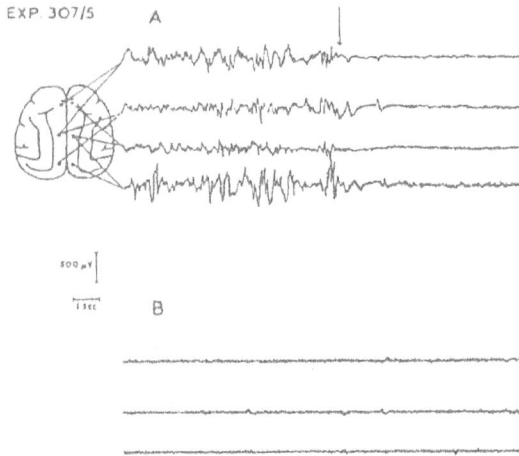

Fig. 4. A: Control record of normal conscious cat showing an arousal response. B: seventeen minutes after the injection of 300 mg. of atropine sulphate into the lateral ventricle of the brain.

(1954). These consisted of increased liveliness and restlessness, together with licking, defaecation and vomiting in the early stages, and with the largest doses, there was also an increase in the respiratory rate. In all four experiments the electrical activity was of the alert type associated with the increased liveliness of the animals (Fig. 4B). In none of these experiments was any slow activity, similar to that seen when the drug was injected intraperitoneally, observed.

(v) *d-Hyoscyamine sulphate.* This drug was given in two experiments in doses of 5.0 and 10.0 mg/kg, by intraperitoneal injection. In neither case did it have any effect on behaviour or electrical activity (Fig. 5B).

(vi) *l-hyoscyamine sulphate.* This was used in four experiments in doses of 1.0 to 4.0 mg/kg, given intraperitoneally. It produced very similar changes in electrical activity to those observed with atropine sulphate (Fig. 5C). There was never any change in behaviour, and in no case was any excitement seen.

(vii) *Combinations of atropine or l-hyoscyamine.* In three experiments atropine sulphate (2.0 mg/kg) was given first, and followed by physostigmine (0.7 to 2.0 mg/kg). In another three experiments *l*-hyoscyamine (1.0 to 2.0 mg/kg) was given first and this was also followed by physostigmine in similar doses. In all of these experiments the slow activity was abolished after the physostigmine had been given, and the record was similar to that seen when the drug was used alone, although somewhat larger doses were required (Fig. 3D). No peripheral effects were observed.

In one of these experiments physostigmine was given in divided doses and it was found that the effect of a small dose was not to abolish the slow activity altogether, but to make it less persistent and also more responsive to sensory stimuli. The arousal stimulus, however, would produce only a brief alerting of the electrical activity, and the slow waves very soon reappeared (Fig. 3C). A further injection of physostigmine abolished the slow activity altogether (Fig. 3D).

In one experiment physostigmine was given first in a normal dose (0.08 mg/kg) and then followed by atropine sulphate. It was found that the slow activity could still be obtained, but that a larger dose of atropine (3.0 mg/kg) was required (Fig. 2C). In another experiment a similar result was obtained when physostigmine was followed by l hyoscyamine.

(viii) *Combinations of atropine, l-hyoscyamine and neostigmine.* In one experiment neostigmine was given after atropine (3.0 mg/kg), and in the other after *l*-hyoscyamine (2.0 mg/kg). In each case the dose of neostigmine was 0-4 mg/kg. It was found to have no effect on the slow activity induced by either of these drugs.

(ix) *Combinations of barbiturates, physostigmine and atropine.* The effects of physo-stigmine on the electrical patterns induced by barbiturates were studied in five experiments. Pentobarbitone was used in three of these experiments and- sodium amytal in the other two. In each case the barbiturate was given in a dose sufficient to produce moderate anaesthesia. With pentobarbitone the dose. required was of the order of 30 to 35 mg/kg by intraperitoneal injec-tion. The characteristic "spindle burst" activity was then seen (Fig. 6A). This usually ranged over a frequency of 10 to 15 c/s and was more prominent in areas of the cortex which were not primary sensory or motor. They were also present in the medial thalamic nuclei, and the caudate nucleus. After physostigmine sulphate (in doses of 0.1 to 0.2 mg/kg) had been given intraperitoneally, the spindle bursts disappeared and the electrical activity was dominated by a continuous rhythmic activity at a frequency of 5 or 6 cycles per second. This appeared in all regions but was largest in amplitude in those areas in which the spindles had been most marked (Fig. 6B). The frequency of this rhythmic activity was noticeably constant.

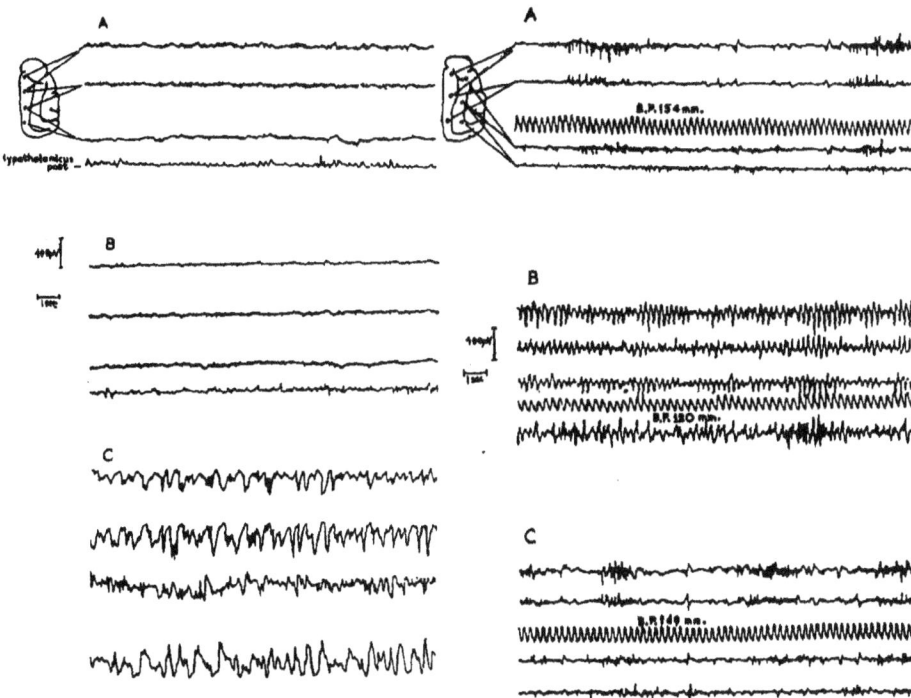

Fig. 5. A: Control record of normal conscious cat in the alert state. B: twenty minutes after the injec-tion of 10 mg/kg of d-hyoscyamine sulphate intra-peritoneally; C: ten minutes after the injection of 1.0 mg/kg of l-hyoscyamine sulphate intraperi-toneally.

Fig. 6. Records from an experiment in which phy-sostigmine and atropine were given to a cat under pentobarbitone anaesthesia and in which blood pressure was also recorded. A, control record of pentobarbitone anaesthesia (30 mg/kg); B: three minutes after the intravenous injection of 0.2 mg/kg of physostigmine sulphate; C: two minutes after the subsequent injection of 1.0 mg/kg of atropine sulphate.

In four experiments it was 6 per second, and in the other one 5 per second. The animal remained fully anaesthetized after physostigmine had been injected, and showed no sign of recovery. In two of these experiments physostigmine was followed by atropine sulphate in doses of 1.0 and 2.0 mg/kg. In both cases the continuous rhythmic activity disappeared within three minutes of the atropine injection, and the spindle bursts characteristic of barbiturate anaesthesia returned (Fig. 6C). The animals made normal recovery from the anaesthetic.

(b) In Acute Preparations. Encéphale isolé and cerveau isolé

The method by which these were prepared has been described. In encéphale isolé the brain receives afferent impulses from the cranial nerves only and the preparation shows periods of drowsiness or sleep which alternate with periods of wakefulness or apparent alertness, indicated by the behaviour of the eyes, ears and pupils (Bremer 1936). The electrical activity of the cortex is different in these two states. In the waking state, in which movements of the ears and eyes, together with a pupillary response to light are seen, the electrical activity consists mainly of low amplitude fast activity in all regions, similar to that seen in the intact animal in the alert state (Fig. 7B). In the sleeping state the eyes are rotated upwards and the pupil is fixed and constricted. The cortical activity in this state is dominated by bursts of spindle activity somewhat similar to those seen in the drowsy intact animal, and in barbitone anaesthesia, together with some slow activity (Fig. 7A). The frequency range of the spindle activity is from 10 to 15 per second. When the *encéphale isolé* preparation is in the sleeping state it can still be roused by sensory stimulation, auditory stimuli (such as taps or clicks) being very effective in the cat. In the acute experiments in which monkeys were used, visual stimuli were also found to be effective.

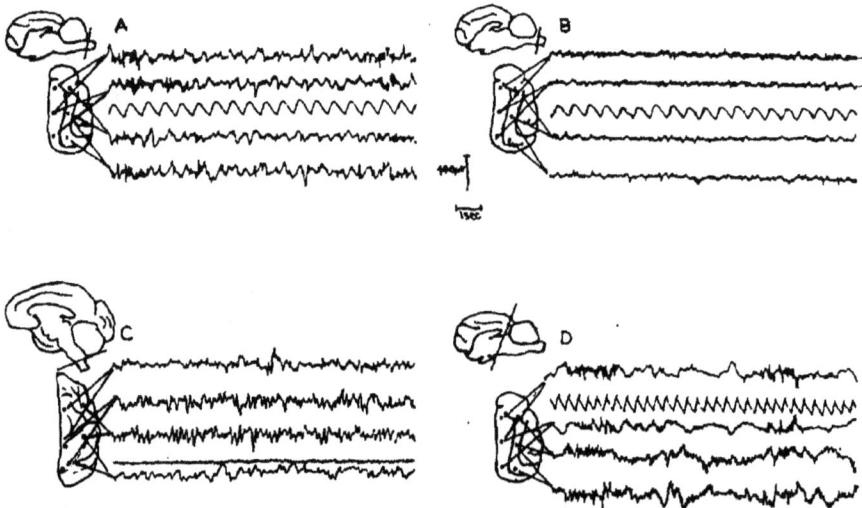

Fig. 7. Normal records of acute preparations. A: encéphale isolé preparation (cat), "sleeping"; B: the same, "waking"; C: encéphale isolé preparation (monkey), "sleeping"; D: cerveau isolé preparation (cat).

In the *cerveau isolé* preparation the mid-brain is transected and this preparation has the appearance of being permanently asleep (Bremer 1935). The eyes and ears no longer move and slow waves and spindle bursts are permanently present (Fig. 7D). This preparation does not respond to afferent stimulation.

(i) *Physostigmine.* In seven experiments in the encéphale isolé preparation, five of which were cats and two monkeys, physostigmine sulphate was given intravenously in doses of 0.1 to 0.5 mg/kg. In all seven experiments, the spindle and slow wave activity of the sleeping state was abolished after the drug had been given, and did not reappear (Fig. 8B). No change in the behaviour of the preparation was, however, observed. In all except one cat experiment blood pressure was recorded simultaneously with electrical activity. The slight blood pressure changes which occurred following physostigmine were transient, and the general level of blood pressure remained unchanged (Fig. 8B). The rate of respiration in these experiments was controlled artificially, and retrained constant.

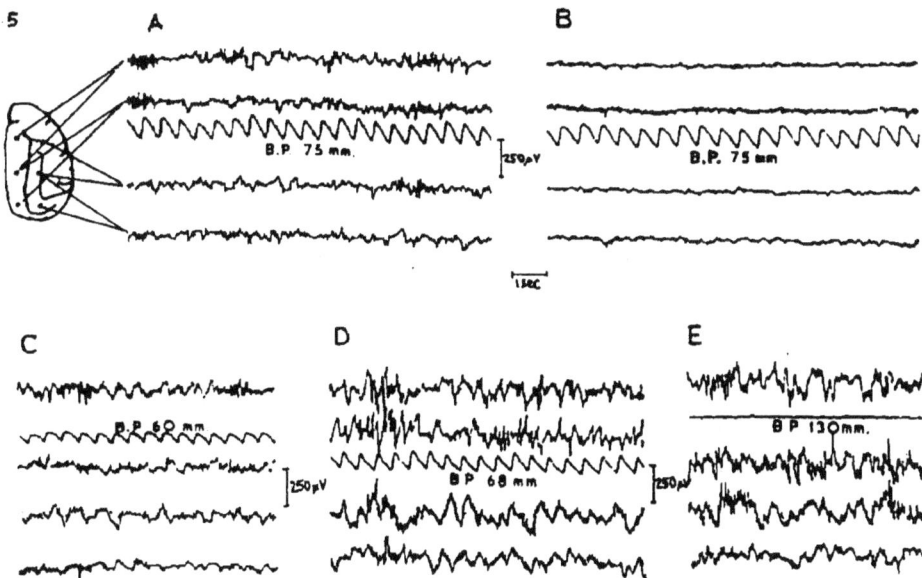

Fig. 8. Records from an acute experiment (encéphale isolé cat preparation) in which blood pressure was recorded. A: control record with the preparation "sleeping"; B: forty seconds after 0.1 mg/kg of physostigmine sulphate had been injected intravenously; C: five minutes after the subsequent injection of 2.5 mg/kg of atropine sulphate; D: six minutes after a total dose of 4.0 mg/kg of atropine had been given; E, sixty seconds after the intravenous injection of 2 mg. of noradrenaline showing the peak of the blood pressure rise.

Physostigmine was given intravenously to the cerveau isolé preparation in four experiments in cats, the doses ranging from 0.1 to 0.5 mg/kg. Here, too, the spindle and slow activity was abolished and did not reappear (Fig. 9B). In two of these experiments blood pressure was recorded simultaneously with the electrical activity. The changes in blood pressure which occurred were again transient, though the electrical effects persisted (Fig. 9B).

(ii) *Atropine and l-hyoscyamine.* Atropine (1.5 to 4.0 mg/kg) was given in four experiments to the *encéphale isolé* and *l*-hyoscyamine (2.0 mg/kg) in one experiment. In each case the slow activity, similar to that seen in the conscious intact animal, was observed (Fig. 10B). No changes in the behavioural state of the preparation were, however, seen, although in one case the drug was injected when the preparation was in the waking state. As was observed with physostigmine, the time course of the blood pressure changes following these drugs did not correspond to the changes in electrical activity (Fig. 10B).

Atropine and /-hyoscyamine were not used in experiments in the *cerveau isolé* preparation except following the administration of physostigmine.

In the acute experiments there was an antagonism between physostigmine and atropine (or *l*-hyoscyamine) similar to that observed in the experiments in the conscious animal, Thus when atropine or *l*-hyoscyamine was given after physostigmine, the effects of the latter were abolished. This was seen with atropine (2.0 to 5.0 mg/kg) in four of the experiments in the *encéphale isolé*, and with *l*-hyoscyamine (2.0 to 4.0 mg/kg) in two. The effect of a small dose of atropine (2.5 mg/kg in Fig. 8C) was to restore the spindle and slow activity of this preparation, whilst a larger dose (Fig. 8D after 4.0 mg/kg) caused the appearance of slow waves of high amplitude as seen when atropine was given alone. Very similar effects were observed in the two experiments in which *l*-hyoscyamine was used.

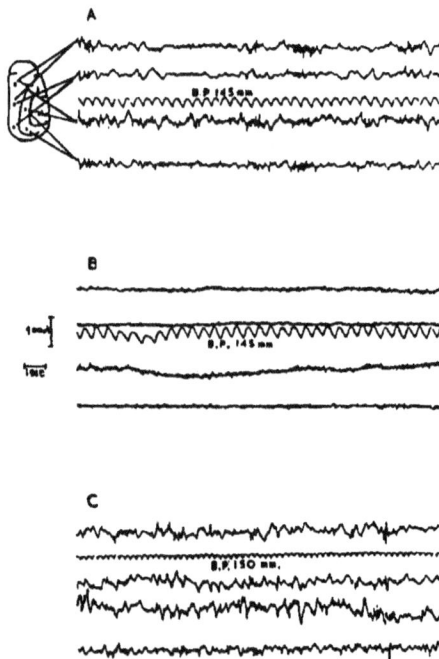

Fig. 9. Records from an acute experiment (cerveau isolé cat preparation) in which physostigmine was followed by atropine. A: control record; B: three minutes after 0.1 mg/kg of physostigmine sulphate had been injected intravenously; C, five minutes after the subsequent injection of 2.0 mg/kg of atropine sulphate.

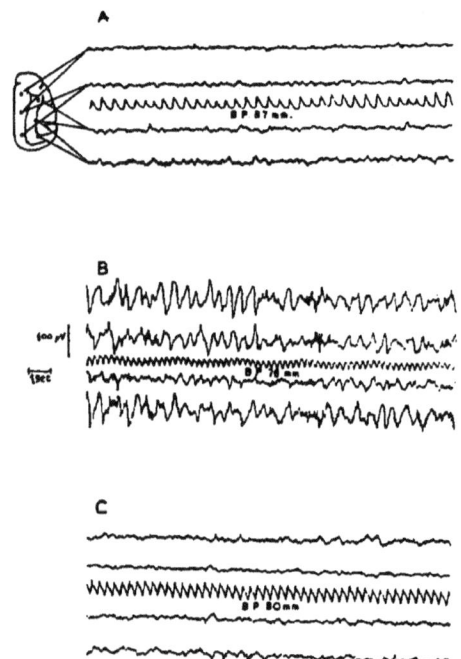

Fig. 10. Records from an acute experiment (encéphale isolé cat preparation) in which atropine was followed by physostigmine. A: control record with the preparation "awake"; B: one and a half minutes after 2.0 mg/kg of atropine sulphate had been injected intravenously; C: seven minutes after the subsequent injection of 0.4 mg/kg of physostigmine sulphate.

In the four experiments in the *cerveau isolé* in which physostigmine had been given, this drug was followed by atropine or *l*-hyoscyamine. The effects were similar to those seen in the *encéphale isolé*. In two experiments atropine (2.0 and 2.5 mg/kg) was used, and in the other two, *l*-hyoscyamine (2.0 and 4.0 mg/kg). In all four the spindle and slow wave activity which had been abolished by the administration of physostigmine reappeared (Fig. 9C).

Conversely, in the experiments in which atropine and I-hyoscyamine were injected intravenously into *encéphale isolé* preparations, it was noted that their effects could be subsequently blocked by physostigmine (Fig. 10C) although in some cases larger doses were required (0.4 to 2.0 mg/kg).

In two experiments with *encéphale isolé* preparations in which atropine had been given following physostigmine in a sufficiently large dose to cause the appearance of the irregular slow waves, the blood pressure had fallen slightly as compared with the level at the beginning of the experiment (Fig. 8D). In these experiments an infusion of *nor*-adrenaline, given into the femoral vein, raised the blood pressure to a level considerably in excess of that observed previously; despite this, the character of the electrical activity remained unchanged, and the slow waves persisted (Fig. 8E).

III. THE EFFECTS OF SYMPATHOMIMETIC, SYMPATHOLYTIC AND RELATED COMPOUNDS ON ELECTRICAL ACTIVITY AND BEHAVIOUR

(a) In the Conscious Animal

(i) *r-amphetamine.* In eighteen experiments in the conscious preparations this drug was given, either alone, or preceded by other drugs. It was usually administered intraperitoneally in doses of 1.0 to 5.0 mg/kg, but in some experiments it was given orally in similar doses. Doses between 1.0 and 2.0 mg/kg had little or no effect on electrical activity or behaviour, whereas doses between 2.0 and 5.0 mg/kg regularly changed the electrical activity to the alert pattern, i.e. low amplitude, fast acclivity (Fig. 11B). This change was seen in all regions of the cortex and in leads from both the medial and lateral thalmic nuclei, the hypothalamus and the caudate nucleus. At the same time the behaviour of the animals was altered. They appeared much more restless and alert. Very often they could be seen to explore the corners of the constant environment box in which they had not previously shown any interest. In some cases they showed excitement; involving circling movements and escape reactions. The pupils were dilated and the respiratory rate increased. In none of these experiments did the animals become drowsy or fall asleep after amphetamine had been given, and the electrical and behavioural effects of the drugs ware still present after five or six hours. However, these effects usually wore off in twenty-four hours. Owing to the extreme restlessness of these animals after amphetamine it was often very difficult to obtain a recording of the electrical activity which was free from movement artefacts.

r-amphetamine also had an effect on the amplitude of the cortical response to rhythmic photic stimulation. When photic stimulation was applied to the normal animal, using an electronic stroboscope lamp which was arranged to give flashes of light at regular intervals, it was possible to record from the primary visual area in the conscious animal a rhythmic response at the same frequency as the stimulus (Fig. 12A). The response was always in the form of a wave and was not a discrete response to each flash, provided the frequency of stimulation was above 4 flashes per second. If the stimulus was maintained, it was found that the response had a steady amplitude and that this did not vary appreciably with the position of the animal relative to the stroboscope lamp (the walls of the constant environment box, being light in colour, gave good reflection of the flash). It was therefore thought that changes in the amplitude of the response were not likely to be due to changes in the position of the animal, though, where the responses were being measured, they were checked as far as possible with the animal in the same position. Changes in the amplitude of the response with changes in the behavioural state of the animal were, however, observed. When the stroboscope lamp was first switched on it usually alerted the animal and the maximum response was then obtained. If the lamp was then left on, the animal sometimes remained alert, but very often, after a while, lapsed into a quiet or drowsy state and the amplitude of the response then diminished. It could be restored by switching the lamp off and on again. Thus the best assessment of the response to photic stimulation at different frequencies was obtained by switching on the lamp at each frequency to be examined, and measuring the response after a given time interval in each case.

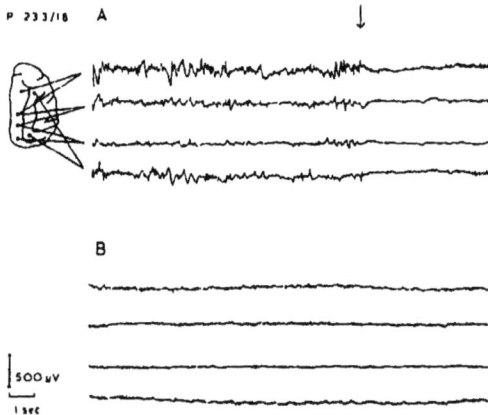

Fig. 11. A: Control record of normal conscious cat with arousal response; B: twenty minutes after an intraperitoneal injection of 2.3 mg/kg of r-amphetamine sulphate.

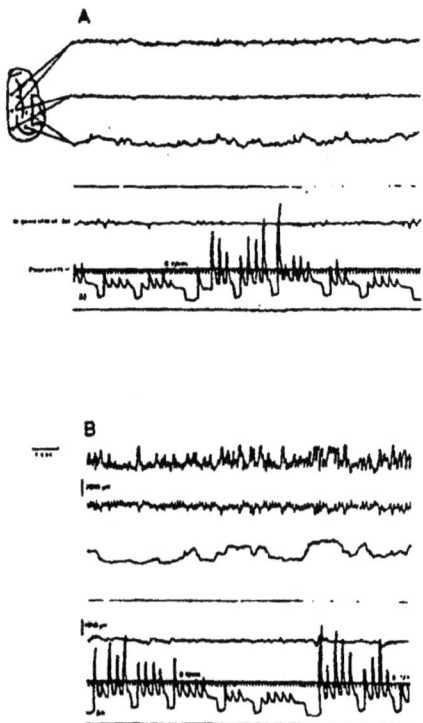

Fig. 12. Records of the response recorded from the visual cortex to rhythmic photic stimulation. A: in the normal conscious animal; B: after 4.0 mg/kg of r-amphetamine sulphate (intraperitoneally). In record B the gain of the wave analyser has been reduced by one-half.

A cortical response to photic stimulation was observed at all frequencies between about 4 and 25 cycles per second and if the stimulus frequency was varied continuously between these limits, the frequency of the response followed in the same way. With stimulation at frequencies below 4 per second there was usually a discrete response to each flash of light. The amplitude of the rhythmic response was usually greatest at lower frequencies an decreased progressively as the stimulus frequency increased. In the normal animal the response was usually too small to be measured above 25 flashes per second.

After 3.0 to 5.0 mg/kg of *r*-amphetamine, this rhythmic response was increased in amplitude, particularly at frequencies between three and ten second (Fig. 12B). This is illustrated in Fig. 13., in which the amplitude of the response recorded from the visual cortex has been plotted against frequency in one of these experiments. The amplitude at the lower frequencies was more than doubled after amphetamine and at higher frequencies a response could be detected up to 24 flashes per second. Similar curves were obtained in the other experiments but in some cases the restlessness of the animals after amphetamine made it difficult to measure the responses accurately.

Since amphetamine also caused dilation of the pupils, the effect of this on the photic response had to be checked. In two experiments the eyes were treated with a 5 per cent solution of cocaine until the pupils were fully dilated and the control recording was then taken. In these experiments, the increase in the photic response was still obtained after the administration of *r*-amphetamine.

(ii) *d-amphetamine.* Experiments on four animals with this substance showed that in similar doses it had the same effect on electrical activity and behaviour as did *r*-amphetamine.

(iii) *l-amphetamine.* This was used in four experiments and was found to have similar effects to *r*-amphetamine but larger doses (10 to 15 mg/kg) were required.

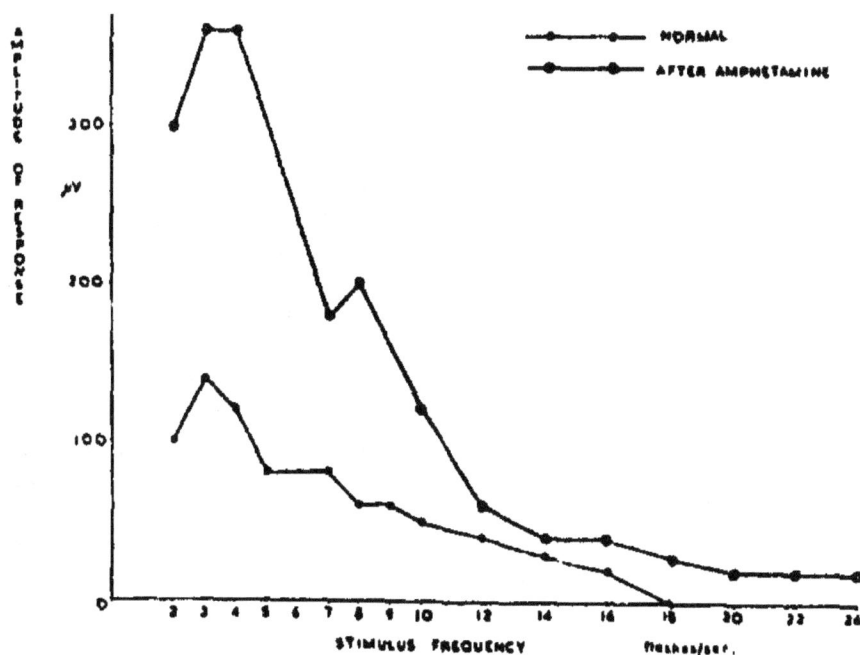

Fig 13. Graph showing the amplitude of the response to rhythmic photic stimulation recorded from the visual cortex in the conscious animal, plotted against the frequency of stimulation. A: in the normal animal; B: after 4.0 mg/kg of r-amphetamine sulphate.

(iv) *Combinations of r-amphetamine and other substances.* Since amphetamine was found to produce alerting of electrical activity, and of behaviour, its effect on the states induced by barbiturates and on the slow activity induced by atropine were tested:

(1) *Barbiturates.* In three experiments, sodium amytal, thiopentone and dial were used respectively, and were given in doses sufficient to produce a state of moderately light anaesthesia: *r*-amphetamine was then administered in increasing doses. It was found that even with large doses (20 mg/kg), amphetamine had no effect on the depth of anaesthesia, or on the electrical patterns induced by the barbiturates.

In one experiment, a large initial dose of *r*-amphetamine (20 mg/kg) was followed by thiopentone. A normal dose of thiopentone (20 to 25 mg/kg) was required to produce anaesthesia and the alert pattern of electrical activity was replaced by the spindle burst activity of barbiturate anaesthesia.

(2) *Atropine.* In three experiments in the conscious preparations, in which *r*-amphetamine had been given in doses of 3.0 to 5.0 mg/kg and alerting of electrical activity and of behaviour had been produced, atropine sulphate was given in doses of 2.0 to 3.0 mg/kg. In each case the premedication with amphetamine did not prevent the appearance of the slow wave activity after atropine, and the usual dose of the latter drug was sufficient to produce this activity. However, behaviourally the animal remained in the excited or hyperactive state induced by amphetamine. In another series of three experiments the order of the drugs was reversed, atropine (2.0 to 3.0 mg/kg) being given first, followed by *r*-amphetamine (3.0 to 5.0 mg/kg). The latter did not modify the slow wave activity, although the animals became excited in the usual way.

(v) *Mescaline.* Eight experiments were carried out with this drug, which was given either by mouth or intraperitoneally in doses between 10 and 25 mg/kg. No change in electrical activity or behaviour were observed with these doses. In two other experiments larger doses (50 mg/kg) were used, and in these vomiting and defaecation occurred within thirty minutes of the drug being given. The vomiting went on at intervals for about one hour, and during this time the electrical activity tended towards the alert type of pattern, as the animals were becoming restless. About an hour and a half after the mescaline had been given, the animals passed into a stuporous state, in which they lay taking little notice of the environment. In this state, the electrical activity was dominated by rhythmic waves at 4-6 c/s from all areas (Fig.

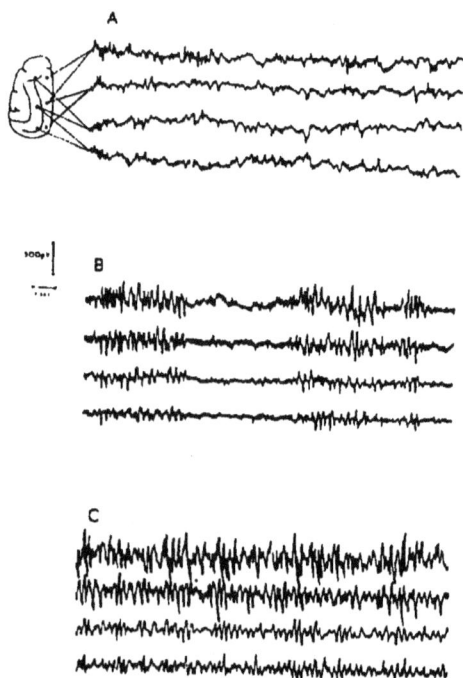

Fig. 14. Records from an experiment in which a large dose of mescaline was given to a conscious animal. A: control record of normal animal in drowsy state; B: eighteen minutes after 50 mg/kg of mescaline sulphate had been injected intraperitoneally; C: two hrs after the administration of mescaline.

14C), although this activity was more prominent in areas of the cortex not primary sensory or motor. Whilst the animals were in this state, they did not respond to the usual sensory stimuli (e. g. noise or light) nor did the electrical activity change. Handling, however, did rouse the animals, and they would then move about for a while before relapsing into the stuporous state. During this active period the electrical activity changed to the alert pattern.

Mescaline was not used in combination with any other drugs.

(vi) *Lysergic acid diethylamide (LSD-25).* This drug was used in eighteen experiments, either alone or preceding other drugs in the conscious animal. The doses were between 7. 5 and 100 µg/kg. Doses of less than 15 µg./kg. appeared to have no effect on electrical activity or behaviour. Doses of 15 to 25 µg./kg were observed in an early series of eight experiments to produce similar changes in electrical activity to those seen with amphetamine, although the change was not always so marked. Thus there was a tendency towards the alert type of activity, but some rhythmic activity often remained, although its amplitude was small and the frequency relatively high (15 to 20 c/s) (Fig. 15B). The animals were always more restless and alert after these doses of LSD-25. In a later series of experiments in which slightly larger doses of LSD-25 were used (35 to 43 µg/kg.), somewhat different electrical effects were observed. Here more rhythmic activity was present in the record. This activity usually occurred in bursts, at a frequency between 4 and 7 c/s. It could be blocked by sensory stimulation in the same way as the rhythmic activity of the normal animal Similar changes in behaviour to those seen in the previous series of experiments were observed.

In this later series, the experimental conditions had been changed slightly inasmuch as the constant environment chamber had been moved into a sound-proofed room. The possible significance of this factor and the differences in the results in the two series of experiments in relation to the possible mode of action of this drug are discussed below.

No change in the cortical response to photic stimulation was observed following administration of LSD-25.

(vii) *Combinations of LSD-25 and other drugs.*

(1) *Barbiturates.* In three experiments LSD-25 was given following administration of barbiturates in doses sufficient to produce a state of moderately light anaesthesia (Fig. 16B). Pentobarbitone was used in two experiments and sodium amytal in the third. When LSD-25 was given in doses between 100 and 150 µg/kg, the characteristic spindle burst activity of the barbiturate anaesthesia disappeared (Fig. 16A). This activity did not change, although the depth of anaesthesia was unaltered, and recovery from the anaesthetic was normal. In one of these experiments LSD-25 was followed by an intravenous injection of 2.0 mg/kg of SKF 688, an adrenaline blocking agent. This drug had

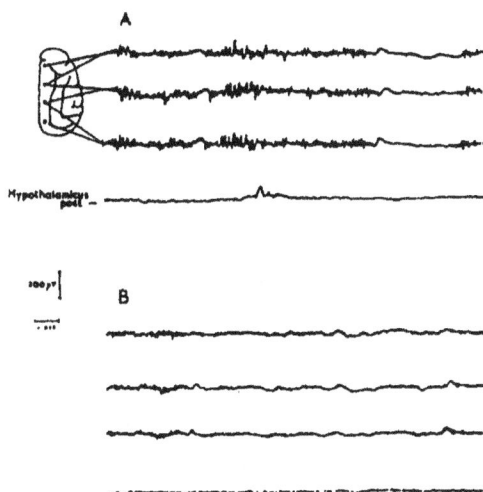

Fig. 15. A: Control record of normal conscious cat in quiet state; B: twenty minutes after an intraperitoneal injection of 15 mg./kg. of LSD-25.

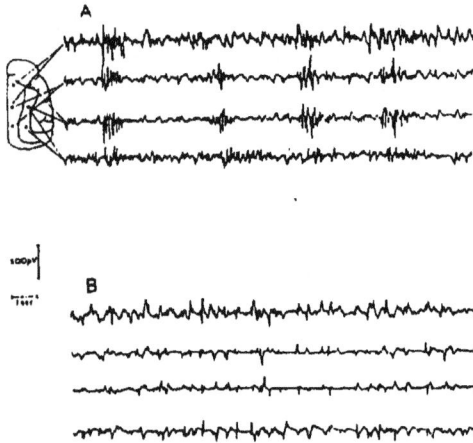

Fig. 16. A: Record of pentobarbitone anaesthesia (30 mg/kg) in a cat. B: minutes after 100 g/kg of LSD-25 had been injected intravenously.

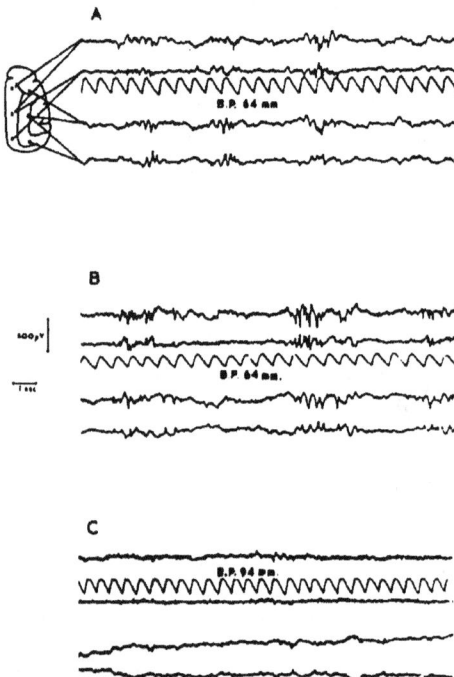

Fig. 17. Records from an acute experiment (encéphale isolé cat preparation) where LSD-25 was followed by r-amphetamine A, control record with the preparation "sleeping"; B: three minutes after 35 mg/kg of LSD-25 had been given intravenously showing no effect on the electrical activity or blood pressure; C: two minutes after the subsequent intravenous injection of 1.0 mg/kg of r-amphetamine sulphate.

no effect on the electrical activity, and did not restore the spindling. In another series of three experiments, LSD-25 was administered in doses of 100 to 150 µg/kg and then followed by sodium amytal. Although the usual dose of amytal produced anaesthesia, the spindle burst activity never appeared.

(2) *Atropine and l-hyoscyamine.* In two experiments, atropine sulphate (3. 0 and 3. 3 mg/kg) and in one experiment, *l*-hyoscyamine (2.0 mg/kg) were administered before LSD-25. Although in each case the dose of LSD-25 was increased to 100 µg./kg, no change in the electrical pattern of slow waves induced by atropine or *l*-hyoscyamine was observed. In every case, however, the animals became more restless and alert.

(b) In Acute Preparations: encéphale isolé and cerveau isolé

(i) *Amphetamine.* In thirteen experiments in the encéphale isolé' preparation (eleven in cats and two in monkeys), *r*-amphetamine was injected intravenously in doses of 1.0 to 3.0 mg/kg (Figs. 17C, 18C and 19C). In all cases the spindle and slow activity was abolished, and did not reapper. The preparations also showed behavioural signs of arousal, i.e. the eyes opened and moved, and the pupils responded to light. In some cases, movements of the ears, jaw and vibrissae were noted. In six cat, and both monkey preparations, blood pressure was recorded from the carotid artery simultaneously with the electrical activity. A rise in blood pressure occurred following the injection of amphetamine and this was maintained throughout the experiment. In two experiments, therefore, smaller quantities of amphetamine (0.2 and 0.5 mg/ kg) were injected initially. These doses were sufficient to produce a blood pressure rise (Fig. 18B), together with a temporary blocking of the spindle activity. The latter, however, returned after about half a minute, whilst the higher level of blood pressure was maintained. A second injection of a larger quantity of amphetamine (1.0 to 2.0 mg/kg) was then given, and the spindling abolished completely and permanently without further blood pressure change. The alerting effects of amphetamine in this type of preparation did not therefore appear to be related to its general circulatory effects.

Amphetamine was also used in eight experiments in the *cerveau isolé* preparation. Six of these were cats and two monkeys. Three of these (cats), were prepared from *encéphale isolé* preparations to which amphetamine had already been given, causing alerting of electrical activity and behaviour, as described above. When the mid-brain transection was made in these preparations, the spindle and slow activity, characteristic of the *cerveau isolé* (Fig. 7D) appeared. This activity could not be abolished by further injections of amphetamine, although doses up to 20 mg/kg were used. At the same time, the eyes and pupils became fixed and showed no change following further administrations of amphetamine. All the other *cerveau isolé* preparations were prepared by the later method, using suction, and without the spinal

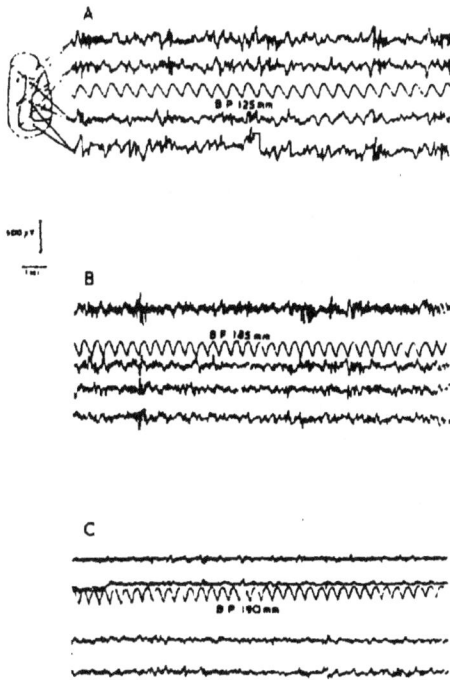

Fig. 18. Records from an acute experiment (encéphale isolé cat preparation) in which r-amphetamine was given initially in a very small dose.
A: control record with the preparation "sleeping";
B: nine minutes after 0.2 mg/kg of r-amphetamine sulphate had been given intravenously showing a rise in blood pressure; the spindle bursts are still present; C: eight minutes after 2.0 mg/kg of r-amphetamine showing alerting of the EEG with little further change in the blood pressure.

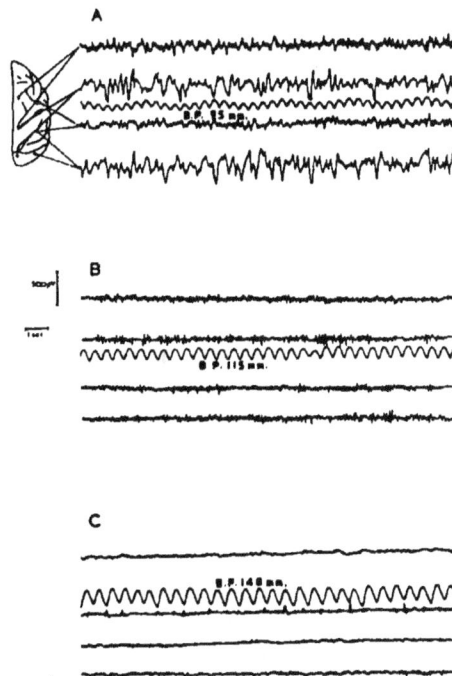

Fig. 19: Records from an acute experiment (encéphale isolé monkey preparation) in which LSD-25 was given first and followed by r-amphetamine.
A: control record with the preparation "sleeping";
B: three minutes after 20 g/kg of LSD-25 had been injected intravenously; C: one minute after the subsequent injection of 1.5 mg/kg of r-amphetamine sulphate intravenously.

cord being sectioned first. In these, too, amphetamine was found to have no effect on electrical activity or behaviour, although doses as high as 50 mg/kg were used.

(ii) *LSD-25*. This drug was used in two experiments in *encéphale isolé* (cat) preparations, and in two experiments in *cerveau isolé* (cat) preparations. No effects on either electrical activity or behaviour were observed in these experiments, despite high doses (up to 300 μg/kg). In the two *encéphale isolé* preparations the administration of LSD-25 (Fig. 17B) was followed by an injection of amphetamine (1.0 mg/kg). An alerting of electrical activity (Fig. 17C) and of behaviour was obtained, following this drug.

In the three experiments in which monkey *encéphale isolé* preparations were used, LSD-25 was found to exert some effect on electrical activity. The monkey preparation was characterized by slow and intermittent rhythmic activity (Figs. 7C and 19A) rather than by the spindle activity seen in the cat. Following LSD-25, given intravenously in doses of 20 to 30 μg/kg, this activity was replaced by bursts of rhythmic activity at a frequency of 7 to 8 c/s, waxing and waning in amplitude (Fig. 19B). This change could be interpreted as a partial alerting of cortical activity, but no change in behaviour was noted. In one of our experiments, 1.5 mg/kg of amphetamine was given subsequently. All rhythmic activity was then abolished (Fig. 19C).

DISCUSSION

The above experiments, the results of which are summarized in Table 2 allow a preliminary grouping of the effects of the drugs investigated and some tentative conclusions as to their likely mode of action. It wilt have been observed that the correlation between the effects on electrical activity of the brain and on behaviour was closer in the case of some drugs than in others. This serves to emphasize the need for recording electrical activity simultaneously with behaviour, and hence, for studying wherever possible, the effects of drugs in suitable chronic, as well as in acute preparations.

In the conscious animal amphetamine produced low voltage fast electrical activity, and excitement (Bradley and Elkes 1953a). This is in agreement with the observations of Shallek and Walz (1953) who noted that *d*-amphetamine, given to unanaesthetized dogs, caused an increase in motor activity and an increase in the frequency of the EEG. The effects of LSD-25 were somewhat similar. In our experiments this drug brought about behavioural alerting of the conscious animal, and a corresponding change in the electrical activity. Unlike amphetamine, however, the extent of these changes varied with the precise experimental conditions, the animal under LSD-25 being strikingly susceptible to environment, and to slight changes in it.

Physostigmine produced an electrical pattern similar to that seen in the alert state; but here (provided small doses were used) no corresponding change in behaviour could be observed. Atropine and *l*-hyoscyamine produced rhythms similar to those seen in sleep. In no case, however, were sleep or drowsiness noted, and occasionally atropine led to excitement. This dissociation between behaviour and electrical activity following atropine was first pointed out by Wikler (1952) who recorded "sleep patterns" in unanaesthetized dogs showing excitement after the administration of the drug. Funderburk and Case (1951) reported corresponding changes in the curarized cat preparation. They were, however, unable to determine whether the slow waves they observed were due to normal sleep, or the effects of atropine. More recently Rinaldi and Himwich (1955a) working with. the curarized rabbit preparation and using atropine and an anticholinesterase (DFP) have reported similar effects on electrical activity. Again, however, the experimental conditions precluded observation of behaviour.

TABLE 2

Conscious animal			Electrical activity of encéphale isolé	Electrical activity of cerveau isolé
Drug	Behavior	Electrical activity		
Physostigmine	normal	fast, low amplitude activity	fast, low amplitude activity	fast, low amplitude activity
Atropine or l-hyoscyamine	normal or excited	slow waves and spindles	slow waves and spindles	slow waves and spindles
Amphetamine	excited	fast, low amplitude activity	fast,, low amplitude activity	no effect
LSD-25	excited	fast, low amplitude activity	no effect	no effect

Neostigmine in our experiments. did not have any effect on electrical activity even in relatively high doses. *l*-Hyoscyamine caused effects similar to atropine, while *d*-hyoscyamine was ineffective. The lack effect of neostigmine is in agreement with its lack of effect in the cord (Schweitzer, Stedman and Wright 1939), although, using this, Bremer and Chatonnet (1949) noted a reduction in voltage and in frequency in the electrocorticogram of the *encéphale isolé* preparation.

The drugs used in our experiments thus fall into two distinct groups those which affected activity and behaviour in the same way (the amphetamines and LSD-25) and those which produced effects on electrical activity which did not result in a corresponding change in behaviour (physostigmine, atropine and *l*-hyoscyamine). Furthermore, wherever combinations of drugs from these two groups were employed, the behavioural effects appeared to be dominated by members of the first group (amphetamine and LSD-25) and the electrical effects by members of the second (physostigmine, atropine and *l*-hyoscyamine). Thus, for example, when atropine was given following *r*-amphetamine, the animals remained excited and hyperactive, but the slow wave activity attributable to atropine invariable appeared; nor could this activity be abolished by amphetamine if the order of the drugs was reversed, despite the fact that amphetamine still produced its characteristic effects on behaviour.

The acute preparations allowed only very limited observations of behavioural change. Within these limits, however, the distinction between the two groups of drugs was maintained. When amphetamine was administered intravenously to the *encéphale isolé* preparation, both behavioural and electrical alerting could be observed. Physostigmine, atropine and *l*-hyoscyamine on the other hand, produced their characteristic electrical effects without behavioural change, and here, too, dose level was found to be important. A small dose of physostigmine would produce a change in electrical activity without a change in behaviour. A larger dose did produce behavioural alerting, which, however, was always accompanied by some peripheral signs, such as salivation. The predominance of the behavioural effects of amphetamine and the electrical effects of atropine could still be seen in the *encéphale* preparation, since, when amphetamine was administered first, and followed by atropine, the preparation remained behaviourally alert, but the electrical activity showed the slow waves usually associated with atropine.

The *encéphale isolé* served one further purpose. By recording blood pressure simultaneously with electrical activity, it could be shown that the central effects of the drugs studied were not related to changes in systemic blood pressure. Thus, although *r*-amphetamine caused a rise in blood pressure, this effect could be produced with a dose much smaller than that required to cause alerting. Similarly, the slow activity induced by atropine did not depend on the fall of blood pressure sometimes seen in these experiments, since the blood pressure level could be restored, or even raised above its original level, by an infusion of *nor*-adrenaline without affecting the electrical pattern in any way. These observations, however, have no bearing on a possible effect of the drugs on local cerebral vascular tone and on local cerebral circulation. The possibility of such effects must be very clearly borne in mind.

In the *cerveau isolé* preparation similar effects on electrical activity were observed with physostigmine, atropine and *l*-hyoscyamine; here, too, the effects could not be related to blood pressure changes, which were recorded in all the later experiments.

The distinction between the two groups of drugs is still further emphasized by a new and different factor, namely, the effect of the plane of section on the response of the electrical activity to the drug under investigation. Thus, physostigmine, atropine and *l*-hyoscyamine still produced their characteristic effects on the electrical activity irrespective of whether the brain was transected at the level of the spinal cord (*encéphale isolé*) or at the level of the superior colliculus (cerveau isolé). These drugs also affected the barbitone anaesthetized preparation. On the other hand, amphetamine, while exerting an effect on the intact animal and on the *encéphale isolé,* had no effect on the *cerveau isolé*; and in the cat, LSD-25 exerted no effect on either of the acute preparations (fig. 20). It did, however, affect the activity seen in barbiturate anaesthesia.

These results, together with the recent studies of Rinaldi and Himwich (1955a), confirm our previous findings (Bradley and Elkes 1953a and b). They also extend these findings to other species. Our own experiments included six monkeys. Rinaldi and Himwich studied the effect of drugs on spontaneous and evoked activity in the curarized rabbit. They observed that DFP led to persistent low voltage fast activity, whereas atropine "evoked an EEG pattern of sleep," and "inhibited all alerting reactions produced by physiological stimuli and the direct stimulation of the mid-brain reticular substance." They also noted that the alerting of the electrocorticogram by DFP was not prevented by transection of the mid-brain. These authors observed a transitory alerting of electrical activity following intracarotid injections of small amounts (0.5-15 µg.) of acetylcholine in both the intact curarized rabbit, and following mesencephalic section. This is in keeping with the observations of Bonnet and Bremer (1937) who used the *encéphale isolé* preparation, and with our own observations on the *encéphale isolé, cerveau isolé*, and the barbiturate anaesthetized preparation (Bradley 1953).

The similarities between DFP and physostigmine suggest that their effects may be due to their anticholinesterase activity, and therefore to an endogenous accumulation of acetylcholine, or a related ester. The effects of atropine and *l*-hyoscyamine may similarly be due to a blockade of cholinergic receptors. There are, however, two differences between the central and the peripheral effects of these drugs. Firstly, the mutual antagonism in central action between physostigmine and atropine or. hyoscyamine is maintained despite relatively high doses of either; secondly, whereas the doses of physostigmine required to produce effects on the electrocorticogram are smaller than those which produce peripheral effects, those of atropine an *l*-hyoscyamine are considerably higher. Despite these differences it seems probable that the central effects of these drugs involve a cholinergic pathway within the central nervous system (Feldberg 1951). Since the effects of these drugs could still be observed after mesencephalic section, it seems unlikely that these receptors are localised below the level of

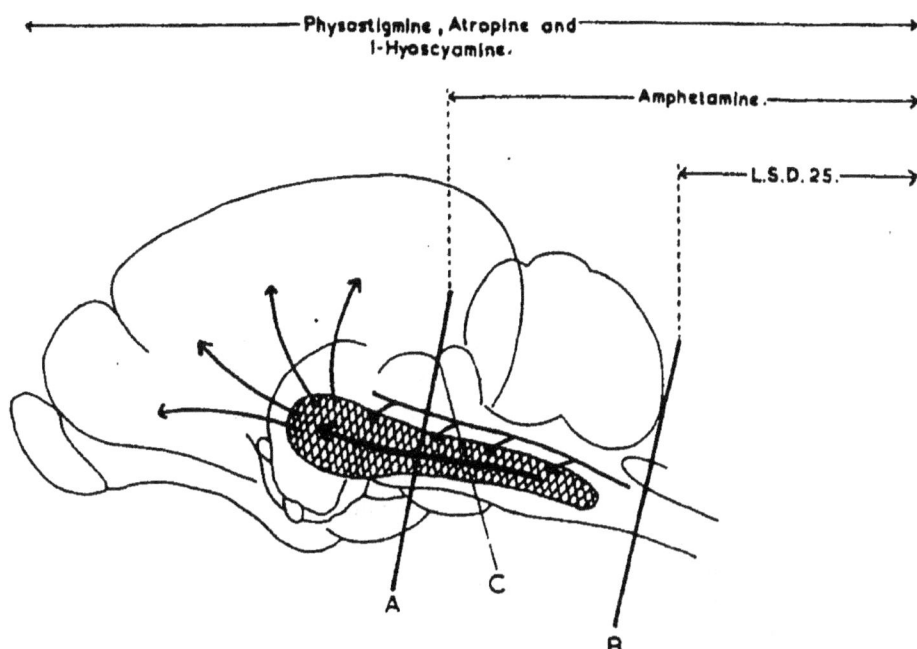

Fig. 20. Diagram through the medial sagittal plane of the cat brain (after Stark, Taylor and Magoun 1951b), showing the reticular activating system of the brainstem (cross-hatched) its afferent collaterals from the sensory pathways and ascending influence on the diencephalon and cortex. A: indicates the plane of transection of the mid-brain for the cerveau isolé and B: the level of section of the spinal cord for the encéphale isolé. C: is the plane which was found by Bonvallet et al. (1954) to be critical for the arousal produced by adrenaline. The susceptibility of the various preparations to the drugs mentioned in the text is indicated.

the section. Equally, the lack of correlation between the effects on electrical activity and behavioural effects in the conscious animal suggests that a cholinergic mechanism is unlikely to be dominant in the mechanisms concerned with wakefulness and arousal.

On the other hand, the effects of amphetamine which produced both the behavioural and electrical signs of arousal, were susceptible to mesencephalic section. The work of Moruzzi and Magoun (1949), Lindsley et al. (1949, 1950) and Starzl et al. (1951a,b) has defined the role played by the reticular formation and tegmentum of the lower brain-stem in the electrical and behavioural arousal response, and the maintenance of wakefulness. As is well known, in their hands, electrical stimulation of this region produced the electrocortical signs of arousal (Moruzzi and Magoun 1949). Lindsley et al. (1949, 1950) noted that acute lesions in this region blocked the effects of stimulation, whilst chronic lesions in the same area led to somnolence and to slow waves in the EEG which could be only transitorily blocked by afferent stimuli. The work of Starzl et al. (1951a,b) has suggested that the activity in this region is maintained by impulses reaching it by way of medical collaterals from the main sensory pathways. When relating our own findings with amphetamine to those of Magoun, Moruzzi et al. (fig. 20), two aspects seemed of interest. First, the behavioural arousal following amphetamine was, like the one following stimulation of the reticular activating system, accompanied by desynchronization of the electrocortical activity; and second, the behavioural and electrical effects of the drugs were apparently dependent on intact mesencephalic connections. This led to the suggestion that the effect of this drug might be exerted on receptors related to, or possibly located in, the brain-stem reticular activating system (Bradley and Elkes 1953a). The recent results of Hiebel et al. (1954) are in keeping with this suggestion. They studied the effect of *d*-amphetamine in curarized preparations subjected to lesions at various levels, and found the critical level of section for this drug was somewhat higher than our own. However, in these experiments the electrocortical activation produced by the drug, rather than the behavioural effect, served as criteria of arousal.

The alerting effect of LSD-25 in the cat was lost following section of the spinal cord at the level of the first cervical vertebra. On the other hand, in the monkey it could still be seen following high spinal section, though this was not as marked as the alerting seen following amphetamine. Unfortunately, it was not possible to determine whether a higher level of section would abolish this effect in the monkey. LSD-25, however, had no effect on the *cerveau isolé* preparation in the cat.

In the conscious cat the degree of alerting obtained with LSD-25 was rather variable and seemed to be dependent on slight variations in the environment. Thus, for example, in early experiments where the animal was placed in the constant environment chamber and housed in the open laboratory, almost complete alerting of the electrical activity was regularly obtained. Here, some noise must have got through the walls and the openings of the box. When in later experiments, the constant environment box was placed in a rigorously sound-proofed room, the degree of alerting of electrical activity was strikingly reduced and some rhythmic activity at 4-6 c/s could be seen in many experiments. Similarly, in one of the *encéphale isolé* experiments in the monkey in which a small portion of the spinal cord had escaped section, more complete alerting was observed than in those experiments where the transection was complete. The alerting produced by amphetamine on the other hand was seen regularly, appeared independent of environment, and depended on dosage only. The effects of *r*-amphetamine in producing an increase in the cortical response to rhythmic photic stimulation in the conscious animal may be related to its alerting effects.

It would thus seem possible that whereas amphetamine may affect some element in the reticular activating system directly, the effects of LSD-25 may be exerted on other elements more closely related to the inflow of medial collaterals from the great afferent pathways. The activation of the symptoms of LSD-25 intoxication by sensory stimulation (Bradley, Elkes and Elkes 1953) and the sequence of development of symptoms observed in typical LSD-25 intoxication, where sensorium and body image arc affected well before motor involvement, are in keeping with this view.

The experiments outlined above suggest the existence of two or possibly three types of receptors within the central nervous system. One is almost certainly cholinergic in nature and its activation or blockade leads to effects on electrical activity which, in the conscious animal, are not necessarily related to behaviour. Rinaldi and Himwich (1955b) concluded that the alerting of electrical activity obtained with DFP and acetylcholine was due to an action on the reticular activating system at the mesencephalic level, and that atropine was a "specific depressant of that system." This was suggested to them by the fact that the slow, atropine-induced electrical activity could not be abolished by sensory stimulation, or stimulation of the mid-brain reticular activating system. In our experiments in the conscious animal receiving atropine, not only was behaviour unaffected, but sensory stimulation produced a normal behavioural response despite persistent high voltage slow, activity. It is therefore difficult to accept the view that the reticular activating system is preponderantly cholinergic in nature, though a cholinergic element may well be represented in that area, and is almost certainly dominant in the pathways leading rostrally from the reticular formation towards the cortex. It may in fact be that the diffuse thalamic projection system (Jasper 1953) may hold such an element, and that it is the effect on these receptors which produces effects on electrical activity without necessarily producing changes in behaviour. Equally, as mentioned above, cholinergic receptors may well be important in regulating local cerebral vascular tone.

The non-cholinergic receptors susceptible to amphetamine may be situated at a fairly high level of the brain-stem reticular formation. The recent work of Bonvallet, Dell and Hiebel (1954) stressing the importance of adrenaline in the function of facilitatory and inhibitory mechanisms would certainly be in keeping with the suggestion. Both *nor*-adrenaline and adrenaline have recently been identified in the upper brain-stem (Vogt 1954). The central action of amphetamine may be due to an action on receptors in this area, though the precise relation to the peripheral sympathomimetic action of the drug must remain an open question.

LSD-25 may act on receptors at the mesencephalic and diencephalic levels specially related to the medial collaterals of the great afferent pathways. The presence of serotonin in the brain (Amin Crawford and Gaddum 1954), the chemical relationship between LSD-25 and serotonin (Woolley and Shaw 1954) and the antagonism between LSD-25 and serotonin (Gaddum 1953), make the existence of receptors for tryptamine derivatives in the central nervous system likely. It is however difficult in the light of recent evidence (Cerletti and Rothlin 1955, Bradley and Hance 1956) to accept the view that the effect of LSD-25 is due solely to its serotonin antagonism.

Perhaps rather than thinking in unitary terms, it may at this stage, be advisable to think in terms of the possible selection by chemical evolution of small families of closely related compounds, which by mutual interplay would govern the phenomena of excitation and inhibition in the central nervous system. Acetylcholine, nor-adrenaline and 5-hydroxytryptamine may be parent molecules of this kind; but one has only to compare the effects of acetylcholine with succinylcholine, or *nor*-adrenaline with its methylated congener to realize how profound the effects of even slight changes of molecular configuration can be. The astonishing use which chemical evolution has made of the steroids is but another example of the same economy. It is likely that neurones possessing slight but definite differences in enzyme constitution may be differentially susceptible to neurohumoral agents. Such neurones may be unevenly distributed in topographically close, or widely separated areas in the central nervous system, these differences probably extending to the finest level of histological organisation. Phylogenetically older parts, and perhaps, more particularly, the mid-line regions and the periventricular nuclei may, in terms of cell population and chemical constitution be significantly different from parts characteristic of late development.

As yet little information is available of the chemistry of the mosaic of cells, and cell groups making up the so-called reticular activating system. The neurones of this system, which is really a system of systems, bear a somewhat special and reciprocal relation to the afferent pathways which impinge upon them by way of collaterals. They are activated by these, but equally, through their activity, determine the ultimate perception of the signal arriving at the cortex by way of the sense-linked pathways (French, Verzeano and Magoun 1953, Arduini and Arduini 1954). The translation of afferent signals into perception may well depend on the interaction of cortical and reticular elements, and may have its neural counterpart in the three dimensional apposition, and patterning of excitatory and inhibitory states in a very large cell population. The reticular formations are distinctive for the diffuseness of their connections and of their effects. Equally, in this dense reticular field self-excitatory phenomena may predominate (Fessard 1953) and the powerful operation of vectorial and spatial influences is likely. Slight variation in local titre of a neurohumoral agent in these key mid-line areas may thus profoundly affect the excitability of large neurone pools at a distance. It would perhaps be permissible to speak of the operation of chemical fields in these regions, which would depend on the rate of liberation, diffusion and destruction of locally produced neurohumoral agents. The agents in question may be either identical with or, more likely, derived from neuro-effector substances familiar to us at the periphery. Their number is probably small, but their influence upon integrative action of higher nervous activity may be profound. The basic states of consciousness may well be determined by variations in the local concentration of these agents.

The suggestion of the existence of three types of receptors within the brain must be regarded as but a first crude approximation in a study in which cytochemistry, pharmacology and electrophysiology are mutually complementary and interdependent. The recent refinement of cytochemical and microchemical techniques (Lowry et al. 1954, Hydén 1955, and Pope 1955); of micro-electrode techniques within the central nervous system (Moruzzi 1953); the development of methods for studying changes in local cerebral circulation (Kety 1954); the growing number of data on the effects of punctuate lesions, and of local electrical stimulation of selected areas on animal behaviour patterns; the ever-increasing range of natural and synthetic compounds exerting selective effects on higher mental function, form an inviting field for such combined studies. The pharmacology of behaviour must, of necessity, draw from each of these fields.

Advances in knowledge, though by no means solely dependent on methods are often inseparably linked with them; and present-day methods are well advanced.

SUMMARY

(1) The effect of various drugs on the electrical activity of the brain has been studied in the conscious animal carrying permanently implanted electrodes, in acute preparations sectioned at high spinal or mid-brain level (*encéphale* and *cerveau isolé* respectively), and in the barbitone anaesthetized preparation.

(2) The importance of studying the effects of drugs in conscious chronic preparations (in which changes in electrical activity can be observed simultaneously with behaviour) is emphasized.

(3) In the conscious animal, atropine and physostigmine caused dissociation between electrical activity and behaviour. Atropine induced slow wave activity. This was similar to that seen in sleep; sleep, however, was never observed. Physostigmine led to an electrical pattern similar to that seen in the alert state, without a corresponding alerting of behaviour. The two drugs were mutually antagonistic.

(4) *l*-Hyoscyamine produced effects similar to those of atropine. *d*-Hyoscyamine and neostigmine were ineffective, except when the latter drug was given in high enough doses to induce peripheral symptoms.

(5) Amphetamine and LSD-25 in the conscious animal led to an alerting of the EEG, and behavioural excitement, there being, in the case of these two drugs, close correlation between

electrical activity and behaviour. The effects of amphetamine were independent of the environment, and depended on dosage only. The effects of LSD-25 depended on factors in the environment, as well as upon the dosage.

(6) In the acute preparations the effects of atropine were similar to those seen in the conscious animal, and were still present when either the upper spinal cord, or mid-brain were transected. Amphetamine caused alerting both of behaviour and electrical activity in the *encéphale isolé*, but had no effect on the *cerveau isolé*. LSD-25 had no effect on either of these preparations in the cat, but ha d some effect on the *encéphale isolé* preparation in the monkey.

(7) Atropine, physostigmine and LSD-25 modified the electrocortical patterns seen under barbitone anaesthesia. Amphetamine had no effect on barbitone induced activity. The depth of anaesthesia remained apparently unaffected by these drugs.

(8) None of the effects described could be correlated either with changes in respiration, or changes in systemic blood pressure.

(9) The grouping of the drugs in relation to their effects on electrical activity and on behaviour in the conscious animal and levels of section in acute experiment, is discussed. An attempt has been made to relate the findings to the known distribution of the reticular- activating system, and the physiology of the brain-stem. It is suggested that three types of receptors are present in the brain. The receptors for LSD-25 may be specially related to the medial collaterals of the great afferent pathways.

(10) The possible operation of chemical fields within selected areas of the brain is discussed.

REFERENCES

Adrian, E. D., and Matthews, B. H. C. (1934) J. Physiol. 81, 440.
Amassian, V. E. (1952) Res. Publ. Ass. Nerv. Ment. Dis. (1950), 30, 371.
Amin, A. H., Crawford, T. B. B., and Gaddum, J. H. (1954) J. Physiol. 126, 596.
Arduini, A., and Arduini, M. G. (1954) J. Pharmacol. 110, 76.
Beckett, S., and Gellhorn, E. (1948) Amer. J. Physiol. 153, 113.
Berger, H. (1933) Arch. psychiat. Nervenkr. 101, 452.
Bonnet, V., and Bremer, F. (1937) C. R. Soc. Biol. Paris, 126, 1271.
Bonvallet, M., Dell, P., and Hiebel, G. (1954) Electroenceph. Clin. Neurophysiol., 6, 119.
Bradley P. B. (1952) Ph.D. Thesis, Birmingham University.
Bradley P. B. (1953) Electroenceph. Clin. Neurophysiol., Supplement III, 21.
Bradley P. B., Elkes, C., and Elkes, J. (1953) J. Physiol., 121, 50 p.
Bradley P. B., and Elkes J. (1953a) J. Physiol. 120, 13 p.
Bradley P. B., and Elkes J. (1953b) J. Physiol. 120, 14 p.
Bradley P. B., and Elkes J. (1953c) Electroenceph. Clin. Neurophysiol. 5, 451.
Bradley P. B., and Hance, A. J. (1956) J. Physiol. 132, 50p.
Bremer, F. (1935) C. R. Soc. Biol., Paris, 118, 1235.
Bremer, F. (1936) C. R. Soc. Biol., Paris, 122, 460.
Bremer, F., and Chatonnet, J. (1949) Arch. Int. Physiol. 57, 106.
Brenner, C., and Merritt, H. H. (1942) Arch. Neurol. Pyschiat. Chicago, 48, 382.
Cerletti, A., and Rothlin, E. (1955) Nature, London, 176, 785.
Chatfield, P. O., and Dempsey, E. W. (1942) Amer. J. Physiol. 135, 633.
Cooke, P. M., and Sherwood, S. L. (1954) Electroenceph. Clin. Neurophysiol. 6, 425.
Delay, J., Lhermitte, F., Verdeaux, G., and Verdeaux, J. (1952) Rev. Neurol. 86, 81.
Essig, C. F., Adkins, F. J., and Barnard, G. L. (1953) Proc. Soc. Exp. Biol. N. Y., 82, 551.
Feldberg, W. (1951) Arch. Int. Physiol. 59, 544.
Feldberg, W., and Sherwood, S. L. (1953) J. Physiol. 120, 3 p.
Feldberg, W., and Sherwood, S. L. (1954) J. Physiol. 123, 148.

Fessard, A. E. (1953) In: Council for International Organizations of Medical Sciences. Brain Mechanisms and Consciousness, Oxford.

Forster, F. M. (1945) Arch. Neurol. Psychiat., Chicago, 54, 391.

Forster, F. M., Borkowski, W. J., and Mccarter, R. H. (1946) J. Neuropath. 5, 364.

Forster, F. M., and Mccarter, R. H. (1945) Amer. J. Physiol. 144, 168.

Freedman, A. M., Bales, P. D., Willis, A., and Himwich, H. E. (1949) Amer. J. Physiol. 156, 117.

French, J. D., Verzeano, M., and Magoun, H. W. (1953) Arch. Neurol. Psychiat., Chicago, 69, 505.

Funderburk, W. H., and Case, T. J. (1951) Electroenceph. Clin. Neurophysiol. 3, 213.

Gaddum, J. H. (1953) J. Physiol. 121, 15p.

Gerard, R. W., and Libet, B. (1940) Amer. J. Psychiat. 96, 1125.

Gibbs, F. A., Gibbs, E. L., and Lennox, W. G. (1937) Arch. Intern. Med. 60, 154.

Grinker, R. R., and Serota, H. (1938) J. Neurophysiol. 1, 573.

Hampson, J. L., Essig, C. F., Mccauley, A., and Himwich, H. E. (1950) Electroenceph. Clin. Neurophysiol. 2, 41.

Hess, R. Jr., Koella, W. P., and Akert, K. (1953) Electroenceph. Clin. Neurophysiol. 5, 75.

Hiebel, G., Bonvallet, M., Huvé, P., and Dell, P. (1954) Sem. Hop. Paris, 30, 1880.

Hyde, J., Beckett, S., and Gellhorn, E. (1949) J. Neurophysiol. 12, 17.

Hydén, H. (1955) In: Waelsch's Biochemistry of the Developing Nervous System. New York, p. 358.

Jasper, H. H. (1953) In: Council for International Organizations of Medical Sciences. Brain Mechanisms and Consciousness. Oxford.

Kety, S. S. (1954) Josiah Macy, Jr., Foundation. Trans. First Conference on Neuropharmacology. New York, p. 13.

Lindsley, D. B., Bowden, J. W., and Magoun, H. W. (1949) Electroenceph. Clin. Neurophysiol. 1, 415.

Lindsley, D. B., Schreiner, L. H., Knowles, W. H., and Magoun, H. W. (1950) Electroenceph. Clin. Neurophysiol. 2, 483.

Lowry, O. H., Roberts, N. R., Wu, M. L., Hixon, W. S., and Crawford, E. J. (1954) J. Biol. Chem., 207, 19.

Miller, F. R., Stavraky, G. W., and Woonton, G. A. (1940) J. Neurophysiol. 3, 131.

Moruzzi, G. (1953) In: Council for International Organizations of Medical Sciences. Brain Mechanisms and Consciousness. Oxford.

Moruzzi, G. and Magoun, H. W. (1949) Electroenceph. Clin. Neurophysiol. 1, 455.

Pope, A. (1955) J. Neuropath. 14, 39.

Rheinberger, M. B., and Jasper, H. H. (1931) Amer. J. Physiol. 119, 186.

Rinaldi, F., and Himwich, H. E. (1955a) Arch. Neurol. Psychiat., Chicago, 73, 387.

Rinaldi, F., and Himwich, H. E. (1955b) Arch. Neurol. Psychiat., Chicago, 73, 396.

Schaller, W., and Walz, D. (1953) Proc. Soc. Exp. Biol. N. Y. 82, 715.

Schweitzer, A., Stedman, E., and Wright, S. (1939) J. Physiol. 96, 302.

Starzl, T. E., and Magoun, H. W. (1951a) J. Neurophysiol. 14, 133.

Taylor, C. W., and Magoun, H. W. (1951b) J. Neurophysiol. 14, 479.

Toman, J. E. P., and Davis, J. P. (1949) Pharmacol. Rev. 1, 425.

Tower, D. B., and Elliott, K. A. C. (1952) J. Appl. Physiol. 4, 669.

Vogt, M. (1954) J. Physiol. 123, 451.

Wikler, A. (1952) Proc. Soc. Exp. Biol. N. Y., 79, 261.

Woolley, D. W., and Shaw, E. (1954) Science, 119, 587.

PAPER 11

DRUG EFFECTS IN RELATION TO RECEPTOR SPECIFICITY WITHIN THE BRAIN: SOME EVIDENCE AND PROVISIONAL FORMULATION

J. Elkes

Reprinted with the kind permission of John Wiley & Sons from Ciba Foundation Symposium on the Neurological Basis of Behavior (pp. 303-332). London, Butterworth, 1958

> *"The body of a worm and the face of a man alike have to be taken as chemical responses. The alchemist dreamed of old that is might be so. The dream, however, supposed a magic chemistry. There they were wrong. The chemistry is plain everyday chemistry. But it is complex. Further, the chemical brew in preparation for it time has been stirring unceasingly throughout some millions of years in the service of a final cause. The brew is a selected brew." (Sherrington 1951)*

Thus in a way all his own, Charles Sherrington expresses his adherence to selectivity, specificity and evolution in biochemical process. At a time when the chemical brew in being so vigorously stirred in a thousand pots, holding high promise to many, yet threatening the very flavour and tang of life itself, it is difficult to escape two simple conclusions. First, that chemicals of the most diverse structure can and do affect the "brew" of the brain, and its mental and behavioral attributes and second, that they do so in strangely ordered and specific ways. To be sure, we cannot at yet speak of a science psychotropic agents. A Linnéan natural history of their properties must precede the beginnings of such a science. Nevertheless, with mounting experience, the phenomena are beginning to group themselves, and the first silhouette of a classification is emerging. The symptoms, for example, of mescaline and lysergic acid diethylamide (LSD-25) intoxication, of morphine addiction, and withdrawal, the changes induced by amphetamine, chlorpromazine or reserpine in man have sequence, rank, order and pattern; they are sensitive to dose, to precise environmental conditions, to potentiation or attenuation by each other. They exhibit both overlap and polarity. In sum, the number of variables affected seems finite, and suggests finite ways by which a particular molecular configuration loosens, imbalances and disturbs ordered and integrated process within the central nervous system. It is already evident that specificity is high, and one is tempted to speculate as to the precise functional or morphological level at which this biochemical specificity operates. Here the questions abound, but they are important questions for upon their definition will depend the precise fashioning of a particular experimental approach. Thus, for example, one may justifiably ask whether factors of access to the brain play a part in the action of these drugs. We know as yet little of the statistical, physicochemical equilibrium, misleadingly named the blood-brain barrier, which regulates the selective interchange between the central nervous system and its environment, or, for the matter, of the factors affecting intracerebral small vessel tone. Again, it is possible to conceive of highly specific effects on a particular metabolic pathway within the energy economy of neuronal or non-neuronal elements. We know that metabolic gradients exist in the brain. Metabolism, too, must be clearly borne in mind; as the effects of lithium (Schou 1957) sharply remind one. But the aspect which, it is proposed to consider below is the relationship of the psychotropic effects of some drugs to the possible existence and function of neurohumoral transmitter substances within the central nervous system. This choice is deliberate, and is made for several reasons. First, a good deal is known of such transmission at peripheral neuro-effector sites, and, used with due caution, these sites may provide useful reference points for the study of the very different central phenomena. Secondly, two neurohumoral substances (acetylcholine and noradrenaline: Feldberg 1945, Vogt 1954), have been identified in the brain, and others, much less defined in their general or local properties (5-hydroxytryptamine [5-HT]: Amin, Crawford and Gaddum 1954) and γ-aminobutyric acid (Bazemore, Elliott and Florey 1956) are coming to light. Thirdly, some drugs (e.g. mescaline and LSD-25) possessing marked psychotropic effects are chemically related to substances present. in the brain. These, however, are exceptions and anyone who has followed the recent lively controversies on the possible relationship of adrenochrome and adrenolutin to naturally occurring catecholamines (Rinkel 1956), or the lack of correlation between anti-5-HT and psychotropic effects in the LSD-series (Rothlin 1957) must be puzzled by the equivocal character of the findings to date. Here the discrepancies and contradictions are the most interesting by far, and invite, and indeed compel, further study.

It is, therefore, proposed to begin with a brief statement of the properties of neurohumoral transmitter substances within the central nervous system; to consider the effects of some drugs, chosen for their possible relation to such substances, on the behavior and the electrical activity of the brain in the. conscious unrestrained animal; to examine some evidence from acute experiments bearing upon the findings obtained in the conscious preparation; and to consider finally the effects of some psychotropic drugs on other highly patterned nervous mechanisms not related to overall behavior, but sharing with them a suggestive susceptibility to these agents. A reflex within, and one outside the central nervous system (the carotid sinus reflex and peristaltic reflex, respectively) will be chosen as examples here. The studies have, in most part, been previously reported {Elkes 1953, 1957; Elkes, Elkes and Bradley 1951; Elkes and Todrick 1955; Ginzel 1955, 1957; Bayliss and Todrick 1955; Bradley and Elkes 1957; Bradley and Key 1956; Bradley and Hance 1957) and are based upon the work of my colleagues P.B. Bradley, K.H. Ginzel, A. Todrick, A.J. Hance and B.J. Key. To them my gratitude is due.

NEUROHUMORAL TRANSMISSION WITHIN THE CENTRAL NERVOUS SYSTEM

The subject has been admirably reviewed by Feldberg (1951), but continues to be fluid and controversial. It would be well to agree upon four minimal desiderata for a substance claiming a transmitter role within the central nervous system. First, the agent should be identifiable in the central nervous system and should vary in concentration with the precise functional state of the tissue. Second, enzymes both for the synthesis and the destruction of the substance to, should be present in those areas of the central nervous where the substance is found. Third, these enzymes should be susceptible to specific inhibition, and the effects of such inhibition should be clearly discernible both in chemical and in functional terms. Fourth, the effects of the application of the hypothetical agent to the central nervous system, either topically or by a selected vascular route, should be early, demonstrable in terms of an effect on function.

In surveying the claims of the substances so far identified in the central nervous system, some of the above desiderata are met only with very important reservations, and some not at all. The gaps are widest in the case of the substances most recently discovered. Thus, for example, it is well known that acetylcholine is present in the central nervous system. Its concentration in the brain is higher in sleep (Richter and Crossland 1949) and in anaesthesia (Tobias, Lipton and Lepinat 1946) than in wakefulness (Richter and Crossland 1949, Wajda 1951). It shows a phasic variation in content following electrical stimulation (Richter and Crossland 1949). Its precise state (whether "bound" or "free") has been implicated in the genesis of epileptogenic discharge (Tower and Elliott 1902). Nevertheless, the enzyme system for acetylcholine shows a curiously uneven distribution within the central nervous system (Feldberg and Vogt 1948) and in development. Although in the assay of acetylcholine synthesis one may well not be dealing with a single enzyme, but rather with a complex enzyme system, and an uneven distribution of cofactors may thus account for differences in net yield in *in vitro* experiments, there is good evidence for regional differences between acetylcholine-synthesizing power in different area of the central nervous system. The low synthesizing power in some parts may he as significant as the high synthesizing power in others. Our knowledge of choline acetylase is incomplete. More particularly, we know little of its precise relationship to cell population, and especially to non-neuronal elements. This may be very relevant when viewed against data on other enzymes governing the turnover of acetylcholine.

A similar doubt pervades the universal function of the acetylcholine-hydrolysing enzyme. Two enzyme systems, the so-called "specific" acetylcholinesterase and the non-specific ("pseudo") cholinesterase must be clearly distinguished. In the rat brain these enzymes develop at different rates and assume different concentrations in different, regions (Elkes and Todrick 1955). There is little doubt of the autonomous existence of "pseudo" cholinesterase in the adult brain (Ord and Thompson 1952). Similarly the specific susceptibility of these enzymes to specific inhibitors is very real (Bayliss and Todrick 1956). For example, 1:5(4-tri-methylammonium)-phenylpentan-3:1-di-iodine (Wellcome 62C47) will inhibit acetylcholinesterase very specifically, where as ethopropazine methylsulphate (Lysivane) will leave this enzyme almost unaffected, yet be a highly selective inhibitor of the "pseudo" esterase. This specificity will operate in mixtures, and can, therefore, be used for the detection of one enzyme in the presence of excess of another (Bayliss and Todrick 1956). Nevertheless, even high, sustained and irreversible inhibition of the cholinesterases from birth will not materially affect the rate of emergence of automatic innate behavior patterns (the eye opening, body righting, placing and startle reactions) in the rat (Elkes, Eayrs and Todrick 1955). On the other hand, the intracarotid injection of very small doses of a specific "pseudo" esterase inhibitor will desynchronize the corticogram much more than a corresponding, or even higher, dose of a specific inhibitor of acetylcholinesterase (Desmedt and LaGrutta 1955). The above gaps (in terms of four minimal desiderata) therefore seriously question the universal transmitter role of acetylcholine within the central nervous system. An ester other than acetylcholine may well be physiologically present, and the role of the non-;specific enzyme may be much more than the provision of a buffer reserve. As yet, little is known of the precise elements, neuronal or non-neuronal, with which the non-specific enzyme is associated. Glia and small blood vessels may the implicated (Koelle 1952). And it must remain an open question whether enzyme, or its unknown substrate, play part in regulating strictly local conditions (Elkes 1953, Desmedt and LaGrutta 1955). It is, however, likely that the striking differences in enzyme content between widely separated areas may extend to the finest level of histological organization. Cellular elements possessing slight but definite differences in enzyme constitution may have differentially populated various areas and layers in the brain and, by virtue these differences, may meet the functional i.e. excitatory and inhibitory needs of a particular neuronal net.

The evidence concerning possible non-cholinergic transmitters poses even more questions than acetylcholine. Adenosine triphosphate (ATP) has been suggested as playing a part along the sensory pathway (Holton and Holton 1953), and the posterior roots, with low acetylcholine synthetising power, have been studied for presence of a depressor substance, substance P (Lembeck 1953). Equally significant is the discovery of noradrenaline and 5-HT in the brain and differential distribution of these substances in various areas of the brain. Midline structures (the hypothalamus, the area postrema, the mesencephalon, the medial thalamic nuclei) appear to be richer in these agents than other areas (Vogt 1954). Furthermore, hypothalamic and adrenomedullary noradrenaline vary *pari passu* under the influences of such drugs as caffeine, leptazol and ergometrine (Vogt 1954). Also stimulation of discrete areas of the hypothalamus will make the adrenaline medulla yield differential proportions of adrenaline and noradrenaline (Folkow and von Euler 1954). Adrenaline will modulate the response to given doses of acetylcholine in the perfused superior cervical ganglion or the spinal cord (Bülbring 1944, Bülbring and Burn 1941). It exerts an inhibitory effect in a central monosynaptic pathway (Marrazzi 1953). Equally, the intraventricular injection of adrenaline or 5-HT results in striking effects on behaviour (Feldberg and Sherwood 1954). The chemical relationship between mescaline and the catechol amines, between 5-HT and LSD-25 and reserpine, is well known. Equally, there is evidence of the release of 5-HT by reserpine (Pletscher, Shore and Brodie 1955) but, significantly enough, of noradrenaline also (Carlsson et al. 1957).

Despite the above evidence several of the minimal desiderata postulated above remain unfulfilled for noradrenaline and 5-HT. We know relatively little of the precise mechanism of synthesis and destruction of the catechol amines and indoles in the brain; and we know little because, as yet the chemical precision tools (in the shape of the powerful and specific enzyme inhibitor" such as are available for the study of the metabolism of the metabolism of acetylcholine) are not available. The effects of amine oxidase inhibitors such as inproniazid (Brodie 1957) may he helpful in this respect. 5-HT (Gaddum and Giarman 1956) and the administration of the precursor of serotonin, 5-hydroxytryptophan, will lead to striking central symptoms (Udenfriend, Weissbach and Bogdanski 1957) emphasizing the role of *local* manufacture and accumulation within certain areas of the brain. As yet little is known of the storage and release of serotonin in the brain (Brodie 1957) though there are powerful indications that the different proportions of "bound" and "free" 5-HT may be related to different functional states. A similar concept to that applied to acetylcholine (Tower and Elliott 1952) may well be operating here. A further remarkable development in a rapidly moving story is the discovery of the inhibitory properties of γ-aminobutyric acid, quantities of which have been identified in the brain (Bazemore, Elliott and Florey 1956).

Despite their inherent limitations, the above considerations supply useful reference points in a study of drugs known to affect behaviour; and it was thought useful in the first instance to confine these investigations to agents either chemically or functionally related to substances present in the brain. Accordingly, the drugs examined were firstly those whose effect was related either to acetylcholine accumulation, or acetylcholine block (physostigmine, neostigmine, di-*iso*propylfluorophosphate [DFP], atropine, *d*-hyoscyamine, *l*-hyoscyamine); second, those related to catecholamines (*dl*-amphetamine, *d*-amphetamine, *l*-amphetamine and mescaline); third; serotonin and some serotonin antagonists, viz. LSD-25, its 2-brom derivative (BOL 148), and monocthylamide (LAE 32), the pyrolidine derivative (LPD 824), the 1-methyl derivative (MLD 41) and the 1-acetyl derivative (ALD 52); and fourth; a so-called tranquillizing agent, chlorpromazine, and its derivative methopromazine. The order of these groups was intentional since it was felt advisable to clarify the effects of familiar agents first, to establish their interaction, and upon the basis of this information to proceed to an examination of the less familiar.

The areas in which these drugs were studied were essentially two. First, their effect on behaviour in the conscious unrestrained animal preparation, with special reference to the relation between effects on behaviour and effects on the electrical activity of the brain. These studies were subsequently extended in suitable acute preparations, which employed both stimulation and recording. Second, in view of the marked representation of autonomic function within the central nervous system, and the known influence of these drugs on autonomic function, their effect on some central and peripheral autonomic reflexes was also examined. The vasomotor response and the peristaltic reflex were selected as representative examples of these reflexes.

THE EFFECT OF DRUGS ON THE ELECTRICAL ACTIVITY OF THE BRAIN IN THE CONSCIOUS UNRESTRAINED ANIMAL, AND IN SOME ACUTE PREPARATIONS (Bradley and Elkes 1957, Bradley and Hance 1957, Bradley 1958)

To avoid the vitiating effects of anaesthetics, and to make for long-term experiment in the individual conscious unrestrained animal, a technique for the permanent implantation of cortical and subcortical electrodes was developed (Bradley and Elkes 1953). Animals thus prepared could be kept for periods of up to six months and this made possible repeated observation of the effect of drugs on electrical activity as well on behaviour. Observations were carried out in a constant environment chamber (Bradley and Elkes 1958) which, at a later stage, was transferred to a sound-proof room. These conditions, coupled with a thorough familiarity on the part of the experimenter with the individual behaviour pattern of individual animals, were designed to reduce the number of variables operating in a particular experiment on the effects of the pharmacological variable only. The route of injection used was generally the intraperitoneal one, though a series of experiments employing the intraventricular cannula in the conscious preparation (Feldberg and Sherwood 1954) was also carried out. In addition, a number of acute preparations were employed. These included the *encéphale* and *cerveau isolé* (Bremer 1935), and also an *encéphale* preparation where behavioural and electrical arousal thresholds in response to electrical stimulation in the midtegmental region could be measured (Bradley and Key 1956). The advantage of these acute preparations was that drugs could be administered by either intravenous, close arterial (intracarotid) or intraventricular injections; and that both blood pressure and respiration could be controlled in these experiments and their effect on the phenomena noted.

The electrical activity of the brain of the conscious unrestrained animal regularly exhibits the so-called alerting response (Rheinberger and Jasper 1937), characterized by low-voltage, fast activity in all leads when the animal's attention is attracted. In this, as in the so-called slow-wave, "drowsy" activity, there is consistent and striking correspondence between the electrical activity and the behaviour of the animal.

This correspondence between electrical activity and behaviour was lost when certain drugs were employed. Thus, physostigmine in doses of 0.05–0.3 mg/kg intraperitoneally resulted in the appearance of low-amplitude, fast activity in all regions similar to, though perhaps not identical with, that seen in the fully alert animal. There was, however, no corresponding behavioural alerting, the animals remaining quiescent, and even apparently asleep. Neostigmine in doses of 0.2 mg/kg produced little change of the electrical activity. Larger doses led to marked parasympathomimetic effects. The effects of DFP bore a resemblance to those of physostigmine (Bradley, Cerquiglini and Elkes 1953). Atropine, on the other hand, when administered in doses of 1–2 mg/kg resulted in high-voltage, slow activity which in general form was not unlike that seen in deep sleep, though the amplitudes were apt to be larger. The animals, however, remained strikingly awake and in some instances showed overactivity and excitement. The application of an arousal stimulus in these preparations would lead to normal behavioural alerting without producing any change in electrical activity. With lower doses of atropine the slow activity was decreased, less persistent and could still be blocked by sensory stimuli. If, however, the drug (atropine sulphate) in doses of 300 mg was administered by the intraventricular route, a marked changing both the electrical activity and behaviour could be noted. Behaviourally the changes were those described by Feldberg and Sherwood (1954) consisting of increased liveliness, hyperpnoea, together with licking, incontinence and vomiting. The electrical activity was very much that associated with alert behaviour. The route of the drug will thus powerfully affect not only the behavioural pattern produced, but the electrical activity associated with a particular behavioural pattern. *l*-Hyoscyamine produced effects very similar to those of atropine, the dose being roughly one-third that of atropine. *d*-hyoscyamine remained ineffective even in high doses (5–10 mg/kg). When atropine or *l*-hyoscyamine was used in combination with physostigmine, an interaction between these drugs became apparent, irrespective of the order in which these drugs were administered. Thus, for example, if atropine (2 mg/kg) was given first and physostigmine administered subsequently in small divided and cumulative doses the slow activity seen with atropine, though not completely abolished, became less persistent and more responsive to sensory stimuli. The arousal response, however, would only be brief and transient, and was soon supplanted by the slow activity seen with atropine. On the other hand, When physostigmine was administered first, a much larger dose of atropine was required to establish the characteristic slow activity. Neostigmine in combination with atropine and *l*-hyoscyamine exerted no effect on the electrical activity produced by these two drugs. An interaction between barbiturates and physostigmine was also seen. The effects of atropine were in keeping with those observed earlier in the corticogram of the dog (Wikler 1952).

Amphetamine, in doses of 2–5 mg/kg intraperitoneally, regularly led to low-voltage, fast activity in all leads. Unlike the effects with physostigmine and atropine, however, there was; with this drug, a striking and sustained correspondence between electrical activity and behaviour, the animal being easily aroused; restless, exploring and excited. These effects were usually present at six hours after the beginning of the experiment and did not wear off until twenty-four hours afterwards. An enhancement of the response to photic stimulation was also noted. *d*-Amphetamine exerted the same effects as *dl*-amphetamine. *l*-Amphetamine required roughly three times the dose to produce corresponding result when used in combination with a barbiturate, large doses of amphetamine were found to exert little additional effect on the electrical activity of the brain. Equally, premeditation with a full dose of amphetamine (3–5 mg/kg) did not prevent the appearance of slow-wave activity after a dose (2–3 mg/kg) of atropine. Behaviourally, however, the animal remained excited irrespective of the order in which these two drugs were administered. Mescaline produced little effect when given intraperitoneally in doses of 10–15 mg/kg. Larger doses (50 mg/kg) led to vomiting and incontinence and were followed within an hour of administration by a strange passive state in which the electrical activity was dominated by rhythmic waves of 4–6 cyc./sec. from all areas. In this state the animal showed little behavioural or electrical response to sensory stimuli. Handling, however, would transitorily arouse the animals, and during this active period the electrical activity changed to the alert pattern. LSD-25 in doses of less than 15 µg/kg. appeared to have little effect on the electrical activity or behaviour. Doses of between 15–25 µg/kg. produced, both in behavioural and electrical terms, effects similar to those seen with amphet~amine, though, quite often, some low-voltage, rhythmic activity (at about 15 cyc./sec.) was seen. A striking feature of LSD-25, however, was the dependence of the patterns seen on the precise environmental setting of the experiment. Thus, with the constant environment chamber placed in an open laboratory, the effects noted were those just described. If, however the experiments were carried out in a sound-proof room, much more rhythmic activity at a slower rate (4–7 cyc./sec.) was observed. This activity could be blocked by sensory stimuli. Under LSD-25 the animal appeared to be inordinately sensitized to its environment.

LSD-25, injected intraventricularly in doses of 100–200 µg, produced high-amplitude, rhythmic activity at 4–7 cyc./sec. (Bradley and Hance 1956). This was only transitorily blocked by sensory stimuli. Behaviourally, the immediate effects were restlessness, licking, twitching, particularly of the ears. This was later followed by retardation. Serotonin administered intraventricularly in doses of 200–250 µg. produced effects previously described by Feldberg and Sherwood (1954). An intraperitoneal injection of LSD-25 failed to antagonize the effects of serotonin. However, given in combination, these two drugs produced an electrical pattern resembling that seen following LSD-25 alone when given intraventricularly. This effect was independent of the order in which the drugs were administered. BOL 148, a powerful inhibitor of serotonin, led only to mild sedation when given in equipotent doses. Similarly, no effects on the electrical activity characteristic of LSD-25 were observed. The result, therefore, suggested a synergism rather than an antagonism between the effects of LSD-25 and 5-HT.

Thus, when considered in terms of relationship between electrical activity and behaviour, the drugs appeared to fall into two groups. First, those (physostigmine, atropine, *l*-hyoscyamine) which, within the very crude framework of gross behavioural change, showed a lack of correlation between effects on electrical activity and behaviour; and second, those (the amphetamines, LSD-25, mescaline) where the correlation between the effects of electrical activity and behaviour was much closer.

This distinction was born out further by acute experiments in the *encéphale* and *cerveau isolé* preparations, severed respectively at high spinal or mesencephalic level (Bradley and Elkes 1957). As is well known the *encéphale isolé* preparation, which receives afferent impulses from the cranial nerves only, alternates both behaviourally and electrically between periods of drowsiness and alerting. The *cerveau*, on the other hand, is a preparation showing drowsiness or sleep only, and does not respond to afferent stimuli.

When examined in these preparations physostigmine, atropine and *l*-hyoscyamine in doses used in the conscious preparation, and in even higher doses, produced effects which closely resembled those seen in the conscious preparation, there being again marked effects on electrical activity and relatively little on the behaviour of this isolated preparation. Equally, it could be shown by suitable cannulation, and simultaneous recording of blood pressure, that these effects were independent of the slight and transient effect on blood pressure produced by these drugs, though an effect on local cerebral vascular tone cannot be excluded and may, in fact, be very important. The effects of amphetamine, however, although readily reproducible in the *encéphale isolé*, could no longer be obtained in the *cerveau isolé* preparation even when very high doses (20 mg/kg) were used. LSD-25, even in doses of up to 300 µg/kg., produced no effect on the electrical activity and on behaviour of the *encéphale* and *cerveau* preparation in the cat. It did, however, exert some effect on the corresponding preparation in the monkey. This was as marked as the effects of even a small dose (1–5 mg) of amphetamine.

The differences between these two groups of drugs further borne out in experiments in which their interaction with chlorpromazine was studied (Bradley and Hance 1957). Both chlorpromazine and methopromazine (administered in varying and divided doses of up to 4 mg/kg intravenously or up to 20 mg/kg intraperitoneally) in the conscious restrained animal led to striking behavioural changes it effects on the electrical activity. Previously friendly and affectionate animals showed marked indifference to both environment and observer and, on occasion, became slightly aggressive when disturbed. Some ataxia was also noted with the larger doses. The electrical activity reflected the changes in behaviour, the record being usually dominated by regular waves at 5–8 cyc./sec., interspersed by slow waves at 2–4 cyc./sec. Neither behavioural nor electrical arousal response could be elicited in these animals. When given in combination with other drugs it was noted that whereas both the behavioural and EEG effects of amphetamine and LSD-25 (given in full doses) could be blocked by chlorpromazine, the effect of atropine and physostigmine on the electrical activity of the brain persisted in the presence of high doses of chlorpromazine; nor did these drugs modify the characteristic behaviour pattern attributable to chlorpromazine. When used in small doses (0.2–1 mg/kg) in the *encéphale* preparation, chlorpromazine led to a transient blocking, within 30 seconds, of the spindle and slow-wave activity characteristic of the *encéphale isolé*. This effect usually passed within 120 seconds: Larger doses (1.5–4 mg/kg) produced an increase in the slow spindle activity in the preparation and at the same time made it more difficult to rouse. Chlorpromazine had no effect on the *cerveau isolé* preparation other than the effects associated with a fall in blood pressure.

The experiments in which the reticular formation was stimulated, and behavioural and electrocortical arousal thresholds determined, served to extend these findings further (Bradley and Key 1956). Concentric, bipolar, stainless steel electrodes were used in these experiments, the pulses being of square wave form and delivered at a rate of 300 cyc./sec. and applied for ten seconds. The arousal threshold was expressed in volts.

Barbiturates had a marked effect on the EEG electrical and behavioural arousal threshold (Arduini and Arduini 1954) and on behaviour threshold, 2–3 mg/kg of phenobarbitone causing a marked rise of both, whilst 10 mg/kg. blocked arousal responses completely. Chlorpromazine even in large doses (25 mg/kg produced only a slight rise in both thresholds, but very small doses (0.1–0.2 mg./kg.) led to a fall of thresholds. *d*-Amphetamine in quite small doses (0.4–1.5/kg.) caused a progressive fall in both EEG and behavioural arousal thresholds until, with the larger doses, the preparation remained permanently awake. It was of interest that LSD-25 caused no change in the thresholds to direct stimulation of the reticular formation in doses of up to 60 µg/kg ;.however, even quite small doses led to marked fall in the threshold to arousal produced by afferent (auditory) stimulation. Atropine led to n progressive increase in the EEG thresholds, but did not affect the threshold for behavioural arousal, the maximum divergence between the two thresholds being reached with dose of 2–3 mg/kg of atropine. If physostigmine (0.1–0.8 mg/kg) was administered after atropine the EEG threshold could be returned to normal and even to zero, still without change in the behavioral threshold. Similar results were obtained when the order of these drugs was reversed. These findings were thus not out of keeping with the observations in the conscious animal noted above (Bradley and Elkes 1957).

THE CENTRAL EFFECTS OF SOME PSYCHOTROPIC DRUGS ON A VASOMOTOR REFLEX PATHWAY (Ginzel 1955, 1957)

The symptoms induced by some psychotropic drugs often include fluctuating vasomotor changes. It seemed, therefore of interest to examine the effects of a drug such as LSD-25 and some of its congeners on a vasomotor reflex, the physiology of which was well known. The carotid sinus response was chosen for the purpose since, in this reflex, chemoreceptor and baroreceptor components can be specifically distinguished. It seemed of interest to determine whether a drug could selectively affect these two component pathways at a high central level. To minimize possible peripheral effects, the drugs were administered by the intraventricular route using a Feldberg-Sherwood cannula (Feldberg and Sherwood 1954), as well as by the intravenous route. Chloralose anaesthesia was employed, the vagi were cut, and the animal was kept under artificial respiration to reduce this particular variable. According to the requirements of a particular experiment, the carotid arteries, asphyxia, electrical stimulation of the carotid sinus nerve or close arterial injection of a nicotine-like substance (sebacinyl bis-choline: Ginzel, Klupp and Werner 1952) leading to stimulation of the carotid body receptors. The drugs examined included LSD-25 itself, and some derivates possessing equal or even higher antiserotonin effects, though not sharing the psychotropic powers of LSD-25. These included BOL 148, LAE 32, LPD 824, MLD 41, ALD 52.

LSD-25 administered in doses of 100–200 µg/kg intraventricularly, regularly reduced or abolished the carotid pressor response. The effects became apparent within 1–3 minutes of administration, lasted between 30–60 minutes and were followed by complete recovery of the reflex. Control injections of equivalent volumes (0.1–0.3 ml) of Ringer solution had no such effect. BOL 148 (possessing similar anti-5-HT action, but lacking the psychotropic properties of LSD-25) was half as powerful, and LPD 824 equipotent with LSD-25. LAE 32, possessing in terms of dosage only onetenth the psychotropic effects of LSD-25, proved at least twice as powerful as LSD-25 when tested against the carotid sinus response. ALD 52 exerted no effect. 5-HT itself administered intraventricularly in divided, but ultimately very large, doses (as high as 1 mg) neither influenced the carotid sinus response nor prevented its subsequent inhibition by LSD-25.

To determine the contribution of the chemo- and baroreceptor components to the effects observed following LSD-25, the animals were allowed to breathe air and oxygen alternatively. As is well known, with pure oxygen inhalation the baroreceptor component of the reflex predominates (von Euler and Lijestrand 1943, Landgren and Neil 1951). It was found that the difference in height of the carotid occlusion pressor response seen during ventilation with air and oxygen, respectively, was reduced or abolished by LSD-25. This difference normally indicates the contribution of the chemoreceptor component to the reflex, and its reduction or abolition therefore suggested a preferential blockade, at high central level, of the chemo-receptor pathway by LSD-25. This was borne out in experiments where the chemoreceptors were directly stimulated by close arterial injection of a nicotine-like substance, or nicotine itself. The response normally elicited by this manoeuvre was either reduced or abolished by the intraventricular administration of LSD-25.

THE EFFECTS OF SOME PSYCHOTROPIC DRUGS ON THE PERISTALTIC REFLEX (Ginzel 1957)

In view of the marked effects of a drug, so specifically psychotropic as LSD-25, on the central component of an autonomic (i.e. vasomotor) reflex, it seemed of interest to examine the effects of this drug and some of its congeners on a highly patterned autonomic reflex in a *peripheral* organ. The peristaltic reflex was chosen deliberately for several reasons. First, it represented a highly organized autonomous reflex depending upon a neuronal net built into the organ itself. Its physiology was known (Trendelenburg 1917). Second, centrally acting drugs such as morphia were known to have a marked effect on this reflex (Schaumann, Giovannini and Jochum 1952); and third, the high content of 5-HT in the gut suggested the investigation of 5-HT antagonists such as LSD-25 and other members of the group. It seemed, in sum, the neuronal network of the myenteric plexus, subserving as it does the highly patterned, regular and reciprocal play of excitation and inhibition which makes up the peristaltic wave might serve as a convenient model for the more complex neuronal nets of the autonomic centres of the brain.

Fresh pieces of guinea-pig lower ileum were mounted in 50-ml Tyrode bath at $37°$ by the method of Trendelenburg (1917). The bath was aerated by a mixture of 95 per cent oxygen and 5 per cent CO_2. The peristaltic reflex was elicited by raising the intraluminal pressure from zero to about 2–3 cm. of water. As has been shown (Trendelenburg 1917), the first response to a rise in intraluminal pressure is the contraction. of the longitudinal muscle fibres. This is termed the "preparatory" phase. W hen a threshold value of about 1.5 cm. water in intraluminal pressure is reached, rhythmic contractions of the circular muscle layer ensue. These sweep down the gut as peristaltic waves, and make up the so-called second "emptying" phase of the preparation.

LSD-25 in concentrations of 5×10^{-6}, while leaving the "preparatory" phase unaffected was found to abolish the emptying phase. BOL 148 was more effective than LSD-25 the range here being 5×10^{-7} to 3×10^{-6}. LAE 32 was equipotent with LSD-25, while MLD 41 and ALD 32 were less regular and weaker than LSD-25. Ergotamine and *d*-hydroergotamine inhibited the emptying phase in concentrations of about 2×10^{-5}. Dibenamine, a potent 5-HT antagonist, blocked the emptying phase in the same concentrations as LSD-25. Of particular interest was the exceedingly powerful effect of chlorpromazine. This drug was effective in concentrations varying from 10^{-8} to 10^{-12}, the precise effective. concentration varying, tantalizingly, and perhaps significantly from preparation to preparation. All the above substances inhibited the contractions produced by nicotine and barium chloride in concentrations which paralysed the emptying phase. They did, however, (with the exception of chlorpromazine) only slightly reduce the contractions elicited by acetylcholine.

Since most of the substances examined were powerful antagonists of 5-HT, the effect of 5-HT itself on the reflex was also studied. It is known that the contraction of the guinea-pig ileum elicited by small doses of 5-HT is abolished after saturation with larger doses (Gaddum

1953) although the response to other substances in the preparation remains unaffected. In keeping with this it was found that 5-HT, in doses of 10^{-5} to 10^{-7}, blocked the emptying phase of the reflex. It was also found that tolerance developed very rapidly, though, in contrast to the effects of LSD-25, the nicotine induced contractions were not suppressed when the peristaltic reflex was paralysed by 5-HT. Thus, LSD-25 apparently could block the reflex in a dose which did not abolish the contraction produced by 5-HT. 5-HT, on the other hand, within a certain dose range appeared to be capable of blocking its own effect on the longitudinal muscle without inhibiting the reflex. If, therefore, the effects of 5-HT antagonists on the peristaltic reflex were attributable to their anti-5HT effect, two different types of receptors for 5-HT in the gut must be assumed (Ginzel 1957). One of these may play a part in the peristaltic reflex and may be susceptible to blockade by large doses of 5-HT. Whether the large stores of 5-HT in the gut are, in fact, physiologically related to this highly organized autonomous local reflex must remain an open question. The evidence is certainly suggestive; and the ready accessibility, regularity and reproducibility of this preparation invites biochemical, physicochemical and electrophysiological investigations alike. We may, perhaps, learn something of the properties of the brain-stem reticular formation by looking at an "electro-ileo-gram".

COMMENT

The above findings permit a provisional survey and some tentative suggestions as to possible modes of action of the agents studied so far. It will have been noted that some drugs showed much closer correspondence than others between their effects on the electrical activity of the brain and on overt behaviour, though it must be stressed that only crude and obvious components of behaviour were studied and a refinement of techniques may well reveal differences not noted hitherto.

In the conscious animal, amphetamine led to low-voltage, fast activity and behavioural excitement. The effects of LSD-25 were less regular; at times they resembled those of amphetamine, at others exhibited a type of rhythmical activity never seen with that drug. Moreover, these variations could, with some confidence, be attributed to slight changes in the precise environmental setting of the particular experiment: Under LSD-25, animals appeared strikingly more susceptible to their environment.

Physostigmine led to changes in electrical activity closely resembling (though not necessarily identical with) those seen in the fully alert state; yet (provided the dose was suitably adjusted) no corresponding change in behaviour could be noted. Atropine and 1-hyoscyamine led to changes in electrical activity which bore a broad resemblance to those seen in sleep. Yet the animals were fully awake, and, in the case of atropine, on occasion showed excitement. Two groups of drugs were therefore clearly distinguished by these experiments. the first comprised amphetamine. and LSD-25, the second physostigmine, atropine and *l*-hyoscyamine. Moreover, whenever these drugs were used in combination with each other, the gross behavioural effects were always dominated by members of the first group, whereas the effects on the electrical activity were dominated by members of the second. The interaction between atropine and amphetamine, for example, showed this quite clearly.

The acute preparations used (the *encéphale* and *cerveau isolé*) made possible some, though limited, observations of behavioural change, as well as the recording of blood pressure and respiration. They were also designed to study the effect of high spinal and mesencephalic section upon the response pattern to individual drugs. Within the limits imposed by the physiology of these preparations, the distinction between the two groups of drugs was maintained. Thus, in the *encéphale isolé*, amphetamine would lead to a limited behavioural alerting, such as is seen in this preparation, whith a corresponding change in the electrical activity; physostigmine, atropine and *l*-hyoscyamine would lead to a change in electrical activity without a corresponding change in behaviour. Nor were these effects attributable to changes in systemic blood pressure, although changes in local vascular tone could not be excluded. Moreover, the existence or severance of spinal or mesencephalic connections profoundly affected the responses to these drugs, and served to sharpen the distinction between the two groups compounds. Thus, whereas, physostigmine,. atropine and *l*-hyoscyamine still exerted their effects in the *encéphale* and *cerveau isolé*, amphetamine, while exerting its effect in the intact animal and the *encéphale isolé*, had no effect on the *cerveau isolé*. LSD-25 (in the cat) exerted no effect on the electrical activity of either of the two acute preparations.

The interaction between the above drugs and chlorpromazine, and their effect on electrical and behavioural arousal thresholds in the *encéphale isolé* preparation, contributed further differences between these two groups. The behavioural and EEG effects of amphetamine and LSD-25 were blocked by chlorpromazine. Atropine and physostigmine still led to changes in electrical activity characteristic of these drugs in the presence of high doses of chlorpromazine, irrespective of an effect on overt behaviour which was always dominated by a given dose of chlorpromazine. In the stimulation experiments, amphetamine caused a progressive fall in both electrocortical and behavioural alerting thresholds until, with larger doses, the preparation remained permanently awake. Atropine led to a progressive increase in EEG threshold without affecting the threshold for behavioural arousal. Physostigmine counteracted this effect of atropine, and led to a diminution of the EEG arousal threshold without affecting the behavioral threshold. The effects of LSD-25 differed in important respects from both amphetamine and the atropine/physostigmine group; for, while causing no change in thresholds to direct stimulation of the reticular formation, small doses (1–2 µg/kg.) given intravenously caused a marked fall in the behavioural and electrocortical threshold for arousal by afferent (auditory) stimulation.

It is now possible to examine very briefly the relevance of the above observation to what has been said earlier concerning neurohumoral transmission within the central nervous system. The effects of physostigmine are presumably linked to its anticholinesterase activity and due to the endogenous accumulation of acetylcholine or a related ester. The effects of atropine or *l*-hyoscyamine may, similarly, be due to blockade of cholinergic sites. Both in terms of dosage and reversibility of effects, there are striking differences between the central and the peripheral effects of atropine and physostigmine. Nevertheless, it would seem fair to assume that cholinergic element is involved in these central effects; though the lack of correlation between effects on electrical activity and behaviour, and their independence of mesencephalic and spinal connections, would suggest a diffuse distribution of this element, a representation at high subcortical and possibly cortical level, and a non-dominant role in the mechanisms governing wakefulness and rousing. The effects of amphetamine were distinguished from those of physostigmine and atropine by the correlation between electrical activity and behaviour, and by their susceptibility to a mesencephalic. (though not spinal) lesion. In both these respects these findings could be related to the now classical observations of Moruzzi and Magoun (1949) which defined the part played by the reticular formation and tegmentum of the lower brain stem in the electrical and behavioural arousing response, and the maintenance of wake-fulness. It was therefore suggested (Bradley and Elkes 1953) that the effect of this drug might be exerted on receptors either related to, or located in the brain-stem reticular activating system. The old German term "Weckamine", i.e. waking amines, would certainly seem appropriate to a drug exerting its effect in elements within the arousal system. The findings of Bonvallet, Dell and Hiebel (1954) are in keeping with this suggestion. However, the intimate play of corticofugal fibres upon the reticular system (French, Hernandez-Péon and Livingston 1955) would potentially make that system susceptible to an effect of the drug exerted at cortical as well as subcortical levels, and it may perhaps be an alteration in *inhibitory* tone in this two-way system which brings about the alteration in sensory thresholds that we know as arousal. Here, too, it would be well to bear in mind the remarkable observations of Ingvar (1955) suggesting the involvement of extraneuronal mechanism in the alerting response.

The alerting effects of LSD-25 in the cat (though to a lesser extent in the monkey) were lost following high spinal section, and could in no circumstances be observed in the *cerveau isolé* preparations. Unlike amphetamine in the conscious cat, the alerting effect of LSD-25 appeared to depend on slight variation in the animal's environment, the animal apparently being strikingly susceptible to cues which it had not previously noted. The striking fall in arousal threshold to afferent (auditory) stimuli, though not to direct stimulation of the reticular formation (Bradley and Key 1956), following LSD-25 has already been noted and has served to differentiate further LSD-25 from amphetamine. Relevant here, too, are the effects of LSD-25 on geniculate transmission (Evarts et al. 1956).

The above evidence tentatively and provisionally suggests the existence of three types of receptors within the brain, related to and dependent upon the natural turnover of three types of substrates within the central nervous system. The first of these is almost certainly cholinergic in nature, though the greatest care has to be exercised in relating it to acetylcholine itself. For the reasons already given, an ester other than acetylcholine may be more important than acetylcholine, and a possible role in regulating local small vessel tone or in the activity of another non-neuronal component cannot be excluded. In any event, the receptor, be it a type of neurone or nn active electrogenic patch of special configuration on the surface membrane of a neurone, would appear to have a diffus distribution. It is unlikely to play a dominant part in the great centrencephalic steering mechanisms governing the basic states of arousal and attention; though, of course, it may well play a part in the more discriminate and delicate forms of behaviour not susceptible to analysis within this crude framework.

The non-cholinergic receptors susceptible *inter alia* to amphetamine may involve elements high in the reticular formation, as well as the cortex; and recent observations of Dell and co-workers (Bonvallet, Dell and Hiebel 1954, Dell 1958, this symposium, p. 187) stressing the role of these elements in the organization of the facilitatory and inhibitory mechanism governing autonomic responses is not out of keeping with this suggestion. Both noradrenaline and adrenaline have recently been identified in midline structures of the upper brain system (Vogt 1954). The role of adrenaline in the functional organization of the hypothalamic pituitary axis is as yet indeterminate but, as has been shown using a discrete stimulation technique (Folkow and von Euler 1954), there appears to be an interplay between hypothalamus and adrenal medulla at a biochemical level. The virtually complementary functions of noradrenaline and adrenaline in peripheral homeostatic autonomic responses have been extensively studied, and an attempt has also been made to relate differential proportions of these two catechol amines to patterns of emotional expression and experience in man (Funkenstein, Greenblatt and Solomon 1953). This may be premature, and may need drastic revision in the light of a refinement of methods and the availability of fresh data. But it is at least conceivable that a naturally occurring catechol amine (or a group of catechol amines) may modulate the play of inthihitory tone in key cell assemblies, and thus govern the release or the storage of the old, diffuse and firmly coded processes which we know as emotion; for, in their simplest form, the patterns of emotional expression and experience would appear to be highly integrated sets of neural activity involving, basically, the acceptance or avoidance of objects, or their secondary equivalents. The peripheral autonomic apparatus is the outer instruments in such attitudes, and the limbic system (MacLean 1950) its inner counterpart. The posterior hypothalamic nuclei have a neural, and quite possibly chemical, connection with both. Yet the regulation of levels of excitability and "set" in neural nets may involve the interaction of a diffuse, and a strictly circumscribed and a local, process; "release" may well depend upon precisely this interaction between a *humoral* and a *local* chemical element. The rule may apply with equal force to the neural nets governing the play of the highly patterned process we know as the peristaltic wave, as those governing muscle tone, or stance, or posture, or "thought". It may be the same rule. The possible operation of chemical fields within certain key areas of the brain has been referred to earlier (Elkes 1953).

The third type of receptor, which may form the biochemical target of LSD-25, may depend upon the natural turnover of an indole or related derivative with which LSD-25 specifically interferes. We have already noted the peculiar susceptibility of LSD-25 effects to environment; equally, in the cat, the effects were abolished by high spinal section with its massive reduction of afferent tone; moreover, in man the subjective effects of LSD-25 were found to be enhanced by rhythmic photic stimulation (Elkes, Elkes and Bradley 1954), and these effects involve perceptual, affective and cognitive areas, and only later overflow into motor function. Moreover, one can recall here the affinity of the symptoms of LSD-intoxication with those induced by massive sensory isolation (Hebb 1955) or with hypnagogic imagery experienced physiologically between wakefulness and sleep (see Müller 1848). It may be that LSD-25 acts on a receptor particularly and peculiarly related to the afferent pathways, and that it possibly interferes with the physiological liberation and turnover of a naturally occurring indole which, in the brain, plays a dominant part in the organization of sensory experience. It is as if a mechanism which forms a fluctuating, though ever present, part of normal adaptive behavior became chemically locked by a psychotropic drug. The receptor in question might be related to the medial (i.e. the non/sense linked) collaterals of the great afferent pathways, and also be built into thalamortical or strictly cortical nets. Its essential feature may be its relation to the afferent system, and its role essentially that of highly patterned inhibition. There is good evidence for the role of organized inhibition in perceptual process. We know, for example, how at the level of the Cochlear nucleus (Allanson and Whitfield 1955) inhibition of fibres lying between the two active arrays plays a part in the so-called "squaring process" and the probable transformation of information at the level. Furthermore, Purpura's work (1957) suggests the activation by LSD-25 of inhibitory synapses, which are also available to transmitter or transmitters released by reticular stimulation of the brain stem. This inhibitory process would therefore appear to be very finely set, and would be modulated by the interplay of related substances of distant and of local origin. It is built into the neuronal net at its finest level of organization. It is this chemical suppresor mechanism which, by matching fresh information against stored patterns, and by reciprocal suppression or "banking" of some, may play a part in the organization of temporal and spatial experience, or in the selective exclusion inherent in the process of logic and abstraction. It is this suppresor mechanism which may be defective is schizophrenia.

SUMMARY

(1) The claims of some substances so far identified in the central nervous system (acetylcholine, noradrenaline, adrenaline, 5-hydroxytryptamine and γ-aminobutyric acid) for a possible central transmitter role are briefly examined in terms of four criteria. None satisfy these criteria in full. It is suggested that, rather than thinking in unitary terms, it might be appropriate to consider the possible selection by chemical evolution of three or four families of closely related compounds which by mutual interplay may pattern the phenomena of central excitation and inhibition. Acetyl*l*-choline, noradrenaline, 5-HT, may be parent molecules of this kind. Centrally occurring congeners of these substances may well exert functions not shared by related molecules at peripheral effector sites.

(2) The effect of a number of drugs (atropine, *l*-hyoscyamine, physostigmine, the amphetamines and LSD-25) on the electrical activity of the brain, and on behavior in the conscious cat preparation, are briefly considered. Two groups of drugs could be distinguished. LSD-25 rendered the animals susceptible to the precise environmental setting of the individual experiment. The distinction between the groups was further sharpened by a study of the effects of mesencephalic and spinal lesions in acute preparations; a study of the interaction between chlorpromazine and these drugs; and by an examination of the effects of these drugs on arousal thresholds.

(3) The effects of LSD-25 on two autonomic pathways, the carotid sinus reflex and the peristaltic reflex, have been studied. LSD-25 reversibly blocked the carotid sinus reflex by a central action. It also inhibited the emptying phase of the peristaltic reflex in the isolated guinea-pig ileum.

(4) The above results provisionally suggest the existence of three types of receptors within the brain, possibly related to and dependent on the physiological turnover of three types of substrates within the central nervous system. The first of these may be cholinergic in nature, though an ester other than acetylcholine may well be more important than acetylcholine itself. This receptor may have a diffuse distribution and is unlikely to play a dominant part in the great centrencephalic steering mechanisms governing basic states of arousal and attention; it may, however, well play part in the more discriminate and delicate forms of behaviour. The noncholinergic receptors susceptible to amphetamine and other catechol amines, my involve elements high in the reticular formation as well as the cortex, and may depend upon the turnover of a naturally occurring catechol amine (or group of catechol amines) which through the possession of some special properties may modulate the play of inhibitory tone in key cell assemblies governing the storage or release of old and firmly coded integrating patterns, including those making up patterns of emotional expression and experience. The peripheral autonomic system is the outer instrument of these patterns, and the limbic system may be its inner counterpart.

The third type of receptor, which may form the biochemical target of LSD-25 may depend upon the natural turnover of an indole derivative with which LSD-25 specifically interferes. This receptor may be particularly and peculiarly related to the afferent system, and may play a dominant part in the maintenance of a highly patterned reciprocal inhibitory process which plays a key part in the organization of temporal and spatial experience, as well as in the selective exclusion inherent in the processes of logic and abstraction. It is possibly this suppresor mechanism that may be defective in schizophrenia.

(5) The dependence of levels of excitability inherent in such concepts as "set" and "release" upon an interaction between humoral and strictly local chemical events is stressed. The possible operation of chemical fields within certain key areas of the brain is suggested.

(6) The lack of any precise data relating intracerebral chemical events to peripheral chemical change is emphasized.

REFERENCES

Allanson, J. T., Whitfield, I. C. (1955). In: III Lond. Symp. Information Theory, p. 269. London: Butterworth.
Amin, A. H., Crawford, T. B. B., and Gaddum, J. H. (1954). J. Physiol. 126, 596.
Arduini, A., and Arduini, M. G. (1954). J. Pharmacol. 110, 76.
Bayliss, B., and Todrick, A. (1956). Biochem. J. 62, 62.
Bazemore, A., Elliott, K. A. C., and Florey, E. (1956). Nature, Lond., 178, 1052.
Bonvallet, M., Dell, P., and Hiebel, G. (1954). EEG clin. Neurophysiol., 6, 119.
Bradley, P. B. (1958). To be published.
Bradley, P. B., Cerquiglini S., and Elkes, J. (1953). J. Physiol. 121, 51P.
Bradley, P. B., and Elkes, J. (1953). J. Physiol. 120, 13P; EEG clin. Neurophysiol. 5, 451.
Bradley, P. B., and Elkes, J. (1957). Brain, 80, 77.
Bradley, P. B., and Hance, A. J. (1956). J. Physiol. 132, 50P.
Bradley, P. B., and Hance, A. J. (1957). EEG clin. Neurophysiol. 9, 191.
Bradley, P. B., and Key, B. J. (1956). XX Int. Physiol. Congr., Abstracts of Communications, p. 124.
Bremer, F. (1935). C. R. Soc. Biol. Paris, 118, 1235.
Brodie, B. B. (1957). Trans. III Conf. The Josiah Macy Jr. Found. N. Y., p. 323.
Bülbring, E. (1944). J. Physiol. 103, 55.
Bülbring, E., and Burn, J. H. (1941). J. Physiol. 100, 337.
Carlsson, A., Rosengren, E., Bertler, A., and Nilsson, J. (1957). Psychotropic Drugs, p. 363. Ed. Garattini, S., and Ghetti, V. Amsterdam, Elsevier.
Desmedt, J. E., and Lagrutta, G. (1955). J. Physiol. 129, 46P.
Elkes, J. (1953). In: Prospects in Psychiatric Research, ed. Tanner, J. M. p. 126. Oxford: Blackwell.
Elkes, J. (1957). Trans. III Conf. The Josiah Macy Jr. Found. N. Y. p. 203.
Elkes, J., Eyars, J. T., and Todrick, A. (1955). In: Biochemistry of the Developing Nervous System, ed. Waelsch, H. p. 499. N. Y.: Academic Press.
Elkes, J., Elkes, C., and Bradley, P. B. (1954). J. ment. Sci. 100, 125.
Elkes, J., and Todrick, A. (1955). In: Biochemistry of the Developing Nervous System, ed. Waelsch, H., p. 309. New York: Academic Press.
Euler, U. S. von, and Liljestrand, G. (1943). Acta physiol. scand., 6, 319.
Evarts, E. V., Landan, W., Freygang, W. H., and Marshall, W. H. (1956). Amer. J. Physiol. 182, 594.
Feldberg, W. (1945). Physiol. Rev., 25, 596.
Feldberg, W. (1951) Arch. int. Physiol., 59, 544.
Feldberg, W., and Sherwood, S. L. (1954). J. Physiol. 123, 148.
Feldberg, W., and Vogt, M. (1948). J. Physiol. 107, 372.
Folkow, B., and Euler, U. S. von (1954) Circulat. Res. 2, 191.
French, J. D., Hernandez-Péon, R., and Livingston, R. B. (1955). J. Neurophysiol. 18, 74.
Funkenstein, D. H., Greenblatt, M., and Solomon, H. C. (1953). Ass. Res. nerv. Dis. Proc. 31, 245.
Gaddum, J. H. (1953) J. Physiol. 119, 363.
Gaddum, J. H., and. Giarman, N. J. (1956). Brit. J. Pharmacol. 11, 88.
Ginzel, K. H. (1955). J. Physiol. 129, 61P.
Ginzel, K. H. (1957). Psychotropic Drugs. p. 48. Ed. Garattini, S., and Ghetti, V. Amsterdam: Elsevier.
Ginzel, K. H., Klupp, H., and Werner, G. (1952). Arch. int. Pharmacodyn. 89, 160.
Hebb, D. O. (1955). Amer. J. Psychiat. 111, 826.
Holton, F. A., and Holton, P. (1953). J. Physiol. 119, 50P.
Ingvar, D. (1955). Acta physiol. scand., 33, 169.
Koelle, G. B. (1952). J. Pharmacol. 106, 401.
Landgren, S., and Neil, E. (1951). Acta physiol. scand., 23, 152.
Lembeck, F. (1953). Arch. exp. Path. Pharmak. 219, 197.
MacClean, P. D. (1950). Psychosom. Med. 11, 338.
Marrazzi, A. S. (1958). Science, 118, 367.

Moruzzi, G., and Magoun, H. W. (1949). EEG clin. Neurophysiol. 1, 455.

Müller, J. (1848). The Physiology of the Senses. Taylor.

Ord, M. G., and Thompson, R. H. S. (1953). Biochem. J. 51, 245.

Pletscher, A., Shore, P. A., and Brodie, B. B. (1955). Science, 122, 374.

Purpura, D. P. (1957). Trans. III Conf. The Josiah Macy Jr. Found. N. Y., p. 297.

Rheinberger, M. B., and Jasper, H. H. (1937). Amer. J. Physiol. 119, 186.

Richter, D., and Crossland, J. (1949). Amer. J. Physiol. 159, 247.

Rinkel, M. (1956). Trans. II Conf. The Josiah Macy Jr. Found. N. Y.

Rothlin, E. (1957). Ann. N. Y. Acad. Sci. 66, 688.

Schaumann, D., Giovannini, M., and Jochum, K. (1932). Arch. exp. Path. Pharmak. 215, 460.

Schou, M. (1957). Pharmacol. Rev. 9, 17.

Sherrington, C. S. (1951). Man and his Nature. p. 104. Cambridge Univ. Press.

Tobias, J. M., Lipton, M. A., and Lepinat, A. A. (1946). Proc. Soc. exp. Biol., N. Y., 61, 51.

Tower, D. B., and Elliott, K. A. C. (1952). J. appl. Physiol. 4, 669.

Trendelenburg (1917). Arch. exp. Path. Pharmak. 81, 55.

Udenfriend, S., Weissbach, H., and Bogdanski, D. F. (1957). Ann. N. Y. Acad. Sci. 66, 602.

Vogt, M. (1954). J. Physiol. 123, 451.

Wajda, I. (1951). The Metabolism of Acetylcholine in the Central Nervous System. Ph.D. Thesis. University of Birmingham.

Wikler, A. (1952). Proc. Soc. exp. Biol. N.Y., 79, 261.

PAPER 12

EFFECTS OF CHLORPROMAZINE ON THE BEHAVIOUR OF CHRONICALLY OVERACTIVE PSYCHOTIC PATIENTS

J. Elkes[*] and Charmian Elkes[**]

*Department of Experimental Psychiatry, University of Birmingham
and Winson Green Hospital, Birmingham*

Reprinted with the kind permission of the BMJ Publishing Group
from the British Medical Journal II: 560-576, 1954

Reports of the varied central effects of chlorpromazine hydrochloride ("Largactil") (Laborit and Huguenard 1951, Courvoisier et al. 1952, Brand et al. 1954), its reputed potentiating action on central depressants (Laborit and Jaulmes 1952, Courvoisier et al. 1953), and the clinical response observed in various psychiatric states (Delay, Deniker, and Harl 1952a,b; Delay, Deniker, Harl, and Grasset 1952, Delay and Deniker 1953, Sigwald and Bouttier 1953) have encouraged a limited trial of this drug in regard to its effect on the behaviour of a small group of chronically overactive psychotic patients in a large and overcrowded mental hospital.

Clinical Material

The material (Table 1) consisted of 12 male and 15 female patients drawn from the disturbed ("refractory") wards of the hospital. These patients were chosen less according to diagnostic category than because of the degree of overactivity they exhibited, which was sufficient to make them a persistent and difficult nursing problem. Of the 27 patients, 10 were diagnosed as schizophrenics and 3 as paraphrenics. These are grouped together in our assessment as suffering from schizophrenic disorders. Seven cases (Nos. 2, 5, 8, 9, 10, 11, and 14) suffered from recurrent or chronic hypomania, one (Case 13) was a manic-depressive, and three cases (Nos. 4, 7, and 24) were chronic agitated melancholics; these formed the affective group. The remaining three (Cases 20, 21, and 22) were confused, restless, overactive female senile dements. Three cases (Nos. 5, 13, and 14) in the affective group and one paraphrenic (Case 15) showed signs of organic cerebral deterioration, and one chronic melancholic (Case 24) had had a leucotomy performed six years ago, after which she had become more destructive and even incontinent.

The medical and nursing staff were thoroughly familiar with the pattern of each patient's illness, and this was taken into account when assessing results.

---

[*] Professor of Experimental Psychiatry, University of Birmingham
[**] Clinical Research Fellow, University of Birmingham

TABLE 1. Clinical Material

	Male	Female	Total
Affective Disorders	3	8	11
Schizophrenic Disorders	9	4	13
Senile Disorders	0	3	3
Total	12	15	27

Design of Trial

The patients were mostly observed in their own wards, but where they were transferred from one ward to another an equilibration period of two weeks was allowed. During this time patients were given an opportunity to adjust to their new environment, and full account was taken of any day-to-day variation shown. Within seven days of the beginning of the trial all sedatives were withdrawn. Chlorpromazine tablets and inert control tablets were then administrated to the same patient in alternating periods for the duration of the trial. Only one observer (C.E.) and the dispenser knew which patients were receiving the active or the inactive preparation at any given time; the medical staff and the day and night nursing staff taking part in the assessment of results were not in possession of this information.

Dosage

To begin with, the effective dose of the drug and the length of the period of continuous medication were a matter of trial and error. Weekly alternation between the active and inert control tablets was tried first; this was followed by the administration of active and placebo tablets in blocks of three weeks at a time. As the trial progressed, however, it was found that clinical changes, in terms of both improvement and relapse, were slow to develop, and a six-weeks period appeared more adequate, for judging the effects of the preparation. Consequently, from the seventh and eighth weeks onwards most of the patients received the drug in six-week blocks. The total dosage of drug and placebo are given in Table I. Although administration usually began with 75 mg, by mouth – one 25-mg tablet tds. – up to 300 mg a day was given transitorily in most cases. These high dosages led to undesirable side-effects, and ultimately 150 mg (two tablets t. d. s.) was found to be both safe and (in those cases in which response was noted) effective. A smaller maintenance dose has not been tried in the present series. The only exception to this was Case 4, in which signs of relapse were noted when the dose was reduced from 150 mg to 100 mg a day. The trial lasted for 22 weeks.

In only three cases (Nos. 2, 10, and 11) was the drug given by the intramuscular route. These cases were included in the trial somewhat later than the others, and at the time were suffering from acute hypomanic states. Each received three injections (of 25 mg) daily for one week, and a total of 100 mg daily during the second and third weeks. No pain was complained of, but as there was some induration at the site of the injection; this route was abandoned and medication by mouth (at 150 mg a day) substituted.

Clinical Assessment and Recording of Results

Each patient was seen daily by the observer in charge of the trial (C.E.), and at weekly intervals by two medical officers. The day and night nursing staff also took part in the trial, the aim being to cover the relevant aspects of the patient's behaviour "round the clock." The day nursing staff were asked to write a daily note on each patient. This covered their general behaviour in the ward, their social attitudes, eating habit, work, and particularly their periods of overactivity and impulsiveness. The night nurses noted restlessness, noisiness, and sleep. The medical observers' findings were recorded in two ways. The first was the usual clinical note, which was made at a weekly interview and did not take into account the day-to-day behaviour in the ward. In addition, however, an attempt was made to itemize (though not score) the various relevant aspects of the patient's mental state and behaviour. „Pro-forma" sheets covering these items were designed in consecutive discussions with the medical staff and used as the patients were seen week by week. These „pro-forma" are still undergoing trial, and will be the subject of a separate communication when complete. Nevertheless, even in their present form they ensured that certain aspects of the clinical picture were always looked for, and no information was lost by default. Assessment was made by one of us (C.E.) at the end of each week on the basis of daily personal observation and of these daily (nurses') and weekly (medical observers') reports; and a final assessment was made again at the end of the trial – that is, after 22 weeks. It is well to remark here that it was the nurses' daily written reports which were found to be particularly useful when analysing results in retrospect. They often served to emphasize changes which might otherwise have been overlooked.

The combination of the "blind" nature of the trial, the fact that the patient was used as his own control, and agreement among the different observers, all contributed towards some confidence in a field in which assessment is notoriously difficult. Our findings so far suggest that chlorpromazine may have its place in the symptomatic treatment of a limited proportion of chronically agitated psychotic patients.

Results

During the first two weeks of the trial nearly all the patients seemed better, irrespective of whether they were receiving the active or inert preparation. They became quieter and more responsive, and one patient (Case 24) ceased to be incontinent and destructive of clothing. This effect, however was transient, and relapse to the behaviour usual for each patient was not long in forthcoming, except in those in whom a genuine response to the drug was observed. It seems likely that this illusory improvement was due to the unaccustomed daily attention which the patients were getting, and their knowledge that they were undergoing a new kind of treatment. The staff's enthusiasm, too, soon found its own level, and as the weeks went by the effects of chlorpromazine could be more clearly distinguished.

In the responses grouped in Table 3 the term "definitely improved" is applied to those cases in which the improvement was undoubtedly attributable to the drug. This was judged by the improvement as medication proceeded, the relapse when placebo therapy was substituted, and the reappearance of improvement when the active preparation was reinstated. The patients became quieter, less tense, and less disturbed by their hallucinations and delusions during the weeks they were receiving chlorpromazine; their eating, sleep and social habits changed for the better, and two (Cases 3 and 6) could be allowed privileges or enjoy occupations which they could not have followed before. In three cases (Nos. 3, 4, and 5) parole was considered – in one of them (Case 5) for the first time in fifteen years. As the inert control tablets were substituted, the behaviour of the patients gradually became more disturbed, although, with the exception of two cases (Nos. 1 and 7), overactivity never quite reached its former level. In one instance, however (Case 4), the patient, after two weeks on placebo tablets, became so unmanageable that chlorpromazine had to be resumed. This patient improved within one week. The cases subject to recurrent attacks of mania (Cases 2 and 5) were given chlorpromazine at a time coinciding with the onset of their overactive phase; this reduced their overactivity to below the level usual for these patients.

TABLE 3

	Definitely improved		Slightly improved		Not improved	
	Male	Female	Male	Female	Male	Female
Affective disorders	1	3	2	4	0	1
Schizophrenic disorders	2	1	4	1	3	2
Senile disorders	0	0	0	0	0	3
Total	7		11		9	

The cases designated "slightly improved" did not show the same clear-cut response. In one group (Cases 9, 12, 15, 16, 17, and 18) there was a gradual lessening of overactivity during chlorpromazine medication, although noisy outbursts in response to hallucinations continued. It was only after prolonged periods (four to six weeks) on placebo that it was noticed that the periods of overactivity during active medication had been less frequent and far less intense than during the placebo period. The other group included five patients (Cases 8, 10, 11, 13 and 14) subject to cyclic disorders. The phasic nature of their overactivity remained basically unaltered; but the extent of their overactivity was somewhat reduced.

The term "not improved" was applied to those cases in which no improvement of any kind could be attributed to chlorpromazine. Included in this group are five schizophrenics (Cases 19, 23, 25, 26, and 27) and the only three cases of senile dementia (Cases 20, 21, and 22) in the trial. There was also one patient (Case 24) in whom the trial was cut short after eight weeks owing to the patient's poor physical state; although, in retrospect, and in the light of further experience with the drug, continued medication would have seemed permissible.

It is important to stress that in no case was the content of the psychosis changed. The schizophrenic and paraphrenic patients continued to be subject to delusions and hallucinations, though they appeared to be less disturbed by them. Those patients who suffered from recurrent attacks of hypomania became less excitable and aggressive during these phases, though their affective swings continued at intervals normal to each patient. The chronically agitated melancholics, while becoming less tense and at times apparently less miserable, did not themselves admit to any improvement in their mental state. Few of these chronic psychotic patients showed improvement which enabled them to become more useful members of the mental hospital society. Others became less difficult nursing problems. Three were considered fit for parole, but none were thought fit for discharge. The relief afforded by chlorpromazine thus appears to be principally symptomatic.

The following notes illustrate the type of change observed.

Improved Cases

Case 3. A 32-year-old schizophrenic man had been in this hospital for six years. He was on escape caution, and was unemployable. His behaviour was greatly disturbed by terrifying visual and auditory hallucinations. He referred to them as "bogies", and, when present, they occupied his whole attention. He spent a great deal of time writing inconsequential sentences, or drawing to "ward off the bogies" and he would often shout abuse at them, banging the furniture, and marching about the ward. His sleep was disturbed, and he required sedation nearly every night. Socially he was very withdrawn and solitary. After three weeks on chlorpromazine he gradually became more accessible and friendly. He worked on the ward, took charge of Christmas decorations, and escape caution was discontinued. Finally, he was able to attend occupational therapy for the first time since his admission. Here he practised his talent for painting. He received no medication apart from chlorpromazine, and had only occasional restless nights despite this. Sporadically he would shout at his hallucinations, but he said that the "bogies did not worry him so much." He relapsed when on placebo tablets, and was graded as definitely improved. By the end of the trial he had gained 11 lb. (5 kg) in weight.

Case 5. A 69-year-old man who was subject to recurrent attacks of mania first became ill at the age of 18 years. He had been admitted four times, and had spent a total of 23 years of his life in this mental hospital. He now showed signs of organic cerebral deterioration. His behaviour was usually quiet, though somewhat elated, but he had regular periods of extreme overactivity when he would constantly run round the ward singing and shouting until he was hoarse. At these times he was quite incapable of maintaining any contact or of any connected conversation. After chlorpromazine medication it was noted that, although his affective swings were not altered, his manic phases were less acute. He was less overactive and less constantly noisy; and, although still garrulous and showing flight of ideas, his attention could be held for very brief periods. During his quiet periods his affect seemed normal. His wife, who knew nothing of the trial, spontaneously remarked on how well he was. He was thought fit for parole for the first time in 15 years. He was graded definitely improved. Weight gain here was negligible.

Case 6. A 46-year-old schizophrenic man fell ill when he was 22 years old. He had been admitted three times, and the length of the present admission was nine years. In the wards he was aimlessly overactive, often aggressive to other patients and staff, and frequently involved in fights and quarrels. At one time he had worked on the hospital farm, but had to be removed because of his impulsive behaviour. In conversation he appeared fairly well orientated but disconnected, and chattered away irrelevantly, using bizarre pseudo-psychiatric neologisms. He was domineering and often interfered with other patients, and his manner suggested hallucinations. After chlorpromazine medication, improvement was noticed only slowly. Although he continued to be rather domineering, he became much less aggressive, and was involved in no violent incidents after the first three weeks of the trial. He started working again on the farm, and did very well. His manner of speaking, however, was unchanged. Although he did not fully relapse on placebo tablets, he was graded as definitely improved because of the social change in him. He gained 17 lb. (7,7 kg) in weight.

Case 4. A 52-year-old chronic agitated melancholic woman, first admitted at the age of 41, was extremely tense and was tortured by delusions of guilt and persecution. Her mental state had not fluctuated for four years, except for temporary improvement after E.C.T. She had to be spoon-fed, refused to occupy herself, and spent a great deal of time weeping, and had once swallowed her wedding-ring in a suicidal attempt. After one week on chlorpromazine she became less tense, and, although often still depressed, there were frequent days when she was cheerful and sociable, helped with the ward work, and knitted for her grandchildren. Her relatives remarked on the change in her, although (as in Case 5) they knew nothing of the treatment she was having. She ate her meals spontaneously and with no difficulty, and gained 34 lb. (15,4 kg) in weight. She relapsed quickly when on placebo medication and showed signs of relapse when the dose of chlorpromazine was reduced from 150 to 100 mg during one week. She was graded definitely improved.

Case 7. A 54-year-old chronic agitated melancholic woman, who had been in hospital for eighteen years, was extremely tense and miserable, and continually wandered round the ward wringing her hands in anguish. She was irritable, occasionally impulsive, and negativistic, and often had to be spoon-fed. She was often incontinent of urine. Within two weeks of chlorpromazine medication she became, at times, more talkative and cheerful and appeared less agitated. Although she continued to grumble eternally about the food, and continued to be incontinent, her appetite increased greatly, she required no spoon-feeding, and she gained 23 lb. (10,4 kg) in weight. She relapsed on placebo tablets, and was graded definitely improved.

Case 2. A 54-year-old woman, who was subject to recurrent attacks of hypomania, had been observed in hospital for one year. Just before treatment was begun she had been allowed home on a month's trial, but was returned to hospital in a state of acute overactivity. She was noisy, impulsive, and aggressive, and had to be nursed in a side room. Chlorpromazine was administered intramuscularly at first; during the second week on the drug she became more subdued in her overt behaviour, although her mood remained elated. At the first sign of her next overactive phase, chlorpromazine (by mouth) was reinstated. The patient continued to be elated and garrulous and to show flight of ideas; nevertheless, her behaviour was changed, and she was able to continue ward work for the whole of this time, a state quite unusual for her. She gained 30 lb. (13,8 kg) in weight, and was graded definitely improved.

Case 1. A 62-year-old paraphrenic woman was greatly disturbed in her behaviour by auditory hallucinations. She used to scream abuse in response to these, particularly to a "Mr. Knock", who put "filthy thoughts into her mind". She was deluded against some members of the staff, whom she habitually screamed at and threatened, and often was impulsive and aggressive when annoyed by other patients. She spent most of her time scrubbing the floor in an obsessional manner, and talking and shouting almost continuously. After three weeks of chlorpromazine medication her overactivity continued, but she was much quieter in response to her hallucinations, and said "she did not bother any more with Mr. Knock", as he "did not annoy her so much." She became quite polite and friendly towards her *bétes noires* among the staff, but was still occasionally stimulated by other patients. She relapsed on placebo tablets, and was graded definitely improved. She lost a negligible amount of weight.

Cases Slightly Improved

Of the slightly improved group, the following may serve as examples.

Case 16. A 43-year-old schizophrenic man, admitted to this hospital 22 years ago, was extremely withdrawn, and barely answered questions in monosyllables. He was never still, but continuously paced or ran up and down the ward, clapping his hands together, and frequently reaching a pitch of such wildly screaming excitement that E.C.T. was needed to calm him. After the beginning of chlorpromazine medication his endless pacing and mannerisms were unaltered, and he was often noisy, but at no time did he reach a degree of excitement at which

E.C.T. would have been considered necessary. He did not relapse during the placebo period, and was graded slightly improved. The gain in weight was negligible.

Case 12. A 48-year-old paraphrenic woman, admitted four years ago, was subject to wildly excited outbursts of aggression against patients and staff in response to hallucinations. After three weeks of chlorpromazine medication she still continued to talk to her hallucinations, and was sometimes noisy in doing so; there were, however, no acute uncontrollable outbursts of aggression. There were signs of more disturbed behaviour during the sixth week after chlorpromazine had been withdraws. She was graded slightly improved. Weight increase was negligible.

Case 8. A 49-year-old woman, readmitted 2,5 years ago, was subject to recurrent attacks of hypomania. During these periods she was continuously overactive, mischievous, and aggressive. When on chlorpromazine she seemed less aggressive during her overactive phases, and less scattered; on some days she was able to carry out ward work. When on placebo she did not relapse to the intensity of her usual manic attacks. She was consequently graded slightly improved. Weight increase was negligible.

Side-effects

With high doses of chlorpromazine (up to 300 mg daily) slight depression and lethargy were noted in some patients (Cases 1, 3, 5, 8, 8, 12, 14, 17, 18, and 27). The patients did not appear well, moved slowly, and their faces bore a greyish drawn look. There was no cyanosis of the extremities, and no marked or consistent change in blood pressure could be detected. Subjectively, the patients complained only of slight and vague malaise. Somewhat similar symptoms were observed in Cases 3, 14, 17, and 27 during the second and third weeks of medication on moderate doses (150 mg a day). These symptoms, however, lasted for only a few days, and no reduction of the dose was thought necessary. Although our patients were not instructed to lie down after taking their tablets, no symptoms attributable to postural hypotension were noted.

One patient (Case 13) developed transient jaundice during the sixth week of the trial. He had received progressively increasing doses of chlorpromazine (75 mg rising to 300 mg a day) for four weeks, and this was followed by two weeks placebo medication. It was during this second week on placebo that jaundice was noted. Laboratory findings at the height of jaundice were: serum bilirubin, 6 mg per 100 ml (van den Bergh direct reaction); thymol turbidity test, 1 unit; zinc sulphate test, 1 unit; cephalin cholesterol (24 hours) negative, (48 hours) negative; total serum proteins, 6.4 g% (albumin 4.4 g, globulin 2 g). The trial was temporarily suspended for six weeks; the jaundice cleared within ten days, and liver-function tests returned to normal within three weeks. At the end of six weeks it was thought safe to resume chlorpromazine medication at the level of 150 mg a day. There was no recurrence of symptoms. No jaundice was seen in any other patient, and liver-function tests, which were performed fortnightly in all patients, showed no abnormality. The cause of this single incidence of jaundice must remain obscure.

Full blood counts were performed in all patients at fortnightly intervals during the trial. In only two cases was abnormality noted. Case 11 showed some polychromatic cells and basophilic stippling in the ninth week of the trial – that is, after seven weeks on chlorpromazine and two weeks on placebo control. The red count was 3,840,000; haemoglobin, 78% (11.5 g); total white count 8,400, This change was transient and was not noted in subsequent blood counts.

Another patient (Case 8) showed slight transient neutropenia during the thirteenth week of the trial, after three weeks of chlorpromazine and six weeks of placebo. The blood count, however, returned to normal and chlorpromazine medication was continued.

Changes in Weight

Nine patients put on weight steadily during the trial, the increase ranging from 11 to 34 lb. (5 to 15.4 kg), gained in 22 weeks. All these patients belonged either to the definitely or to the slightly improved groups (Table 1). They included two cases of chronic agitated melancholia (Cases 4 and 7), three cases of chronic or recurrent hypomania (Cases 2, 10 and 11), one case of chronic hypomania with schizoid features (Case 9), ant three cases of schizophrenia (Cases 3, 6, and 18). The remaining eight patients showed fluctuation in their monthly weights within a range of –5 lb. to +6 lb. (–2.3 to +2.7 kg). This was not regarded as significant. One patient (Case 19) had gained 13 lb. (5.9 kg) by the end of the trial; but this increase had to be discounted, as his record showed a regular fluctuation by this amount for the last five years.

Comment

The limited aim of the above small trial was to determine the usefulness of chlorpromazine in the management of the overactive chronic psychotic patient in the overcrowded disturbed wards of a mental hospital. As mentioned above, the 27 patients comprising the clinical material were chosen, not according to diagnostic category, but solely on the strength of the overactivity which they exhibited. Nor were they segregated in a "chlorpromazine ward." It seemed to us important, at first, to establish the effect of the drug on the individual patient in his normal ward environment, where he mixed with and was exposed to the often provocative behaviour of untreated overactive patients. Also, rather than use matched groups, we have used the patient as his own control, and alternated the active with the inactive preparation. There is a good deal to be said for either method of conducting a clinical trial; nevertheless the somewhat smaller group made possible by the self-controlled design permitted the frequent, continuous, and independent observation of the material on on which the assessment hinged.

In our experience the effects of chlorpromazine usually did not become fully apparent until after three to six weeks of continuous medication (at or around the level of 150 mg a day). The results were not dramatic, but were often subtle and not fully appreciated until after the effect of the drug had worn off (either following substitution by placebo or discontinuation at the end of the trial). They do, however, warrant further study. Statistical analyses of our small numbers in terms of diagnostic category, mean age, and length of hospitalization are hazardous. Nevertheless, we can but remark that, with the exception of one patient who had undergone leucotomy (Case 24), all cases in the affective group responded either definitely of slightly in terms of our criteria, whereas the unimproved group included five schizophrenics out of a total of thirteen, and the only three cases of senile dementia in the trial. A relatively young schizophrenic, however (Case 3), showed definite improvement, although two others of about the same age (Cases 25 and 26) did not.

The essentially symptomatic nature of the response has already been stressed, and cannot be overemphasized. Although affect became more subdued, and attitude and behaviour reflected this improvement, the ingrained psychotic thought disorder seemed to be unchanged. The patients in the definitely and slightly improved groups became quieter and more amenable to suggestion and guidance by the nursing staff, and could carry out simple ward tasks with some degree of enjoyment. None required extra sedation when on chlorpromazine. In two cases relatives spontaneously remarked upon the patients' improvement. Three were considered fit for parole, though none were thought fit for discharge. The reply to the question whether the drug may be useful in te management of the chronically overactive psychotic would thus appear to be a qualified "yes".

A further point of interest was the increase in weight of nine patients. All belonged to the definitely or slightly improved group. For the present we are inclined to attribute this to improved eating habit as the patients became less tense, less preoccupied, or less assaultive; though more direct metabolic effects of the drug cannot be excluded.

In terms of reduction of overactivity, our results are broadly in keeping with those reported from the Continent (Delay, Deniker and Harl 1952a,b; Delay, Deniker, Harl, and Grasset 1952; Delay and Deniker 1952), though the more chronic nature of our material makes detailed comparison somewhat difficult. The transient and partial response in chronic schizophrenics has been commented on (Lehmann and Hanrahan 1954). The response in Case 48, reported in another paper (Sigwald and Bouttier 1953), in which "there was no disappearance of hallucinations, but the interpretation became less acute and there was no longer any complaint of menace or revenge", certainly calls to mind our own experience in Cases 1 and 3.[*] The calming effect in manic-depressive disorders has also been observed by others (Staehelin and Kielholz 1953, Lehmann and Hanrahan 1954). More recently, in this country, the effect of chlorpromazine in chronic schizophrenics has been examined by J. Carse and D. W. Kay (personal communication), with whom we have exchanged information throughout the conduct of our own trial. In a controlled „blind" trial they used 62 patients, one group of which (32 patients) received chlorpromazine and another (30 patients) a placebo over five weeks. These authors conclude that there was improvement, significant at the 5% level, in the chlorpromazine-treated group, as compared with the group receiving control tablets, and that „there was a case for further investigation." In view of the chronic nature of both their material and ours, it should certainly be of interest to examine the effect of full doses of the drug (used both alone and in one-by-one combination with other drugs) in cases of recent psychotic illness. A systematic trial in neurotic tension states is also called for, and the effect on eating habit would suggest trial in anorexia nervosa.

Perhaps we may be allowed to draw attention to one last point – namely, the lessons we feel we have learnt from the trial itself. The research instrument in a trial of this sort being a group of people, and its conduct being inseparable from the individual use of words, we were impressed by the necessity for a "blind" and self-controlled design, and independent multiple documentation. Furthermore, we were equally impressed by the false picture apt to be conveyed if undue reliance was placed on interview alone, as conducted in the clinic room. The patients' behaviour in the ward was apt to be very different. For that reason the day and night nursing staff became indispensable and valued members of the observers' team. We were warmed and encouraged by the energy and care with which they did what was requested of them, provided this was clearly and simply set out at the beginning. A chronic "back" ward thus became a rather interesting place to work in. There may well be a case for training senior nursing staff in elementary research method and in medical documentation. This would make

---

[*] Since submitting this paper for publication we have seen the paper by D. Anton-Stephens (J. ment. Sci. 1954, 100, 543). The "psychic indifference" cited by this author is in keeping with our own observations.

for increased interest, increased attention to, and respect for, detail, and the availability of a fund of information, all too often lost because hit has not been asked for.

As the present trial was half-way completed, Professor Hogben was good enough to show us the manuscript of his joint paper (Hogben and Sim 1953), which has since appeared. This account of a simple experiment in human pharmacology admirably summarizes all salient features of this type of trial, and we commend it to all interested.

Summary

The effect of chlorpromazine was studied in 27 chronic agitated psychotic patients. Of these, 13 were schizophrenics, 11 belonged to the affective group, and 3 to the senile group. The patients were used as their own controls, chlorpromazine and identical inert placebo tablets being alternated in the same patient over varying periods. Records were kept independently by the medical and day and night nursing staff. The code of the trial was known to only one of those taking part in it, and assessment was based on the retrospective examination of the records of each patient.

Seven patients were considered definitely and 11 slightly improved. Improvement often did not become apparent until after three to six weeks of continuous medication (at or around the level of 150 mg a day). The affective group appeared to respond slightly better than the schizophrenics. The patients became quieter, less tense, and less disturbed by their hallucinations and delusions, and more amenable to the suggestions and care of the nursing staff. Three patients were thought fit for parole, though none were thought fit for discharge.

Nine patients showed an increase in weight ranging from 11 to 34 lb. (5 to 15.4 kg) in 22 weeks. All were members of the definitely or slightly improved group. This increase probably reflects improved eating habit.

One case developed transient jaundice, and two cases showed slight and transient blood changes. Apart from this, the drug appeared to be tolerated well in the dosage ultimately adopted (150 mg a day). None of the patients required extra sedation when on chlorpromazine.

It is concluded that this drug may have its place in the management of the chronically overactive psychotic patient, and that controlled trial in other psychiatric conditions is called for.

We wish to express our thanks to Dr. J.J. O'Reilly, physician-superintendent of Winson Green Hospital, for facilities generously put at our disposal at that hospital; to Drs. A.B. Hegarty, P.M. Jeavons, E. Jacoby, and C. MacDermott, and the day and night nursing staff of the hospital for taking part in the assessment of results; to Dr. W.R. Thrower, of Messrs. May and Baker, Ltd., for advice and a liberal supply of chlorpromazine and placebo tablets; and to the Birmingham Regional Hospital Board and the United Birmingham Hospitals Endowment Fund for financial support.

REFERENCES

Brand, B. D., Harris, T. D., Borison, H. L. and Goodman, L. S. (1954) J. Pharmacol., 110, 86.
Courvoisier, S., Fournel, J., Ductot, R., Koisky, M., and Koetschel, P. (1953), Arch. Int. Pharmaco dyn., 52. 305.

Delay, J. and Deniker, P. (1953) Therapie, 8, 347

Delay, J. and Hart, J. M. (1952a) Ann. Médico-psychol., 110, 112.

Delay, J. and Hart, J. M. (1952b) Ibid. 110, 267.

Hogben, L., and Sim, M. (1953) Brit. J. prev. Soc. Med., 7. 163.

Laborit, H., and Huguenard, P. (1951). Presse méd., 59. 1329.

Laborit, H. and Jaulmes, C. (1952). Toulouse méd., 53. 821.

Lehmann, H. E. and Hanrahan, G. E. (1954). Arch. Neurol. Psychiat. Chicago, 71, 227.

Sigwald, J. and Bouttier, D. (1953). Ann. Méd., 54. 150.

Staehelin, J. E., and Kielholz, P. (1953). Schweiz. Med. Wschr. 83. 581.

Part Four

REVIEWS

PAPERS

13. J. Elkes: *Psychopharmacology: The need for some points of reference.*
Reprinted with the kind permission of Charles C. Thomas Publisher from R. M. Feather-stone and A. Simon (eds.), *Pharmacological Approach to the Study of the Mind* (pp. 26–37). Springfield, Charles C. Thomas Publisher Ltd., 1960

14. J. Elkes: *Drugs influencing affect and behavior: Possible neural correlates in relation to mode of action.*
Reprinted with the kind permission of Charles C. Thomas Publisher from A. Simon, C.C. Herbert and R. Strauss (eds.) *The Physiology of Emotions* (pp. 95–150). Springfield, Charles C. Thomas Publisher Ltd., 1961

15. J. Elkes: *Behavioral pharmacology in relation to psychiatry.*
Reprinted with the kind permission of Springer Verlag from H.W. Gruhle, R. Jung, W. Mayer-Gross and M. Muller (eds.) *Psychiatrie der Gegenwart* (pp. 929–1038). Berlin/Heidelberg/New York, Springer Verlag, 1967

ARGUMENT

These three papers engage in more detail in the area of functional neuroanatomy, electro-physiology, neurochemistry, animal behavior, and the clinical trial, as they emerged to Elkes as footings of an evolving science of psychopharmacology. They converge on a plea for a deeper understanding of regional process in the brain as it subserves its integrative function (Paper 14 – 1961). Paper 14 also contains references to synaptically active amino acids, and the interaction between neurotransmitters and hormones.

The length of Paper 15 (1967), and its 500 references, reflect Elkes' attempt to represent the scope of the field, as it appeared to him in 1966. It examines, in some detail, the four foot-ings of a science of psychopharmacology: functional neuroanatomy, electrophysiology, ani-mal behavior and the human experiment and clinical trial. Seymour Kety, at the time Director of the Laboratory Clinical Science, at the National Institute of Mental Health (USA), and Joel Elkes were responsible for the Fourth International Neurochemical Symposium, held in Varenna, Italy, in June 1960. The theme was "Regional Neurochemistry". The *Proceedings* of this Symposium were published by Pergamon Press, Oxford, in 1961.

PAPER 13

PSYCHOPHARMACOLOGY: THE NEED FOR SOME POINTS OF REFERENCE*

Joel Elkes

Reprinted with the kind permission of Charles C. Thomas Publisher
from R.M. Featherstone and A. Simon (eds.), *Pharmacological Approach to the Study of the Mind* (pp. 26–37). Springfield, Charles C. Thomas Publisher Ltd., 1960

It is difficult to know where to begin within the wide span of the topic assigned to me by the Program Committee. To be sure, the roots of our latter-day-subject go deep; and it may, perhaps, be appropriate to begin by inquiring, very briefly, why a field so well known, and so deeply embedded in the culture of the race should have been shrouded in silence for so long, and why Western science should have quickened to its present interest only in the middle of the twentieth century. To say that two empirical findings in the late forties – the discovery of the psychosomimetic effects of LSD-25, and of the tranquilizing powers of some of the phenothiazines – should, in themselves have initiated the current period in psychiatry would, at best, be only a partial answer; the reasons for this delay go deeper, and into the very substance of the subject. Among these, thought has to be given to the essentially subjective and personal nature of the phenomena induced by psychotropic drugs in man, and the setting in which they were originally observed; their affinity with other subjective phenomena, studied by Western science; the relation of both to the development of the experimental behavioural disciplines; and to the recent growth of cognate basic neurological sciences. It is these which make up the climate of the subject, and it is their interplay which may well have made for its delay, and is now making for its growth.

At a time the clinician is assailed by an ever changing array of new compounds, it is well to remember that markedly psychotropic effects were first observed in a religious ceremonial setting where the drugs (such as, for example, mescal) formed a cardinal part of a local culture; that some elements in these drugs induced states made them particularly suitable for the purposes for which they were being used; and that, in some central and essential characteristics, these elements were strongly personal, subjective, averbal and incommunicable. All observers who, since Lewin's (1) and Hoffmann's (2) original discoveries, have used mescaline and LSD25 on themselves, or on others, agree that the most important areas of disturbed function lie in the affective:, perceptual, and cognitive fields; that alteration in overt behavior need

---

* The first part of this paper includes material originally presented in Working Paper No. 1, Study Group on Ataractic and Hallucinogenic Drugs, World Health Organisation, Geneva 1957. It was subsequently incorporated in the Report of the Group (WHO, Technical Report No. 152) and reproduced in this paper with the permission of the Chief Editor, Technical Publications, WHO, Geneva, in 1961, and with the kind permission of Information Management and Dissemination, WHO, Geneva, in 2001..

not necessarily accompany striking subjective change, and if it does, can form only the crudest counterpart of the subjective experience. Equally, the intensity, variation, speed, and fluctuating, kaleidoscopic play of the phenomena is such as to defy ordinary language. The mere act of description may, in fact, alter the phenomena. Thus even the most dispassionate and objective observers are compelled in their protocol to resort to simile and allusion in an. attempt to describe what is, by common consent, outside the range of normal human experience. But even in more homely examples, the same difficulties apply. A great deal, for instance, has been written on the so-called tranquillisers; we all know that they "quiet" the "disturbed." But how much, or how little; do we know of the meaning, or the shades of meaning of this chemically induced tranquillity to the individual patient, or the normal individual, in whom dose range alone suggests the effects may be quite different? Again, it is one thing to observe a Parkinsonian syndrome in the course of reserpine therapy; it is a totally different matter to inquire into the mental state of the patient at the same time and discover (or attempt to measure) the affective and perceptual changes inseparable from this state. In all psychotropic drug effects, therefore, overt behaviour, including the ordinary currency of language., can be but a segment of the evidence; the larger portion lies within, and requires special and in many ways novel techniques for its adequate description, let alone understanding.

The above remarks may indicate one group of reasons for the isolation and the lag of this field despite its long recognised existence. The phenomena were first observed in culturally remote regions, and were of a nature which, in the first instance, was inclined to appeal more to the cultural anthropologist and the student of comparative religion than to the psychologist or physician; they were strongly subjective, and were reflected only very inadequately in overt behaviour; they contained central elements which, being well outside the range of normal conscious observation, were very difficult to describe without the fashioning of special linguistic tools; and by their similarity with some varieties of religious experience moved on to ground which nineteenth century science was reluctant to enter. In the human psychological sciences we are only gradually recovering from the limitations of the purely behavioural method: we do so by recognising what it can describe and measure, and what, so far, it cannot. In the area under discussion the behavioural approach is self-limiting, and one which loses information. On the other hand, such information as is accessible to subjective inquiry is apt to be descriptive, anecdotal, and, in the absence of adequate calibration, very difficult to measure. It is out of the discrepancies, dissatisfaction and tensions of this dilemma that new methods of inquiry into these highly subjective states arc likely to emerge. The territory of experience they are to survey and map is indeed large; and in this territory the clinical needs and states arc but a province.

It is perhaps not surprising that subjective phenomena such as these should have seemed strange fare to the scientific culture of the mid-nineteenth century. In a science preoccupied with the properties of solid matter, and not yet exposed to the loosening and expansion which, within a few decades, were to lead to the refashioning of physics, only the staunchest spirits would publicly acknowledge their interest in the subjective psychology of the individual, or attempt to define its phenomena, and its laws. Mentioned here may perhaps be Humphrey Davy's experiments with nitrous oxide; but one could also add in this context, Johannes von Müller's enquiries into the hypnagogic phenomena (3), or Galton's essays on the *Visions of Sane Persons* (4) or his *Statistics of Mental Imagery* (5) or William James' *Varieties of Religious Experience* (6); and it is perhaps well to compare Weir Mitchell's clear and concise account of mescaline intoxication (7), published in 1896, with Ladd's account of the so-called visual dreams, published four years earlier (8). The affinity then, between the phenomena of normal mental life and drug induced states was quite apparent even at this early stage. It seemed, even then, that certain functional modalities used transitorily, falteringly, and sparingly in the normal repertoire of human behavior and experience could, as it were, be locked, or modified, by the drugs into more persistent manifestations. Quite early thus, there seemed little doubt of. the enrichment which the study of chemically induced mental changes was likely to derive from a comparison with cognate phenomena outside the strictly chemical domain. Today's speculations on the relation of the Sensory Isolation Experience to the drug-induced experience thus raises familiar questions: questions which Sherrington (9) saw quite plainly, and which Freud, in one of his last masterly essays, posed with equal clarity (10). And with good reason. For the techniques of psychoanalysis and, most particularly, those of free association, and the analysis of transference, have familiarized the analyst, almost like no one else, with a range of manifestations not readily accessible to other methods, but having in common with the drug-induced phenomena already mentioned their central, subjective and private aspects, which at the most important phases of the analytic experience, may well the outside the range of the ordinary currency of language.

Related to these areas of human psychology, however, there is a further area, the uneven development of which may have contributed to the further isolation and alienation of our subject. Despite the revolutionary inventiveness of Pavlovian theory and method, the animal behavioral sciences were, to begin with, confined to the study of very simple modalities within strictly controlled and highly artificial laboratory situations. Much less emphasis was laid, in those initial stages, upon the cues in an animal's natural environment governing its behavior in the free state, or the forces operating in the organization of an animal community, or the evolution of response patterns with ontogenetic development. Yet all of these factors are important in assessing agents which, by common consent, not only affect perception or learning, but profoundly govern social attitudes within the species. The over-simplification of a problem thus tended to make the answers irrelevant to the larger questions which are now being posed. Yet, here too, things are changing. The operant conditioning techniques (11, 12), the self-stimulation studies, (both electrical and chemical – 13) linked to the anatomical and endocrinological studies are providing data on the basic steering mechanisms which govern appetitive or aversive behavior within the nervous system. And the great ethological schools (14, 15) are going a long way towards establishing strong and regular relationships between precepts in an animal's natural environment, and the affectively charged patterns of motor behavior which they elicit. The firmness and specificity of these innate release mechanisms (IRM) is truly astonishing, and would appear to be as firmly coded in a species as, for example, claws and plumage. These findings are sure to be linked with the pleasure and pain motivational systems before very long. Moreover, the factors making for hierarchical structure in an animal community are being defined, and the critical dependence of drug effects upon the precise social settings is becoming very apparent. Even so mundane a quantity as effective dose is related to numbers of a animals in the group in which a particular drug is being studied (16). Again, the plasticity of the nervous system during certain critical phases of its early development may be related to intense biochemical change during this period (17) and thus, perhaps, in time provide links with learning theory also. Slowly, thus, the animal behavioral sciences are breaking the constraint imposed upon them by an all too mannered design; and the contact and communication between them and empirical findings of the clinic is steadily increasing.

There is, a third area whose lag has been felt by the young subject we are here discussing; for, surprisingly, the Basic Neurological Sciences have only recently been able to assume their full share, and stature in relation to the development of a pharmacology of behavior. In a curious way, the areas in question lie at opposite extremes, being concerned, on the one hand, with the fine structure of subcellular building blocks of the nervous system; and, on the other, with the nature and properties of those systems making for integrative functioning within the nervous system as a whole. Techniques of electron microscopy and x-ray diffraction, micro-fluorimetric and spectrographic techniques, are defining the basic structural plan along which highly ordered protein and lipoprotein systems, so prevalent in the nervous system, are built; and are already going a long way towards establishing the macro-molecular organization of the active electrogenic sub-organs of the neurone concerned with synaptic transmission. The chemistry of the interneuronal proteins is being defined, and is yielding. The layer by layer geological map of the brain, in terms of its enzyme constitution is in the making, and the principle of the chemical *in*homogeneity and suborganization of the brain is clearly emerging as a universal in all such studies. Chemical gradients and differences, hitherto assumed on the basis of psychological experiment, are becoming apparent; and at a finer level of organization, a chemical topology at sub-cellular, macro-cellular level is now distinctly possible.

Parallel with this, however, and in a way at the other extreme, has been the increasing preoccupation of the Neurological Sciences with the nature and properties of those systems concerned with integration of function within the central nervous system, and subserving the states of consciousness, and the patterns of affective response. The apparatus of the hypothalamic nuclei, the intermediate cable systems and coding stations comprised by the Limbic System, and the complex system of systems gathered under the name Reticular Activating System have defined a wealth of anatomical, electrophysiological and behavioral data, and thus prepared the ground for chemical and pharmacological inquiry. In this the context, the existence, and differential and uneven distribution, of the catecholamines and indoles, and gamma amino butyric acid (18), and the enzymes concerned in their manufacture and disposal are but early examples. The existence of humoral factors, and the possible operation of chemical fields in the brain have also been postulated (19), and the existence of three types of processes (excitation, inhibition and modulation), depending on the interplay of three families of metabolites has been provisionally put forward (20, 21).

In taking stock, therefore, it would seem that three separate and related trends may have colluded in making for delay and isolation of the subject up to present. The essentially personal and subjective nature of the phenomena made for their isolation in an intellectual climate preoccupied with description and measurement in the physical and natural sciences; the animal and behavioral techniques were apt to center on conditions and situations only indirectly and partly applicable to the problems posed by the psychotropic drug effects in man; and the basic neurological sciences were ill-prepared to receive the wealth of essentially empirical findings coming from the clinic. They are still wanting; and it may, perhaps, be permissible to inquire where they are wanting, and where they promise most.

In the most obvious sense we lack the models of language to describe and measure those uniquely human phenomena which are our business; the linguistic tools remain crude and uncalibrated, and the assessment of the non-verbal element rudimentary. The outer shell of behavior can be described; there serviceable rating scales (some forty in number) are available. Some of these have stood the test of preliminary trial; yet their robustness, accuracy, reliability and economy in the very varied settings in which drugs are being used still remain to be established. They may tell us a great deal about the behavioral change in the patient; and if properly applied in a different context, about the environment in which he/she functions; their yield may be greatly increased by being coupled to modern data reduction procedures. But of those large behaviorally silent pools within, where so much happens with such uncanny speed, behavior rating scales, or schedules of reinforcement will tell us little. The value of introspective process is brought home by even the simplest experiment. Equally, anyone who has worked with drugs is aware of the highly personal equation which runs through each drug-induced experience, however mundane. For the same drug, in the same dose, in the same subject will lead to very different effects according to the events, which precede or accompany, or follow, a particular medication. It will be affected profoundly by the interpersonal and motivational situation in which it is given. Inherent in our linguistic model, therefore, there must be the vector of time; or of anticipatory or retrospective set, and of the matching and coding of what is actual, against the templates of the innate; they may go some way towards slowly defining the chemical parameters of psychodynamic process.

I now come to the second of our models, the animal behavioral model, in whose very concept lay both their high promise, and their most serious limitation. The outer shell of behavior can only go so far and no further, and, as was pointed out recently by Evarts (22), the same nuclear mental disturbance, be it chemically induced, be it idiopathic, may outwardly manifest a variety of behavioral patterns, which, though disparate and even opposed, may be related in the same central disturbance. Of the conditioned avoidance reaction, of enhanced or reduced conflict tolerance, of undue tameness, or aversive, or appetitive behavior, we see a great deal in the laboratory. This is the repertoire the animal organism plays in response to information, which has been grouped and polarized in terms of its appetitive or aversive connotation; but how little do we know of an animal's serial ordering of behavior in time, of the sequental organization, on a priority basis of simultaneously presented stimuli; or of the cues in an animal's natural environment, which lead to inhibition, or storage, or release of those patterns with which laboratory conditions have made us all too familiar. Yet it is this central coding and ordering and arrangement of information, in a formal and technical sense, which would appear most significantly, affected by the psychotropic drugs. To rely on the several behavioral syndromes therefore may not be enough. New tests are needed, and may well group the drugs in quite novel and unexpectedly meaningful ways.

The third neural and biochemical model is one now in the process of being fashioned, and has been admirably covered by the previous speakers. It, too, has its history, as readers of Campion and Elliot Smith's, *Neural Basis of Thought* (23, published in 1934) are apt to discover. The neuroanatomical basis of the great steering mechanism is being defined, and the three great systems – the Hypothalamic, the Limbic and the Reticular Activating Systems – are already beginning to resolve into individual functional components. Corticofugal, as well as corticopetal influences are becoming apparent, and the enigma of the Caudate, Striatal and Lenticular masses is at long last being explored through the drug-induced extrapyramidal motor disorders.

Yet, superimposed upon the anatomical and cytological map, there now steadily emerges a chemical map, not only in terms of the differential distribution of components, and the appropriate enzyme systems, but in terms, also, of differential development. A concept of *regional* and *local* economy in some areas is emerging, and tracer studies with selected metabolites are steadily adding to this view. Two questions, related to each other, are, however, linked to these concepts. The first is the adequacy of the concept of the blood-brain barrier as a general membrane equilibrium, maintaining identical gradients at any point between plasma and the extracellular fluid of nervous tissue: this may not necessarily be so, some areas of the brain (for example, the hypothalamus) being more permeable to some metabolites of systemic origin, or possibly allowing the transfer of a few special metabolites from selected sites into the systemic circulation. To the concepts of a general blood-brain barrier, one may this be compelled to add the possibility of *local* differences and gradients; differences not only determined by the polar and other physicochemical characteristics of the molecules concerned, but also by considerations of vascular patterns, and differential small vessel and capillary tone, so notoriously susceptible to local conditions. We may have to think of brain-brain barriers, as well as blood-brain barriers: and seriously weight the possibility of whether, while the synthesis, function and fate of some modules may be a strictly local and intracerebral event, others, of analogues configuration, may be able to cross the barrier and modulate intracerebral and peripheral events in relation to each other. The roles of hormones in regulating such strictly local transfers, and the possible release of neurohumoral substances from their unknown anchoring surface, is still very much an open question: yet it is evident that minute quantities of hormones locally applied to the hypothalamus in critical concentrations can, and do, release patterns of behavior (24), though the biochemical correlates of such observations are totally lacking.

Linked to this question there is the second question to which both previous speakers have already alluded. This is the relationship of systemic biochemical events to events within the central nervous system and the accuracy with which such peripheral biochemical indicators may reflect what, possibly, are quite local intracerebral events. Naturally, data in this respect can be more readily obtained in the animal experiment than in the human situation, though even here radioactive tracer techniques can be of value. It is, perhaps, not too much to hope that the sustained study of the effects of a few selected drugs on endocrine and biochemical responses in the individual patients over long periods may, in time, contribute to a definition of prognostic indicators in the choice of individual drugs for particular syndromes. Furthermore, it is equally possible that drugs, discriminately used, may lead to the recognition of pharmacological and biochemical cleavage planes between syndromes bearing a superficial clinical resemblance, and thus contribute to a clearer and more rigorous classification of the phenomena of mental disorder than has been possible on clinical grounds alone. Such responses linked to genetic factors may be particularly relevant in this context.

There remains one other (and, I suppose, an ultimate) model of whose advent into the field I personally have not doubt. The ability to recognize relationships in time, is the essential function of mathematics; and if mathematics and information theory have hesitated on the edge of the behavioral and the physiological sciences for so long, it is, perhaps, because, with certain notable exceptions, they have never really been tempered against the precise requirements of the physiological experiment. The intellectual history of such distance and alienation is common enough; yet the history of physics suggests, in some measure, that sooner or later such isolation is broken; and that as experiments become more precise, their conceptual, mathematical models become more feasible, possible, and productive. Cybernetic theory, although drawing heavily on biological models, has nor returned to the parent science what it drew from it. The climate, however, is now changing slowly and unmistakably. The time vector and the probability of events in time are invading theories of perception and of learning, just as they did the physical sciences of a century ago. Moreover, the essentially random nature of the assembly of units making up an information carrying system, or of systems capable of adaptation in the face of change, is receiving steadily increasing recognition. The "wiring" theories of old are giving place to less rigid, more statistical and, yet apparently, more correct models. Information theory has so far only tenuously interacted with genetics or immunochemistry, where its implications are obvious. In the central nervous system it has proved particularly valuable in the understanding of the coding process along sensory pathways (25, 26), and very gradually the theoretical framework is being expanded to accept and manipulate data in other areas, such as the process of recognition of universals in language, and cognate secondary signalling systems. It would therefore seem advisable to give early thought to the bringing of mathematical talent into the physiological and neurochemical, as well as the psychological laboratory; and to exposing individuals so endowed to data at the bench level. It may perhaps be not too much to hope that concepts only partly and inadequately covered by the linguistic tools now employed will find their precise and compact mathematical expression through such a process of mutual exposure. The concept of the nervous system as a chemically mediated organ of information may thus be made a little more real. For unless we understand the code and cipher in which the brain constructs and stores, silently and with uncanny speed, its models of reality, and the distortion of this coding, by controlled chemical means, we will, whatever language we choose to employ, and whatever chemical aspect we wish to follow, be standing outside the phenomena: our language will be descriptive, and do justice merely to some properties of the process, rather than the process itself. Yet a careful contemplation of the clinical phenomena plainly makes demands higher than this; and whether we like it or not, we shall be faced with these demands in the light of the very experiments which clinical observations compel.

REFERENCES

1. Lewin, L.: Phantastica, narcotic and stimulating drugs: Their use and abuse. New York, Dutton 1931.
2. Stoll, W.A.: LSD, ein Phantasticum aus der Muttterkorngruppe. Schweiz. Arch. Neurol. Psychiat., 60:279-323 1947.
3. Müller, J.V.: Physiology of the senses. Voice and muscular motion and the mental faculties (Müller's Elements of Physiology, and supplement). London, Taylor, Walton & Maberly, 1848.
4. Galton, F.: The visions of sane persons (from Fortnightly Review), Pop. Sci. Month., New York, 29:519-531, 1881.
5. Galton, F.: Statistics of mental imagery. Mind, 5:301-318,1880.
6. James, W.: The varieties of religious experience: A study in human nature. (Gifford Lectures on Natural Religion 1901-02), New York, Longmans 1928.
7. Mitchell, S.W.: Remarks on the effects of anhelonium lewinii. (The Mescal Button), Brit. M. J., 2:1625-1629, 1896.
8. Ladd, G.T.: Contributions to the psychology of visual dreams. Mind (new series), 1:299-304, 1892.
9. Sherrington, C.S.: Man on his nature (Gifford Lectures 1937-8). New York, MacMillan 1941.
10. Freud, S.: An outline of psychoanalysis. New York, Norton 1949.
11. Skinner, B.F.: Am. Psychol., 8:69 1953.
12. Hunt, H.: Some effects of drugs on classical (Type S) conditioning. Ann. N. Y. Acad. Sc., 65:258-267 1956.
13. Olds, J.: Selective effects of drives and drugs in "Reward" systems of the brain. Ciba Foundation. Neurological Basis of Behavior. London 1958, pp. 124-148.
14. Lorenz, K.Z.: The comparative methods in studying innate behaiour patterns. Physiological Mechanisms in Animal Behaviour. London, Cambridge Univ. Press 1950. Pp. 221-268.
15. Tinbergen, N.: The hierarchical organization of nervous mechanisms underlying instinctive behaviour. London, Cambridge Univ. Press 1950. Pp. 305-312.
16. Chance, M.R.A.: Factors influencing toxicity of sympathomimetic amines in solitary mice. J. Pharmacol & Exp. Therap., 89:289-296, 1947.
17. Waelsch, H. (ed.): Biochemistry of the developing nervous system. New York, Academic Press 1955.

18. Roberts, E., Harman, P.J. and Frankel, S.: γ-aminobutyric acid content and glutamic decarboxylate activity in developing mouse brain. Proc. Soc. Exp. Biol. & Med., 78:799-803 1951.

19. Elkes, J.: Effect of psychosomimetic drugs in animals and in man, in Abramson, H. A., Ed., Neuropharmacology. Trasactions of Third Conference. New York, Josiah Macy, Jr. Fnd. 1957, pp. 205-296.

20. Bradley, P.B. and Elkes, J.: The effect of some drugs on the electrical activity of the brain. Brain, 80:77-117 1957.

21. Elkes, J.: Drug effects in relation to receptor specificity within the brain: Some evidence and provisional formulation. Ciba Foundation Symposium on Neurological Basis of Behaviour, London 1958. Pp. 303-332.

22. Evarts, E.V.: A discussion of the relevance of effects of drugs on animal behavior to the possible effects of drugs on psychopathological processes in man. In press 1959.

23. Campion, G.G. and Smith, Elliot: The neural basis of thought. London 1934.

24. Harris, G.W., Michael, R.P. and Scott, P.P.: Neurological site of action of stilbestrol in eliciting sexual behaviour. Ciba Foundation Symposium on Neurological Basis of Behavior, London 1958. Pp. 236-257.

25. Galambos, R. and Davis, H.: The response of single auditory nerve fibres to acoustic stimulation. J. Neurophysiol., 6:3957 1943.

26. Allanson, J.T. and Whitfield, I.C. In: Cherry, C. Ed.: Third London Symposium on Information Theory. The Cochlear Nucleus and its Relation to Theories of Hearing. London, Butterworth 1956. p. 269.

PAPER 14

DRUGS INFLUENCING AFFECT AND BEHAVIOR: POSSIBLE NEURAL CORRELATES IN RELATION TO MODE OF ACTION*

Joel Elkes

Reprinted with the kind permission of Charles C. Thomas Publisher
from A. Simon, C.C. Herbert and R. Strauss (eds.) *The Physiology of Emotions* (pp. 95–150).
Springfield, Charles C. Thomas Publisher Ltd., 1961

> *"It is interesting to notice that the different nervous centres of the body manifest elective affinities for particular poisons... That medicinal substances do display these elective affinities is a proof, at any rate, that there are important intimate differences in the constitution or composition of the different nervous centres, notwithstanding that we are unable to detect the nature of them; and it may be we have in these different effects of poisons on the nervous system the promise of a useful means of investigation into the constitution of the latter."*
> *(1)*

It is curios, yet in keeping with all we know of him, how this passage, written by Henry Maudsley nearly one hundred years ago should set the theme of much that is new and fresh in the pharmacology of the brain and of behavior – a subject which, by way of uneasy travail, is slowly transforming a terrain of empirical natural history into the growing edge of a new science. It does so by resolving more and more into the disciplines which compound it; and equally, by compelling, as does no other branch of the neurological sciences, a fusion of these various disciplines. It ranges from behavior, including the swift nonverbal transactions of thought, to the neural substrate of behavior. This, indeed, is a wide span. Yet it is the steady extension of the subject to the limits of its cognate disciplines which, already, is leading to the evolution of a pharmacology of behavior of total organisms very different from a pharmacology preoccupied with the behavior of tissues and organs. In these advances – empirical and experimental – the action of drugs on the affective systems has taken pride of place. Man's feeling states obtrude themselves incessantly in his social transactions, and have consistently compelled a seeking out of means for their attenuation or enhancement (1) or change. The tranquilizers and stimulants are as old as alcohol and opium, tea or coffee. Familiarity, however, has blunted our curiosity about these old established remedies; and many excellent re-

---

* In: The Physiology of Emotions. Report of the Third Annual Symposium of the Kaiser Foundation Hospitals in Northern California, San Francisco

views already cover the agents, which have come down to us in recent years in empirical profusion (2–6). It is therefore the limited purpose of this paper to examine some correlates of the action of psychotropic drugs which may bear upon their influence on the affect systems and which – to borrow Maudsley's phrase – may perhaps shadow out some trends for future enquiry. These correlates will be considered at the neuroanatomical, electrophysiological, and neurohumoral levels.

I. NEUROANATOMICAL CONSIDERATIONS:
THE SUBORGANIZATION, INTERCONNECTEDNESS AND MUTUAL
OCCLUSIVENESS OF THE SYSTEMS SUBSERVING AFFECTIVE BEHAVIOR

The steady shift in emphasis from the form and function of the cerebral cortex to a mounting emphasis on subcortical centers has singled out three, or perhaps four, systems which, as emphasized by other speakers (7), by mutual interplay steer the patterns of affective behavior in the discharge of their adaptive, homeostatic functions. The system in question are the hypothalamus, the reticular activating system, and the rhinencephalic formation; with perhaps a fourth group, the caudate and lentiform masses (the so called "corpus striatum") now moving into focus also. Each of these has received its share of extensive review (8–15) but in the case of each, cumulative experience with a variety of techniques has steadily emphasized three separate, though related, trends. The first is the discrete neuroanatomical and cytological suborganization of these systems; the second, the interconnectedness of elements within these systems with each other, and with relatively distant elements at high cortical and high spinal level; and the third, the reciprocal, complementary, yet mutually occlusive relationship which some patterns bear to each other. These trends may be relevant when considered against the action and the mode of action of drugs on these systems.

There is little doubt in the light of even older studies of the anatomical inhomogeneity and cytological differentiation of the hypothalamus (8–10). Similarly, more recent studies have emphasized a remarkable anatomical and cytoarchitectonic (16, 17) differentiation within the reticular activating system (18) where, as Olszewski put it "the variety of cells found within a few cubic centimeters of the mesencephalon is greater than in any other part of the central nervous system" (10). The elements entering into the paleocortical and subcortical structures which comprise the so-called "limbic system" (13), show similar differentiation. Each of the systems thus encompasses a mosaic of subsystems, which, in a manner only poorly understood at present, are related and fitted into each other.

This understanding, however, is being steadily enhanced by the connections now being established between the various subsystems, and between them and various regions of the cortex. These connections are reticulofugal as well as reticulopetal, corticofugal as well as corticopetal. Rich connections have been shown to exist between a widespread area in the mesencephalom, and the hypothalamus (20). These projections originate in the ventral part of the periaqueductal grey substance, including Gudden's dorsal tegmental nucleus, and the paramedian and medial tegmental cell groups. They extend to the hypothalamus by way of the dorsal longitudinal fasciculus of Schutz (wich terminates in the periventricular region of the hypothalamus) and the system of the mammillary peduncle (which though feeding principally into the mamillary body, also projects to the lateral hypothalamus, as well to the preoptic and septal regions). The lower midbrain, so richly exposed to nonspecific ascending afferent influences, is thus put into a dicert connection with areas bearing upon endocrine and autonomic regulation. It is, incidentally, also of interest that direct projections from the more rostral midbrain tegmentum travel to the caudate and lentiform nuclei. The story of these latter structures, and their relation to behavior, remains to be written.

The above pathways, connecting the midbrain with the hypothalamus however, find their descending counterpart in the rich and varied connections of the limbic system to the midbrain. Their description forms a landmark on the subject (21). The projections are both direct and indirect. The direct hippocampomesencephalic projections distribute only to the rostral part of the central grey substance. The indirect hippocampal pathways "in part interrupted by further relays, and probably also representing indirect projections of the amygdaloid complex, originate in the septum and in the lateral preoptic and hypothalamic regions, as well as in the mammillary body. Such pathways reach the midbrain in three fibre systems, viz., the medial forebrain bundle, the fasciculus retroflexus, and the mammillo-tegmental tract. Each of these three bundles has a dual distribution in the midbrain: part of their fibres terminate in extensive central lateral regions of the tegmentum, while the remaining component distributes to various subdivisions of a paramedian midbrain region encompassing the ventral part of the central grey substance, Tsai's ventral tegmental region, interpeduncular nucleus, Bechterew's centralis tegmenti superior, and Gudden's dorsal and deep tegmental nuclei." (22)

Three points emerge from the above studies. First, they demonstrate a striking and reciprocal two-way apposition of the connections linking the limbic forebrain structures with midline areas in the midbrain, the arrangement amply justifies the term "limbic system midbrain circuit" (21), introduced to describe this two-way path. Secondly, it is well to note the inordinately widespread efferent routes emanating from this system. These "escape pathways" (21) over and above the closed loops already mentioned, include projections to the medial hypothalamic region, to the anterior and intralaminar nuclei of the thalamus, as well as the diffuse ascending and descending conduction systems of the midbrain tegmentum. Thirdly, the septal and lateral preoptic regions and the medial hypothalamus would appear to be specially placed in this intricate reciprocal arrangement. Both are nodal areas, for the septal area shares primary projections from the hippocampus and the amygdala, and projects on to the midbrain by way of the medial forebrain bundle and, less directly, by way of the stria medullaris,, the habenula, and the fasciculus retroflexus. The medial hypothalamic region receives (downward) fibres from the limbic forebrain structures via the stria terminalis as well as the bundle of Schutz. Short fibres from the same circuit probably connect with the supraoptic nucleus of the hypothalamus. Thus, on anatomical grounds alone, the septal and hypothalamic regions are in a peculiarly favorable position to balance and translate influences within the limbic-midbrain circuits into endocrine and visceromotor responses. The suborganization of the paleocortical structures (12–14, 23), their differential responsiveness (in terms of latency) following electrical stimulation of the amygdala (24), and their role in behavioral motivation have been recently fully reviewed (25, 26). Here, again one is impressed by the richness of the afferent connections of the limbic-midbrain system and the limited, fast, cable-like efferent connections which it forms with the midline areas known to mediate affectively charged motor responses. In a way yet poorly understood this system would appear to be intermediate between the discrete analysis of diverse signals at "high" level and the discharge of the limited, genetically coded, stereotype responses known as affective behavior. It appears to participate in both, and to modulate the wide range of one against the limited repertoire of the other. It is possible that this limbic-midbrain circuit may play a part in the several simultaneous transactions concerned with the apposition and matching of new information against motivationally charged stored patterns; in determining the positive (appetitive) or negative(aversive) connotation of a given stimulus situation; and in mediating the discharge of the most appropriate affective responses. The speed at which these transactions occur must presumably be very high.

There is, however, a third feature which characterizes the organization of the deeply ingrained, genetically coded response patterns which participate in the operation of the motivational systems. This is their reciprocal, mutual occlusiveness, despite a close juxtaposition of cell assemblies which subserve and selectively release them. That this is a fairly general principle is apparent in the older findings on the distribution of the cell groups subserving temperature control in the diencephalon (27), where the opposing modalities of heat loss (vasodilatation and increases respiration) and heat conservation (vasoconstriction, release of epinephrine) appeared to be regulated by an interplay between elements situated within a short distance of each other. The central neural regulation of food intake shows a similar pattern. The demonstration of "appetite" and "satiety" centers within the hypothalamus (28) suggests the existence of closely related mechanisms for the initiation and for the suspension of eating behavior, and a mutually appropriate interlocking of these two mechanisms. It the areas of motor activity and patterns of emotional expression, a series of major and now classical stimulation studies (29) has defined the so-called "ergotropic" areas, concerned with increased motor excitability, activation of respiration, rise of blood pressure and pulse rate. These have been contrasted with the so-called "trophotropic" areas leading to inhibition of motor activity, diminution of muscle tone, slowing of respiration, and fall in blood pressure. Whereas the former are principally distributed in a relatively broad area of the posterior subthalamus, posterior hypothalamus, and anterior midbrain, the latter is more likely to be encountered in the anterior hypothalamic field, and an area between the habenulointerpeduncular tract and the mammillothalamic bundle. The same studies also drew attention to the predominantly sympathetic autonomic responses associated with stimulation of the ergotropic areas, and the predominantly parasympathetic responses elicited by stimulation of the trophotropic areas. Yet caution has to be exercised in an unqualified acceptance of this distribution. The parameters of electrical stimulation are important and in certain instances (such as lower frequencies of stimulation) may, for example, elicit parasympathetic effects in the posterior (ergotropic) areas of the hypothalamus (30), or elicit both parasympathetic and sympathetic discharge (31) upon stimulation of an area. The recent extension of these stimulation studies to self-stimulation techniques (32) has further contributed toward a broad topography of the so-called "motivational systems." In the rat, the positive motivational systems (33) include most of the rhinencephalic cortex as well as part of the thalamus, tegmentum, and basal hypothalamus. The negative motivational system is far smaller. It invades the subthalamus and the dorsal hypothalamus, and its relationship to the recognized pain systems is far from clear. It is difficult at present to assess the full physiological meaning, of these far reaching studies. Their important implications, though recently considered (34), require further step-by-step enquiry. They do, however, suggest a broad binary grouping of the patterns of affective behavior, and also the possibility of a discrete suborganization of other patterns within this double frame of reference. Discrete stimulation studies (35, 38) have demonstrated the fractionation of such patterns, and the remarkable way in which one "bit" of behavior can be selected and made to manifest out of context with the program of behavior of which it is part. It is obvious that to serve the adaptive purposes for which they were presumably intended, these various subsystems must be guided in their comprehensive performance by further integrating systems. These have been sought particularly at the paleocortical level, whose contribution to the control of motivational systems has recently received comprehensive review (25, 26). The cumulative evidence is in places contradictory. Yet it strongly suggests that elements in the limbic system can both restrain and activate the patterns of discharge associated with affective behavior. Mentioned here may be the early and lucid studies on the influence of temporal lobe deficits on emotional behavior in monkeys (37), these studies included lesions in the fronto-temporal cortex, the pyriform lobe, the amygdaloid complex, the presubiculum and the hippocampus. Equally important were the ablation studies in the cat (38) which furnished strong suggestive evidence of the role of the amygdaloid complex or the cingulate gyrus, or both, in restraining gross affective discharge in the neodecorticate preparation. In these, as in subsequent series (39, 40) species differences loomed large. They did, however, stress the modulating function of discrete and highly localized areas in the rhinencephalic formation on the patterns of emotional expression and, moreover, drew attention to the association of some areas with the discharge of broadly pleasurable responses.

Recent studies in which chemical stimulation (by means of locally applied crystals of carbaminoylcholine) was substituted for electrical stimulation (41) have particularly emphasized this aspect. These demonstrated a high incidence of enhanced pleasure and grooming reactions following the induction of discharges from the hippocampus, as against a low incidence following chemical stimulation in other regions. Taken in conjunction with the anatomical evidence cited above it is possible to subsume, in a tentative and far from satisfying way, the existence of two systems concerned respectively with pleasurable or aversive behavior. What, however, has to be constantly borne in mind is the remarkable balance between excitation and inhibition, tonic restraint and release, which operates in these delicate and swiftly changing equilibria. It is difficult to speak of diffuse influences in systems which sweep and in places overlap and interlock with one another in this remarkable way. Overactivity and underactivity, attack or avoidance, "pleasure", or "fear", or "indifference" may apparently play and flow into each other according to delicate shifts in balance in certain nodal cell groups. The septal region, the median eminence of the hypothalamus, the periaqueductal grey, and other as yet unidentified regions may comprise nodal points in maintaining these equilibria. Yet we know little of the switchgear and the discriminate and selective gating mechanisms which quite automatically operate within the various systems in arriving at the appropriate homeostatic response. As in the case of other modalities (for example, muscle tone, or posture, or fine voluntary movement), the deliberate selection (by experimental intervention) of one "bit" of behavior from a larger repertoire in no way reflects the elegance, smoothness, and flow of the normal operation. What normally manifests, what finally is selected out, or, as we say, what we "experience" represents in fact, a final common path. Yet the activation of such an affective response, and the genetically programmed cell assembly which subserves it, is presumably preceded, within fractions of a second, by several simultaneous transactions involving the temporal apposition, convergence, and coding of neural patterns at widely separated topographical levels. It may, for example, involve the taking in of sensory cues (or the activation of a memory trace); the analysis and matching of these in terms of cognate traces, or, as we say "experience"; a grouping and further condensation of these transforms in terms of their appetitive (YES) or aversive (NO) connotation; and the final activation of the appropriate motor-somato-endocrine response. The reasons for mentioning these aspects here are, first, to point to the dependence of the affective response on the history of the nervous system at any particular time: what it will put out will, to a large extent, depend on what it has "experienced"; and secondly, to show that pharmacological interference at the level of final commom path of response can be but one of several ways in which a drug may influence motivational behavior. The stages preceding the final response may be as important as the response itself.

There is one last point which will be briefly considered, inasmuch as it may bear upon the interplay and balance between the various subsystems comprised within the affective apparatus. It has been known for some time that motor activity and a number of autonomic functions may be subject to periodic and self-limiting fluctuations. Thus, for example, in the rat (42) activity and food intake show regular four to five day peaks, coinciding with oestrus. This stable and rhythmic behavior, however, is markedly distorted by even a single exposure to severe stress, such as forced swimming or prolonged fighting. The five-day cycle is replaced by a cycle very much longer (of the order of 20 to 22 days); food intake is markedly increased, though its relation to motor activity is inverted. There is marked increase in weight; and there are signs strongly suggestive of hypothalamic and pituitary involvement. A pituitary tumor has been described in such cases. (42)

A single severe stress thus appears capable of producing irreversible damage in an area which, as almost no other, acts as a governor or regulator of autonomic discharges. One wonders what the role of these cell masses and of those feeding into them, in the adaptation to stresses of a more mundane, more subtle, and more clinical nature, may be. For the present, blood hormones, and particularly 17-hydroxycorticoid levels, most readily reflect these responses; and here again, an interaction between the amygdala, the hippocampus, and the hypothalamus becomes evident. In the conscious monkey, stimulation of the amygdala leads to a striking rise in plasma 17-hydroxycorticoid levels and transection of the fornix markedly affects the diurnal fluctuation in the excretion level of the hormone (43). In a way yet no be fully determined, the endocrine system is thus locked to the great modulator systems which by reciprocal interaction guide the motivational systems in their appropriate response. It is even conceivable that the rhythmic fluctuations in excitability noted above may reflect shifts in balance between systems which figuratively may be referred to as coupled oscillators. Such systems are used with great advantage in the discharge of some simple, autonomic functions in the brain stem, such as the rhythmic discharge of the respiratory center (44), and would appear to depend upon reciprocal inhibition within a closely knit neural net for their effective operation. There seems little doubt of the operation of reciprocal inhibitory influences within the nets subserving the motivationals systems, though it is equally evident that a remarkable modification of this interaction at the hands of modulator systems must have also occurred. By and large, this favors delay in place of immediate discharge; fractioned, graded performance in lieu of display at open throttle. Yet this modulation breaks down under stress. We do not normally laugh and cry at the same time; but we may do so after a catastrophe. We do normally display the extreme excitement or inordinate muscular power readily observed in an active manic patient or in any one of us when "blinded" by rage. Yet such performance is evidently within the capacity of the ordinary human frame. One should thus not be deceived by appearances, and postulate stimulation wherever one sees overactivity. Stress response may travel in different guises. It may manifest equally as overactivity resulting from the faltering of a physiological braking mechanism, or as underactivity resulting from excessive inhibitory tone, fired, in turn, by a runaway excitatory process. Ideally (though rarely) the balance is neat, and guided by the demands of the "here" and the "now". In stress states, this neat modulation is lost. The balance is more autonomous and more dependent on self-limiting fluctuations. Put another way, the steering mechanisms are set at "automatic".

These three principles, then – the anatomical and cytological suborganization of the systems subserving affective behavior, their interconnectedness, and the balanced, yet mutually, occlusive nature of their operation – may give one some indication of the complexities which face a pharmacological approach to this field. This is borne out by several simple, yet telling experiments, of which only three will be cited.

In a study reported in 1957 (45) it could be shown that in rats carrying permanently implanted electrodes in the medial forebrain bundle, near the fornix, dual effects from stimulation via the same electrode could be regularly observed. The animal would press a bar to turn on the stimulation, and thus show an initial reward effect. This, however, would be followed, by the turning off of the stimulus (brought about by the turning of a wheel), and presumably signified an escape from "punishing" effects as the stimulus continued. The sequence would be regularly repeated. It was suggested that it reflected a differential rate of recruitment of the patterns of reward and punishment behavior when the systems subserving them were stimulated simultaneously.

It was if interest in these experiments that drugs with effects as opposite as those of methamphetamine (2 mg/kg.) and chlorpromazine (4 mg./kg.) produced roughly similar effects on the overall rate of bar pressing. However, when the positive and negative components were measured separately, striking qualitative differences could be shown. Methamphetamine increased the average time to turn the stimulation off. Chlorpromazine, on the other hand, had its largest effects on the opposite measure; namely, the time the animals waited before the stimulation was turned on. The time to turn the stimulation off was also increased, but much less. Thus, an overall measure (bar pressing) may, in fact, obscure two measures related to different effects possibly exerted on different systems; and do so despite a single electrode placement, which may be mistakenly associated with a single effect.

That such differential effects are likely is brought out by a second series of studies (33) in which the electrode location was varied and the effects of drugs on self-stimulation rates were examined. With electrodes placed in the anterior hypothalamus, self-stimulation rates were little affected by chlorpromazine; but with electrodes in the ventral posterior hypothalamus, there was striking inhibition. There were similar indications of the relation of electrode placement to the effects of other drugs, though the role of stimulus duration and the possibility of biphasic responses should be borne in mind in these experiments. Yet the indications of a preferential effect of some drugs on the appetitive and aversive systems are, at least, suggestive. This is also borne out in yet another study where operant conditioning techniques were employed. It could, for example, be shown in both the rat and the monkey (46) that, whereas pentobarbitone exerted an early effect on avoidance behavior (i.e., reduced the number of responses, which if preserved, prevented the delivery of a shock to the animal), the same drug exerted relatively little effect on appetitive behavior (i.e., while the animal was lever-pressing for a sugar pellet reward). Hyoscine, on the other hand, had the observed effect: even in small doses; it led to an immediate depressant effect upon reward behavior, while leaving avoidance behavior was relatively less affected.

II. SOME ELECTROPHYSIOLOGICAL CORRELATES

Numerous other examples including some early studies (47) could be added to the instances given above. They illustrate the delicate balance between the cell groups governing affective behavior, and the susceptibility to drugs of these actively maintained equilibria. The indicators of shifts in these subsystems in relation to behavior are, at present, few and far between. Some electrophysiological correlates will now be briefly considered.

In inquiries of this kind, particularly when concerned with agents of a complex and multiple action, one is apt to be assisted (even though at times misled) by drugs whose action can, with some confidence, be attributed to one or other overriding property. The anticholinesterases, (such as physostigmine and DFP) or the acetylcholine blocking agents (such as atropine and its analogues) are compounds of this kind. It is for that reason that, when some years ago in Birmingham, England Dr. P.B. Bradley and I (and later, Dr. A.J Hance and Dr. B.J. Key) began to examine the effects of drugs on the electrical activity of the brain and their relation to behavior in the conscious animal, it was thought advisable to begin with drugs related to acetylcholine, an to extend these studies subsequently to agents known or suspected to interact with other substances in the brain. Such drugs included the group of amphetamines, LSD-25, and some related compounds. The interaction between a number of tranquilizers and the patterns established for these drugs was examined as a further step.

The Effect of Some Drugs on the Electrical Activity of the Brain in the Conscious Animal, and in Some Acute Preparations

The results, which are published (48–53) will be only briefly reviewed here. Observed in the conscious cat preparation, carrying permanently implanted cortical and subcortical electrodes (48), the effects of the drugs were found to fall into two broad groups. Physostigmine (an anticholinesterase), used in relatively small doses (0,05–0,3 mg./kg. i.p.), led to low voltage fast activity closely resembling (though not entirely identical with) that seen in the fully alert animal. However, provided the dose of the drugs was kept suitably low, no corresponding "alerting" of overt behavior could be detected. The animals appeared quiet and resting despite an incongruous low-voltage electrocorticogram. On the other hand, atropine (1–2 mg./kg.) and l-hyoscyamine (0,4–0,8 mg./kg.), led to high voltage slow activity which, in some respects resembled the activity seen in deep sleep. However, here again there was no correspondence between electrical activity and behavior. The animals were fully awake and, in some instances, showed motor excitement. It should be stressed, however, that in those early experiments no psychological test situations were employed; and that subtler deficits in performance may have therefore gone undetected. The discrepancy between electrical activity and overt behavior, however, was quite striking, and in the case of atropine was in keeping with observations noted independently in the corticogram of the dog (54).

In contrast to the above three drugs (all related to the action of acetylcholine), amphetamine (1–5 mg./kg.) in both its optically active and inactive forms regularly led to low voltage fast ("alert") activity in the conscious animal. This was accompanied by behavioral excitement. The effects of LSD-25 (in doses of 15–25 μg./kg.) were less regular. At times they resembled those of amphetamine; at others they showed rhythmic activity (at about 15 cycles/sec.). A striking feature of the effects of LSD-25 was the dependence of the patterns seen on the precise environmental setting of the experiment. For example, when carried out in a constant environment chamber placed in an open laboratory where, presumably, noises from other rooms could penetrate, the effects noted were the ones just described. However, if these experiments were carried out in a soundproof room, rhythmic activity at a rather slower rate (4–7 cyc./sec.) was noted. This activity could be blocked by sensory stimuli. It thus appeared that one effect of LSD 25 was to sensitize the animal inordinately to its environment.

When considered in terms of the relationship of electrical activity to overt behavior, the drugs thus appeared to fall into two groups. The first comprised those drugs (physostigmine, atropine, and l-hyoscyamine) which, within the crude framework of gross behavioral change, showed a lack of correlation between the effects on electrical activity and on behavior. The second group covered drugs (the amphetamines, LSD-25, and, to a lesser extent, mescaline – 51) where the correlation between the effects on electrical activity and behavior was much closer. Moreover, when the drugs were used in combination with each other, the gross behavior effects were always dominated by the second group (the amphetamines and LSD 25), whereas the effects on electrical activity were dominated by the first. The interaction for example, between atropine and amphetamine showed this quite clearly.

The distinction between these two groups of drugs was borne out further by acute experiments in which the effects of high spinal and mesencephalic section were studied. These experiments were carried out in the *encéphale* and *cerveau isolé* (55) preparations long found useful in enquiries concerned with the mechanisms subserving sleep and arousal. The *encéphale isolé* (severed at the level of the first cervical vertebra) receives afferent impulses from the cranial nerve only. It alternates, both behaviorally and electrically, between periods of drowsiness and a limited form of alerting (as shown by eye movement, retraction of the nictitating membrane, and movement of the vibrissae). The *cerveau isolé* is severed at the level of the midbrain. It shows drowsiness or sleep only, and responds to afferent stimuli in a much more limited way.

When examined in these preparations, physostigmine, atropine, and l-hyoscyamine, used in doses comparable to the conscious preparation, led to effects closely resembling those seen in the conscious preparation; there being, again, marked effects on electrical activity with relatively little effects on the admittedly limited behavior of the preparation. The effects were independent of the transient effects of the drugs on blood pressure. Effects on *local* cerebral vascular tone, however, were not excluded by these experiments.

In contrast to the above three drugs the effects of amphetamine, although readily obtainable in the *encéphale isolé* preparation, could no longer be observed in the *cerveau isolé* preparation, even where relatively large doses of the drugs were used. LSD-25, on the other hand, produced no effects on either the electrical activity or the behavior of either of these acute preparations. Some effects in the monkey, however, were noted.

In the absence of evidence to the contrary it was assumed that the effects of physostigmine were related to its anticholinesterase activity, and presumably due to the endogenous accumulation of acetylcholine or a related choline ester within the central nervous system. Similarly, the effects of atropine and l-hyoscyamine were thought to be due to a blockade of cholinergic sites. There are, of course, differences between the central and the peripheral effects of atropine and physostigmine in terms of both dosage and reversibility of effects; nevertheless, a cholinergic element may be presumed to be involved in these central effects. The lack of correlation between electrical activity and behavior, and the independence of the effects observed of mesencephalic and spinal connections would, however, suggest a diffuse distribution of this element and a possible representation of it at high subcortical and/or cortical (as well a mesencephalic) levels.

In this respect, amphetamine differed from the drugs just considered. In the case of this agent, there appeared to be a closer correlation between electrical activity and behavior; furthermore the effects on electrical activity and behavior were modified by mesencephalic (though not by spinal) transection. In view of the striking part played by the tegmental reticular substance in behavioral and electrical arousal (56, 57) it was suggested (19, 51, 58) that the effect of this drug might be exerted on elements either intimately related to, or located in the brain stem reticular activating system. The presence of *nor*epinephrine in this area of the brain (59) the extensive studies on sympathetic humoral influences in this area (60) and the direct demonstration of epinephrine sensitive elements in brain stem (61) were all in keeping with this suggested mode of action of this powerful centrally acting sympathomimetic amine.

The effects of LSD-25 were somewhat different, and in their susceptibility to and dependence on afferent input suggested the involvement of an element particularly and peculiarly related to the afferent pathways. This element had to be distinguished from the element involved in the action of amphetamine. It was judged to play a key part in the organization of sensory experience and to do so primarily by way of a discrete, highly patterned inhibitory mechanism, reciprocating with, and dependent on afferent input (51, 53). Whether this mechanism was linked to the natural turnover of an indole (with which LSD-25 interfered) seemed uncertain at the time. Present day evidence has hardly contributed to a satisfactory solution.

The grouping established for the above six drugs was found to obtain also when the study was extended to an examination of the interaction between them and chlorpromazine (62). Both chlorpromazine and methopromazine were administered, in divided doses, alone and in combination. Given alone, chlorpromazine led to striking behavioral changes and effects on the electrical activity. Previously friendly and affectionate animals showed marked indifference to both environment and observer and, on occasion, became slightly aggressive when disturbed. The electrical activity reflected these changes in behavior, the record usually being dominated by regular waves at 5–8 cycles/sec. interspersed by slow waves at 2–4 cycles/sec. Neither behavioral nor electrical arousal response could be obtained in these animals. When chlorpromazine was given in combination with the drugs mentioned, it was noted that whereas both the behavioral and the electroencephalographic effects of amphetamine and LSD-25 (administered in full doses) could be blocked by premedication with chlorpromazine, the effects of atropine and physostigmine on the electrical activity of the brain persisted in the presence, even, of high doses of chlorpromazine; nor did these latter drugs appreciably modify the behavior patterns attributable to chlorpromazine. When administered in small doses (0,2–1 mg./kg.) in the *encéphale isolé,* chlorpromazine led in some (though not all) experiments to a transient blocking of the spindle and slow-wave activity often seen in this type of preparation. This effect usually passed within about two minutes. Larger doses, however (1,5–4 mg./kg.), produced an increase in the slow spindle activity in the preparation, and also made the preparation more diffcult to rouse. Chlorpromazine had little effect on the *cerveau isolé* preparation; such effects as were seen were associated with a fall in blood pressure, and could thus not be readily distinguished from the circulatory effects of the drug on this preparation.

The Effect of Chlorpromazine and Some Other Drugs on Arousal Responses

The grouping suggested by the above findings could be carried a little further by studies of the effect of a number of drugs on arousal responses. A distinction must be made between behavioral and electrocortical arousal; and, equally, between arousal produced by direct stimulation of elements in the reticular formation, and indirect stimulation by way of one of the sensory pathways. The *encéphale isolé* is suitable for such studies. As mentioned earlier, a waking state in this preparation can be readily distinguished from the drowsy or "sleeping" state. The first state is accompanied by low voltage, fast activity not unlike that seen in the intact alert animal; the second, by slow waves at 1–4 cycles per second, or spindle activity at 6–12 cycles per second. The correspondence between electrical activity and behavioral states in these preparations is maintained throughout, although individual variations in patterns of sleep activity can often be encountered. Furthermore, because of the intact cranial nerve connections, such a preparation is susceptible to arousal by tactile or auditory stimuli. It is, of course, also aroused by direct electrical stimulation of the brain stem reticular formation; here sharp behavioral arousal is reflected in a corresponding activation of the electrocorticogram.

In such experiments, the arousal thresholds can be determined by applying a stimulus (rectangular pulses of 1 m.sec. duration at frequency of 300 cycles per second) for fixed period (10 sec.), and by gradually increasing the stimulus voltage to a point where behavioral and electrocortical arousal can be independently noted. Similarly, arousal thresholds to sensory (auditory) stimulation can (though somewhat crudely) be expressed in terms of the voltage which, when applied to a loudspeaker delivering a note of constant frequency, results in arousal. Responses to single clicks can also be determined at the auditory cortex in the same experiment.

The results obtained with the drugs so far mentioned further emphasized the grouping which the experiments in the conscious animal had previously suggested (63). Thus, for example, amphetamine in doses of 01–1 mg./kg. led to a progressive lowering of both the threshold for electroencephalographic arousal, and behavioral arousal in response to direct stimulation of the reticular formation; similarly, there was also a fall, at much same rate, in the threshold for arousal by auditory stimulation, while the threshold for single click responses recorded at the cortex remained comparatively unchanged. In doses of 1 mg./kg., there was permanent alerting of the preparation, both in terms of electrical activity and behavior. LSD-25, on the other hand while exerting (in doses of 1–20 µg./kg.) relatively little effects on arousal to direct stimulation of the reticular formation, caused a marked fall in the threshold for arousal by auditory stimulation. This could be seen in doses of the order of 1–2 µg./kg. Atropine (in doses of 0,2–4 mg./kg.) led to the usual appearance of the characteristic slow wave activity in the electrocorticogram, but left the behavioral threshold (as judged by the criteria enumerated above) relatively unchanged. Although both tactile and auditory stimuli could still produce behavioral alerting after atropine, they did not modify electrical activity. There thus appeared a wide divergence between the threshold for electrocortical arousal and that for arousal in terms of behavioral response.

Physostigmine produced effects opposite to those of atropine, leading to a fall of threshold for electrical activity with relatively little change in behavioral threshold. If injected after atropine (in doses 0.1–0.8 mg./kg.) this drug would lead to a progressive lowering of the electroencephalogaphic arousal threshold, as the slow activity induced by atropine gradually gave way to the low voltage fast activity seen with physostigmine. The behavioral threshold, however, was not markedly affected by this drug.

The above parameters were found useful in a subsequent examination of the effects of chlorpromazine and some ten other tranquilizing drugs on the arousal responses in the *encéphale* preparation (61). Earlier and important (65) experiments, though suggesting an action of chlorpromazine at the level of the reticular activating system, had also emphasized the paradoxical nature of some of these responses. Used in relatively large doses (up to 5 mg./kg.),65 it could be shown that the drug exerted only slight effects on electroencephalographic and behavioral arousal brought about by stimulation of the reticular formation, while markedly elevating the behavioral arousal threshold to stimulation of the diffuse thalamic projection system. Furthermore, unlike pentobarbital (which diminished conduction time in the reticular formation), chlorpromazine was found to increase reticular input and conduction (65). Dose and parameters of stimulation may well be critical in such studies. Thus, for example, in experiments where electrical and behavioral arousal to direct electrical stimulation of the reticular formation were recorded (64), chlorpromazine in very small doses (0.1–0.5 mg./kg.) caused a slight fall in the behavioral and electrocortical arousal thresholds, in about one third of such experiments. However, with a total dose of 0.8 mg./kg. there was a return to the original threshold. This effect could not be seen with a number of other drugs tested (see below). In the same experiments, doses 2.0–4 mg./kg. caused a slight rise in threshold for both electrocortical and behavior arousal. Larger doses caused no further change in threshold.

In contrast to the above relatively slight effects on arousal responses produced by direct stimulation of the reticular formation, the effect of chlorpromazine on arousal responses produced by sensory (auditory) stimulation were quite marked. Small doses (0.1–0.3 mg./kg.) of chlorpromazine produced relatively little effect on these parameters; however, with lager doses (0.5–1.8 mg./kg.) both electrocortical and behavioral thresholds showed a marked rise. Moreover, the arousal responses themselves became less marked, both in terms of extent and duration. In doses of 2.0–4.0 mg./kg. the evoked auditory arousal response was blocked completely. At the same time the preparation became unresponsive to other types of sensory stimulation, although pain (pinching of ears) still produced some response. Interestingly enough, the threshold for single click response recorded at the auditory cortex remained unchanged throughout the experiment.

Since these earlier studies, similar techniques have been applied to an examination of some other drugs (64). These included promazine, acepromazine, hydroxyzine, benactyzine, imipramine, hyoscine, reserpine, rescinnamine, deserpidine, meprobamate and azacyclonal. According to the responses observed, the drugs were found to fall into four groups. The results are summarized in Table 1.

Group I included drugs which caused only slight diminution of the arousal responses to direct stimulation of the brain stem reticular formation, but a rise threshold to arousal by indirect sensory (auditory) stimulation. Included in this group are chlorpromazine, promazine, acepromazine and hydroxyzine. It should be noted that the interaction between these drugs and amphetamine, atropine, and physostigmine was in keeping with previous findings. Whereas chlorpromazine appeared to block the effects of amphetamine, the latter drug still produced some effects when given after promazine, acepromazine and hydroxyzine; though it never led to complete alerting. Atropine and physostigmine, on the other hand, when superimposed on chlorpromazine, produced their marked effect on electrical activity of the brain, but did not modify overt behavior. Most of the drugs in this group share antiepinephrine properties, though some also show an action against 5-hydroxytryptamine, histamine, and acetylcholine.

TABLE 1. The Effects of Some Drugs on Arousal Thresholds
(After Bradley & Key, 1959 [64])

Group	Principal Characteristics	Drugs Included in Group
I.	Slight rise in threshold for arousal through stimulation of the brain stem reticular formation. Marked rise in threshold to arousal to indirect (auditory) stimulation.	Chlorpromazine Promazine Acepromazine Hydroxyzine
II.	Marked rise in electrocortical activation threshold through direct stimulation of brain stem reticulalr formation; "dissociation" between electrocortical and behavioral arousal.	Benactyzine Imipramine Hyoscine
III.	Little effect on arousal thresholds to direct stimulation. "Fast" electrocortical activity in large doses.	Reserpine Rescinnamine Deserpidine
IV.	Little effect on arousal thresholds.	Meprobamate Azacyclonal

Group II. Drugs in this group led to an increase in arousal thresholds, but at the same time produced dissociation between electrical activity and behavior. Comprised in this group are benactyzine, impramine, and hyoscine. These drugs did not antagonize the alerting effects of amphetamine on behavior; moreover, they did not markedly affect thresholds for behavioral arousal induced by sensory stimulation. It is well to remember that benactyzine and hyoscine are atropine analogues; and that imipramine, closely allied to promazine, also shares some weak antiacetylcholine properties. Drugs in this group exert a comparatively weak antiepinephrine action, and appear more effective in blocking the blood pressure and antispasmodic effects of acetylcholine than do drugs in the other groups.

Group III. This group comprises drugs which have relatively little effect on arousal thresholds, but which, in full doses cause marked changes in the electrocorticogram towards the "activation" pattern. Included in this group are reserpine and two related compounds, rescinnamine and deserpidine. These drugs produces no charge in the threshold for arousal by stimulation of the brain stem although they did, in large dose, lead to a change in the electrocorticogram towards a faster frequency. This, however, appeared unrelated to the behavioral state, the preparation usually showing little evidence of arousal. Drugs in this group, although possessing some antispasmodic activity against epinephrine, acetylcholine, and histamine, share a depleting action on the stores of serotonin and of catecholamines in the brain (see below).

Group IV. Drugs in this group could not be shown to exert any marked effect either on electrocortical activity or on the behavioral arousal threshold. Included in this group are meprobamate and azacyclonal. Meprobamate (in doses of 20–40 mg./kg.) had no effect on thresholds of arousal induced by direct stimulation of the reticular formation. Equally, the responses to afferent stimulation showed little change, and even with large doses, the electrocorticogram remained relatively unaltered. Somewhat similar effects were observed with azacyclonal.

The above studies give an indication of the broad and empirically crude nature of any grouping so far possible on the basis of neurophysiological evidence. It is obvious that the electrophysiological effects of the diverse tranquilizers are not necessarily related to their clinical effectiveness, and that they can at best give only a very inadequate indication as to their mode of action. This is borne out by two further sets of observations not unrelated to the above studies; these concern so-called stimulating (rather than tranquilizing) agents.

It has been suggested that dimethylaminoethanol (DMAE) owes its central stimulant effects to a possible role as a precursor of acetylcholine within the central nervous system (66). In a recent study the effects of this drug, and of amphetamine have been compared (67). DMAE was indeed found to lower the threshold for electroencephalographic arousal elicited both by stimulation of the reticular formation and also following thalamic stimulation. The increased activity of the latter was found to be insufficient to increase the low-voltage fast electroencephalographic activity in the absence of ascending influences from the reticular formation. DMAE was thus presumed to have a tonic effect on the entire reticular formation. The compound was found to antagonize the depressant effects of barbiturates on the pathways subserving wakefulness. The action of DMAE on the reticular activating system was thus similar to, but not as striking as that of amphetamine.

Another study (68, 69) has compared the effects of drugs used in the treatment of depression in terms of their effect on electrocortical (though not behavioral) arousal. The drugs were found to fall into two groups. The first, which included amphetamine, pipradrol, methylphenidate, iproniazid and DMAE, was found to lead to electrocortical "arousal". The second group did not share this property, and was thought to block the mesodiencephalic arousal system (MDAS). Inasmuch as this group included benactyzine and imipramine it presumably corresponded to Group II in the series previously cited.

The equivocal position of the last two drugs should, incidentally, be noted. Benactyzine, which started as minor tranquilizer (70), can also, apparently, be viewed as a stimulant; and imipramine, though an antidepressant, is closely related to promazine, a tranquilizer (71).

Viewed in terms of possible modes of action, amphetamine and chlorpromazine have some slight advantage over the other drugs so far considered. In the case of both, there is some circumstantial evidence for the involvement of a catechol amine mediated mechanism. The evidence for a possible central adrenergic mechanism in the action of amphetamine has been briefly referred to above. The obverse, in a sense, appears to be true for chlorpromazine and allied drugs, where a central antiepinephrine effect is not out of keeping with the evidence. These drugs would appear to act less by a direct depression of the arousal mechanism than by an effect on an element or mechanism intermediate between afferent input and the arousal mechanism, or on tonic inhibitory influences playing upon the reticular core from high subcortical cell masses. The relatively slight effect on arousal thresholds to direct stimulation; the marked effect on threshold to arousal by indirect sensory (auditory) stimulation; the marked antagonism to amphetamine, and the antiepinephrine properties of this group of drug would suggest an interference with a central adrenergic process which in some way regulates the balance of inhibitory tone governing conduction within the reticular formation. Two other curious findings concerning chlorpromazine may be quoted. The first is the slight fall of threshold brought about by small doses (61). The second is the increase in conduction time following chlorpromazine (65). The shifts within the system are thus subtle and dose dependent; and a change in response to afferent stimulation (as reflected in the discrepancy between the responses to direct and indirect stimulation) may in some manner reflect an increased capacity of the reticular core to "filter" (65) sensory input without necessarily engaging the reticular-hypothalamic mechanisms. One must surmise that the catecholamines may play a part in maintaining the balance between excitation and inhibition in key areas of the reticular system, which, indeed is a system of systems.

Unit Activity in the Reticular Formation as Studied by Microelectrode Techniques

There is a further kind of experiment, which can be used to study interaction at the level here considered. The microelectrode studies of spontaneous and evoked activity of units in the reticular formation (72) invite an extension of such studies into to pharmacological field. In one such preliminary study (73, 74) recordings were obtained from single units in the mesencephalon and medulla, using floating microelectrodes. Blood pressure was recorded simultaneously to control for vasomotor effects. The units selected for observation were classified as reticular in character from the fact that they showed convergence responses, and from the effects observed by stimulation through microelectrodes after recordings had been completed. Observations were also made on a number of units belonging to specific sensory projection systems, such as for example units situated in the mesencephalic nucleus of the fifth nerve, or the superior colliculus. The drugs were administered by the intravenous or intracarotid route.

The studies concerned primarily the effects of epinephrine, acetylcholine, and chlorpromazine, and it is for this reason that they are mentioned in the present context. With epinephrine variable effects were observed. The activity of units was either unaffected, or showed an increase or a decrease in the rate of discharge. Following intravenous injection, the effects were usually seen only during a rise in blood pressure; but following intracarotid injections (1–5 µg.) the effects were similar, though no change in blood pressure could be observed. The effects of acetylcholine (which was applied in doses of 0.2–1.0 µg. by the intracarotid route only) were somewhat different. These responses were of two kinds; first, a primary increase or decrease in frequency, starting within a few seconds of the injection and lasting only a few seconds; second, a response of much longer latency. The latter appeared more constant and was observed in every unit tested; whereas the primary effect was not always seen. The secondary effect was invariably accompanied by a slight fall in blood pressure, through no change in blood pressure was observed during the primary effect. These effects were still present after bilateral denervation of the carotid sinus and also following the injection of a paralyzing dose of tubocurarine. These units, therefore, were capable of being either facilitated or inhibited following the intracarotid administration of these drugs. It was of interest, also, that units belonging in the specific sensory systems of the brain stem were not affected by the injections of epinephrine. This striking difference in susceptibility, which is in keeping with more recent findings on other specific sensory systems (73) may well be of significance to a theory of the interaction-in-time of the specific and the nonspecific projection systems.

Chlorpromazine, when applied in doses of 2 to 4 mg./kg., led to a marked decrease in the frequency of the spontaneous activity of units; moreover, the units became much less responsive to peripheral stimuli. Thus, "a unit which previously responded to light stabbing or stroking of one of the legs with a burst of 9 to 10 spikes consistently produced only 2 or 3 spikes in response to a similar stimulus after chlorpromazine had been injected." (73) This effect was observed to occur with doses of 2 to 4 mg./kg. intravenously (a dose which, as noted above, is effective in blocking arousal to afferent stimulation). Further increase in this dose did not increase the effect, and even with the largest doses some response to tapping of the legs was always obtained. If pentobarbitone or sodium pentothal was administered after chlorpromazine, all spontaneous activity disappeared and no responses from the unit could be obtained. The activity reappeared within twenty or thirty minutes after injection, and eventually recovered fully when the effect of the barbiturates had worn off. The effect was not observed with barbiturates alone. It suggested a synergism between chlorpromazine and barbiturates.

III. SOME NEUROHUMORAL CORRELATES

The above instances have been chosen to illustrate the hybrid nature of the type of compounds dealt with so far, which cuts through much that is tacitly implicit in the older concepts of stimulation and depression. As in the case of morphia, behavioral and affective under-responsiveness may well be an active state. It is at present impossible, nor is it conceptually permissible, to locate the action of the psycho-active drugs to any particular area or any particular cell group. All one can assume is a shift within the balancing processes, which normally regulate the interaction-in-time between widely scattered neural nets converging in several nodal areas. The interconnectedness of the various subsystems concerned with affective response has already been emphasized. Fibre length and thickness, precise dendritic arrangement and synaptic delay will determine the timing and coincidence of patterns in these widely separated cell lattices. Yet, assuming that certain standard processes determine the primary synaptic events within such vast cell assemblies, we have still to account, somehow, in chemical terms for the altered threshold which lead to the selective suppression or release, the gating, in terms of storage or flow of the highly organized patterns of activity which we know as affective behavior. It has been suggested (53) that the regulation of levels of excitability in such neural nets may involve the interaction of humoral field effects and highly localized synaptic events in certain trigger areas of the brain stem. Cholinergic as well as noncholinergic elements may be involved in this interaction. The regional and local economy, in terms of neurohumoral mediation, may therefore be relevant in the action of the drugs discussed so far. Some of these neurohumoral correlates will now be considered.

A rich literature has grown around the subject of central synaptic transmission, and only a few aspect will be mentioned within the present context. It may be useful to begin by agreeing on four minimal desiderata (52) which should be fulfilled by a substance claiming the role of a neurohumoral mediator within the central nervous system. First, the substance should be present in the central nervous system and should vary in concentration with the functional state of the tissue. Second, enzyme systems (both for the synthesis and for the destruction of the substance in question) should be present in the areas of the central nervous system where the substance is normally found. Third, these enzymes should be susceptible to inhibition by specific inhibitors or antimetabolites and the effects of such inhibition should be clearly demonstrable in chemical or functional terms. Fourth, the application of the hypothetical agent or its precursor to the central nervous system, either directly or by a physiological route, should exert clear effects on function.

These criteria are met in part by a number of substances, though, significantly, in the case of each, important reservations obtain. Thus, for example, though acetylcholine is present in the central nervous system, the enzyme system concerned in its synthesis (the choline acetylase system) has a curiously uneven distribution, some areas of the central nervous system being strikingly low in the enzyme (76). The central role of acetylcholine, and related choline esters have been more fully considered elsewhere (52, 53, 77). Recent attention has been directed towards substances other than acetylcholine; these include epinephrine, *norepi-*

nephrine, and related catecholamines; serotonin, and a group of related indoles; and surprisingly, a number of amino acids which have been found capable of markedly affecting synaptic transmission.

Norepinephrine, Epinephrine, Serotonin and Related Substances

It has been shown that *nor*epinephrine (with an admixture of 5–20% epinephrine) has a differential pattern of distribution within the brain (59). This pattern is different from that of acetylcholine. The highest concentration of *nor*epinephrine are found in the hypothalamus, the area postrema, and the periventricular grey substance; other parts of the mesencephalon and the medulla also contain sizeable concentrations. A third catecholamine, dopamine (a probable precursor of epinephrine), has also been shown to be present in the brain; though, significantly, its distribution is different from that of *nor*epinephrine, the highest concentration being found in the lentiform and the caudate nucleus (78, 79).

The tissue catecholamines appear to be associated with particulate cell constituents, and microsome-like granules, rich in ATP (80, 81). The synthesis of catecholamine proceeds by way of several distinct steps. The parent substance is the amino acid, tyrosine, from which 3,4-dihydroxyphenylalanine (DOPA) is formed by oxidation DOPA is changed to dopamine by the action of an enzyme, dopa decarboxylase, in the presence of pyridoxal phosphate, which acts as a coenzyme. This enzyme has been identified both in the sympathetic ganglia and in the grey matter of the central nervous system (82); though, to date, its regional distribution is relatively unknown. The subsequent step of oxidation of dopamine to *nor*epinephrine has been demonstrated by the use of isotopically labeled precursors *in vivo* (83), and in perfusion experiments (84). The nature and the catalysts involved in this reaction are relatively unknown at present. The final step is the N-methylation of *nor*epinephrine to epinephrine. It is likely that adenosyl methionine acts as a methyl donor in this reaction (85).

Two points are worthy of note in regard to the possible synthesis of the substance in the brain. It has been shown that isotopically (tritium) labeled epinephrine does not readily cross the blood-brain barrier, except possibly in small amounts in the region of the hypothalamus (86); on the other hand, dopa, its precursor, can readily enter the central nervous system (79). Moreover, the intravenous injection of dopa in rabbits can cause large increases in the concentration of dopamine in the brain, whereas the levels of *nor*epinephrine and epinephrine may not be significantly changed (87). However, after catecholamine depletion by reserpine, dopa restores catecholamine levels within a matter of hours. This strongly suggests that the brain possesses the enzymes necessary for the synthesis of catecholamines from its precursors.

The inactivation of epinephrine by way of O-methylation through catechol-O-methyltransferase, an enzyme present in the brain, has been considered in detail in the preceding paper (88). The speed of the reaction should be noted. The disposition of the methylated metabolite is carried forward further by mono amine oxidase to 3-methoxy-4-hydroxy mandelic acid (vanillyl mandelic acid, VMA – 89). Although it is highly probable that the catecholamines are, for the greater part, O-methylated before they are oxidized, it is also possible that some exidation may precede O-methylation to a limited extent. In this context, however, the relative slowness of the reaction, of mono-amine oxidase, with epinephrine is of interest. Both, the precursor (dopamine) and the methylated product (metanephrine or *nor*metanephrine) would appear to form better substrates for the action of this enzyme than does epinephrine itself. Though a direct protective action of mono-amine oxidase inhibitors, such as iproniazid and beta phenylisopropylhydrazine (JB 516), on *nor*epinephrine and epinephrine cannot be excluded, it is at least equally likely that the action may be exerted by increasing the stores of dopamine and thus, possibly, the source material for *nor*epinephrine. Be this as it may, *nor*epinephrine, epinephrine, and their precursor, dopamine, apparently possess the enzymes for both the manufacture and the disposal of these powerful amines. Equally, there is suggestive evidence, mentioned above and reviewed elsewhere (90) for a central action of these substances.

The third agent implicated in the central action of psychotropic drugs is 5-hydroxytryptamine (serotonin). Its occurrence in the brain was demonstrated quite early (91), and its distribution parallels that of *nor*epinephrine, the highest yields being obtained in the hypothalamus, the area postrema, and the periventricular grey (92, 93). However, high values are also found in the amygdala, thalamus and certain areas of the limbic system (93), such as the hippocampal gyrus, orbital gyrus, the cingulate and retrosplenial cortex, the septal nuclei, and the habenula.

Serotonin is derived from the amino acid tryptophan, from which its immediate precursor 5-hydroxytrytophan is formed by oxidation. The conversion of 5-hydroxytryptophan into serotonin is brought about by way of decarboxylation. The enzyme concerned, 5-hydroxytryptophan decarboxylase, has been shown to have a distribution similar to serotonin (94) and in its requirement for pyridoxal phosphate as coenzyme, and in its distribution in the cytoplasmic fraction of brain homogenate, closely resembles dopa decarboxylase. There is a further similarity between the catecholamine systems and the system here considered. For, though serotonin itself does not appear to transfer readily through the blood brain barrier, as evidenced by the lack of accumulation of serotonin in the brain following infusion and the lack for example, of central symptoms in carcinoid tumors, the administration of 5-hydroxytryptophan increases brain 5-HT levels significantly and leads to marked central effects (95). Here again, there is thus indirect evidence of the local manufacture of serotonin from its immediate precursor, though it must remain undetermined what proportion of these effects may be due to the immediate effect of 5-hydroxytryptophan, or to 5-hydroxytryptamine.

Unlike epinephrine and *nor*epinephrine, however, there would appear to be good reason for believing that mono-amine oxidase may be responsible for the disposition of serotonin in the central nervous system. Inhibition of amine oxidase by iproniazid leads to an increase of brain serotonin level (95, 96). The product of deamination (5-hydroxy-indole acetic acid, 5-HIAA) is the main urinary metabolite of serotonin; after inhibition of amine oxidase there is sharp fall of 5-hydroxy-indole acetic acid (97, 98). In fact, this fall of 5-HIAA excretion can be used as a guide in evaluating the efficiency of an amine oxidase inhibitor in man (98). Furthermore, in the presence of an amine oxidase inhibitor (for example, iproniazid, or JB 516), the injection of 5-hydroxytryptophan leads to marked rise in brain serotonin. Amine oxidase inhibitors can also be used to study the turnover of serotonin in the brain. Preliminary experiments suggest this to be high (99). Thus, in the case of serotonin, (as in the case of epinephrine) the principal criteria appear to be met; though the precise effects of administration differ considerably according to where, how, and how much of the substance is applied at any particular time.

The Synaptically Active Amino Acids

There is a fourth group of substances which has recently been shown to exert an effect on synaptic transmission within the central nervous system. This includes a series of amino acids, such as the ω-guanidino acids and, to a lesser extent, the α-guanidino acids (100), but is best represented in the striking distribution and effects of γ-amino butyric acid (GABA, 101–103). This substance is found in readily extractable from in large quantities in the central nervous system of a number of species. It is formed from glutamic acid by the action decarboxylase (GAD). Both GABA itself and the decarboxylase are found in higher yield in gray than in white matter, and both are laid down very rapidly in the brain during early postnatal development. The decarboxylation of glutamic acid to γ-aminobutyrate requires the presence of pyridoxal phosphate, and thus brings the formation of this acid into intimate relationship with cellular oxidation.

The disposition of GABA is carried through by GABA transaminase (GABA-T), an enzyme found in the brain and other tissues, which brings about the transamination of GABA with α-ketoglutarate to from l-glutamic acid and succinic acid in the brain, the succinate entering the tricarboxylic cycle. The distribution of GABA-T and GAD in the nervous system of the monkey is uneven (104, 105). The relatively high concentration of GABA-T, *inter alia*, in the hypothalamus and the olivary nucleus is noteworthy.

As is the case with *nor*epinephrine and serotonin, GABA itself does not readily penetrate the blood brain barrier, but depends for its presence in the brain on local manufacture from its precursor, glutamic acid. A number of other findings should also be noted. The enzymes concerned with the synthesis (GAD) and the disposition (GABA-T) of GABA show a remarkable sensitivity to pH, GAD showing maximal activity at pH 6.5, and GABA-T at pH 8.2 (103). Small shifts in intracellular pH (occasioned for example by CO_2 shifts and differences in the activity of carbonic anhydrase) could thus be envisioned to affect profoundly the levels of intracellular GABA. The amount of GABA present in any particular area must thus reflect a balance between the rate of formation and the rate of utilisation of the material, and the level of enzyme activity in a particular area (and the ratio between the activity of the two enzymes) may thus be a much more accurate indicator of GABA activity in a particular area than is the actual amount of GABA presents at a particular time. Fortunately, the activity of these enzymes can be affected. The semicarbazides, by interfering with pyridoxal phosphate activity (an essential coenzyme factor in the action of the decarboxylase) can inhibit decarboxylase activity, leading to fall in GABA levels in the central nervous system. Hydroxylamine, on the other land, can be shown to inhibit GABA – transferase (GABA-T) more than the decarboxylase, and thus leads to an endogenous accumulation of GABA *in vivo* (106).

The first indication of a possible physiological role of GABA in the mammalian nervous system stems from the demonstration of the convulsive properties of the semicarbazides (107), the application of which *in vivo* was found to lead to repetitive seizures following a significantly long latent period. This presumably resulted from the fall in endogenously produced GABA, and was borne out by the fact the topical application of low does of GABA reduced or blocked electrically induced seizures in the hippocampus (108). Hydroxylamine, on the other hand, led to a marked reduction in the duration and spread of electrically induced after – discharges in the cat in acute experiments, and in conscious monkeys carrying indwelling electrodes (109). The monkeys appeared more placid without being sedated, and were much easier to handle for as a long as seven hours after the administration of hydroxylamine (109). The predominantly inhibitory role of GABA on synaptic transmission has been stressed in a number of studies (110), though its universal role as a principal inhibitory substance in the mammalian central nervous system can by no means regarded as settled (111).

The above findings are mentioned because they present a significant break in a tradition which, up to quite recently, has unduly emphasised a distinction between the power economy, the protein synthesis, and the process and agents affecting the electrogenic properties, and the permeability, of the neurone membrane. Distinctions such as these are no doubt convenient, and can be readily made in the mind, they help to delimit one's problems and to guide one's experiment. They are, however, unlikely to be made in the cell, where the various phases appear functionally linked and interdependent. Thus, for example the rate of protein synthesis in the brain and the rate of turnover of amino acids is known to be very high (112). Glutamic acid (the parent substance of GABA) has been long known to play a part in energy metabolism and protein synthesis (113). Yet its derivative, GABA, together with other amino acids, can be shown to exert effects on synaptic transmission which, to say the least, are quite respectable. One thus assumes that if, indeed, such substances do naturally occur in the central nervous system, their effect must be both local and transient, and that some subcellular compartmentalisation (114) carefully regulates the manufacture, storage, release, and inactivation of the various agents, quite possibly in different proportions and at different rates. One is also struck by certain common features shared by the agents considered so far. In the case of each (acetylcholine, *nor*epinephrine, serotonin and GABA), the active agent, though readily formed in the brain, does not readily penetrate the blood brain barrier; their precursors (dopa, 5-hydroxytryptophan, glutamic acid) do so fairly readily, and are found in some instances (such as in the case of dopamine) to have a distribution pattern rather a different from their products. Again, the enzyme systems for their synthesis and disposition have a differential distribution pattern throughout the brain; and though sharing certain features in common (for example dependence upon decarboxylation in the case of dopamine, 5-hydroxytryptophan and glutamic acid), also show marked differences in respect to other enzyme activity (for example, their differential susceptibility to mono-amine oxidase, or O-methyltransferase). Furthermore, there is some suggestive evidence of susceptibility in some cases, to strictly local conditions (for example, local pH in the case of GAD and GABA-T). The picture, which thus emerges is one of convergence and interaction between a number of highly localised processes, proceeding at different rates and, possibly, at a different subcellular sites in the same segment of time. Their coincidence and relative overlap may profoundly determine the final sequence of events leading to discharge in a particular cell assembly.

Some Interactions Between Drugs and Neuroeffector Substances Within the Central Nervous System

The interrelatedness and the importance of relative and local shifts within a relatively small area is borne out by the complex and multiple effects of drugs on levels of neuroeffector substances within the nervous system. This can be observes at both central and peripheral sites. In a series of early experiments, it was shown that depletion of hypothalamic catecholamines could be brought about by a variety of drugs, some of which were convulsants (such as caffeine, leptazol, nicotine and picrotoxin) and some which were accounted as behaviorally depressant (such as morphine). There was excellent correlation between the loss of hypothalamic *nor*epinephrine and adrenal medullary *nor*epinephrine. Furthermore, there was a correlation between loss of *nor*epinephrine in the hypothalamus and in the midbrain. These experiments suggested that depletion of hypothalamic *nor*epinephrine was related to the stimulation of the symphatetic center of the brain stem; though it should be noted in passing that both stimulants and depressants were apparently capable of inducing such chemically judged stimulation; and that, though morphine had a depleting effect on hypothalamic catecholamine levels, this property was shared by such diverse agents as insulin, and ether (115).

The situation was found to be somewhat different in the case of reserpine. This drug leads to a release of large amounts of serotonin from body depots, and strikingly lowers brain 5-HT levels within four hours of administration. These effects may persist for several days (116, 117). During this period of low serotonin levels, the excretion of 5-hydroxy-indole acetic acid also rises. This suggests that, in the reserpinized animal, serotonin continues to be formed at a normal rate; but that there is an inability on the part of the tissues to bind the substance, with a consequent vulnerability of serotonin to oxidation by mono-amine oxidase. The inhibition of mono-amine oxidase by iproniazid prior to the administration of reserpine converts the sedative action of reserpine to a stimulant one (117, 118, 119) there being, on the face of it a beguilingly direct correlation between a lowering of brain serotonin levels and the sedative action of reserpine.

The complexity of the matter, however, is illustrated by a number of further observations. First, reserpine not only depletes serotonin, but also lowers the levels of *nor*epinephire in the brain (120), a property, which it shares with a number of drugs already mentioned. Secondly, dopamine (a precursor of epinephrine) also disappears from the brain following treatment with reserpine (87, 121). Thirdly, when considered quantitatively there is, in contrast to other cathecholamine depleting drugs, no parallelism in the case of reserpine between the central sympathetic activities (as judged by, adrenal medullary cathecholamine depletion) and the loss of catecholamines from the brain (115, 120). Lastly, the striking reduction of brain catecholamines by reserpine does not (in keeping with the above findings) result in direction of the electrical activity of the sympathetic outflow the preganglionic fibres (115), despite the marked reduction of the excitability of postganglionic fibres in the sympathetic chain. This would rather lead one to believe that a low residue of catecholamines or serotonin is not necessary related to a loss of central sympathetic activity. Furthermore, it was found that animals sedated by reserpine could be aroused by a number of drugs, such as morphia, amphetamine, and LSD-25 (115).

Discrepancies such as these suggest that one may be dealing with rather local and relative shifts, possibly at intracellular level. Some recent experiments are in keeping with this view.

In these studies (87, 121), the intracellular distribution of epinephrine, *nor*epinephire, and hydroxytyramine (dopamine) was examined in terms of partition between mitochondria and cytoplasm of the substances concerned. The brain stem of the rabbit was used. The normal distribution was compared with that following reserpine and the effect of administration of dopa was also studied. It was found that in the untreated animal, epinephrine, *nor*epinephrine, and hydroxytyramine (dopamine) were present in the ratio of 1:4:5, and that each was distributed approximately evenly between the particulate fraction (consisting mainly of mitochondria) and the cytoplasm. Reserpine was use in doses which brought about the disappearance of approximately 50% of the cathecholamines within four hours; it was found the rate of disappearance for all three amines was similar. However, the cytoplasmic fraction was depleted more rapidly than the particulate fraction, and this depletion was maintained irrespective of whether the amine-oxidase had been inhibited by prior injection of iproniazid. The intravenous injection of dopa in the reserpinized animal was found to restore the concentration of epinephrine and *nor*epinephrine to normal levels within an hour. Interestingly enough, the level of hydroxytyramine (dopamine) was increased far beyond the control level. The concentration of all amines was raised in both cellular fractions, suggesting that reserpine did not prevent the uptake of amines by the particulate components. The effect of dopa on brain catecholamines in untreated animals was similar. It, too, caused a striking rise in hydroxytyramine, though epinephrine and *nor*epinephrine were not significantly raised above their normal level. This suggested that the brain stem tissue was capable of rapid synthesis of epinephrine, provided dopa was supplied; and that normal concentrations were close to saturation level. The above study did not examine the effect of similar procedures on the intracellular distribution of serotonin, which, presumably (because of its greater susceptibility to monoamine oxidase) might have shown a rather different pattern. However, there is now some evidence that following reserpine, serotonin, in contrast to the catecholamines, disappears more rapidly from the particulate than the soluble fraction (122). This would not be out of keeping with the original suggestion that the action of reserpine depends on "free" serotonin.

Many more facts could be added to the ones already cited. They would, however, merely confuse an already tangled issue, and by their own accumulation point to the urgency of inquires of a rather different kind. It is regrettable that though many excellent studies have centered on single substances and single neurohumoral systems, very few studies have considered the effects of graded doses of the same drugs on the *relative* concentration of suspected key substances and their associated enzyme systems in discrete areas of the brain, or have weighed the possible *inter*action between substances in relation to chemically induced behavioral states or chemically induced electrophysiological change. Yet, it is submitted that it is the *relative* ratio of one substance to another – the ratio of, say a choline ester, a catecholamine, or an indole amine, or GABA in a particular place at a particular time – which may profoundly affect the net effect at a particular site. *Change* in concentration would thus seem to matter as much as absolute amount, and rate of reaction may be at least as important as the kind of reaction one is considering. It is, in fact, the relative interaction between reactions proceeding at rather different rates, which may affect the anchoring or release of a particular substance from its binding site, and thus modulate the opening or closure of the switchgear at some of the nodal points in the brain considered above.

That such relative shifts in concentration may, in fact, decisively influence the physiological effects of neuroeffector agents is illustrated by a second, and much older, set of experiments (123–126) which has been quoted previously in a cognate discussion (127). In 1941 it was shown that even small amounts of epinephrine applied in experiments which allowed separate perfusion of the spinal cord, could markedly affect the response to a given dose of acetylcholine, applied to the perfusate. Small doses of epinephrine steadied the muscle responses to acetylcholine; large doses (of the order of 100 μg) increased the (knee jerk) reflex, and very large doses (of the order of 300 μg) led to a prolonged diminution (126). In somewhat similar experiments, carried on a few years later, the interaction between acetylcholine and epinephrine was examined in the superior cervical ganglion preparation (124, 125). In both situations the balance of evidence suggested that whereas epinephrine had relatively little effect by itself, it was capable of profoundly modifying the response to acetylcholine. Small doses usually led to facilitation; larger doses, to inhibition. It was of interest, also, that in observing the effect of these agents on spinal movement patterns in the decerebrate preparation (128) the effects of epinephrine on flexors appeared opposite to its effects on extensors, and usually opposed those of acetylcholine. Though the variety of responses elicited in this particular series was inordinately wide, one cannot but again be struck by the reality of interaction between these two agents, and the wide repertoire of responses elicitable by this interaction. It would appear that epinephrine can modulate responses to acetylcholine (129) and that the net resultant of this interaction depends upon the relative proportions of the two substances, at particular sites at a particular time.

Possible Hormonal Factors Affecting Binding and Release to Neuroeffector Agents

The above examples are cited merely to indicate the kind of subcellular level of organization which seems to be the business level of the shifts and transactions so far considered. Little is known of the physiological (rather than pharmacological) factors which govern the storage and release of substances at theses subcellular sites. One would naturally suspect ionic shifts, though the evidence in this respects, so far, is very circumstantial. Equally, the role of hormones in these transactions is, at present, hardly more than suggestive.

There is a respectable body of evidence, recently admirably reviewed (130) which indicates a close physiological interaction between the cortical steroids and the epinephrines. The two groups of hormones would seem to operate physiologically as one functional unit. The steroids maintain the integrity and responsiveness of tissues in the process of reacting to the epinephrines; many actions of the epinephrines are not elicitable in the absence of steroids. Equally, and perhaps more significantly, however, many actions attributed to the steroids may, in fact, be more cogently ascribed to the action of the epinephrines (130). It is therefore of particular interest that there are at present some early indications of the effects of hormones on levels of neuroeffector substances in the brain. Adrenalectomy leads to an increase of brain serotonin (131). Exposure of rats to stress both of a cold ($0°C$) and a warm ($37°C$) environment prevents the release of serotonin by reserpine; it also prevents sedation by this substance (132). Also, more recently it has been shown that a marked depletion of *nor*epinephrine (though not of serotonin) follows exposure of rats to cold stress (133). A differential response of this kind is of interest, and may point to an as yet totally unexplored dependence of drug effects on hormonal equilibria within the brain itself. It would indeed be well to explore systematically the effect of graded hormone concentrations both on drug responsiveness and on the effects of drugs on the binding of amines at their unknown subcellular anchoring sites. This problem can perhaps be approached at a local as well as a systemic level. It can, for example, be shown that very small stereotactically placed implants of a hormone (stilbestrol dibutyrate) in the posterior hypothalamus will release a stereotyped form of behavior (sexual behavior) in the cat (134). The effect shows some specificity for both the hormone and the placement of the hormone. Little is at present known of the precise neural mechanism governing this release of a behavioral pattern. Earlier studies (135), however, would make on suspect a participation of neuroeffector substances in the ultimate mediation of a pituitary response, and it is conceivable that in the above experiments in the immediate vicinity of the implant may lead to significant changes in the balance of neuroeffector substances at a regional level.

The scanty clinical data so far available on the relation of plasma hydrocortisone level to affect give further pause for thought. There is a significant and linear relationship between an increase in anxiety, anger, and plasma hydrocortisone levels (136). Moreover, and perhaps less expected, it has been shown that severe depression it also accompanied by elevated plasma hydrocortisone levels (137), and that deeply retarded and underactive patients show hormone levels higher than those in a less depressed group. Depression would thus appear to be an active stress response; and the retarded, tearless state a final phase, as an active, adaptive process. This phase is largely inhibitory, as against the excitatory components commonly seen in the so-called "agitated depressive syndromes." It would be idle to speculate at present as to the possible effects of these various degrees of pituitary-adrenocortical mobilization on the binding and release of neuroeffector substances in nodal (or trigger) areas of the brain. It may even be that the reverse is true, and that differential proportions of catecholamines within the brain may affect the degree of adrenocortical mobilization. Yet there is some evidence, quoted in an adjoining paper (138) for the influence of purely situational factors on the relative pro-portions of *nor*epinephrine and epinephrine in the plasma. Lability or overactivity or under-activity may, however, have its neurohumoral correlates in the brain, as well as in the plasma. The data to date are scanty. Many more are needed before a rational hypothesis to account for these various states can be put forward.

IV. TOWARDS AN ANALYSIS OF REGIONAL PROCESS WITHIN THE BRAIN

The above findings and many others, of necessity omitted, serve to emphasize the impor-tance of regional and local economy in the function of the brain as a detector and organizer of spatiotemporal change in the course of adaptive behavior. The anatomical and cytological suborganization of even quite small areas of the brain has been mentioned; it is reflected by sharp regional differences in chemical constitution at cellular and, quite possibly, subcellular (139) levels. Nor would it be appropriate to assume that local and, in some areas, rather spe-cific chemical properties are not reflected in differences in local permeability of the blood brain barrier or in changes in small-vessel tone. There are, in fact, early indications that the converse may be true; that some areas (for example, the hypothalamus) may be differentially permeable to some metabolities (86), and that change in local function may be related to change in local blood flow (140). The principle of shielding, and of metabolic autonomy, so strikingly reflected in the existence of the blood brain barrier, may well have deeper meaning, and have to be carried into the chemical architecture of the brain itself. For all one knows, there may be pericellular barriers in some areas (for example the so-called "specific" lateral pathways); and local vascular shunts may well meet varying local needs. It may no longer be sufficient to look for differences in enzyme constitution between gross cell masses to account for a differential susceptibility of the nervous system to neuroleptic agents. Such differences must be sought at a more discrete level. As no other organ in the body, the brain has evolved as an aggregate of suborgans, resulting in – if one may so put it – an assembly of chemically me-diated homeostats. The chemical imprints of this evolution are becoming evident with time. A principle of metabolic compartmentalization (141) is emerging, of which the highly localized synthesis, storage, release, and disposition of neuroeffector substances at subcellular sites is but one instance. The convergence, relative ratio, and turnover-in-time of a few relatively sim-ple interlocking chemical reactions may profoundly affect excitability thresholds at particular sites at a particular time. The nodal midline areas appear to be peculiarly susceptible to such chemical shifts. Only overall data are so far available of the nature of these shifts; they do, however, suggest some similarity with mechanisms employed in neurohumoral mediation elsewhere.

It has been felt by the writer for some time (127, 142, 51–53) that these and cognate interac-tions may depend upon the presence and uneven distribution in the central nervous system of small families of compounds, derived from neuroeffector substances long familiar for their peripheral effects, yet possessed of special properties in the central nervous system, not shared in peripheral autonomic nets. Acetylcholine, epinephrine and serotonin may be prototypes of this kind. But behind acetylcholine there now stand esters other than acetylcholine; behind epinephrine there is hydroxytyramine; and behind serotonin melatonin (143). Hypotheses linked solely to one or other of these agents have not stood the test of time. It is upon distribution gradients of these and cognate substances that some of the modulating and gating mechanisms in the central nervous system may well depend.

It is therefore encouraging that methods for the analysis of regional transactions within the brain are now becoming available. The quantitative histochemistry of some enzyme systems in relation to cell population is feasible (144–147) and is bound sooner of later to be related to the action of drugs (148) at subcellular sites. Equally, the effects of drugs (149) and of hormones (134) applied to discrete areas of the brain are now being studied in relation to behavior; and though the interpretation of such effects is an admittedly hazardous undertaking, it is bound to become more discrete and precise with growing experience of the field. Furthermore, the electrophysiological correlates of such procedures are bound to be explored, and to be increasingly related to the electrophysiological correlates of conditioning, viewed in terms of the coding and transformation of signals within the brain. The shadows of which Maudsley spoke are thus sharpening into silhouettes; and in this process of growing understanding, the drugs influencing affect and behavior may play a part far beyond their empirical yield.

REFERENCES

1. Maudsley, Henry: The Physiology and Pathology of the Mind. Third Edition, Part 2. New York, D. Appleton & Co., 1882. p. 195.
2. Kety, S.S., Editor: The Pharmacology of Psychotomimetric and Psychotherapeutic Drugs. Ann. New York Acad. Sc. 66 (3):417, 1957.
3. Wikler, A.: The Relation of Psychiatry to Pharmacology. Baltimore, Williams & Wilkins, 1957.
4. Cole, J. O., and Gerard, R.W., Editors: Psychopharmacology Problems in Evaluation; Proc. Conf. On the Evaluation of Pharmacotherapy in Mental Illness. Washington, D.C. 1956. Washington, D.C., Nat. Acad. Sc. Nat. Res. Council Pub. 583, 1959.
5. Kline, N. S., Editor: Psychopharmacology Frontiers: Proc. of Psycho-pharmacology Symposium, Internat. Congr. of Psychiatry, Zürich 1957, Boston, Little, Brown & Co. 1959.
6. Bradley, P. B., Deniker, P., Radouco-Thomas, C., Editors: Neuro-Psychopharmacology, Proc. of 1st Internat. Congr. of Neuropharmacology, Rome 1958. Amsterdam, Elsevier, 1959.
7. Magoun, H. W. (p .26), Beach, F. S. (p. 151), Gerard, R. W. (p. 163), Pribram, K. H. (p. 173), Ganong, W. F. (p. 64): Present volume.
8. Ingram, W. R., Hanner, F. I., and Ranson, S. W.: The topography of the nuclei of the diencephalon of the cat. J. Comp. Neurol. 55:333, 1932.
9. Ingram, W. R.: Nuclear organization and chief connections of the primate hypothalamus. Proc. A. Res. Nerv. & Ment. Dis. 20:195, 1940.
10. Clark, W. E. L.: Beattie, J., Reddock, G., and Dott, N.M.: The Hypothalamus; Morphological, functional, Clinical and Surginal Aspects. Edinburgh, London, Oliver & Boyd, 1938.
11. Jasper, H. H., Proctor, L.D., Knighton, R. S., Noshay, W. C., and Costello, R. T., Editors: Reticular Formation of the Brain. Henry Ford Hospital Internat. Symposium, Boston, Little, Brown & Co. 1958.
12. Papez, J. W. A proposed mechanism of emotion. Arch. Neurol. & Psychiat. 38:725, 1937.
13. MacLean, P. D. The limbic system ("visceral brain") in relation to central gray and reticulum of the brain stem. Psychosom. Med. 17:355, 1955.
14. Adey, W. R.: Organization of the rhinencephalon. In Reticular Formation of the Brain. Henry Ford Hospital Internat. Symposium, H. H. Jasper et al., Eds. Boston, Little, Brown & Co. 1958. p. 621.
15. Putnam, T. J., Frantz, A. M., Ranson, S. W., Editors: The Diseases of the Basal Ganglia, Proc. A. Res. Nerv. & Ment. Dis., Vol. XXI, Baltimore, Williams & Wilkins, 1942.
16. Nauta, W. J. H., and Whitlock, D. G.: An anatomical analysis of the non-specific thalamic projection system. In Brain Mechanisms and Consciousness: A Symposium. Council for Internat. Organizations of Medical Sciences. J. F. Delafresnaye, Ed., Oxford, Blackwell Scientific Publications, 1954, p. 81.
17. Olszewski, J.: The cytoarchitecture of the human reticular formation. In Brain Mechanisms and consciousness: A Symposium. Council for Internat. Organizations of Medical Sciences. J. F. Delafresnaye, E., Oxford, Blackwell Scientific Publications, 1954. p. 54.
18. Scheibel, M. F., and Scheibel, A. B.: Structural substrates for integrative patterns in the brain stem reticular core. In Reticular Formation of the Brain. Henry Ford Hospital Internat. Symposium, H. H. Jasper et al., Eds., Boston, Little, Brown & Co. 1958, p. 31.
19. Olszewski, J. Loc. cit. (ref.17) p. 72.

20. Nauta, W. J. H., and Kuypers, H. G. J. M.: Some ascending pathways in the brain stem reticular formation. In: Reticular Formation of the Brain. Henry Ford Hospital Internat. Symposium, H. H. Jasper et al., Eds., Boston, Little, Brown & Co. 1958, p. 3.

21. Nauta, W. J. H.: Hippocampal projections and related neural pathways to the mid-brain in the cat. Brain 81:319, 1958.

22. Nauta, W. J. H.: Loc. cit. (Ref. No. 21), p. 339.

23. Pribram, K. H. and Kruger, L.: Functions of the "olfactory brain." Ann. New York Acad. Sc. 58:109, 1954.

24. Gloor, P.: Electrophysiological studies on the connections of the amygdaloid nucleus in the cat. II. The electro physiological properties of the amygdaloid projection system. Electroencephalog. & Clin. Neurophysiol. 7:243, 1955.

25. Brady, J. V.: The paleocortex and behavioral motivation. In Biological and Biochemical Bases of Behavior. Symposium on Interdisciplinary Research, Univ. of Wisconsin 1955 II. F. Harlow, and C. N. Wooolsey, Eds., Madison, Univ. of Wisconsin Press, 1958, p. 193.

26. Olds, J.: Adaptive functions of paleocortical and related structures. In Biological and Biochemical Bases of Behavior. Symposium on Interdisciplinary Research, Univ. of Wisconsin 1955. H. F. Harlow, and C. N. Woolsey, Eds. Madison, Univ. of Wisconsin Press, 1958, p. 237.

27. Ranson, S. W.: Regulation of body temperature. Proc. A Res. Nerv. & Ment. Dis. 20:342, 1940.

28. Brobeck, J. R.: Neural regulation of food intake. Ann. New York Acad. Sc. 63:44, 1955.

29. Hess, W. R.: Das Zwischenhirn: Syndrome, Lokalisationen, Funktionen. Basel, Schwabe, 1949.

30. Hare, K., and Geohegan, W. A.: Influence of frequency of stimulus upon the response to hypothalamic stimulation. J. Neurophysiol. 4:266, 1941.

31. Gellhorn, E., Cortell, R., and Murphy, J.P.: Are mass discharges characteristic of central autonomic structures? Am. J. Physiol. 146:376, 1946.

32. Olds, J., and Milner, P.: Positive reinforcement produced by electrical stimulation of septal area and other regions of rat brain. J. Comp. Physiol. 47:419, 1954.

33. Olds, J.: Selective effects of drives and drugs on "reward" systems of the brain. In Neurological Basis of Behaviour, Ciba Foundation Symposium, London 1957. G.F.W. Wolstenholme, C. M. O'Connor, Eds., London, J.& A. Churchill, 1958. p. 124.

34. Olds, J.: Studies of neuropharmacologicals by electrical and chemical manipulation of the brain in animals with chronically implanted electrodes. In Neuro-Psychopharmacology. Proc. of 1st Internat. Congr. of Neuropharmac ology, Rome 1958. P.B. Bradley, P. Deniker, and C. Radouco-Thomas, Eds., Amsterdam, Elsevier, 1959. p. 20.

35. Kaada, B.R., Andersen, P., and Janssen, J., Jr.: Stimulation of the amygdaloid nuclear complex in unanesthetized cats. Neurology 4:48, 1954.

36. Andersson, B., Jewell, P. A., and Larsson, S.: An appraisal of the effects of diencephalic stimulation of conscious animals in terms of normal behaviour. In Neurological Basis of Behaviour. Ciba Foundation Symposium, London 1957. G.E.W. Wolstenholme, and C.M. O'Connor, Eds., London, J. and A. Churchill, 1958, p. 76.

37. Klüver, H., and Bucy, P. C.: "Psychic blindness" and other symptoms following bilateral temporal lobectomy in Rhesus monkeys. Am. J. Physiol. 119:352, 1937.

38. Bard, P., and Mountcastle, V. B.: Some forebrain mechanisms involved in expression of rage with special reference to suppression of angry behavior. Proc. A. Res. Nerv. & Ment. Dis. 27:362, 1948.

39. Schreiner, I., and Kling, A.: Behavioral changes following rhinencephalic injury in cat. J. Neurophysiol. 16:643, 1953.

40. Fuller, J. I., Rosvold, H. E., and Pribram, K. H.: The effect on affective and cognitive behavior in the dog of lesions of the pyriform-amygdala-hippocampal complex. J. Comp. & Physiol, Psychol. 50:89, 1957.

41. MacLean, P. D.: Chemical and electrical stimulation of hippocampus in unrestrained animals. I. Methods and electroencephalographic findings. A.M.A. Arch. Neurol. & Psychiat. 78:113, 1957.

42. Richter, C. P.: Neurological basis of responses to stress. In: Neurological Basis of Behavior. Ciba Foundation Symposium, London 1957. G.E.W. Wolstenholme, and C. M. O'Connor, Eds., London, J. & A. Churchill, 1958. p. 204.

43. Manson, J. W.: The central nervous system regulation of ACTH secretion. In Reticular Formation of the Brain. Henry Ford Hospital Internat. Symposium. H.H. Jasper et al., Eds., Boston, Little, Brown & Co. 1958, p. 546.

44. Salmoiraghi, G. C., and Burns, B. C.: Localization and patterns of discharge of respiratory neurones. J. Neuro physiol. (In press.)

45. Miller, N. E.: Objective techniques for studying motivational effects of drugs on animals. In: Psychotropic Drugs. S. Garattini and V. Ghetti, Eds., Amsterdam, Elsevier, 1957. p. 83.

46. Brady, J. V.: Differential drug effects upon aversive and appetitive components of a behavioral repertoire. In: Neuro-Psychopharmacology, Proc. of 1st Internat. Congr. of Neuro-pharmacology, Rome 1958. Amsterdam, Elsevier, 1959.

47. Masserman, J. H. and Yum, K. S. An analysis of the influence of alcohol on experimental neuroses in cats. Psychosom. Med. 18:36, 1946.

48. Bradley, P. B., and Elkes, J.: A technique for recording the electrical activity of the brain in the conscious animal. Electroencephalog. & Clin. Neurophysiol. 5:451, 1953.

49. Bradley, P. B., and Elkes, J.: The effect of amphetamine and D-lysergic acid diethylamide (LSD 25) on the electrical activity of the brain of the conscious cat. J. Physiol. 120:136, 1953.

50. Bradley, P. B., and Elkes, J.: The effect of atropine, hyoscyamine, physostigmine and neostigmine on the electrical activity of the brain of the conscious cat. J. Physiol. 120:148, 1953.

51. Bradley, P. B., and Elkes, J.: The effects of some drugs on the electrical activity of the brain. Brain, 80:77, 1957.

52. Elkes, J.: Discussion in J.M. Tanner (ed.) Prospectsin Psychiatric Research (pp. 126-135). Oxford, Blackwell Publications, 1957

53. Elkes, J.: Drug effects in relation to receptor specificity within the brain: some evidence and privisional formulation. In Neurological Basis of Behavior. Ciba Foundation Symposium, London, 1957. G.E.W. Wolsten holme, and C.M. O'Connor, Eds., London, J. & A. Churchill, 1958. p. 303.

54. Wikler, A.: Pharmacologic dissociation of behavior and EEG "sleep patterns" in dogs: morphine, N-allyl normorphine, and atropine. Proc. Soc. Exper. Biol. & Med. 79:261, 1952.
55. Bremer, F.: Cerveau isolé et physiologie du sommeil. Compt. Rend. Soc. de biol. 118:1235, 1935.
56. Moruzzi, G. and Magoun, H.W.: Brain stem retucular formation and activation of the EEG. Electroencephalog. & Clin. Neurophysiol. 1:455, 1949.
57. Magoun, H. W.: The ascending reticular activating system. Proc. A. Res. Nerv. & Ment. Dis. 30:480, 1952.
58. Hiebel, G., Bonvallet, M., Huve, P., and Dell, P.: Analyse neurophysiologique de l'action centrale de la d-amphétamine (maxiton). Semaine h"p. Paris. 30:1880, 1954.
59. Vogt, M.: The concentration of symphatin in different parts of the central nervous system under normal conditions and after the administration of drugs. J. Physiol. 123:451, 1954.
60. Dell, P. C.: Humoral effects on the brain stem reticular formations. In Reticular Formation of the Brain. Henry Ford Hospital Internat. Symposium. H. H. Jasper et al., Eds., Boston, Little, Brown & Co. 1958. p. 365.
61. Rothballer, A. B.: Studies on the adrenaline-sensitive component of the reticular activating system. Electro encephalog. & Clin. Neurophysiol. 8:603, 1956.
62. Bradley, P. B. and Hance, A. J.: The effect of chlorpromazine and methopromazine on the electrical activity of the brain in the cat. Electroencephalog. Clin. Neurophysiol. 9:191, 1957.
63. Bradley, P.B. The central action of certain drugs in relation to the reticular formation of the brain. In: Reticular Formation of the Brain. Henry Ford Hospital Int. Symposium. H.H. Jasper et al., Eds., Boston, Little, Brown & Co. 1958. p. 123.
64. Bradley, P. B., and Key, B. J.: A comparative study of the effects of drugs on the arousal system of the brain. Br. J. Pharmacol. 14:340, 1959.
65. Killam, K. F., and Killam, E. K.: Drug action on pathways involving the reticular formation. In Reticular Formation of the Brain. Henry Ford Hospital Internat. Symposium. H.H. Jasper et al., Eds., Boston, Little, Brown & Co. 1958. p. 111.
66. Pfeiffer, C. C., Jenney, E. H., Gallagher, W., Smith, R.P., Bevan, W., Jr., Killam, K.F., Killam, E.K. and Blackmore, W.: Stimulant effect of 2-dimethylaminoethanol; possible precursor of brain acetylcholine, Science 126:610, 1957
67. Killam, K. B., Gangloff, H., Konigsmark, B., and Killam, K. E.: The action of pharmacologic agents on evoked cortical activity. In Biological Psychiatry. Proc. of Scientific Sessions of Soc. of Biol. Psychiat., San Francisco 1958. J. H. Masserman, Ed., New York, Grune & Stratton, 1959. p. 53.
68. Himwich, H.E., Van Meter, W. G., and Owens, H.: Drugs used in the treatment of the depressions. In Biological Psychiatry. Proc. of Scientific Sessions of Soc. of Biol. Psychiat., San Francisco 1958. J.H. Masserman, Ed., New York, Grune & Stratton, 1959. p. 27.
69. Elkes, J.: Discussion of Himwich, H., et al., (Ref. No.68.) p. 50.
70. Jacobsen, E., and Skaarup, Y.: Experimental induction of conflict-behaviour in cats: the effect of some anti cholinergic compounds. Acta pharmacol. Et toxicol. (KbH) 1I:125, 1955.
71. Sigg, E.B.: Pharmacological studies with tofranil. Canad. Psychiat. A. J. 4:75, 1959.
72. Amassian, V. E., and Waller, H. J.: Spatiotemporal patterns of activity in individual reticular neurons. In Reticular Formation of the Brain. Henry Ford Hospital Internat. Symposium. H. H. Jasper et al., Eds., Boston, Little, Brown & Co. 1958. p. 69.
73. Bradley, P. B.: Microelectrode approach to the neuropharmacology of the reticular formation. In Psychotropic Drugs. S. Garattini and V. Ghetti, Eds., Amsterdam, Elsevier, 1957. p. 207.
74. Bradley, P. B., and Mollica, A.: The effect of adrenaline and acetylcholine on single unit activity in the reticular formation of the decerebrate cat. Arch. ital. biol. 94:168, 1958.
75. Whitfield, I. C., Schwartz, A., and Fotheringham, J. B.: unpublished findings
76. Feldberg, W., and Vogt, M.: Acetylcholine synthesis in different regions of central nervous system. J. Physiol. 107:372,. 1948.
77. Feldberg, W.,: Present views on mode of action of acetylchloine in central nervous system. Physiol. Rev. 25:596, 1945.
78. Weil-Malherbe, H., and Bone, A. D.: Intracellular distribution of catecholamines in the brain. Nature (London), 180:1050, 1957.
79. Carlsson, A.: The occurrence, distribution and physiological role of catecholamines in the nervous system. Pharmacol. Rev. 11:490, 1957
80. Blaschko, H., Hagen, J. M., and Hagen, P.: Mitochondrial enzymes and chromaffin-granules. J. Physiol. 139:316, 1957.
81. Falck, B., Hillarp, N. A., and H"gberg, B.: Content and intracellular distribution of adenosine triphosphate in cow adrenal medulla. Acta physiol. Scand.
82. Holtz, P. and Westerman, E.: šber die Dopadecarboxylase und Histidindecarboxylase des Nervengewebes. Arch. Exper. Path. U. Pharmakol. 227:538, 1956.
83. Udenfriend, S., and Wyngaarden, J. B.: Precursors of adrenal epinephrine and *nor*epinehprine "in vivo". Biochem. et biophys. Acta 20:48, 1956.
84. Rosenfeld, G., Leeper, L. C., and Udenfriend, S.: Biosynthesis of *nor*epinephrine and epinephrine by the isolated perfused calf adrenal. Fed. Proc. 16:331, 1957.
85. Kirshner, N., and Goodall, M. C.: Formation of adrenaline from noradrenaline, Fed. Proc. 16:73, 1957.
86. Weil-Malherbe, H., Axelrod, J., and Tomchick, R.: Blood-brain barrier for adrenaline. Science 129:1226, 1959.
87. Weil-Malherbe, H., and Bone, A. D.: The effect of reserpine on the intracellular distribution of catecholamines in the brain stem of the rabbit. J. Neurochem. 4:251, 1959.
88. Kety, S. S.: The possible relationships between the catecholamines and emotional states. (p.77) Present volume

89. Armstrong, M. D.: McMillan, A., and Shaw, K. N. F.: 3-Methoxy-+-hydroxy-D-mandelic acid, a urinary metabolite of *nor*epinephrine. Biochim. et biophys. Acta 25:422, 1957.
90. Symposium on Catecholamines. Pharmacol. Rev. 11 (2-Part 2): 232, 1959.
91. Twarog, B. M., and Page, I. H.: Serotonin content of some mammalian tissues and urine and a method for its determination. Am. J. Physiol. 175:157, 1953.
92. Amin, A. H., Crawford, T.B.B., and Gaddum, J.H.: The distribution of substance P and 5-hydroxy-tryptamine in the central nervous system of the dog. J. Physiol. 126:596, 1954.
93. Paasonen, M. K., MacLean, P. D., and Giarman, N. J.: 5-Hydroxytryptamine (serotonin, enteramine) content of structures of the limbic system. J. Neurochem. 1:326, 1957.
94. Gaddum, J. H., and Giarman, N. J.: Preliminary studies on the biosynthesis of 5-hydroxytryptamine. Brit. J. Pharmacol. 11:88, 1956.
95. Udenfriend, S., Bogdanski, D.F., and Weissbach, H.: Biochemistry and metabolism of serotonin as it relates to the nervous system. In Metabolism of the Nervous System, Internat. Neurochemical Symposium, Aarhus, Denmark 1957. D. Richter Ed., New York, Pergamon Press, 1957., p. 566.
96. Shore, P. A., Mead, J. A., Kuntzman, R. G., Spector, S., and Brodie, B.B.: On the physiologic significance of monoamine oxidase in brain. Science 126:1063, 1957.
97. Corne, S. J., and Graham, J. D.: The effect of inhibition of amine oxidase "in vivo" on administered adrenaline, noradrenaline, tyramine and serotonin. J. Physiol. 135:339, 1957.
98. Sjoerdsma, A., Gillespie, L., Jr., and Udenfriend, S.: A simple method for the measurement of monoamine oxidase inhibition in man. Lancet 2:159, 1958.
99. Udenfriend, S., and Weissbach, H.: Turnover of 5-hydroxytryptamine (serotonin) in tissues. Proc. Soc. Exper. Biol. & Med. 97:748, 1958.
100. Purpura, D. P., Girado, M., Smith, T. G., Callan, D. A., and Grundfest, H.: Structure-activity determinants of pharmacological effects of amino acids and related compounds on central synapses. J. Neurochem. 3:238, 1959.
101. Roberts, E., Harman, P. J., and Frankel, S.: γ-Aminobutyric acid content and glutamic decarboxylase activity in developing mouse brain. Proc. Soc. Exper. Biol. & Med. 78:799, 1951.
102. Roberts, E.: Formation and utilization of γ-aminobutyric acid in brain. Progress in Neurobiology 1:11, 1956.
103. Roberts, E.: The biochemistry of gamma aminobutyric acid in the central nervous system. Proc. of the Western Pharmacology Soc. (Seattle, McCaffrey Dogwood Press) 1:29, 1958.
104. Salvador, R. A., and Albers, R. W.: The distribution of glutamic γ-aminobutyric transaminase in the nervous system of the rhesus monkey. J. Biol. Chem. 234:922, 1959.
105. Albers, R. W., and Brady, R. O.: The distribution of glutamic decarboxylase in the nervous system of the rhesus monkey. J. Biol. Chem. 234:926, 1959.
106. Baxter, C. F., and Roberts, E. (In press.)
107. Killam, K. F.: Convulsant hydrazides. II. Comparison of electrical changes and enzyme inhibition induced by administration of thiosemicarbazide. J. Pharmacol. & Exper. Therap. 119:263, 1957.
108. Dasgupta, S. R., Killam, E. K., and Killam, K. F.: Drug action on rhinencephalic seizure activity in the cat. J. Pharmacol. & Exper. Therap. 122:16A, 1958.
109. Eidelberg, E., Baxter, C. F., Roberts, E., Saldias, C. A., and French, J. D. In: Inhibition in the Nervous System and γ<Φ255Δ>−Αμινοβυτψριχ Αχιδ. Προχ. οφ Σψμποσιυμ Σπονσορεδ βψ Αιρ Φορχε Οφφιχε οφ Σχιεντιφιχ Ρεσεαρχη, Δυαρτε, Χαλιφ. 1959. Ε. Ροβερτσ, Εδ., Νεω Ψορκ, Περγαμον Πρεσσ. (Ιν πρεσσ.)
110. Florey, E., and McLennan, H.: Effects of an inhibitory factor (factor I) from brain on central synaptic transmission. J. Physiol. 130:446, 1955.
111. Roberts, E., Editor, Inhibition in the Nervous System and γ-Aminobutyric Acid. Proc. of Symposium Sponsored by Air Force Office of Scientific Research, Durarte, Calif. 1959. New York, Pergamon Press (In press)
112. Waelsch, H. W.: Metabolism of proteins and amino acids. In Metabolism of the Nervous System. Internat. Neurochemical Symposium, Aarhus, Denmark 1956. D. Richter, Ed., New York, Pergamon Press, 1957, p. 431.
113. Strecker, H. J.: Glutamic acid and glutamine. In Metabolism of the Nervous System. Internat. Neurochemical Symposium, Aarhus, Denmark 1957. D. Richter, Ed., New York, Pergamon Press, 1957. p. 459.
114. Waelsch, H. W. New aspects of amine metabolism. In The Chemical Pathology of the Nervous System. J. Folch-Pi, Ed., London, Pergamon Press. (In press)
115. Vogt, M.: Catecholamines in brain. Pharmacol. Rev. 11:483, 1959.
116. Brodie, B. B., Pletscher, A., and Shore, P. A.: Evidence that serotonin has a role in brain function. Science, 122:968, 1955.
117. Brodie, B. B., Pletscher, A., and Shore, P. A.: Possible role of serotonin in brain fuction and in reserpine action. J. Pharmacol. & Exper Therap. 116:19, 1956.
118. Pletscher, A., Shore, P. A., and Brodie B. B.: Serotonin as a mediator of reserpine action in brain. J. Pharmacol. & Exper. Therap. 116:84, 1956.
119. Pletscher, A., Shore, P. A., and Brodie, B. B.: Release of brain serotonin by reserpine. J. Pharmcol. & Exper. Therap. 116:46, 1956.
120. Holzbauer, M., and Vogt, M.: Depression by reserpine of the noradrenaline concentration in the hypothalamus of the cat. J. Neurochem. 1:8, 1956.
121. Weil-Malherbe, H.: Personal communication
122. Giarman, N. J., and Schanberg, S.: The intracellular distribution of 5-hydroxytryptamine (HT; serotonin) in the rat's brain. Biochem. Pharmacol. 1:301, 1959.
123. Bülbring, E., and Burn, J. H.: Observations bearing on synaptic transmission by acetylcholine in the spinal cord. J. Physiol. 100:337, 1941.
124. Bülbring, E.: The action of adrenaline on transmission in the superior cervical ganglion. J. Physiol. 103:55 1944.

125. Bülbring, E., and Burn, J. H.: An action of adrenaline on transmission in the sympathetic ganglia, which may play a part in shock. J. Physiol. 101:289, 1942.
126. Schweitzer, A., and Wright, S.: The action of adrenaline on the knee jerk. J. Physiol. 88:476, 1937.
127. Elkes, J.: On possible uses of pharmacological method in psychiatric research. In: Prospects in Psychiatric Research. Proc. Oxford conference of Mental Health Research Fund, March 1952. J. M. Tanner, Ed., Oxford, Blackwell Scientific Publications, 1953, p. 126.
128. Bülbring, E., Burn, J. H., and Skoglund, C. R.: The action of acetylcholine and adrenaline on flexor and extensor movements evoked by stimulation of the descending motor tracts. J. Physiol. 107:289, 1948.
129. Burn, J. H.: The relation of adrenaline to acetylcholine in the nervous system. Physiol. Rev. 25:377, 1945.
130. Ramey, E. R., and Goldstein, M. S.: Adrenal cortex and the sympathetic nervous system. Physiol. Rev. 37:155, 1957.
131. De Maio, D.: Influence of adrenalectomy and hypophysectomy on cerebral serotonin. Science 129:1678, 1959.
132. Garattini, S., and Valzelli, L.: Researches on the mechanism of reserpine sedative action. Science 128:1278:, 1958.
133. Brodie, B. B., Finger, K. F., Orlans, F. B., Quinn, G. P., and Sulser, F.: Evidence that tranquilizing action of reserpine is associated with change in brain serotonin and not in brain *nor*epinephrine. 1960. (In press.)
134. Harris, G. W., Michael, R. P., and Scott, P. P.: Neurological site of action of stilboestrol in eliciting sexual behavior. In: Neurological Basis of Behavior, Ciba Foundation Symposium, London 1957. G. E. W. Wolsten holme, and C. M. O'Connor, Eds., London, J. C. A. Churchill, 1958. p. 236.
135. Sawyer, C. H.: Activation and blockade of the release of pituitary gonadotropin as influenced by the reticular formation. In Reticular Formation of the Brain. Henry Ford Hospital Internat. Symposium. H. H. Jasper, et al., Eds. Boston, Little, Brown & Co. 1958. p. 223.
136. Persky, H., Hamburg, D. A., Basowitz, H., Grinker, R. R., Sabshin M., Korchin, S. J., Herz, M., Board F. A., and Heath, H. A. Relation of emotional responses and changes in plasma hydrocortisone level after stressful interview. A. M. A. Arch. Neurol. & Psychiat. 79:434, 1958.
137. Board, F., Wadeson, R., and Persky, H.: Depressive affect and endocrine functions. A. M. A. Arch. Neurol. & Psychiat. 78:612, 1957.
138. Mason, J. W., and Hamburg, d. A.: Quoted by S. S. Kety, present volume.
139. Waelsch, H., Editor: Ultrastructure and Cellular Chemistry of Neural Tissue. Progress in Neurobiology, Vol. II, New York, Hocher-Harper, 1957.
140. Sokoloff, I.: Local blood flow in neural tissue. In New Research Techniques in Neuroanatomy. A Symposium Sponsored by the Nat. Multiple Sclerosis Soc. W. F. Windle, Ed., Charles C. Thomas, 1957. p. 51.
141. Waelsch, H. W.: Personal communication
142. Elkes, J., Elkes, C., and Bradley, P. B.: The effect of some drugs on the electrical activity of the brain, and on behavior. J. Ment. Sc. 100:125, 1954.
143. Lerner, A. B., Case, J. d., Takahashi, Y., Lee, T. H. and Mori, W.: Isolation of melanotonin, the pineal gland factor that lightens melanocytes. J. Am. Chem. Soc. 80:2587, 1958.
144. Nurnberger, J. I., and Gordon, M. W.: The cell density of neural tissues: Direct counting method and possible applications as a biologic referent. Progress in Neurobiology 2:100, 1957.
145. Pope, A., Hess, H. H., and Allen, J. N.: Quantitative histochemistry of proteolytic and oxidative enzymes in human cerebral cortex and brain tumors. Progress in Neurobiology 2:182, 1957.
146. Robins, E., Smith, D. E., and Jen, M. K.: The quantitative distribution of eight enzymes of glucose methabolism and two citric acid cycle enzymes in the cerebellar cortex and its subjacent white matter. Progress in Neurogiology 2:205, 1957.
147. Koelle, G. B.: The localization of acetylcholinesterase in neurons. Progress in Neurobiology 2:164, 1957.
148. Berger, M.: Effect of chlorpromazine on oxidative phosphorylation of brain mitochondria. Progress in neuro biology 2:158, 1957.
149. Olds, J., and Olds, M. E.: Positive reinforcement produced by stimulating hypothalamus with iproniazid and other compounds. Science 127:1175, 1958.
150. John, E. R., and Killam, K. F.: Electrophysiological correlates of avoidance conditioning in the cat. J. Pharmacol. & Exper. Therap. 125:252, 1959.

PAPER 15

BEHAVIORAL PHARMACOLOGY IN RELATION TO PSYCHIATRY[**]

Joel Elkes

Reprinted with the kind permission of Springer Verlag
from H.W. Gruhle, R. Jung, W. Mayer-Gross and M. Muller (eds.) *Psychiatrie der Gegenwart*
(pp. 929–1038). Berlin/Heidelberg/New York, Springer Verlag, 1967

CONTENTS

* * The first part of this paper includes material originally presented in Working Paper No. 1, Study Group on Ataractic and Hallucinogenic Drugs, World Health Organisation, Geneva 1957. It was subsequently incorporated in the Report of the Group (WHO, Technical Report No. 152) and reproduced in this paper with the permission of the Chief Editor, Technical Publications, WHO, Geneva, in 1961, and with the kind permission of Information Management and Dissemination, WHO, Geneva, in 2001..

I. INTRODUCTION

It is more to accident than design that psychopharmacology owes its strange place in the behavioral sciences and in psychiatry today. Lysergic acid diethyl-amide, chlorpromazine and reserpine (see ref. 2 for history) had their beginning in the inspired empiricism of their originators. Yet the impact of the pharmacotherapies, from their humble beginnings a mere decade ago, has been so massive, and the accumulation of data so rapid that many problems requiring scrutiny from the beginning are only now emerging to be faced. Nevertheless, a realization of these problems is essential for the long-term growth of the field.

It is the limited purpose of this paper to draw attention to some gaps in our existing knowledge; to inquire how these ignorances have arisen, and how they may be linked; to weigh their relative importance; to indicate some areas where progress is being made by established methods; and, equally, to point to others still awaiting the development of appropriate techniques. No attempt is made, in any way, to cover the ground comprehensively; or to be up to date with the latest remedy or the latest theoretical formulation. Topics such as addiction, and the effect of barbiturates or anticonvulsants have not been included. Psychopharmacology poses many questions which are relevant to the aspirations of present day psychiatry as an experimental and a clinical science; it is some of these questions which it is intended to examine, and no more. Also, much that is mentioned has been covered in several excellent recent symposia and reviews (1–6). The reader is referred to these for more detailed information.

The Origins of Present Ignorances

The sudden and explosive growth of interest in the psychotropic agents over the past few years should not blind one to their antecedents. The historical roots of the subject go deep, and it is perhaps by viewing these that the present ignorances can be most adequately assessed. The recorded facts up to the beginnings of the present century could, in themselves, make rich reading; yet one suspects that they would merely represent the visible fringe of a vast, old, stream of experience of the race which, essentially unrecorded, yet ever-present, has penetrated and dyed deep the varied fibber and pattern of many cultures. It is a humbling thought that mescaline, cohoba, morphia, marihuana, reserpine or psilocybin owe their discovery at western hands to chance, rather than active search. The search, however, has now begun in earnest; and the skills of the organic chemist are at hand to amplify, supplant and enrich the properties of natural products.

It is pertinent to inquire as to why this field of psychotropic drugs should have been shrouded in silence for so long, and why western science should have quickened to an interest in their effects only in the second half of the 20th century. In assessing possible reasons, cognizance has to be taken of the nature of the phenomena induced by the drugs and the setting in which they were originally observed; their affinity with other phenomena, studied by western science; the relation of both to the development of the experimental behavioural disciplines; and to the recent growth of cognate basic neurological sciences. These will now be briefly considered.

The Essentially Personal and Subjective Nature of Psychotropic Drug Effects in Man

At a time when the clinician is dominated by a mounting literature on the so-called ataractic and stimulant compounds, it is well to recall that some of the earliest drugs to receive intensive study were the psychodysleptic (psychosomimetic, hallucinogenic) agents. The literature on these abounds, and only three aspects need emphasis in the present content. First, that the effects were originally observed in a religious and ceremonial setting which formed a cardinal part of a local culture; second, that some elements in the phenomena induced by these drugs made them particularly suitable for the purpose for which they were being used; and third, that these elements were strongly subjective, personal and, in some essential aspects, averbal and incommunicable. All early observers (7–10) who have used mescaline and LSD 25 on themselves, or on others, agree that the most important areas of disturbed function lie in the affective, perceptual, and cognitive fields; that alteration in overt behaviour need not necessarily accompany striking subjective change, and, if it does, can form only the crudest counterpart of the subjective experience. Equally, the intensity, variation, speed, and fluctuating, kaleidoscope play of the phenomena is such as to defy the ordinary currency of language. The mere act of description may, in fact, alter the phenomena. Thus, even the most objective observers are constantly compelled in their protocol to resort to simile and allusion in an attempt to describe what, by common consent, is outside the range of normal human experience. But even in more homely examples, the same difficulties apply. A great deal, for instance, has been written on the so-called tranquillizers; we all know that they quiet the "disturbed". But how much, or how little, do we know of the meaning, or the shades of meaning, of this chemically induced tranquillity in the individual patient, or in the normal individual, in whom dose range alone suggests the effects may be quite different? Again, it is one thing to observe a Parkinsonian syndrome in the course of drug therapy; it is a totally different matter to inquire into the mental state of the patient at the same time and to discover (or attempt to measure) the affective and perceptual changes inseparable from this state. In all psychotropic drug effects, therefore, overt behaviour, including the ordinary tools of language, can be but a segment of the evidence; the larger portion lies within, and requires special and, in many ways novel, techniques for its adequate description, let alone understanding.

The above remarks may perhaps indicate one group of reasons for the isolation and the lag of this field despite its long recognized existence. The phenomena were first observed in culturally remote regions, and were of a nature which, in the first instance, was inclined to appeal more to the cultural anthropologist and the student of comparative religion than to the nineteenth century psychologist or physician; they were strongly subjective, and were reflected only very inadequately in overt behaviour; they contained central elements which, being well outside the range of normal conscious observation were very difficult to describe; and by their similarity with some varieties of religious experience moved on to ground which nineteenth century science was reluctant to enter. In the psychological sciences we are only gradually recovering from the limitations of the so-called objective method: we do so by recognizing what it can describe and measure and what, so far, it cannot. In the area under discussion the purely behavioral approach is self-limiting, and one which loses information. On the other hand, such information as is accessible to subjective inquiry is apt to be descriptive, anecdotal, and, in the absence of adequate calibration, very difficult to measure. It is out of the discrepancies, dissatisfactions and tensions of this dilemma that new methods of inquiry into these highly subjective states are likely to emerge. The territory of experience they are to survey and map is indeed large; and in this territory the clinical needs and states are but a province.

The Affinity with other Subjective States, including the Psychoanalytic Experience

It is perhaps not irrelevant that the long isolation of psychotropic drugs from the general body of knowledge is shared by a number of other areas whose essential and outstanding characteristic is the subjective and personal nature of the phenomena observed. In a nineteenth century preoccupied with the objective and measurable properties of solid matter, and not yet exposed to the loosening and expansion which followed the emergence of quantum mechanics and the theory of relativity, only the staunchest investigators would publicly acknowledge their interest in the private psychology of the individual, or attempt to define the common components, and individual differences in these phenomena. Noted in this context may be Galton's "The Vision of Sane Persons" (ll) and "The Statistics of Mental Imagery" (12) and James' "The Varieties of Religious Experience" (13), works which draw attention to phenomena apt to be more familiar to novelists than to scientists, and whose everyday manifestations had been assiduously ignored. Changes in perception, affect, and body image during the brief twilight states separating wakefulness from sleep (the so-called hypnagogic imagery), the déja-vu phenomena, the synaesthesias, the ecstatic feelings of "identity" and "fusion" accompanying intense religious experience are met with in these and cognate writings; as are also attempts to group and analyse these phenomena. These papers relate to much that both preceded and followed them. Thus, the hypnagogic phenomena were described quite early by Müller (14), and, much later, by Leaning (15). "Visual Dreams" were analysed by Ladd (16). In 1896 Weir-Mitchell published his classical account of mescaline intoxication (17); and it is well to compare this paper with Ladd's paper on spontaneously induced visual dreams published four years earlier. Havelock Ellis (18) tried to compare both spontaneous and drug-induced imagery; and in his masterly essays (19, 20) Klüver drew attention to form constants, seen not only in mescal intoxication but also in normal subjects under certain conditions in the absence of drugs. Thus it seemed that the drug-induced phenomena contained elements which were well within the frame of normal human subjective experience, though, ordinarily, their incidence was alight, and their range and quality were profoundly affected by the use of drugs. It appeared as if certain functional modalities, part and parcel of the normal adaptive behaviour and normally used only transitorily and sparingly in the waking state, could be chemically locked by the psychodysleptic agents into more persistent manifestations. There is thus little question of the enrichment which psychopharmacology is likely to derive from a study of cognate phenomena outside the limited chemical domain.

This will apply with special force to psychoanalysis, which began its remarkable development in a cul-de-sac of silence, doubt and disapproval. Like no other body of knowledge in the past it described phenomena ranging from the most mundane to the inordinate properties of dreams and the phantasies of the mentally disturbed. Moreover, it attempted to group these phenomena, to device methods for their study, and to build, on the basis of these findings, a coherent theoretical framework the many modifications of which at the hands of its originator only emphasize its tentative and empirical nature. In the context in which the problem is being examined, only three aspects need be stressed. First, that the technique of personal analysis and its tools, those of free association and the analysis of transference, has familiarized the psychoanalyst with a range of manifestations not readily accessible to any other method; second, that these phenomena share with the ones already listed a strongly subjective private element which often (and perhaps at the most important phases of the analytic experience) is outside the normal range of communication by language; and thirdly, that the methodological difficulties in assessing the nature and outcome of the analytic process, far from being solved, are only now being adequately faced (21). In this respect, again, there is some similarity between the problems posed by the subjective drug-induced experience, and the analytic experience; and tools used in one may find a fruitful application in the other. It is, however, significant how isolated and separated the advances in the respective sectors of a common field have been so far: the subject matter fitted ill the brash innocence of a young emerging materialist science. Yet the paradox remains. For why did the same age accept and encourage its inordinately penetrating and sensitive master novelists?

The Uneven Development of the Animal Behavioral Sciences

A further source of weakness lies in the uneven development of the animal behavioral sciences, which promise well for the analysis of drug induced states. The study of the effects of drugs on overt behavior in laboratory animals goes back well into the nineteenth century; for example, a paper on the effects of alcohol on the behavior of the rat, specifying recording methods, is dated 1898 (22). However, again the initial emphases reflect the hopes, and the prejudices of the age; and despite (and, perhaps, because of) the revolutionary inventiveness of the Pavlovian laboratory, and the conceptual fusion of behavior with neurophysiological process which it engendered, these trends continued to shape both experiment and interpretation. Essentially, the areas studied were learning, autonomic function, sensory discrimination and gross behavioral change, observed (for very good reason) in the single animal, in strictly controlled and highly artificial laboratory conditions. Much less emphasis was placed, in those initial stages, upon the step-by-step analysis of patterns of affective response, and the factors leading to their enhancement and attenuation (though here, too great beginnings were being made); the individual differences between animals and the factors making for these differences (though Pavlov was fully aware of both); the cues in an animal's environment which govern its normal behavior in the *free* state; or the forces operating in the social organization of an animal community. Yet each of these factors is important in assessing agents which, by common consent not only affect perception, or learning but profoundly colour motivation, and the social attitudes within the species. The over-isolation of a problem, and an undue emphasis on technique, thus tended to make the answers irrelevant to the larger questions which were being posed.

Pavlov, in studying the so-called "excited" forms of experimental neurosis, was quick to perceive the pharmacological implications of his findings. Quite early he noted the effects of bromides in restoring the negative conditioned response without impairing its "positive" counterpart (23) and suggested an effect of bromides on internal inhibition. A great many studies have stemmed from this experimental approach (24, 25) and have borne fruit in their respective areas. The "Conflict syndrome" forms an engagingly attractive paradigm: the phenomena, both behavioral and autonomic, are readily reproducible, and the conditions in which they are observed readily controlled. Yet it is the discrete analysis of the intermediate steps and components of the complex transaction resulting ultimately in conflict or avoidance behavior which is of moment in the analysis of drug effects upon such behavior. Such analysis must weigh the contribution of sensory cues; the relative strength, and relation to each other, of appetitive drives; the strength of the inhibitory mechanisms, innate or acquired, which normally regulate the release of these drives; and the strength of the motor apparatus normally at their disposal to bring about their discharge. "Tranquillization" or "Stimulation" may thus travel in many guises, and mask a multiplicity of factors compounding a total response.

These issues are being faced at present, and from very different sources. One such notable approach involves the application of a number of different tests and techniques to an identical behavioral situation, in an attempt to weigh the contribution of individual factors to a reproducible response (26). Another is the intensive and careful analysis of temporal patterns in different stimulus and response situations. It is here that the continuous process or free operant techniques offer their major contribution. These have received ample review (27), and their application to the analysis of psychotropic drug effects has been manifold. The techniques of electronic programming of stimulus situations, and the automatic recording of responses make for continuity and permanence of record; and provide ready material for the detection of statistical trends.

The above methods, in most instances, employ single animals. There are not many investigations (28) which make the social setting of the experiment a special point of enquiry. Studies of this aspect grew up separately, and from very different sources.

Patterns of sexual behavior were studied early and intensively (29), and form a model which, because of its stereotype nature and its ready susceptibility to chemical variables, is one of high promise for pharmacological study. Similarly, the hierarchical structure of animals living in groups has received attention, both in the case of rodents (30) and of primates (31); the analysis of aversive, or playful appetitive behavior in terms of the factors which regulate it within the group is now becoming possible. Similarly, maternal behavior has been described in detail in several species, with special attention to the sensory action cues which release a latent trend into overt behavior. It is here that the recent contributions of the great ethological schools (32, 33) become most relevant. For by isolating, albeit in few submammalian species, special stimulus situations which release highly organized and highly specific (yet self-limiting) response, an analysis of the precise perceptual cues operating in such Innate Release Mechanism (IRM) becomes possible. Thus, strong and regular relationships can be established between percepts in an animal's natural environment, and affectively charged motor behavior. The firmness and specificity of these genetically coded patterns is remarkably high, and would appear as deeply ingrained as, for example, claws and plumage.

There is one further aspect which has been brought out by these ethological studies, namely, the susceptibility and plasticity of the nervous system during certain critical phases of its development. The well-known imprinting process merely serves to emphasize the functional counterpart of what is almost certainly intense biochemical change during the developmental period (34). Moreover, its careful experimental scrutiny provides, for the first time, methodological tools for approaching, in an objective experimental fashion, some of the most controversial, yet central, ideas of psychoanalytic theory. There is resistance on both sides to crossing this particular stream. Admittedly, as yet, the stepping stones are few and precarious. Time, however, will compel such a crossing.

It is significant that in none of the areas last mentioned (the built-in response patterns, the susceptibility of the developing nervous system to early environmental cues and the factors governing social norms in a group) have the chemical and pharmacological factors received the attention they merit. It is no doubt felt by the workers concerned that the areas are too new, and the ignorances too many to be weighed down by yet another set of variables. Yet each of these areas compels and commands an examination of precisely these factors. For example, we know very little of the neural and chemical nature of the imprinting process, though there are early indications that the may be affected by some drugs in a striking way (35). A detailed examination of thresholds of action, and of synergism and antagonism between drugs is certainly called for in relation to this function. Similarly a study of the effects of drugs on the emergence of innate patterns of behavior may in time contribute to an understanding of the chemical and hormonal mechanisms subserving these processes. This will particularly apply to the administration of specific enzyme inhibitors from birth (36), and the conflation of biochemical with behavioral techniques. Most particularly, however, the effect of drugs on social behavior and the dependence of drug effects on social setting is relevant, not only because of the theoretical implications of such observations but because of considerations of a strictly mundane and practical nature. It was noted some time ago that the effect of amphetamine in mice varied with the number of animals in a group (37). Subsequent more detailed studies (38, 39) confirmed these observations, it being shown that a single animal would tolerate higher doses of the drug than animals crowded in a group, where mutual activation lead to a fall in the LD 50. Thus a powerful new variable was found to operate even in simple toxicity studies. This factor of number in a group has been investigated further in relation to hormone effects (40), and the interaction of tranquillizing with stimulant compounds (41). Such observations form the logical counterpart of studies centered on the effect of drugs on social behavior, and would have gone undetected, had the studies been confined to the individual, or the restrained, animal. The effect of drugs on socially released responses may thus provide a new and sensitive parameter in the exploration of both.

Despite all that has been said, there is one central weakness running through the areas mentioned so far. It rests in the simple fact that the psychotic process in man, and its most relevant attribute of thought disorder, need not necessarily manifest behaviorally at all; or that when it does it (in verbal, or other, terms) may bring into play a wide and divergent repertoire of response, which, though very different, and even incompatible at their extremes, may reflect the same nuclear pathological process. A thoughtful paper (42) has examined these aspects, and questioned the value of treating a cluster of affective response in the experimental animal as models of disorders of cognitive function in man The ability to maintain delayed responses, to abstract common cues from related items, and to order information serially in time must be judged more relevant to the psychoses, and particularly the schizophrenia, than mere "tranquillization", "activation" or "enhanced conflict tolerance". An undue emphasis on these obvious responses may be totally misleading in regard to the chemotherapy of mental disorder.

Some Recent Trends in the Basic Neurological Sciences

A further group of reasons for the lag of the psychopharmacological field may well lie in the uneven development of the basic neurological sciences. It is only the last two decades, and, most particularly, the last decade, which has seen a sharpening of interest in the areas which, between them, serve to strengthen the groundwork of a pharmacology of behavior. In some ways these areas lie at opposite extremes, being concerned on the one hand, with the finer structure (in submicroscopic and microchemical terms) of the functional units of the nervous system and, on the other, with the nature and properties of those systems making for integrative functioning within the nervous system as a whole. Electron microscopy and X-ray diffraction (43–45) are contributing to some knowledge of the basic structural plan along which the highly ordered lipoprotein systems, so prevalent in nervous tissue, are built. It is possible, for example, that knowledge of the organization of the structural unit of the myelin sheath may furnish insights into the structure of the neurone membrane. Here a comparison of X-ray diffraction and electron microscopy has proved particularly valuable. Furthermore, the structure and properties of the active electrogenic patches in the neurone membrane (which presumably comprise the receptors for naturally occurring neurohumoral transmitter substances) are slowly yielding to microelectrode and micropipette studies; and it is, perhaps, not too much to hope that the dimension of there suborgans of the neurone may, in time yield to direct methods rather than the inferences implicit in a study of the structure/activity relationship of neurotropic compounds.

It is significant too, that the chemical analysis of the nervous system has increasingly called for a refinement of microchemical techniques. The brain is *par excellence* a chemically *in*homogeneous organ; and the analysis of chemical differences at the finest level of cytological organization is becoming a basic necessity in understanding the properties of individual cell groups within the organ. For that reason a mapping of the brain in the terms of broad topographical areas is no longer sufficient. Microchemical techniques make possible a layer-by-layer mapping of enzyme systems in relation to cell population (46, 47), and thus may provide insights not merely into the geography, but, if one may be permitted to use the term, the geology of the brain. Regional differences between various areas in the brain are emerging, and are sure, in time, to contribute to our understanding of the functional relationships between various areas, and between adjacent, but different cellular elements in the same area. The recently developed microfluorimetric and fluorescent staining techniques for the detection of low concentrations of physiologically active compounds will no doubt add further microchemical data. The enzymological map of the central nervous system is thus slowly in the making and chemical gradients within it may, in time, be defined in cytochemical terms. Of necessity, such information form a prerequisite for an understanding of the chemical targets of the psychotropic drugs.

In much the same way as biochemistry and biophysics of the nervous system have moved increasingly in the direction of submicroscopic morphology and cytochemistry, the physiology and, to a much lesser extent, the pharmacology of the nervous system have become increasingly concerned with the nature and properties of the integrative processes within the central nervous system. The ablation and stimulation studies in animals and man, the effects of punctate lesions, the analysis of the arousal system (48) and the mixed, convergent reticular, as well as the lateral sense-linked pathways, the role of the limbic system (49) and, more recently, self stimulation studies (50) have defined a wealth of physiological phenomena relevant to pharmacological inquiry. They have also emphasized three separate, though related, trends. The first is the inhomogeneity, and the discrete neuroanatomical and cytological suborganization of those areas of the brain which, on present evidence, subserve the discharge of patterns of affective behavior; second, the two-way apposition and interconnectedness of a number of each subsystems despite their wide topographical separation; and third, the reciprocal, complementary, yet mutually occlusive relationship which some patterns and modalities represented in these systems bear to each other. The anatomical and cytoarchitectonic differentiation of the hypothalamus, the reticular activating system and the paleocortical structures have received steady attention (51–54) over the last two decades. Similarly, the existence of rich two-way connections between the midbrain and elements in the limbic system [the so-called Limbic-Midbrain Circuit (55)] has served to emphasize the importance of bringing reticular elements into immediate relation with structures and areas mediating visceromotor and endocrine responses. The control of corticopetal input by corticofugal influences (56) is another example of a cognate self-monitoring mechanism. The mutual occlusiveness of the patterns subserving behavior may be viewed as examples of the same economy. The reciprocal inhibitor arrangement governing for example the "stop" and "start" mechanisms of eating (57) or drinking (58) behavior, or the existence of closely apposed "eating and "satiety" centers, serve to illustrate the principle. Opposing patterns thus appear to interlock, and their selective restraint or release, their storage or flow, would seem to depend upon the functional state in relatively limited cell assemblies. On grounds of anatomical connectedness alone, certain midline areas (such as the septal nuclei, the median eminence and, possibly, portions of the periaqueductal grey) would qualify as nodal areas in the balanced operation of these selective gating mechanisms. Little precise information is at present available on the chemical shifts subserving these transactions: yet the effect of drugs (59) on hypothalamic-pituitary hormonal responses would suggest that, at least in part, these shifts must be sought at neurohumoral level.

It is in this context the discovery of the existence of catecholamines (60) and indoles (61) and gamma amino butyric acid (62) in the brain are major events though of necessity these must be regarded as a mere beginning. The existence of humoral influences in the brain has been postulated (63, 64); and on the basis of evidence obtained in the conscious animal, and in suitable acute preparations, the possible existence of three *families* of compounds (related respectively to a naturally occurring choline ester, catecholamine and indole) has been put forward by the author (63, 65–67). The importance of *inter*action between various members has also been stressed (66, 67).

There is another area towards which neurophysiology has been heading in the last two decades, albeit in an unsatisfactory and far from committed manner. Information theory, developed originally to meet the needs of weapon and industrial research, has looked to the nervous system for cellular analogs of assemblies designed to operate high-speed computers. Early attempts to fuse theory, with physiological experiment remained relatively isolated (68), and after an intermittent period in the mid-forties, cybernetic speculation continued to develop relatively independently of physiological experiment to the continued disadvantage of both. It served, however, to move into focus one very important aspect of systems capable of recognition, and of adaptation to change. This was the role of initial randomness of possible connections, and of delay, in the classification of temporal and spatial patterns (69, 70). Such concepts in no way detracted from the role of pre-existing inborn neural patterns and the genetically coded neural connections, which presumably subserved them. They did, however, question the oversimplified "wiring" theories of learning; and steadily emphasize the statistical, probabilistic nature of homeostasis, and of the trial-and-error process of learned adaptive behavior. Careful cytological surveys of cell populations in special areas, and their axonal and dendritic connections (71) provided an insight into the matrix of the information carrying apparatus. However, it is the writer's feeling that a preoccupation with such structural and spatial characteristics may be of only limited value. The synthesis and turnover-*in-time* of the neuroproteine, and their individual building blocks may be more relevant to the physicochemical preservation and coding of experience. These chemical characteristics need not necessarily have a histological counterpart.

It is only relatively recently that a fusion between information theory and neurophysiological experiment has been attempted, particularly in relation to the nature of the coding of information at high sensory levels (72, 73). Significantly, it is the process of highly patterned *inhibition* between adjacent elements which was found to play a key role in the transformation of the information in the visual (74) and auditory (75) pathways. A number of interesting speculation have been put forward as to the precise cellular array likely to meet the demands of such information carrying systems (75). Such studies form a useful beginning, if only by bringing the subject of neurocommunication into the neurobiological laboratory, where, it is submitted, it properly belongs.

It may well be asked why information theory should be introduced into the argument at this particular point. It is, however, felt by the writer that both biochemical and electrophysiological data will remain descriptive and only loosely related to behavior, unless they are linked to information theory, premature though such a linkage may be. The disorders induced by psychodysleptic agents, as well as those states (both physiological and pathological) to which they are related must, sooner or later be viewed as disorders of the brain as a chemically mediated organ of information. Information theory must be tempered against precise physiological and biochemical experiment. Neuropharmacology, and the pharmacology of behavior are thus faced with problems not dissimilar to those faced by genetics and immunochemistry.

In taking stock, therefore, it would seem that three separate though related trends may have colluded in making for delay and isolation of the subject here considered. The essentially personal and subjective nature of the phenomena made for their isolation in an intellectual climate preoccupied with description and measurement in the physical sciences; the animal and behavioral techniques were apt to center on conditions and situations only indirectly and partly applicable to the problems posed by the psychotropic drug effects in man; and the basic neurological sciences were ill prepared to receive the wealth of essentially empirical findings coming from the clinic, and from the laboratories. The lack of facts was thus reflected in a lack of conceptual models; no such lack of facts impedes us today.

II. PSYCHOACTIVE DRUGS:
SOME PROBLEMS FACING A PROVISIONAL CLASSIFICATION

Classification in a field as actively growing as that of the psychotropic agents has special difficulties. The boundaries shift, and the constraints imposed by criteria of undue severity are soon felt and broken. Nevertheless, the attempts made so far at a classification are timely if for no other reason than to draw attention to the problems inherent in the process, and to point out their own deficiencies. The inordinately wide range of action of the psychotropic drugs introduced special difficulties. As is well known their influence on thought process and behavior is but one of their effects. Most (indeed all) have a widespread range of action on physiological targets outside the CNS, making their psychotropic features special instances of more general phenomena. The question of precise and relevant criteria to serve as a basis for a classification therefore forces itself on the subject from the outset; and here, as elsewhere, the lack of positive guidelines only emphasises the lack of definition of the field as a whole. Some of these difficulties will be briefly considered.

A Provisional Classification According to Chemical Constitution

Psychotropic drugs have widespread chemical lineage. Such drugs are found among the amines and related compounds (amphetamine, methamphetamine, and some methoxy derivatives, such as mescaline or tryptamine derivatives such as NN-dimethyltryptamine); the ergot derivatives and antiserotonins (such as LSD 25, and its congeners); the atropine analogs, (such as hyoscine); piperidyl derivatives (such as azacyclonol and the N-substituted piperidyl benzilates, the latter having a marked psychodysleptic effect); the phenothiazines (which, though, principally, so-called tranquillisers, also, by simple substitution of a sulphur atom, may result in an iminodibenzyl derivative, such as imipramine, a "stimulant"); a number of amine oxidase inhibitors of varying specificity; and miscellaneous compounds, such as deanol and methylphenidate. Chemical constitution would thus seem to be a very poor guide to the psychoactive properties of a particular drug. Systematic substitution in the phenothiazine nucleus, however, may hold some important lessons for the future. It has resulted in a number of compounds, varying in their effective dose, in the incidence of extrapyramidal symptoms, and other clinical manifestations. A similar examination of a series of substituted LSD-derivatives has also been reported (76). It is obvious that such careful and systematic substitution studies point the way towards a clearer recognition of the chemical features and properties, which should weigh in any future classification.

A Provisional Classification According to Chemical Effects

The difficulties mentioned in the preceding paragraph are reflected further in the ignorance of biochemical effects *in vitro* and *in vivo*. These effects have been reviewed (77–79). It must, however, be admitted that the evidence is scanty; "in vitro" the utilisation of various substrates (glucose, lactose, pyruvate, hexose monophosphate) has been examined. The effects on oxalacetic carboxylase and transaminase, succinic dehydrogenase and cytochrome oxidase and oxidative phosphorylation, have also been studied, and the effects of the drugs on the cholinesterases has been tested. It is difficult in such a sparse yet confused field to assess which of the findings is significant. The aspects, however, which need emphasis are first, the difference between the effect of some drugs on the resting as against stimulated brain tissue (80) suggesting, for example, that LSD-may interact with a chemical product of activity. Secondly, differences in the effects of chlorpromazine on mitochondria obtained from brain and from liver, which suggests difference in structure in mitochondria obtained from these two sources (81); and thirdly, a number of studies into the intermediate metabolism of such drugs as LSD-25 (82), Dimethyltryptamine (83) and Chlorpromazine (84, 84a, 85, 85a) where an examination of metabolites may perhaps lead to the isolation of more active, rather than less active, compounds. There are some indications that this may be so in the case of Dimethyltryptamine (86). The strange and specific predilection of LSD-25 for the pseudo cholinesterase in human plasma should also be noted (87). Looking at the mounting list of compounds, a systematic study is obviously one of forbidding magnitude, and will have to be confined to drugs showing only the clearest psychotropic effects. However, an examination of a few of such compounds and a definition of their distribution patterns, and the pharmacological effects of their breakdown products may go a long way in assisting one in the classification of other drugs in biochemical terms.

Pharmacological Effects at Peripheral Drug Receptors

The abundant batteries of preparations available for testing the synergism and antagonism of a given drug with naturally occurring substances such as acetylcholine, adrenaline, serotonin, histamine, substance P, and the like, afford a wide terrain for the so-called screening procedures. Such studies no doubt provide some data for classification. Their relevance to the problem in hand, however, must be seriously questioned. The lack, for example, of a relationship between the psychotropic effects of LSD-25 and their anti-serotonin effects (88) is but one special instance where initial over-simplification of a theory has yielded to further experience. On the other hand, no one will deny the wide distribution of systems sensitive to psychotropic drugs in neural nets of varying ontogenetic or phylogenetic development. The question, therefore, arises as to the relative relevance of the various simplified and isolated preparations available for such screening procedures. It is suggested that the neural nets subserving an integrated autonomic function could be useful in this regard. The observations of the effect of psychotropic drugs on the peristaltic reflex are perhaps worthy of mention. As is well known (89) this reflex is essentially a highly ordered stretch response (i.e. a response to a rise of intraluminar pressure) resulting in the organized sweep of an excitatory (i. e. contractile) wave, preceded by an equally ordered (and reciprocal) inhibitory one. This organised reflex phase (and not the contraction of the longitudinal muscle) has been shown sensitive to LSD-25 and some LSD-derivatives, (90). Furthermore, the effects of morphia on gut movement have also been analysed in detail (91). It is, of course, too much to hope for satisfactory model system in such isolated preparations. On the other hand, local reflexes in limited neural nets may provide a firmer basis for analogies than sundry empirical test preparations. These models, however, will have to undergo repeated calibration and matching against other preparations before their usefulness can be clearly defined. Such studies have now been reported (92).

Central Effects other than Behavioral

Here again the evidence far outweighs the theoretical yield. The effects on postural reflexes (93) the respiratory and vasomotor reflexes (94) have been studied, as have the effects on synaptic transmission within the central nervous system (96), on thalamic recovery time (96), on geniculate transmission (97), on spontaneous and evoked (63, 65, 66, 98, 99) electrical activity, as well as activity in the reticular formation recorded by means of microelectrode (see below). Some of these aspects have already been mentioned. It is difficult to pick out any particular features, which shows correspondence between psychotropic effects and objective findings. The effects, however, on geniculate transmission (97) and on behavioral and electrical arousal thresholds in suitable preparations, either in response to direct stimulation of the reticular formation, or to afferent stimulation (99) would seem at this point as near an approximation as can be made. The integrative "set" functions, disturbed or redressed by psychotropic drugs must be viewed in statistical terms. High speed data reduction techniques will be needed to establish relationships between behavioral states, and these third order manifestations.

Classification According to Effects on Patterns of Animal Behavior, including Synergism and Antagonism with other Drugs

Some points in this area have already been raised in another context but may be briefly restated. It is obvious that the requirements will vary according to the particular modality, which the behavioral model is designed to represent. Whether it is the "tolerance" of a conflict situation, or reduction of natural aggressive behavior (as in wild rats), or abolition of a conditioned avoidance reaction, or various social patterns, will depend very much upon the cluster of symptoms on which one tends to focus. At best, however, this can be but a partial approach: the behavioral patterns may not necessarily be related to the pathological process one intends to treat. It has already been pointed out that the animal's behavior tests most directly related to relevant psychological deficits in the psychoses are to be found in tests of reaction time, tests for the serial ordering of behavior, for the immediate organization of behaviour in relation to simultaneously presented stimuli, and above all, in tests assessing what may be called the ability to abstract common items in randomly presenting stimuli. It is conceivable that, in time, such tests may serve to group drugs into quite novel patterns of activity. Discrete stimulation studies, particularly in primates, may greatly contribute to this field. The interaction between psychoactive drugs and the hypnotics (such as Barbiturates) or convulsants forms another area of enquiry.

Subjective and Objective Effects in Man

The limitations of the behavioral method have been briefly mentioned and various difficulties of assessment are examined again below. A classification of the effects of the various drugs in man, of necessity, requires a clear and unequivocal definition of the terms used to describe each of these effects. A carefully calibrated glossary is thus needed. It is, however encouraging to note how useful a classification on clinical grounds alone can be (101).

That the above items represent only a few of the many possible ways in which the subject of classification can be viewed is shown by various proposals for classification, made by a number of authors (102, 102a). Of these one review (103, 104) is particularly noteworthy for the allowance it makes for the difficulties and, at times, irreconcilable differences inherent in the problem. The reader is referred to it as containing valuable source material. In that review, an attempt has been made by the author to group the drugs under a number of headings. These are: (a) some gross behavioral effects in the individual unrestrained animal; (b) some effects on behavior patterns in a controlled experimental setting, such as the free operant and other conditioning techniques; (c) some gross effects on higher mental function in man; (d) effects on polysynaptic reflexes; (e) effects on convulsive thresholds; (f) effects on the so-called autonomic centres of the brain; (g) effects on the vomiting centre, and on clinical motion sickness; (h) effects on the extrapyramidal system; (i) effects on the spontaneous and induced electrical activity of the brain; (j) some examples of synergism and of antagonism between the drugs and selected other compounds. (k) the interaction between the drugs in question, and neurohumoral substances of possible general biological importance. On the basis of these and related findings an (albeit unsatisfactory) provisional classification has been proposed. Some of the properties of the principal compounds may now be briefly reviewed.

A. The Major Psycholeptic Agents (the Major Tranquillizers)

a) The Phenothiazines

Three groups of these compounds can be distinguished, according to the termination of the side chain in a dimethyl-amino group, in a piperazine ring or in a piperidine ring.

1. *Dimethylamine Series.* Chlorpromazine is the most prominent member of this group. It has been suggested (105) that the effect on the inhibition of the conditioned avoidance response in rats and the tranquilizing effect on monkeys increases with substitution in the 2-position. Fluorine substitution, as in the case of trifluopromazine leads to an enhancement of extrapyramidal symptoms. The compound is characterized by marked adrenolytic activity,

moderate to minimal anticholinergic activity, an antihistaminic effect, and some convulsant properties (106).

2. *Piperazine Group.* Substitution by the piperazine nucleus results in the emergence of a powerful group of compounds, about 7 to 10 times more potent than members of the Dimethylamine series. Members of this group exert marked extrapyramidal effects (107). Some (like trifluoperazine) are reported to possess an activating effect in underachieving schizophrenics. The peripheral autonomic effects in this group are somewhat reduced.

3. *Piperidine Series.* Two members – mepazine and thioridazine – may be regarded as representative of this group. They exert relatively slight adrenolytic effects, and slight-to-marked parasympatholytic effects, and are reputed to have less extrapyramidal effects.

The toxic side-effects of the phenothiazines are considered elsewhere. However, mention may be made of the acute toxic symptoms which include drowsiness, confusion, vivid dreaming, ataxia and visual hallucinations. Chronic effects may manifest in terms of agranulocytosis, and leucopenia and photosensitivity of the skin. There may be a lowering of convulsive threshold in epileptics. The hypotensive reaction may be severe (108).

An important point is made in the above attempt at classification (103) in regard to the interaction between neuro-effector substances with the phenothiazines, as compared with the rauwolfia alkaloids. As has been noted, the former group possesses reasonably well developed anti-adrenaline (or anti-acetylcholine or anti-histamine) properties. In members of the rauwolfia group, the action is more related to the liberation of serotonin or catecholamines from their subcellular anchoring sites. Whereas the phenothiazines are therefore described as possessing a so-called "direct" effect, the rauwolfia alkaloids are envisaged as exerting an "indirect" action (103). This may be an oversimplification.

b) Rauwolfia Alkaloids

These include reserpine, rescinnamine, and deserpidine. The mode of action (particularly in regard to serotonin and catecholamine liberation) is considered briefly below. Reserpine exerts no anticonvulsant action. Indeed it antagonizes the anticonvulsant action of diphenylhydantoin and the barbiturates. It prolongs barbiturate sleeping time, though it possesses no analgesic activity. It can block or reduce a rise in blood pressure produced by hypoxia, or by central stimulation of the sciatic or vagus nerves. The over-all autonomic effect is a peripheral sympathetic blockade, probably due to catecholamine depletion at peripheral sympathetic sites. Many components enter into its central action (109). Reserpine can be tolerated in remarkably high doses. Lethargy and prolonged sleep have been reported following 200 mg with complete recovery. Edema, nasal congestion and diarrhoea and depression have been noted with chronic administration. Bleeding from chronic duodenal ulcer has also been reported (110).

B. The Minor Tranquillizers

This group includes such compounds as promethazine (a phenothiazine derivative); benzhydrol and benzhydryl derivatives, such as captodiamine and hydroxyzine. These substances exert effects qualitatively similar though quantitatively less pronounced than the major tranquillizers. They all prolong hexobarbital anaesthesia. On the other hand, like the major tranquillizers, they have no anaesthetic effects when given alone. Some possess an anti-histamine and anti-emetic action. In many ways this group would appear to be at the pharmacodynamic crossroads, "being roughly placed between the anti-histaminic anti-emetic, antimotion-sickness compounds on the one hand, and the major tranquillizers on the other" (111). Promethazine was originally developed as an anti-histamine agent, but also possesses anti-motion-sickness effects. A further substitution results in diethazine, which is an effective anti-Parkinson drug. Captodiamine is a thio-derivative of diphenhydramine having sedative properties. Hydroxyzine is chemically related to an anti-histamine drug, chlorcyclizine, and has marked sedative effects. At the peripheral sites, many of the minor tranquillizers possess anti-histaminic anti-acetylcholine and/or local anaesthetic effects. Occasional skin reactions and drowsiness may be seen with hydroxyzine (112).

C. The Hypnosedatives and Tranquillosedatives

(Phenoglycodol, Azacyclonol, Meprobamate, Zoxazolamine)

This miscellaneous group, represented here by four members could be enlarged and indeed, (were it to include such agents as amylobarbitol urethane, and related substances), could comprise many of the hypnotics commonly listed as sedatives in any textbook of therapeutics. All members in this group exert a sedative action in small and moderate doses and decrease spontaneous activity in the experimental animal. In full doses some lead to sleep and even anaesthesia. For the sake of convenience this group which has properties in common with the hypnotics, may be termed "hypnosedative". Other members possess a marked depressant action on polysynaptic reflex pathways, which action however correlates only poorly with their sedative effects. The members of this group which includes phenoglycodol, meprobamate and zoxazolamine have some effects in common with a minor tranquillizer and may therefore be termed "tranquillosedatives". In terms of structure, azacyclonol is an isomer of pipradrol, but devoid of its stimulant action. Indeed it prolongs hexobarbital sleeping time and antagonizes the psychomotor stimulant actions of pipradrol. It antagonizes hyperactivity caused by cocaine, dextroamphetamine and morphine in mice. It has been reputed to antagonize the hallucinogenic effects of LSD-25 in man, though the clinical results have been inconsistent (113).

As mentioned, the compounds in the tranquillosedative group (phenaglycodol, zoxazolamine and meprobamate) are characterized by a depressant effect on polysynaptic pathways in doses where effects on monosynaptic spinal reflexes are slight. In this sense, they share an important property with mephenesin. They also share a depressant effect on the reticular formation and abolish decerebrate rigidity. The net result of these actions is muscular relaxation when high doses are used. It should, however, be noted that although the depressant effect on interneurones in polysynaptic pathways is shared by all compounds, this property taken by itself, can serve as no guide to the tranquillizing properties of a particular substance. For example, mephenesin and zoxazolamine exert a marked depressant effect on polysynaptic reflexes; yet their tranquillizing effect is only apparent with high doses. Meprobamate, on the other hand exerts definite sedative effects; yet, in terms of its effect on polysynaptic reflexes, it is only slightly more effective than mephenesin. Like mephenesin meprobamate and zoxazolamine have an antagonistic effect on metrazol convulsions. Also, phenaglycodol in addition to its effects on the spinal level, exerts an effect at supra-spinal level. In fact, the substance appears to be sharing some properties with barbiturates, and others with meprobamate.

Certain sharp differences between members of this group and the major tranquillizers should be noted. Full doses of the tranquillo-sedatives lead to ataxia followed by a stage of tranquillization and anaesthesia. Moreover, the centers regulating autonomic function are relatively unaffected by these drugs. Extrapyramidal symptoms are never seen with full doses, nor are any anti-Parkinsonian effects observed. Furthermore, in contrast to the major tranquillizers, the drugs in this group increase the threshold to electrically induced convulsions, and antagonize Pentetrazol convulsions. The major tranquillizers have the opposite effect. In some respects, these drugs also differ from the anaesthetics and sedatives. Sedation by most anaesthetics is preceded by a stage of excitation. The effect of full doses of the tranquillo-sedatives is continued sedation merging into sleep. No taming effect of monkeys has been described in hypnotics, while this effect is pronounced with meprobamate and phenaglycodol. The reactivity patterns of animals, both innate and acquired, also show some differences between the hypnosedatives and tranquillo-sedatives. Also the effect on the electrical activity of the brain is different in the two groups. The recruiting response, for example, is enhanced by barbiturates, and inhibited by mephenesin.

Meprobamate ingested in large doses leads to drowsiness. Continuous use may lead to allergic skin rashes. Withdrawal symptoms have been reported following continuous use (114).

D. Psychoactive Antiacetylcholine Agents

This group includes Atropine, Hyoscine, Benactyzine and N-ethyl-3 piperidyl benzilate and is considered again below. Its common feature, shared by all members is marked anti-acetylcholine effect at peripheral neuro-effector sites. Atropine in high doses leads to over-activity and excitement. Hyoscine, on the other hand, can act as a sedative and, indeed, has been used as such in mental hospital practice. Benactyzine, a more recently discovered member of this group (see below) has no sedative action when taken by itself, although it prolongs hexobarbitone anaesthesia. On the other hand, it markedly affects stress-induced behavior in controlled situations. It is a powerful drug, acting in the same order of dosage as atropine. N-ethyl-3 piperidyl benzilate is a psychodysleptic agent. Thus, within this small group, at least three kinds of actions are represented. It is far from clear whether these involve real qualitative differences. A careful dose/response analysis in man is urgently needed.

E. The Major Psychoanaleptics
("Stimulant" or "Antidepressant" Compounds)

a) The Monoamine Oxidase Inhibitors: Iproniazid, Isocarboxazid, Nialamide, Phenelzine, Phenylisopropylhydrazine

These compounds form a group of special interest, both in terms of their clinical effects, and their theoretical implication. Clinically and pharmacologically they are classified as stimulating compounds, though they share relatively few properties with other "stimulant" drugs, such as the amphetamines and caffeine. Iproniazid is to date the most representative member of the group. Its inhibiting effect on monoamine oxidase was demonstrated in 1952 (115). The effect of such inhibition on brain amine content is referred to elsewhere. Moderate doses of monoamine oxidase inhibitors have relatively little effect on the experimental animal. Signs of central stimulation are seen either following cumulative or convulsive doses (116). Also, the property of monoamine oxidase inhibition is shared to a lesser extent by a number of other compounds.

High doses of Iproniazid may lead to marked fall in blood pressure, sweating, semi-stupor and insomnia. The greatest care should be exercised in the administration of barbiturates, nor-epinephrine or cortisone in the case of acute iproniazid poisoning. Chronic reactions include twitching of extremities, hyperreflexia, vertigo, constipation, drowsiness, xerostomia and delayed starting of micturition. Clonus, orthostatic hypotension, edema, toxic hepatitis resulting in jaundice, hepatocellular necrosis and fatalities have been reported during administration of iproniazid (117).

b) Imipramine

This substance presents interesting features. Chemically it is closely related to a tranquilliser (promazine); yet its place in practice is that of an "antidepressant". Its clinical and experimental uses have been reviewed (118). It is definitely not a monoamine oxidase inhibitor. Its effect on conditioned avoidance response, hexobarbital, sleeping time and alcohol induced sedation in mice, or body temperature is much less pronounced than that of chlorpromazine. There is, however, some slight indication of sensitization by the drug of peripheral sites to noradrenaline as tested in the innervated and denervated nictitating membrane preparation (119), though it is difficult to relate this to its mode of action. It exerts a weak parasympatholytic action; and in terms of its effect on arousal responses, it resembles the effects of hyoscine and benactyzine (see below).

F. The Minor Psychoanaleptic Compounds

(Amphetamine, Methamphetamine, Methylphenidate, Pipradrol and Deanol)

Amphetamine and Methylamphetamine. In their classic paper published in 1910 (120) Barger and Dale reported on the adrenergic action of 57 aliphatic and aromatic amines. Their results concerned, in particular, the pressor effects of the amines in the decerebrate cat. Some twenty years later the therapeutic value of ephedrine was demonstrated (121). The racemic form of amphetamine was introduced in 1933 (122). Many more compounds have followed.

In general, amphetamine shares its adrenergic action with ephedrine, producing mydriasis, inhibition of the gastrointestinal tract, and peripheral vasoconstriction. It lowers the threshold of stimulation of the arousal system and leads to marked electrical and behavioral arousal in the conscious animal (65). It antagonizes the effect of hypnotics and sedatives, and affects a number of autonomic centers, increasing, for example, body temperature, and decreasing appetite. There is suggestive evidence that whatever its peripheral effects, amphetamine exerts a powerful action on elements in the reticular activating system (64, 65). Pipradrol and Methylphenidate are minor stimulants. Their effect is inclined to be more gradual, both in onset and attenuation. Neither compound, however, possesses marked sympathomimetic properties, nor is there any striking effect on autonomic centers (104). Blood pressure and appetite are thus not strikingly affected.

Dimethylaminoethanol (Deanol) (123) is a simple compound belonging to a rather different group. Its chemical similarity to choline has suggested the possibility that the drug might act on a precursor to acetylcholine in the central nervous system. It exerts a mild stimulant effect.

A detailed analysis of the electrophysiological effects of this compound has been recently undertaken (124). The drug was shown to induce low voltage fast activity in the EEG, suggestive of mild stimulation. It lowered the threshold to EEG arousal elicited from the reticular formation and possibly, additionally from the thalamus. Furthermore, the compound antagonizes the depressant influence of barbiturates on pathways subserving wakefulness. A further feature of this particular study was that it is one of the few reports in the literature where the *variability in response of different animals* of the same species (cat) from *experiment to experiment* was taken into account. The action of Deanol was thought to be similar, but not as striking, as amphetamine.

Amphetamine has been combined with barbiturates as a mild euphoriant. Taken in excess it can lead to restlessness, anorexia, hyperreflexia, insomnia and hallucinosis. More interestingly, a series of cases of "amphetamine psychosis" has recently been reported (125). The clinical picture presented by this syndrome resembles, in a striking manner, an acute schizophrenic episode.

G. The So-called Psychodysleptic (Psychosomimetic, Hallucinogenic) Compounds

a) Mescalin and Related Compounds (Methylenedioxyphenisopropylamine (MDA), Trimethoxyphenisopropylamine (TMA)

It is noteworthy how few and far between are the systemic pharmacodynamic studies of mescaline, despite its long recognized existence. Most concern animal behavioral studies (126) or rather specialized electrophysiological effects. Mescaline exerts an inhibitory effect on the transcallosal pathway. Azacyclonal reduces this inhibitory action. The effects of mescaline are reversed by chlorpromazine (127).

The more recently synthesized mescalin analogues (MDA and TMA) are briefly considered below.

b) Lysergic Acid Diethylamide and Related Compounds

Some aspects of this ambiguous and controversial topic are considered elsewhere (I, 1/b, pp. 62/63).

c) Indole Derivatives

Psilocybin. The pharmacology of this active principle of a Mexican mushroom has been recently described (128). Although a powerful dysleptic compound, it is considerably less toxic than, for example, bufotenin. It leads to marked reduction of motor activity; and despite that, a shortening of the reaction time to nociceptive stimulation. In the autonomic area there is marked mydriasis, increase in heart and respiratory rate and a slight but significant rise in rectal temperature. There is also a marked elevation of blood sugar content. There is a fall in mean arterial blood pressure in the dog.

There is little interaction between the drug and adrenaline acetylcholine, histamine and nicotine as studied in suitable test preparations. On the other hand, it is a serotonin antagonist though about 80 times less potent than LSD-25.

Bufotonin and Dimethyltryptamine. These two derivatives are of special interest since both are related to serotonin. Bufotenin is the dimethyl derivative of serotonin, 5-hydroxytrypt-amine being capable of conversion (129) to bufotenin, bufotenidine, hydrobufotenin, or bufothionine. In the monkey, bufotenin leads to behavioral changes, practically identical with the injection of (an albeit heroic) dose of LSD-25 (130). In many bufotenin leads to generalized tingling, changing complexion, pre-cordial discomfort, nystagmus, mydriasis and changes in perception, including visual changes (131).

Dimethyltryptamine differs from bufotenin merely in the fact that it contains no OH group in the fifth position. The effects of this compound have been compared with those of LSD-25 and mescaline and the substance has also been used in psychotics (132). The outstanding characteristic of Dimethyltryptamine is, first, the rapid appearance, of the symptoms, and their equally rapid decay; symptoms fade within an hour or so (133). Secondly, whereas in the case of LSD-25, the autonomic effects precede the mental symptoms, the sensory disturbances are reported to coincide with the appearance of these autonomic effects. Choreiform and athetoid movements are also observed with this substance; they are only rarely seen in LSD-25 intoxication. The 6-hydroxylation of Dimethyltryptamine is mentioned elsewhere (see below).

H. Some Psychoactive Ions: Bromine and Lithium

The reader is referred to standard texts with regard to the action of Bromine. This halogen displaces chlorine in the extra-cellular fluid, though there is evidence, also, of the entry of Bromine into nerve cells (134). Lithium was introduced in the treatment of overactive states in

Fig. 1.

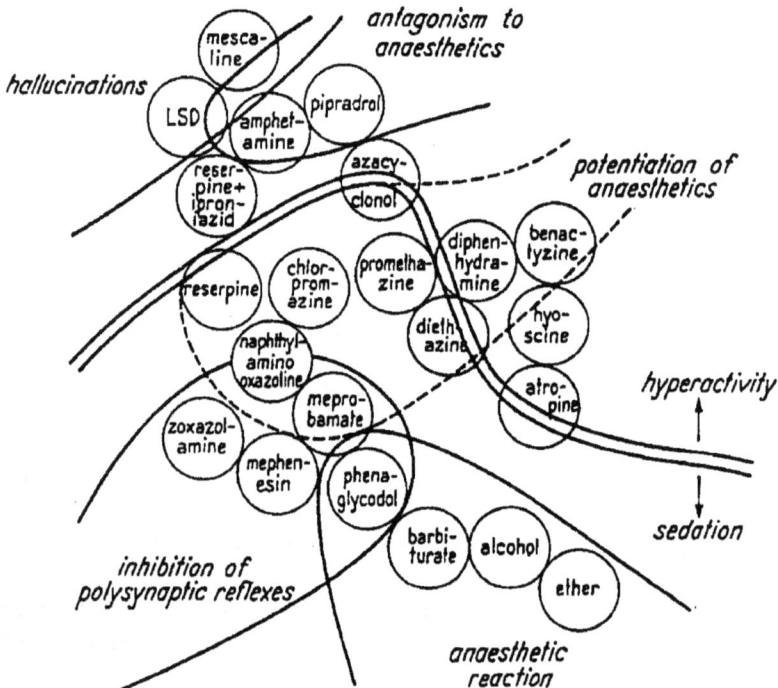

Fig. 2.

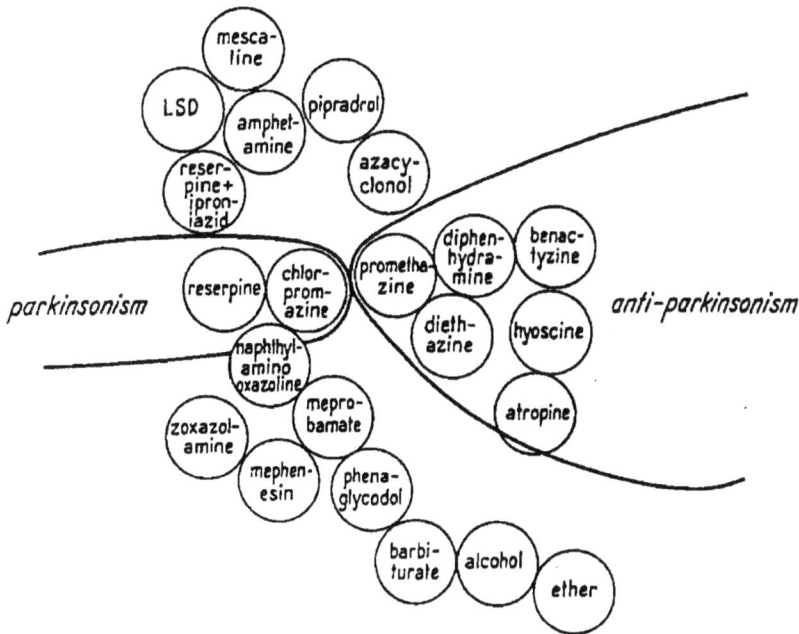

Fig. 2.

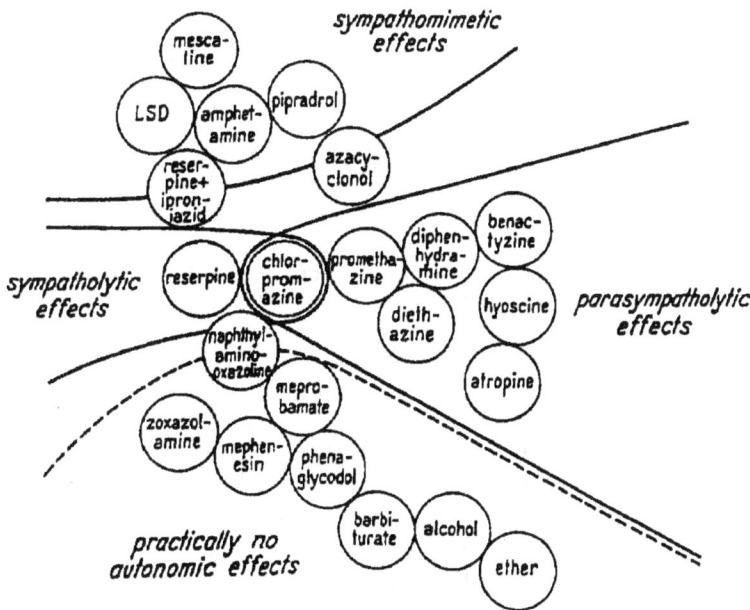

Fig. 3.

1949 (135). The pharmacology (136) and therapeutics (137) of the ion has been reviewed. It is effective against the manic phases of the manic depressive psychosis, and, in protracted or recurrent mania, "offers advantage over all other available therapies". It is a toxic ion and can potentially lead to renal tubular damage. A high sodium intake accelerates renal elimination, and serves to protect against such damage.

Fig. 4.

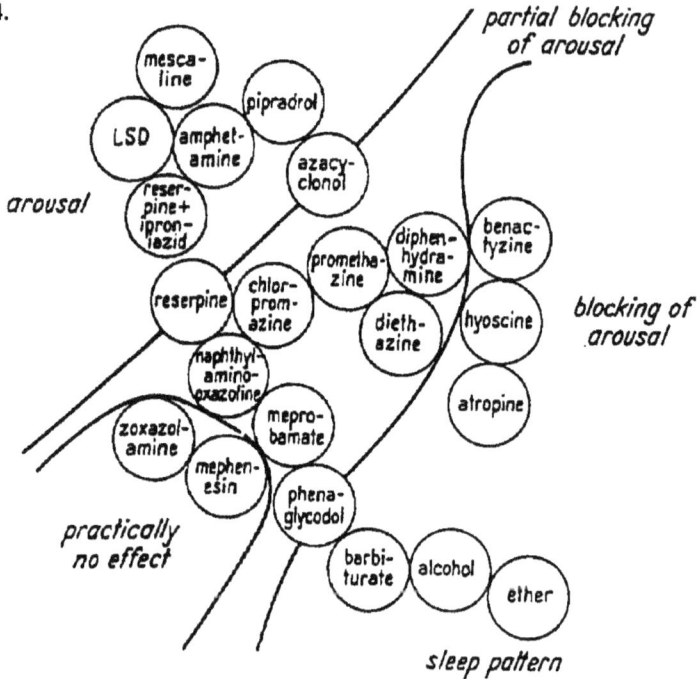

Fig. 1-4. Diagrammatic classification of some psychotropic drugs
according to various types of action (after Jacobsen, 104)

The above outline merely represents one way of classifying psychoactive drugs. It is bound
to be superseded by others. Indeed, with the growth of the field, classification should be subject to continuous review.

III. POSSIBLE NEURAL CORRELATES BEARING ON
THE MODE OF ACTION OF PSYCHOACTIVE DRUGS

A. Neuroanatomical Considerations

The past three decades have seen a steady shift in the attention of those interested in the
neuroanatomical substrate of behavior from the form and function (and particularly, the
so-called higher inhibitory function) of the cerebral cortex to the possible role of subcortical
cell masses in the mediation of the patterns of affective behavior. Three systems, in particular,
have been singled out in these studies. These are the Hypothalamus, the Ascending Reticular
Activating System, and the so-called Rhinencephalic or Limbic Formation; with a fourth
group, the Caudate and Lentiform masses (the so-called Corpus Striatum) belatedly attracting
mounting interest. All have received extensive review. They are mentioned here only because
of their possible bearing upon the mode of action of drugs influencing affect and behavior.

The role of the hypothalamus in the control of patterns of emotional expression has been
explored by a variety of techniques. The controversial subject of hypothalamic pituitary relationships has been considered by several authors (138 59). Stated very briefly, the cumulative
evidence tended to implicate the hypothalamus in the activation and discharge of highly orga-

nized patterns of emotional expression and of autonomic and visceromotor control. During earlier studies, these patterns of overt behavior were thought to be identical with the subjective "experience" of emotion. Later, a distinction between the experience, and overt expression of emotion was made; whether this separation is all that it implies, remains problematical. However, it also became increasingly evident that the hypothalamus by way of the pituitary, powerfully influenced the endocrine correlates of sexual activity, of common affective states, and even diurnal rhythms. The literature around this subject is growing steadily (139).

The second system to be defined was the so-called Reticular Activating (140) or Meso-Diencephalic Arousal System (MDAS, 141) initially postulated on the basis of the electro-cortical and behavioral arousal produced by the electrical stimulation in the midtegmental region (142). This system which, indeed, is a system of systems, comprises elements which ascend from the medullary and pontine regions, inextricably mixed with projections from the midtegmental region, the periaqueductal grey matter, the Superior Colliculus, spreading rostrally into so-called intralaminar thalamic nuclei, the subthalamic region, and thence, by way of the so-called diffuse thalamic projection system, on to the fronto parietal cortex. The various components in these projection systems within the general system have been recently reviewed (143, 144). Of particular interest, however, is the extensive mesencephalic projection from the mesencephalon on to the hypothalamus and the medial septal nuclei. These projections originate in the ventral part of the periaqueductal grey substance; including Gudden's Dorsal Tegmental Nucleus, and the Paramedian and Medial Tegmental cell group. They extend to the hypothalamus by way of the Dorsal Longitudinal Fasciculus of Schütz, (which terminates in the periventricular region of the hypothalamus), and the system of the Mamillary Peduncle (which, though feeding principally into the Mamillary Body, also projects to the lateral region of the Hypothalamus, as well as the Preoptic and Septal region.) The lower midbrain, so richly exposed to non-specific ascending afferent influences is thus put into a direct connection with areas bearing upon endocrine and autonomic regulation. It is, incidentally also of interest that direct projections from the more rostral midbrain tegmentum travel to the Caudate and Lentiform Nuclei. The relation of these structures to behavior must remain enigmatic for the present.

There is one further aspect which should be noted in connection with the above. Far from purely ascending, the reticular system also receives rich projections from the frontal sensorimotor, cingulate and orbito frontal cortex and the entorhinal cortex. The significance of the pattern of distribution of these corticofugal fibres is far from clear at present; though there is good evidence of the influence of these fibres on arousal, on sensory conduction and on modulation of motor control (145).

The third system to receive extensive attention in recent years is the so-called Rhinencephalic or Limbic system, postulated originally on purely anatomical grounds (146). This system includes the Cingulate Gyrus, the Hippocampus, the Amygdala, and the Fornix System and has been shown by a variety of techniques (which includes ablation, electrical and chemical stimulation studies in the conscious unanaesthetized animal) to control and modulate behavior related, in part, to smelling, searching, eating and sexual function, as well as to escape, or acceptance, or attack of objects within the animal's environment. Both aggressiveness and undue tameness, inapproachability and playful behavior have been elicited by appropriate stimulation or ablation of elements within the system (147). It has, in fact, been suggested that whereas the Hypothalamus may be concerned with the expression of emotion, elements within the Limbic system may perhaps be more concerned with its subjective experience. Whether in view of the inter-connectedness of the various systems referred to below, such a separation is indeed permissible must remain an open question. Nevertheless, it would seem that elements within the Limbic system may powerfully determine the aversive or appetitive connotation of a. particular stimulus situation; and be concerned in the mediation of an appropriate homeostatic response. It is as if, what may be termed "Basic Attitudes" were in some way influenced by elements within this system.

It is, therefore, of special interest that the pathways connecting the midbrain with the Hypothalamus, referred to above, find their descending counterpart in the rich and varied connections of elements in the Limbic System with the midbrain. These projections (which have recently received a definitive formulation (143, 144, 144A) are both direct and indirect. The direct Hippocampo-Mesencephalic projections are principally destined for the rostral part of the Central Grey Substance. The indirect Hippocampal pathways "in part interrupted by further relays, and probably also representing indirect projections of the amygdaloid complex originate in the septum, and in the Lateral Preoptic and Hypothalamic regions, as well as in the mamillary body. Such pathways reach the midbrain in three fibre systems, via the Medial Forebrain bundle, the Fasciculus Retroflexus, and the Mammillo-Tegmental Tract. Each of these three bundles has a dual distribution in the midbrain; part of their fibres terminate in extensive central lateral regions of the Tegmentum, while the remaining component distributes to various subdivisions of a paramedian midbrain region encompassing the ventral part of the central grey substance, Tsai's ventral tegmental region, the interpeduncular nucleus Bechterew's n. centralis tegmenti superior, and Gunnerr's dorsal and deep tegmental nuclei. (148)

A number of points are implicit in the above findings. First, they demonstrate a striking and reciprocal two-way apposition of the connections between the Limbic forebrain structures and periaqueductal areas in the midbrain. This arrangement fully justifies the term "Limbic System Midbrain Circuit", used to describe this two-way path (144). Secondly, the rich efferent projections emanating from this system should be noted. These so-called "escape pathways" (144) over and above the closed loops mentioned previously include projections to the Medial hypothalamic region, to the anterior intralaminar nuclei of the thalamus, as well as the so-called diffuse ascending and descending conduction systems of the midbrain tegmentum. Thirdly, the Septal and Lateral Preoptic regions and the Medial Hypothalamus would appear to occupy a. rather special place in this intricate reciprocal arrangement. For both, in a sense, are nodal areas. The Septal area shares primary projections from the Hippocampus and the Amygdala, and projects on to the midbrain by way of the Medial Forebrain Bundle, and, less directly by way of the Stria Medullaris, the Habenula and the Fasciculus Retroflexus. The Medial Hypothalamic region receives (downward) fibres from the Limbic Forebrain structures via the Stria Terminalis as well as the Bundle of Schutz. Short Fibres from the same circuit probably connect with the Supraoptic Nucleus of the Hypothalamus. Thus, on anatomical grounds alone, the Septal and Hypothalamic regions are in a peculiarly favorable position to balance and translate influences within the Limbic Midbrain Circuits into endocrine and visceromotor responses. There are some further principles implicit in these neuroanatomical and physiological findings. The first is the fractionation and suborganizations of cell assemblies previously considered parts of single functional system. There is little doubt, even in the light of some quite early studies (149) of the anatomical inhomogeneity and cytological suborganization of the hypothalamus. Similarly, more recent studies have emphasized the remarkable anatomic and cytoarchitectonic differentiation within the Reticular Activating System, where on histological grounds alone (150) one would suspect a much greater differentiation than is conveyed by the term "Reticular Formation". The elements entering into the paleocortical and subcortical components of the Limbic System show similar differentiation. Each of the systems thus encompasses a mosaic of sub-systems, which, in a manner only poorly understood at present, are related and molded into each other.

The second principle, of reciprocal and mutual interconnectedness has already been stressed. It implies a two-way apposition of cellular masses, considered separate until a few decades also. This principle of interconnectedness, however, may well be related to yet a third feature which characterizes the organization of the deeply ingrained response patterns known as affective behavior. This is their mutual occlusiveness, despite a, close anatomical juxtaposition of the cell assemblies which subserve, and selectively release them. The principle is well illustrated in studies of the central neural regulation of food intake. The distribution of "appetite" and "satiety" centers within the hypothalamus (151) suggest the existence of closely related mechanisms for the initiation, and for the suspension of eating behavior, and a mutually appropriate interlocking of these two mechanisms. In the areas of motor activity and of emotional expression a major series of stimulation studies in the conscious animal (152) has defined the so-called "ergotropic" areas concerned with increased motor excitability, stimulation of respiration, rise in blood pressure and pulse rate. These areas have been contrasted with the so-called "trophotropic" areas leading to inhibition of motor activity, lowering of muscle tone, slowing of respiration and fall in blood pressure. Whereas the former would appear to be principally found in a relatively broad band of the posterior subthalamus, posterior hypothalamus, and anterior midbrain, the latter appeared confined to the anterior hypothalamic field, and a strip between the habenuelointerpeduncular tract and the mamillothalamic bundle. These studies also suggested a predominantly sympathetic autonomic response pattern associated with the stimulation of the "ergotropic" areas, and a predominantly parasympathetic pattern found in the "trophotropic" areas. This distribution, however, can only be accepted with some reservation, there being evidence of the dependence of the predominantly parasympathetic and sympathetic responses on the parameters of stimulation in a particular area (153). The recent extension of these stimulation studies to self-stimulation techniques (see below) has further contributed to the broad topography of the so-called motivational systems. In the rat, the positive motivational systems include most of the rhinencephalic cortex, as well as part of the Thalamus, Tegmentum and the Basal hypothalamus. The negative motivational system is much smaller. It invades the subthalamus, the Dorsal Hypothalamus and its relationship to the recognized pain systems is far from clear. It is hard for the present to assess the full physiological, (as distinct from experimental), meaning of these far-reaching studies. The implications, though reviewed, (154) require further enquiry. They do, however, suggest a broad binary grouping of patterns of affective behavior, and also, the possibility of further discrete suborganization of other patterns within this double frame of reference. There is furthermore, strongly suggestive evidence of the fractionation of such patterns, it being certainly noteworthy how one segment of behavior, can, by appropriate stimulation techniques, be selected out of context of the programme of behavior of which it is a part. Normally, the selection and gating of these patterns is governed by a complex interlocking of higher integrating systems. However, the experimental intervention hardly conveys the smoothness and flow of these control mechanisms. The balance between excitation and inhibition, tonic restraint and selective release would thus seem finely set. "Overactivity" and "underactivity", "attack" or "avoidance", "pleasure" or "fear", or "indifference" would appear to play into each other according to delicate shifts in balance in certain nodal cell groups.

The septal region, the median eminence of the hypothalamus, the periaqueductal grey and other, as yet unidentified regions may comprise nodal points in maintaining these equilibria. To date we know little of the switchgear, and the discriminate and selective gating mechanisms which automatically operate within the various systems in arriving at the appropriate homeostatic response. The final common path of motor "discharge" (or, what we choose to call "experience") must be presumed to be the final stage in a series of extremely rapid transactions involving the temporal apposition; convergence, and coding of neural patterns at widely separated topographical levels. It may, for example, involve the taking in of sensory cues (or the activation of a memory trace); the analysis and matching of these in terms of cognate traces ("experience"); a grouping and further condensation of these transform in terms other appetitive (Yes) and aversive (No) connotations; and the final activation of the appropriate motor-somato-endocrine response. The reason for drawing attention to this aspect is, first, to point to the dependence of the pattern of affective response on the *history* of the nervous system at any particular time; what it will put out will, to a large extent, depend on what it has "experienced"; and secondly to emphasise that pharmacological interference at the level of the final common path of response can but be *one* of several ways in which a drug may influence motivational behavior. Effects on the various transactions preceding the response may be as critical as the response itself. It is the compound effect, which must be borne in mind before proposing unduly simple (or simpleton) schemata for the effects of various drug groups on overt behavior.

B. Problems of Access

Cerebral Blood Flow. Regional Vessel Tone. The Blood Brain, Barrier;
The Perisynaptic Barrier

It is evident that the action of psychotropic drugs on the brain will be conditioned by the ability of the drugs, or their products, to reach target sites within the brain. Consideration of access must of necessity include the possible effect of drugs on the cerebral circulation, both general and local; the penetration of drugs across the blood-brain barrier; and the possible existence of special barriers at subcellular sites. These possibilities will now be briefly considered.

a) The Effect of drugs on the Cerebral Circulation

Two authoritative reviews have considered the effects of drugs on cerebral circulation (155, 156). Moat findings to data refer to measurements of overall cerebral circulation, and rest on the now classical procedure (157) applying the Fick principle to the exchange of an inert gas (Nitrous oxide) between the blood and the brain. More recently an elegant and highly promising technique for the measurement of local cerebral circulation in the experimental animal has also been developed (158).

As pointed out in the reviews just mentioned, a drug may affect cerebral circulation, either by affecting the perfusion pressure (which is largely dependent on mean arterial blood pressure) or by a change in what is termed cerebral vascular resistance which may be viewed as the sum of all the factors which impede the flow of blood through the brain. Blood pressure will only affect cerebral blood flow if it falls below a critical value of the order of 80 mm.Hg. Changes above appear to have little direct effect on cerebral circulation. Such influences must therefore be principally sought in the intrinsic regulation of cerebral circulation; and here by far the most important factor is the cerebral vascular tone.

The role of neurogenic influences in regulating cerebral vascular tone is ill defined at present; though there is evidence of autonomic influences, the effects of stimulation of these pathways are transient and uncertain. On the other hand, there is little doubt of the effects of humoral agents on over-all cerebral circulation. Of these, the moat important by far is carbon dioxide, which, when inspired in concentrations of 5–7% can double cerebral blood flow through a marked decrease in cerebral vascular resistance. No drug has yet been discovered which has effects on cerebral blood flow, which are nearly as potent as those of Carbon Dioxide (159).

Nevertheless some of the general vasodilators exert a powerful effect upon the vascular bed of the brain. Histamine, and the nitrites may serve as examples of drugs of this kind; though the order of dose is too high to make these drugs useful in man. Papaverine however leads to moderate increases in cerebral blood flow when given intravenously in man (160). Surprisingly, alcohol in moderate doses leads to relatively little effect on cerebral blood flow (161). The xanthine group, (particularly aminophylline and caffeine (162) appear to act as cerebral vasoconstrictors. Some hypotensive agents, such as the veratrum alkaloids (163) hydralazine (164) the ganglion blocking agents, (such as tetraethyl-ammonium), some ergot derivatives, (such as dihydroergocornine), although all exerting marked hypotensive effects, lead to no corresponding fall in cerebral circulation. It would thus seem that in those instances the relaxation of the cerebral vessels is just sufficient to maintain normal cerebral circulation, despite a fall in systemic blood pressure. Similarly, no significant fall in cerebral circulation could be observed with dihydroergocornine (165) or reserpine (166), despite the marked hypotensive effects of these substances.

The effects of the catecholamines and related sympathomimetic drugs on cerebral circulation have been the subject of a number of studies. Adrenaline, administered in continuous intravenous infusion at a rate sufficient to produce a significant increase in mean arterial blood pressure, leads to a comparable increase in cerebral blood flow, suggesting a lack of marked vasoconstrictor effects on the cerebral vessels at that dosage (167). There is, however, in such experiments a significant increase in the over-all oxygen consumption of the brain, (of the order of about 20%) which may be associated with feelings of anxiety, usually reported when adrenaline is administered. In the case of *nor*adrenaline, a rise in blood pressure as result of the infusion is accompanied by an increase in cerebral vascular resistance with a moderate decrease in cerebral blood flow. Here no changes are apparent in oxygen consumption; nor does this drug produce significant changes in the mental state. Amphetamine in relatively high doses (of the order of 20 mg) leads to relatively little change in either cerebral blood flow or oxygen and glucose consumption (168). Mescalin has only been studied in very large doses in monkeys; and here led to an increase in cerebral blood flow (169). LSD-25 at the height of its hallucinogenic effect in man did not lead to change in cerebral circulation or cerebral metabolism (170). Similarly, both chlorpromazine and reserpine administered in chronic studies did not lead to measurable change in over-all circulation (171, 172). Of conditions of endocrine imbalance the most marked effects "in vivo" are encountered in thyrotoxicosis (173). Here, strangely, an increase in cerebral blood flow is not accompanied by change in the rate of oxygen consumption by the brain; and this despite a steep rise in oxygen consumption of the rest of the body.

It is thus evident that apart from a few agents, (of which, significantly, two naturally occurring substances, namely Carbon Dioxide and adrenaline are members) drugs exert relatively little effect on over-all cerebral circulation. Effects in terms of access must therefore be sought in changes in local vascular tone and in local distribution. Significantly, the density of the capillary bed (i. e. the length of capillary per unit volume) is not constant throughout the nervous system. These differences are seen in the development of the capillary bed, but are most striking in the fully developed nervous system (174, 175). For example, the least vascular part of the grey matter is nearly one and a half times as vascular as the richest part of white matter (174, 175). Regional differences in the vascularisation of different nuclei also exist (176); thus in the supraoptic and paraventricular nuclei of the hypothalamus, and the locus coeruleus of the medulla are particularly vascular areas. The Globus Pallidus has smaller vascular density than the Putamen; and this, in turn, is less vascular than the Lateral Geniculate body (177).

In the light of these local gradients in vascular density, techniques for the quantitative determination of regional cerebral blood flow are an especially timely and important development. Gross and over-all indications can be obtained by the insertion of thermocouples into various areas of the brain. These, however, allow only measurements in a few areas at a time. More recently a method has been described (158) capable of measuring simultaneously and quantitatively the blood flow in as many as twenty-eight structures of the brain. This method is based on the principle that the uptake of an inert radioactive gas (in this case I^{131} tagged trifluoriodomethane), by tissue is a function of the preceding history of the arterial concentration of the gas, the partition coefficient of the gas between the tissue and blood, the time, and the blood flow to that tissue. During an intravenous infusion of a solution of the radioactive gas, arterial concentration is continuously monitored by means of a scintillation counter; at a specific time the head is removed and frozen, and the concentrations of the gas in the various cerebral structures are determined by a unique radioautographic technique. From these data, as well as from the measured solubilities of the gas in blood and brain tissues, blood flow in the various structures is calculated. The method appears to yield reliable quantitative results but "is obviously limited to applications in laboratory animals" (155).

In a significant application of this procedure (178) it could be shown that during thiopental anaesthesia, the blood flow in a number of cerebral structures was reduced, the greatest reduction occurring in the primary sensory areas of the cerebral cortex which during consciousness had highest perfusion rates of all cortical areas. The results suggested that the differences in blood flow among the various cortical areas, so obvious during consciousness, were eliminated by thiopental anaesthesia, the cerebral blood flow becoming more uniform, and dropping to a lower level.

The possible relationship between local cerebral blood flow and local functional activity was examined in a second study by the same laboratory. Photic stimulation of the retina was used; this gave indication of change in local flow following prolonged photic stimulation. Though, of necessity, preliminary and technically complex, these methods are of the greatest interest to any enquiry into the regional pharmacology of the brain. It is to be hoped that they will be combined with other measures, such as measurement of temperature change, O_2 and CO_2 concentration, and, possibly, even measures of local Direct-Current (D.C.) changes. A study of regional blood flow and regional metabolism is inseparable from a study of regional factors influencing the action of drugs on the brain (179).

b) The Blood-Brain Barrier

Regional and Perisynaptic factors Governing Penetration

A further factor influencing the rate of penetration of drugs into the brain, and the accessibility of its various parts is the complex physico-chemical equilibrium known since 1921 (180) as the "Blood Brain Barrier". The structural connotation of this term disguises the composite and statistical nature of this equilibrium. The subject has been reviewed (177, 188), and only a few aspects will be mentioned in the present context.

In the first place, it would be well to be clear on the elements, which may contribute to the structural substrate of this barrier. The transport of a substance to brain tissue will obviously depend upon general and regional small vessel tone, and the physiological state of the local capillary bed. Within the capillary, the possible role of the endothelial cell, the interendothetical region, the endocapillary layer must be separately considered. Outside the small vessel, the contribution of the reticular perivascular sheath and of the glial element must also be weighed. Last and very pertinent to any discussion of the subject is the finely granular or molecular substance, vastly preponderating over cells and nuclear elements of the neuroglia, known as the cerebral ground substance (181). A neutral mucopolysaccharide may be the main component of the material, and may, in fact, be a principal factor in the regulation of the blood brain barrier effects. Whatever its precise architecture and. chemical constitution, there is little doubt that it is this finely granular colloidal material which may make up the most immediate chemical milieu of the neuron, and powerfully regulate conditions at its special electrogenic sites. Lastly, a clear distinction must also be made between the extracellular fluid of brain tissue, which is presumably embedded in the cerebral ground substance, and the cerebrospinal fluid. Whereas the former has ubiquitous distribution throughout the brain, the latter penetrates the brain substance by way of perivascular spaces, which continue down to arteriolar level only.

A number of theories have been advanced to account for the differences in permeability through the many elements making up the blood-brain barrier. Thus, for example, it has been suggested (183) that the endothelial cell has a low permeability to ion and to lipoid insoluble substances, and a high permeability to oxygen, carbon dioxide and lipoid soluble substances. The inter-endothelial region, on the other hand, has a high permeability to water, ions and large lipoid-insoluble molecules and is thus similar to an artificial porous membrane. A pore radius of $30–45\text{Å}$ and a pore density $1\text{-}2\text{x}10^9 \text{ cm}^2$ per capillary wall would account for the observed rates of passage of water and lipoid insoluble molecules. Attempts have also been made to compare the passage of the two groups mentioned with the conditions prevailing in the non-nervous capillary. As far as they go, the indications are suggestive. Oxygen and gases enter the brain readily, and there is relatively little hindrance to the entry of lipoid soluble substances, such as chloroform, ethyl alcohol and urethane (184). The entry of water is relatively unhindered (185), but many ions and organic crystalloid show characteristic delay or barrier effects. Thus, for example, anions such as bromide, iodide, thiocyanate, phosphate and chloride do not reach equilibrium with the brain extracellular fluid after three hours. Cation penetration is even slower, sodium reaching equilibrium only after sixty-two hours (186) and potassium somewhat more quickly. Among organic crystalloids, urea and glucose appear to have a limited entry. The exchange of isotope labelled ions has been recently reviewed (188).

That lipoid solubility may in some (though not all) instance influence the rate of penetration of a drug into the brain is indicated by some findings (189). In these, the lipoid solubility (in terms of chloroform/water partition coefficient, (at pH 7.4) was examined and related to the time taken to attain a C.S.F./plasma ratio of 1 *in vivo*. The findings are given in Table 1.

TABLE 1. Correlation of Penetration of drugs into Cerebrospinal Fluid of Rabbits and Chloroform to Water Partition Ratio of the Drugs [after Brodie, B. B. (189)]

Compound	Partition ratio at ph 7.4	Time to attain CSF to plasma ratio of 1 minute
Thiopental	102	< 5
Aminopyrine	73	< 5
Antipyrine	28	< 5
Aniline	19	< 5
4-Aminoantipyrine	15	< 5
Barbital	4.8	40
Acetanilide	3.7	120
N-acetyl-4-amino-antipyrine	1.4	> 180
Salicylyc acid	0.02	> 360

It will be noted that whereas, for example, thiopental with a high partition coefficient penetrated into the cerebrospinal fluid relatively readily barbital occupies an intermediate position and salicylic acid was very low in its rate of penetration.

"It is evident that drugs which are highly lipoid soluble at physiologic pH cross the blood-brain barrier rapidly; in fact, all compounds with a certain minimal lipoid solubility penetrate as rapidly that their rate appears to be blood flow limited. Drugs with lower lipoid solubility (salicylic acid, for example), penetrate more slowly, while quaternary compounds which are completely ionised and therefore lipoid insoluble, penetrate in almost negligible amounts, A number of non-lipid soluble substances readily pass into the central nervous system, but these are generally normal substrates for which specialized carrier mechanisms are present. Such a mechanism, for example, is present for glucose but not for *nor*epinephrine." (189)

The latter statement poses many questions. Little information is available to date on the role of plasma proteins in regulating this transfer. It becomes particularly relevant in connection with the transfer of naturally occurring metabolites, such as *nor*adrenaline and adrenaline across the blood brain barrier. *Nor*adrenaline does not readily transfer across the blood brain barrier. This may well be related to its poor lipoid solubility. A number of lipoid soluble congeners of *nor*adrenaline, (for example desoxyephedrine, amphetamine and tetrahydro-beta-phthylamine) penetrate the blood-brain barrier quite readily; though, again, the precise mechanism is far from clear. A somewhat similar state obtains with regard to 5-hydroxytryptamine (serotonin); here the substance itself penetrates the blood brain barrier less readily than its precursor, 5-hydroxytryptophane. In regard to these physiologically present substances, at any rate, the brain appears to preserve not only a selective permeability, but also an apparently regional chemical autonomy. The local manufacture within the brain is, in fact, part of such a regional economy.

There is a further aspect which must be considered in connection with the above, namely the existence of regional differences in accessibility, and the rate of penetration of substances within the brain itself. It has been known for some time that a number of special structures of the brain become stained after parenteral injection of vital dyes. Apart from obviously non-nervous elements, such as the hypophysis, the pineal gland and the choroid plexus, these areas include the tuber cinereum, the supraoptic crest recess, and the area postrema in the medulla. Striking differences in the structure of the ependymal lining can also be shown for certain regions (190). Also, using tritium labelled adrenaline, there is an accumulation of this substance in the hypothalamus at a rate which, though low when compared with other tissues, is measurably higher here than in any other parts of the brain (191).

Differences of accessibility may thus make the hypothalamic mechanisms particularly sensitive to shifts in plasma *nor*adrenaline or adrenaline, and the effect of drugs (191A), and treatment procedures, such as EST, in these transfers are in urgent need of investigation. It has also been shown that the relative secretion of noradrenaline and adrenaline in the adrenal medulla can be discretely influenced by the stimulation of discrete cell groups within the hypothalamus (192). The possibly of a self-limiting and self-setting mechanism in regard to adrenaline secretion must thus be considered.

The behavioral effects of drugs applied by the intraventricular route in the conscious animal have opened up a large and important area of enquiry. The technique has been used in cats (193), in dogs (194), and in mice (195), and suggests that transfer of the drug can indeed occur from the C.S.F. The paradoxical effects of adrenaline (which induces drowsiness when applied by this route) may be due to its reaching areas of the brain normally shielded from it by the blood brain barrier. The important structural differences in the ependyma should be borne in mind here also.

There is, however, a third group of factors of a more hypothetical nature, which may also bear upon the action, and the mode of action of centrally acting drugs upon the individual neurone in the Central Nervous System. Microelectrode studies, particularly those coupled with the electrophoretic local application of synaptically active substances to single units (see below), have suggested the existence of perisynaptic barriers and regional differences at the synaptic junctions (195a). Little accurate information as to the nature of this barrier is at present available. It may be enzymic, or structural in nature. Relevant here, however, may be the presence of distinctive delimiting membrane bounding in the pre-synaptic terminals; and the demonstration of the fine vesicles in the synaptic area by electron microscopy; and the existence of a space of 100–200Å thickness between the opposing pre-synaptic and postsynaptic membrane (196), the so-called intrasynaptic space or synaptic cleft. These structural features may possibly account for the so-called synaptic barrier; though for the present it is uncertain whether such barriers account for differences in susceptibility to chemical agents on the part of various units within the Central Nervous System.

C. Biochemical and Pharmacological Considerations

As is common in the study of the mode of action of chemotherapeutic agents, *in vitro* systems form an accessible paradigm of *in vivo* effects. It is, however, well to realize the special care, which, in the nervous system, has to be exercised in applying *in vitro* models to *in vivo* situations. The barriers shielding nervous tissue from indiscriminate assault of circulating metabolites (or drugs) has already been stressed, and the existence of gradients within the central nervous system itself has also been emphasized. Furthermore there is ample evidence to suggest a chemical and enzymological inhomogeneity within the nervous system itself, extending both to gross topographical as well as on to a finer cytological detail. Unlike a bacterial culture growing in its own nutrient medium, a brain slice is but the crudest approximation of its parent tissue and, in fact, only a relative improvement on a homogenate. A specification of the origin of the sample is always needed: and even then it is well to remember the grossly unphysio-logical state in which the function of such a sheet of neurones is observed, despite every care and precaution which may be taken to the contrary. With these reservations in mind, the *in vitro* effects of some drugs will now be briefly considered.

a) Biochemical Effects of Some Psychoactive Drugs "in vitro"

One of the earliest *in vitro* studies of the effects of psychoactive drugs concerns a series of amines, and, more particularly, mescalin. This drug was found to inhibit the oxidation of glu-cose, lactate, pyruvate and glutamate, but not of succinate by minced guinea pig brain (197). It was suggested by the authors at the time that liver dysfunction might conceivably lead to a faulty detoxication in terms of amines, which in turn might adversely affect brain respiration. However, the concentrations of drugs used in these *in vitro* experiments were higher than those likely to obtain *in vivo*; particularly since the distribution of C^{14} labelled mescaline (198, 201) indicated that only a small fraction of the labelled material was found to enter the Central Nervous System. This disparity was also stressed by others (199). Nevertheless, based on the fact that succinate is not inhibited by mescaline, an attempt was made to attenuate induced symptoms in man by the intravenous administration of sodium succinate. This experiment, however, was not controlled by placebo (200).

Mescaline was found to be without effect on oxaloacetic and oxalosuccinic carboxylase or transaminase activity and, equally, was found to have no effect on succinic dehydrogenase and cytochrome oxidase (202). Mescalin at 10^{-3} M had no effect on oxygen uptake or on phosphorylation in preparations of brain mitochondria respiring *in vitro* in a pyruvate sub-strate (203).

Using an imaginative method which allowed comparison between resting tissue and the ef-fect of electrical stimulation on brain slices suitably arranged in a Warburg vessel, it was found that even high concentrations of mescalin (10^{-2} M) did not affect the uptake of oxygen, or the production of lactate on a substrate of glucose by unstimulated slices. If, however, mes-caline was tested in stimulated slices, a somewhat lower concentration (10^{-3} M) led to 50% in-hibition of extra oxygen uptake, and the formation of lactate resulting from the electrical stim-ulation. The metabolism of the stimulated tissue thus appeared to be more sensitive to this (and other) drugs than the unstimulated metabolism. Significantly however, even a slight fall in concentration (to 10^{-4} M) led to the disappearance of this effect. It should be noted that this concentration is still considerably (about 10 times) in excess of the calculated *in vivo* value. The effect of LSD-25 *in vitro* on oxygen uptake and production of lactic acid in stimulated brain slices were similarly unimpressive. An attempt to reverse these effects with serotonin was not successful (204). Serotonin is a weak uncoupling agent for oxidative phosphoryl-ation, leading to 50% uncoupling with liver mitochondria at 5×10^{-4} M (205).

The reported rise following LSD-25, of acetylcholine in the brain of the guinea pig (206) encouraged a study of the effects of LSD-25 on Cholinesterase activity (207). A strange and rather specific effect of LSD-25 was encountered. In the relatively low concentration of 5×10^{-6} M, LSD-25 was found to produce 50% inhibition of the non-specific (pseudo) cholinesterase of human brain, though even at 10 times that concentration only a 10% inhibi-tion of the true esterase was achieved. The same order of effects was obtained using blood true esterase and pseudo-esterase; again, the sensitivity of the human esterases to these inhibitory effects was particularly noteworthy.

These studies were extended to an examination of the effects of 2-Bromlysergic acid diethylamide (BOL 148) (208) and to a number of other psychoactive drugs, which include Chlorpromazine, Psilocybin, N-Allyl-normorphine, Cocaine, Harmine, Meprobamate, d-Amphetamine and Mescaline. It was found that "while a number of drugs which produce psychosomimetic symptoms in man are reasonably potent inhibitors of human serum cholinesterase, this does not appear to be either a necessary or an adequate characteristic of such activity" (209). Thus, for example, BOL 148 which is not a psychosomimetic drug is almost as potent a cholinesterase inhibitor as is LSD-25, while Chlorpromazine, a neuroleptic agent exceeded the anticholinesterase effects in terms of molar effectiveness. Mescaline was found to be devoid of this effect, as were d-Amphetamine, and Meprobamate. The study, however, served to emphasise the occurrence of an atypical form of human serum cholinesterase differing from normal in its sensitivity to a number of inhibitors.

In considering the biochemical effects of chlorpromazine, it is well to remember that it is not unrelated to another phenothiazine, methylene blue, which has played a significant role in the development of chemotherapy. It acts as hydrogen acceptor in enzymatic reactions, and also as an inhibitor of cholinesterase, a feature already mentioned. The action of phenothiazines has been studied, using the purified enzyme systems, particulate cell components, and tissue slices. In an early examination of the anthelmintic action of the phenothiazines (210) it was found that phenothiazine was a strong inhibitor of over-all oxidation succinate, of hexokinase and cytochrome oxidase. In a substituted phenothiazine like chlorpromazine, the solubility and charge are decisively altered by side chain and rings substitution, and are bound to affect distribution. S-35 labelled chlorpromazine enters the brain quite rapidly (211) though the suggestion that chlorpromazine accumulates preferentially in the hypothalamus must be treated with caution. In this context the observation that chlorpromazine administered to rats results in a significant increase in the concentration of ATP in the brain, particularly in the thalamic-hypothalamic region, (212) is of interest. This has been attributed to the inactivity of the animals, resulting in a decreased utilization of the nucleotide.

The above observations are mentioned in passing, insofar as they relate to the effects of chlorpromazine on oxidative phosphorylation in mitochondria of liver and brain (213). Chlorpromazine is an effective uncoupler of oxidative phosphorylation in rat liver mitochondria, in concentrations of 2×10^{-4} M. This is true for all substrates used, α-Ketoglutarate, succinate, pyruvate and malate and glutamate. "Although the effect of the drug on respiration was slight, if present at all, the yield of ATP, as measured with the hexokinase glucose system as trap, was considerably lower in the presence of the drug" (214). The effect of chlorpromazine, used in similar concentrations on brain mitochondria was considerably less marked. Oxidative phosphorylation was essentially unaffected.

This lack of effect however in no way reflected a lack of reactivity of (guinea pig and monkey) brain mitochondria to other uncoupling agents, such as 2,4-dinitrophenol. The results thus suggested difference between mitochondria in the brain and liver, not only in regard to the effect of chlorpromazine but also in regard to the utilization of added cytochrome. It has been argued that mitochondria obtained from brain in contrast with those from liver are able to metabolize glucose by glycolysis (215). It is possible that mitochondria from these two organs are possessed of structural differences, and that the effects of chlorpromazine on liver mitochondria are only secondarily effects on oxidative phosphorylation. The increase of ATP in the hypothalamus following chlorpromazine (212) is thus not at variance with the effect of chlorpromazine observed *in vitro*.

(b) The Metabolic Fate of some Psychoactive Compounds

It is evident that the *in vivo* effect of a particular drug on the brain may not necessarily be due to the drug itself, but rather to a derivative of the compound originally administered. Distribution throughout the body, the entry of a substance into the brain, and change in the tissues or in particular organs (for example, the liver) may profoundly determine both the activation, and the inactivation of a particular compound. This is not the place to discuss the factors, and particularly the physicochemical characteristics influencing the distribution of compounds throughout the body; the subject has been considered admirably by others (216). Rather is it the intention of this brief account to note some of the metabolic changes undergone by some psychoactive compounds in the body. A recent comprehensive treatment of the subject of detoxification (217) may be found particularly useful by the interested reader.

The metabolic changes undergone by chlorpromazine have been only partly accounted for to date. Little of a given dose of chlorpromazine is found free in the urine. The sulphoxide may account for about 5% (218). The presence of other polar metabolites has been recently suggested (219). The sulphoxide, however, is less active pharmacologically than other possible metabolites whose presence, though suggested, must remain conjectural (220). More recent studies (221, 222) have drawn attention to the excretion of phenolic glycuronides following the administration of chlorpromazine. It may well be that the formation of phenolic derivatives (including phenolic amines) may be an important pathway in the metabolism of chlorpromazine. Such amines could conceivably compete with naturally occurring compounds, and thus be related to the mode of action of chlorpromazine. The identification of chlorpromazine N-oxide is another important step (223). Also, on the basis of a comparison of the pharmacological activity of a number of possible metabolites [Monoethylchlorpromazine (NOR 1 CP), Chlorpromazine N-oxide (CPNO), Chlorpromazine Sulphoxide (CPSO)] and of some derivatives of Promazine, it was suggested that at least in animals, the effects of chlorpromazine may be due to the metabolites of the drug. Demethylated, hydroxylated and demethylated-hydroxylated metabolites seem the most likely (224).

A similar state of affairs obtains in regard to mescalin. Radioactive carbon labelled mescalin can be shown to be incorporated in tissue proteins from which it is subsequently slowly released with excretion in urine and faeces. Significantly little of the material could be traced to the brain, compared with the liver and other organs (198, 201). This was also the case in another study (225) where 28–46% of the administered material was recovered unchanged. In an older study (226) about one third of administered mescaline (in dogs and rabbits) was recovered as the trimethoxyphenyl acetic acid (implying a deamination of the mescaline). This product, however, was not encountered in man.

In two other studies an attempt was made to relate metabolism in man to the time course of clinical effects induced by the drug. In one (227), the failures to show the presence 3,4,5-trimethoxyphenylacetic acid was confirmed; 65% of the amine remained unaccounted for; 1–2% was found to be excreted as the glutamine conjugate of 3,4-dihydroxy-5-methoxyphenylacetic acid. In another study (228) an average of 31% of the drug administered was recovered in the urine within six hours; and an additional 7.4% as trimethoxyphenylacetic acid. Again, the unaccounted portion should be noted; as should be the fact that, in this study, the blood levels and rates of excretion did not fall off asymptotically, but formed a flattening curve, with secondary peaks with some elevation between the third and sixth hours. There was also some delay in the occurrence of maximal behavioral change.

Another psychoactive substance, which has recently undergone investigation in respect to *in vivo* change, is dimethyltryptamine. As noted above, this substance induces "psychoso-mimetic" effects in man; these are characterised by rapid onset and rapid decay. It has been shown by Szara that this agent undergoes hydroxylation, in the 6 position, probably by a microsomal enzyme system in the liver; that the 6-hydroxyl derivative is more, rather than less active in inducing behavioral effects, in the experimental animal; that the rate of 6-hydroxylation may very from animal to animal in the same species (rat); and that the thresh-old for inducing behavioral change in an operant conditioning situation in an individual ani-mal may vary with the rate of hydroxylation in the particular animal. These observations rep-resent to the best of the author's knowledge, one of the few instances where the potency of s psychoactive compound is increased through *in vivo* change (229, 230).

The distribution and metabolism of LSD-25 has been studied in several laboratories. Using a specific and sensitive method of assay for its detection in tissues (231) (cat) it was found that the drug was extensively bound to plasma proteins, and there was no hindrance in the passage of the drug across the blood brain barrier. It was shown to be present in the brain, though the concentration in plasma liver and kidney was higher. The drug was almost completely me-tabolised in the body, only negligible amounts being exerted in urine, and in the stools.

The substance was found to be transformed to 2-oxy LSD-by an enzyme system present in liver microsomes. This derivative did not "possess LSD-like activity in. the Central Nervous System" (232). The contrast between the inactivation of LSD-25 and the relative activation of Dimethyltryptamine should be noted.

c) Possible Intracerebral Target Processes

Interaction between drugs and Neurohumoral Agents

1. General Considerations

The last few years have led to suggestive evidence of the interaction between some psychoac-tive agents, and neurohumoral substances within the brain. The origins of these suggestions are an interesting reflection on the empirical, and even arbitrary, nature of the field. Mescalin bears some chemical relationship to adrenaline, ephedrine and amphetamine. Both LSD-25 and reserpine contain the indole nucleus and can thus, albeit rather loosely, be related to sero-tonin. The psychotropic properties of atropine and of its isomer scopolamine have long been attributed to a central anti-acetylcholine effect. The same applies to N-ethyl-3-piperidyl-benzilate and to benactyzine. As has been pointed out elsewhere in this volume, (see Vol. I, p. 59; Waelsch and Weil-Malherbe) the suggestion for a possible role of acetylcholine in chemi-cal mediation within the central nervous system, preceded the demonstration of *nor*adrenaline and serotonin within the brain by over a decade. The latter discoveries, in fact, coincided, in some measure, and with the discovery of psychotropic effects of some of the compounds here considered. It is these historical links which have made for the present conceptual matrix. As will be apparent from what follows, this remains hybrid, mainly because an all-too-ready transfer of the rules accepted for the autonomic nervous system to a hypothetical pharmacol-ogy of the brain. Yet the evidence must, of necessity, come from within the brain: this truism will brook no compromise.

A good deal has been written on the role of neurohumoral transmission within the brain; since it has also been dealt in another place (Waelsch and Weil-Malherbe loc. cit.) only a few aspects will be mentioned in the present context. In the first place, it would be well to agree upon certain minimal desiderata, which have to be satisfied by a substance claiming the role of a neurohumoral mediator within the central nervous system (233). First, the substance should be present in the central nervous system and should vary in concentration with the functional state of the tissue. Second, enzyme systems should be present both for the synthesis, and for the destruction of the substance in question; these should also be present in the areas of the central nervous system where the substance is normally found. Third, the enzymes should be susceptible to inhibition by specific inhibitors, or antimetabolites, and the effects of such inhibition should be clearly demonstrable in chemical or functional terms. Fourth, the application of a hypothetical agent, or its precursor or product, to the central nervous system, either directly or by a selected physiological route, should exert clear effects on function.

These criteria are met in part by a number of substances, though in the case of each important reservations obtain. To be sure Acetylcholine is present in the brain; variation in content has been reported with sleep (234) and anaesthesia (235). Yet the enzyme system for Acetylcholine synthesis shows a curiously uneven distribution, some areas being richer in the enzyme than others (236). Although in the estimation of Acetylcholine synthesising power one may not be dealing with a single enzyme, but rather with a complex enzyme system, (and an uneven distribution of a cofactor accounting for the differences in yield of *in vitro* experiments) the regional difference between acetylcholine synthesising power in different areas are real. A universal role of Acetylcholine throughout the central nervous system must thus be doubted; and a possible alternation between cholinergic and noncholinergic elements has been tentatively put forward (236).

A similar doubt pervades the universal role of the "true" (i.e. acetylcholine specific) acetylcholinesterase. A non-specific pseudo cholinesterase (hydrolysing benzoyl and butyryl choline at a rate preferential to acetylcholine) has also been demonstrated within the brain (237). In the rat brain these enzymes develop at different rates, and assume different concentrations in different regions (238). The specific susceptibility of these enzymes to specific inhibition is very real (239). This specificity operates in mixtures, and can be used for the detection of low concentrations of one enzyme in the presence of another. Sustained and irreversible inhibition of cholinesterase from birth does not materially affect the rate of emergence of innate behavior patterns in the rat (240). Higher nervous function however was not tested in these experiments, there being indication that this may be affected by cholinergic mechanisms (241). On the other hand, the intracarotid injection of very small doses of a specific pseudo-esterase inhibitor will desynchronise the corticogram much more than a corresponding (or even higher) dose of a specific inhibitor of Acetylcholinesterase (242).

It is discrepancies such as these, which counsel caution in regarding choline as the sole or even principal neurohumoral transmitter in the central nervous system or even in equating "true" cholinesterase activity with the presence of acetylcholine. In looking for complementary chemical mediators numerous substances such as the depressor substance P (243, 244) and even Adenosine triphosphate itself (255) have been variously considered. More significant however, has been the discovery of *nor*adrenaline and serotonin in the brain, and the differential distribution of these substances in various areas of the brain. Midline structures (the hypothalamus, the mesencephalon, the midline thalamic nuclei and the area postrema appear to be richer in these agents than other areas (256, 257). Furthermore hypothalamic and adrenomedullary *nor*adrenaline were found to vary, *pari passu* under the influence of such drugs as caffeine leptazol and ergometrine (256); also it has been reported that stimulation of discrete areas of the hypothalamus could make the adrenal medulla yield differential proportions of adrenaline and *nor*adrenaline (192). That, however, caution is in place in this field is indicated by a number of stubborn paradoxes which continue to come to light. In the first place, serotonin and *nor*epinephrine are not the only members of their respective groups which have been identified in the brain. The presence of a precursor of adrenaline, Dopamine has been clearly demonstrated (257A); moreover this substance has a differential distribution from noradrenaline, being found in relatively high concentration in the putamen and the caudate nucleus (258). Melatonin a substance related to serotonin has remarkably high concentrations in the pineal (259). Again, there is no necessary correlation between the distribution of the decarboxylating enzyme (dopa decarboxylase) and 5-hydroxytryptophane decarboxylase and the *nor*adrenaline or serotonin content of particular nervous sites. For example, sympathetic ganglia contain little serotonin, though their decarboxylase activity may be high; the caudate nucleus, already mentioned, is another exception. It has, in fact, been concluded that in nervous tissue, biosynthesis of catecholamines stops at the *nor*adrenaline level. Here Dopamine is the precursor of the transmitter, and besides this, an effector substance of its own. In the lung, intestine and liver, Dopamine is the end product of biosynthesis. Here it may act as a local hormone (260).

There is a further group of substances, which has recently commanded attention as being capable of affecting central synaptic transmission. This includes a series of synaptically active amino acids (261) and is best represented in the striking distribution and effects of Gamma amino butyric acid (GABA) (262–265). This substance, referred to elsewhere in this volume) is found in large quantities readily extractable from the Central Nervous System of a number of species. It is formed from Glutamic acid by the action of Glutamic acid Decarboxylase (GAD). Both GABA itself and the Decarboxylase are found in higher yield in gray than in white matter, and both are laid down very rapidly in the brain during early postnatal development. The decarboxylation of glutamic acid to Gamma aminobutyrate requires the presence of pyridoxal phosphate, and thus brings the formation of this acid into intimate relationship with cellular oxidation.

The disposition of GABA is carried through by GABA transaminase (GABA-T), an enzyme found in the brain, and other tissues which brings about the transamination of GABA with alpha Ketoglutarate to form L-Glutamic acid and succinic semialdehyde. The latter compound is then oxidized to succinic acid in the brain the succinate entering the tricarboxylic cycle. The distribution of GABA-T and GAD in the nervous system of the monkey is uneven (266). The relatively high concentration of GABA-T, inter alia, in the hypothalamus and the olivary nucleus is noteworthy.

As is the case with adrenaline and serotonin, GABA itself does not readily penetrate the blood brain barrier, but depends for its presence in the brain on local manufacture from its precursor, glutamic acid. A number of other findings should also be noted. The enzymes concerned with the synthesis (GAD) and the disposition (GABA-T) of GABA show a remarkable sensitivity to pH, GAD showing maximal activity of pH 6.5, and GABA-T at pH 8.2 (264). Small shifts in intracellular pH, (occasioned, for example, by CO_2 shifts and differences in the activity of carbonic anhydrase), could thus be envisioned to markedly affect the levels of intracellular GABA. The amount of GABA present in any particular area must thus reflect a balance between the rate of formation and the rate of utilization of the material, and the level of enzyme activity in a particular area. The ratio between the activity of the two enzymes may thus be a much more accurate indicator of GABA activity in a particular area than the actual amount of GABA present at a particular time. Fortunately, the activity of these enzymes can be affected. The semicarbazides, by interfering with pyridoxal phosphate activity (an essential coenzyme factor in the action of the Decarboxylase) can inhibit decarboxylase activity, leading to a fall in GABA levels in the CNS. Hydroxylamine, on the other hand, can be shown to inhibit GABA-Transferase (GABA-T) more than decarboxylase, and thus leads to an endogenous accumulation of GABA *in vivo*.

The first indication of a possible physiological role of GABA in the mammalian nervous system stems from the demonstration of the convulsive properties of the semicarbazides (267), the application of which *in vivo* was found to lead to repetitive seizures following a significantly long latent period. This presumably resulted from the fall in endogenously produced GABA, and was borne out by the fact that the topical application of low doses of GABA reduced or blocked electrically induced seizures in the hippocampus (268). Hydroxylamine, on the other hand led to a marked reduction in the duration and spread of electrically induced after-discharges in the cat in acute experiments, and in conscious monkeys carrying indwelling electrodes (269). The monkeys appeared more placid without being sedated, and were much easier to handle for as long as seven hours after the administration of hydroxylamine. The predominantly inhibitory role of GABA on synaptic transmission has been stressed in a number of studies (270); though its universal role as the principal inhibitory substance in the mammalian central nervous system can by no means be regarded as settled (265).

The above findings are mentioned because they represent a significant break in a tradition which, up to quite recently, has unduly emphasized a distinction between the power economy, the protein synthesis, and the processes and agents affecting the electrogenic properties, and the permeability of the neurone membrane. Distinctions such as these are no doubt convenient, and can be readily made in the mind; they help to delimit one's problem and to guide one's experiment. They are, however, unlikely to be made in the cell, where the various phases appear functionally linked and interdependent. Thus, for example, the rate of protein synthesis in the brain, and the rate of turnover of amino acids is known to be very high (271). Glutamic acid (the parent substance of GABA) has been long known to play a part in energy metabolism and protein synthesis. Yet its derivative, GABA together with other amino acids, can be shown to exert effects on synaptic transmission which, to say the least, are quite respectable. One must thus assume that if, indeed, such substances do naturally occur in the central nervous system, their effect must be both local and transient; and that some subcellular compartmentalization (272), carefully regulates the manufacture, storage, release, and inactivation of the various agents, quite possibly in different proportions, and at different rates. One is also struck by certain common features shared by the agents considered so far. In the case of each (acetylcholine, *nor*adrenaline, serotonin and GABA), the active agent, though readily formed in the brain, does not readily penetrate the blood brain barrier; their precursors (dopa, 5-hydroxytryptophane) do so fairly readily, and are found, in some instances, (such as in the case of Dopamine) to have a distribution pattern rather different from their products. Again, the enzyme systems for their synthesis and disposition have a differential distribution pattern throughout the brain; and, though sharing certain features in common (for example dependence upon decarboxylation in the case of Dopamine, 5-hydroxytryptophane and glutamic acid) also show marked differences in respect to other enzyme activity (for example, their differential susceptibility) to mono amine oxidase, or O-methyltransferase). Furthermore there is some; suggestive evidence of susceptibility in some cases to strictly local conditions (for example local pH in the case of GAD and GABA-T). The picture, which thus emerges, is one of convergence and interaction between a number of highly localized processes, proceeding at different rates, and possibly, at different subcellular sites in the same segment of time. Their coincidence and relative overlap may profoundly determine the final sequence of events leading to discharge in a particular cell assembly. Inasmuch as the net statistical balance within the closed neural loops of the CNS is likely to be affected by interaction of a drug with any single element (be it cholinergic or non-cholinergic), the greatest reservation has to be exercised in ascribing the central effects of a particular drug to its most obvious and predominant property. It is hoped that what follows will be viewed with these reservations in mind.

2. Some Drugs Presumed to Interact with Acetylcholine in the Central Nervous System: Atropine, Hyoscine, Benactyzine and N-ethyl-3-piperidyl benzilate (JB 318)

Atropine and Hyoscine. Atropine, a constituent of belladonna leaves, is a derivative of tropane, a nucleus common to many alkaloids. Esterification of tropanol (hydroxytropane) with tropic acid results in the formation of atropine.

Tropic acid is α-phenyl-β-hydroxypropionic acid. The alpha carbon atom of this acid is asymmetric. Similar asymmetry applies to the mandelic acid radical with which tropanol is esterified to form homatropine. In Hyoscine (scopolamine) (an alkaloid found in belladonna and also in *Datura metel*) the tropanol nucleus contains an ether linkage.

The mode of action of atropine and related compounds in relation to autonomic effectors has been reviewed (273). There is suggestive evidence that it achieves its effect by way of competitive inhibition of acetylcholine; neither choline acetylase nor cholinesterase is markedly affected by atropine. The alkaloid is excreted in greater part unchanged in man; in rabbits, however, there is a remarkable capacity on the part of tissues (and particularly liver and kidney) to hydrolyse atropine (274). This degree of tolerance (275, 276) shows individual (i. e. intra species) variation.

In man full doses of atropine leads to mydriasis, xerostomia, dysphagia, redness of skin, malaise, muscular weakness, and rise in body temperature. Confusion and hallucinosis are frequently seen and disturbances of attention and of short-term memory (forgetting the beginning of sentences as they are spoken) have also been reported. Confusional states have also been reported in children. The principal clinical effect of atropine in man is thus what is usually, and loosely, termed a "stimulant" effect.

In contrast to atropine, scopolamine reduces motor activity. Two phases of the action of the drug have been distinguished. The first is characterized by mainly autonomic effects; the second, setting in later, may manifest in depersonalisation, disturbances of body image, hyperacusis, coupled with the reduction of drive and retardation, drowsiness and sleep. Hallucinations and illusions are observed relatively rarely. There is also reduction in muscle tone. It also possesses antiemetic and antimotion sickness properties. Intramuscularly, scopolamine has been employed as one of the older remedies in the control mania and delirium tremens. It is also being used to promote drowsiness with amnesia in obstetric practice (the so-called twilight sleep). To achieve this it is usually given with a sedative such as morphine, meperidine or even barbiturate. Atropine of course is the remedy of choice in the treatment of poison by the anticholinesterase agents. A recent study has examined the dose response relationship for the autonomic and mental effects of atropine and hyoscine in man (277).

Benactyzine. This substance, a diethylaminoethylester of benzilic acid, was tested for its effects in stress induced behavior in 1955 (278). It exerts a marked antiacetylcholine effect, blocking the spasmogenic effect of acetylcholine in the isolated intestine preparation, the hypotensive effect of acetylcholine, and the effects produced by stimulation of the peripheral stump of the severed vagus nerve (279). It also augments the pressor responses to adrenaline. It is a powerful drug of the order of dose range of atropine. Injected in mice, it leads to hyperexcitability and convulsion, and also increases the incidence of death resulting from electroconvulsive seizures. On the other hand, and perhaps somewhat paradoxically, small doses of the drug increase the hexobarbital sleeping time. In monkeys 1–6 mg/kg of benactyzine leads to mydriasis and decrease in spontaneous movement, without ataxia, or the so-called the taming effect. Large doses, on the other hand, lead to convulsions, which are followed by retardation. In chloralose anaesthetized cats, the knee jerk and flexor reflexes are not altered by a dose of 3 mg/kg; but after 10 mg/kg the reflexes are abolished, followed by respiratory arrest. In curarized unanesthetized cats, 1 mg/kg of bensetyzine leads to slowing and increasing amplitude of electrical activity as recorded from subcortical and cortical areas. This is not unlike the effect observed with atropine (280). The so-called arousal response (i.e. low voltage and fast activity to sensory or thalamic stimulation) is blocked by benactyzine; recruiting responses in the cortex, (evoked by thalamic stimulation) are not affected. Of particular interest are the extensive behavioral studies carried out in cats and rodents using the so-called "experimental neuroses" model (see below). In relatively small doses (0.75 to 2.0 mg) benactyzine was found to "normalize" behavior, to diminish the so-called displacement activities (playful behavior, licking, opening the food box in the absence of signals); it also reduced the duration in the feeding cycle which, in the absence of the drug, is characteristically prolonged after induction of motivational conflict. In the rat, benactyzine in this respect was more active than alcohol. Interestingly enough, scopolamine (though in a much smaller doses of 0.05 to 0.1 mg) did not exert the effect seen with benactyzine. Similar effects of the drug were observed in regard to manifest "tension" in the experimental animal (as judged by bristling fur, arched back, immobility, hiding in corners, raised tail). It was concluded by these investigators that "apparently the relaxation was due to a diminished fear of the coming stimulus" (281).

In man the results have been equivocal. Variable clinical effects with benactyzine have been observed in tension states (282). On the other hand, in the normal, symptoms, such as depersonalization, change in body image, and memory disturbance may be seen.

The N-substituted Piperidyl Benzylates. A number of N-substituted piperidyl benzylates have been recently examined for psychosomimetic effects (283). All share a degree of antiacetylcholine activity (as tested in the guinea pig ileum); some of them (particularly the N-methyl and N-ethyl-3-piperidyl benzilate) exhibit psychosomimetic properties, there being some relation between the antiacetylcholine effects of and the psychosomimetic effects in at least 3 members of the group. This must await further data. The ethyl substituted compound (JB 318) has been tested most extensively.

In rats the drug induces a bobbing and swaying head movement, particularly in the vertical direction. In man muscular weakness, drowsiness incoordination and hyperreflexia were noted. More marked, however, were the mental effects appearing within 1–2 hours after administration. A careful study in 10 subjects using a counterbalanced design, has compared the effects of 15 mg of JB 318 with those of 100 μg LSD-25 (284). A number of psychometric test procedures were employed. The results indicated significant differences between LSD-25 and

JB 318 both in the perceptual and affective responses. JB 318 was judged "a more potent hallucinogenic," LSD-25 leading to more change in affect and body image.

The demonstration of effects such as these in a synthetic antiacetylcholine agent opens a number of possible approaches to the study of structure activity relationships in terms of interaction between various congeners in man. It is to be hoped that this group of compounds will be subjected to systematic enquiry.

3. Drugs Presumed to Exert Central Adrenergic Blockade: Chlorpromazine

The ability of some drugs to block central responses to adrenaline and noradrenaline in the nervous system is far from settled (285) and must await further evidence as to the precise role played by sympathomimetic amines in the mediation, or modulation of central processes. By and large the effects are regarded as stimulant; the old term for some sympathomimetic amines ("Weckamine", "waking amines") indeed implies this type of action. On the other hand, the catecholamines can (at least at local level) also show inhibitory effects (such as following intraventricular injection (193) or in the transcallosal pathway preparation (see below). Such effects need not necessarily be regarded as contradictory, in view of the close functional juxtaposition of stimulation and inhibition within the central nervous system.

A number of adrenergic blocking agents have been shown to antagonize the increased motor activity induced by methamphetamine as tested in the mouse (286). It would however be unjustifiable to attribute these effects to specific adrenergic blockade, since these effects do not correlate at all well with the peripheral blocking action of the compounds studied. Indeed, adrenaline and noradrenaline themselves may produce an antagonism to methamphetamine induced activity (287). Again, a well-known adrenergic blocking agent, such as Dibenamine does not appreciably affect adrenaline induced respiratory stimulation (288). More recently a benzo-dioxine derivative (Ethoxybutamoxane) has been shown to be highly effective in laboratory tests in its neuroleptic properties (289). The compound was deliberately developed for its central adrenergic blocking action. Moreover benzodioxanes exert some paradoxical actions difficult to reconcile with purely central adrenergic blockade. They may, for example, lead to a rise of blood pressure in unanaesthetized animals and in man. A further use of central adrenergic blocking agents has been the attempted elucidation of the role of adrenergic mechanisms in the activation or blockade of hypothalamic pituitary responses. The results, again, have been inconclusive. A number of adrenergic blocking agents have been shown to inhibit ACTH release, induced by the injection of adrenaline, and a number of other sympathomimetic amines. These agents however do not block the release to other types of stress (290, 291). The role of adrenergic mechanisms in the release of gonadotropic hormones is even less defined. For example, in the rabbit, ovulation can be induced by injection of small amounts of adrenaline and noradrenaline into the third ventricle, the hypothalamus or the adenohypophysis. Several relatively specific B-haloalkylamine amine-blocking agents have been shown to block this response to adrenaline and noradrenaline (292, 293).

There is, nevertheless, some tenuous evidence that adrenergic blocking agents may influence central nervous system activity. The B-haloalkylamines lead to mild sedation, and a feeling of lethargy (294). Dibenamine is reputed to induce some disorders of time sense, and of memory function (295). Dibenzyline, administered in relatively smaller doses, apparently does not share in these effects. So far no consistent relationship has been established between adrenergic blocking activity and, the effects on mental function, or motor performance. Another group is the natural or dehydrogenated ergot alkaloids. These may lead to marked central symptoms (296). Interestingly enough these effects are usually seen with doses lower than those required to produce even minimal peripheral adrenergic blockade. It is even likely that central inhibition of the sympathetic centers (297) may be responsible for the peripheral vasodilation and the fall in blood pressure induced by these agents in man. Nausea and vomiting may be due to an action on the chemoreceptor trigger zone in the medulla. Here again, then, the results are suggestive, but equivocal.

A forceful argument to include chlorpromazine in the group of central adrenergic blocking agents has been put forward (298). The following findings are cited in support of this view.

1. Chlorpromazine counteracts the pharmacological effects and the EEG arousal induced by amphetamine and the pharmacological effects induced by Dopa, amphetamine, cocaine, and LSD-25. In regard to the latter, it has been suggested that there is a competitive antagonism between these sympathomimetic agents and chlorpromazine, suggesting that these compounds may act on the same receptors.

2. Chlorpromazine suppresses the centrally mediated rise in blood pressure induced by cocaine.

3. Chlorpromazine lowers blood pressure and antagonizes the carotid pressor reflex when given intracisternally in doses too small to alter the pressor effects of administered adrenaline.

4. Chlorpromazine relaxes the nictitating membrane and leads to miosis and bradycardia following intraventricular injection of a dose too small to be effective intravenously.

5. The failure of the drug to block the peripheral depressor and mydriatic effects of injected noradrenaline. Central effects of chlorpromazine are thus envisioned.

The argument, though suggestive, must still be regarded as circumstantial. It does nevertheless serve the useful purpose in drawing attention to aspects of this intricate problem. First there is the question of dosage. Since it is argued the central adrenaline blocking effects are exerted before the peripheral effects become manifest, this is of obvious import. Yet accurate quantitative data in this respect are lacking at present. Second, there is the question of a preferential blockade for adrenaline over *nor*adrenaline. This, too, needs systematic testing. Thirdly, a careful fractionation of the contribution of afferent pathways (from peripheral baro or chemoreceptor sites) is needed for assessment of the total effect. Lastly, the relative role of chlorpromazine, or a metabolite (possibly a phenolic amine) in adrenergic blockade remains to be determined. Thus, nine years after the first clinical trial of chlorpromazine, its central mode of action continues to mystify and bemuse.

4. Drugs Interfering with the Disposition of Adrenaline and Serotonin: The Monoamine Oxidase Inhibitors

The present interest in the central action of monoamine oxidase inhibitors arose from the observations that the drug Iproniazid, originally used in the treatment of tuberculosis (299), exerted marked central, so called "stimulant" effects (300). Also, Isoniazid has, in fact, been used in the treatment of depression (301). Later studies (302) demonstrated inhibitory effects of Iproniazid on monoamine oxidase. The drug has proven a valuable tool in the systematic study of the properties of monoamine oxidases, and their interaction with various substrates (303).

The renewed interest in the *in vivo* disposition of biogenic amines and their implication for the physiology of the brain however goea back for nearly two decades. It was suggested in

1940 (304) that the stimulant action of amphetamine might, in fact, be based on the inhibition of monoamine oxidase. It was observed in these studies that oxidation of various amines by monoamine oxidase led to the formation of intermediate aldehydes, which, then, underwent further oxidation to form the corresponding acids. The intermediate aldehydes are depresaant in nature; it was therefore suggested that amphetamine might possibly exert its central effect by preventing (by way of monoamine oxidase blockade) the formation of such aldehydes. There was, however, little evidence for monoamine oxidase inhibition *in vivo* in doses in which amphetamine produced stimulation.

For this reason, and in the absence of convincing evidence to the contrary, the stimulant action of amphetamine must for the present be ascribed to a more direct sympathomimetic action.

As has been discussed in detail (see Waelsch and Weil-Malherbe, this vol. I. pp. 54 ff.) the biosynthesis of *nor*epinephrine and serotonin in the brain proceeds by way of decarboxylation of their precursors, (Dopamine and 5-hydroxytryptamine respectively). Upon synthesis, the amines are stored at subcellular particulate storage sites. In this bound form, they are incapable of exerting their physiological effect, nor are they susceptible to degradation by the appropriate enzymes. It is likely that there is normally a constant, but limited release of stored amines from the so-called "bound" to the "free" form; and that it is this released or free form which constitutes the physiologically active agent. Also, it is this free form which is prone to enzymatic attack.

It has been suggested that monoamine oxidase may play an important role in both metabolism of serotonin and noradrenaline in the brain (see 298). The enzyme is found in various areas of the brain. In the normal state its activity must be presumed to affect the balance between the amounts of amine synthesised, stored, and released from its anchoring sites. When a monoamine oxidase inhibitor is administered, this net balance between synthesis, storage and disposition is disturbed; and the levels of free and depot amine are increased in consequence. There is thus little interference with the biosynthesis of the amine in the presence of the inhibitor. That this is likely to be the case is also suggested by the fact that the administration of both 5-hydroxytryptophane and Iproniazid increases the amounts of serotonin in the brain. Similarly, the administration of DOPA increases the level of brain epinephrine and *nor*epinephrine as well as the level of Dopamine.

The monoamine oxidase inhibiting effect of Iproniazid has encouraged the search for a number of analogues. Isocarboxazid, Nialamide, Phenelzine, and B-Phenylisopropylhydrazine are such agents. A large number of others are coming forward. B-Phenylisopropylhydrazine (also known as JB 516, "Catron") may serve as an example. It has a structure not unlike amphetamine; also it is at least 20 times as potent as Iproniazid, *in vitro* and *in vivo.* Compared with iproniazid it shows a greater selectivity *in vivo* for brain monoamine oxidase than for the liver enzyme (305). The difference in the organ selectivity of the two compounds is not due to the special affinities for the brain or liver enzyme, since *in vitro* the monoamine oxidase of both organs shows the same susceptibility to inhibition. Rather does it appear that, JB 516 penetrates the blood-brain barrier more readily. An analysis of the various features of molecular structures, which make for this permeability has been attempted. They appear to be related to the presence of the benzene ring; the alkyl congener of JB 516, isopropylhydrazine showing less predilection for the brain monoamine oxidase. The optimum structure for the aryl-alkyl hydrazines for inhibiting brain monoamine oxidase *in vivo* consists of a non-substituted benzene ring, an isopropyl or ethyl chain and a terminal or unsubstituted hydrazine group (305).

There is suggestive evidence that the central excitation produced by Iproniazid and JB 516 may be related to a rise in brain *nor*adrenaline but not of brain serotonin (298). For example, single doses of 100 mg/kg of Iproniazid in rabbits caused a doubling in the level of brain serotonin and a relatively smaller rise in *nor*adrenaline. However no pharmacological signs were observed. In contrast, daily doses of 25 mg/kg of Iproniazid elevate serotonin levels to the same extent as a single large dose, but elicit appreciably higher *nor*adrenaline levels which reach a maximum by the fourth day. At this time the animal shows signs of hyperactivity. On stopping the drug, the excitation disappears when *nor*adrenaline levels have declined, even though serotonin levels are still elevated. Another item adduced in support of the view that *nor*adrenaline may be an important factor in central excitation is found in the failure of monoamine oxidase inhibitors to produce psychomotor activity in cats even after daily administration of the monoamine oxidase inhibitor up to two weeks (298). In this species, the inhibitors induce a pronounced rise in brain serotonin but have little effect on *nor*adrenaline. JB 516 raises brain serotonin more rapidly than does Iproniazid. A 3 mg/kg dose used in rabbits, raises brain serotonin by 50% in 10–15 minutes, in contrast to several hours required by Iproniazid. Though animals given Iproniazid show only a slow rise in brain serotonin, there is a relatively rapid decline in brain monoamine oxidase activity as measured by the capacity of brain homogenates to metabolize serotonin. This suggests that factors involving the penetration of drugs to the enzyme (in addition to blood-brain barrier) account for the rapidity of action of JB 516, and that the rise of brain serotonin may be the best index of monoamine oxidase inhibition *in vivo*.

Though the position with regard to serotonin is reasonably clear, some doubt exists as to the role of monoamine oxidase in relation to the inactivation of noradrenaline. The importance of the O-methylation pathway (306) is clearly established. The metabolism of the amine by tissue homogenate containing monoamine oxidase is relatively slow. It has, however, been argued that this *in vitro* evidence need not necessarily apply to *in vivo* inactivation. Monoamine oxidase in the body is likely to be concentrated at subcellular sites where the amine is normally released. The disruption of cells (as in any *in vitro* procedure) may "destroy the close spatial relationship between enzyme and substrate" (298). It is also possible that monoamine oxidase inhibition may lead to a rise in the level of Dopamine, the precursor of *nor*adrenaline and thus lead to a rise of *nor*adrenaline indirectly. Furthermore, it is possible that whereas the O-methyltransferase enzyme may be important in the metabolism of circulating catechol amine, it may be only partially involved in the degradation of *nor*adrenaline at adrenergic sites, including the brain. Thus, it can be shown that in rabbit pre-treated six hours earlier with Iproniazid there is a paradoxical reversal of the response to the reserpine; the drug in this instance leading to excitement, increased psychomotor activity, enhanced respiration and elevated level of sympathetic activity. In such animals the reserpine causes a release of brain *nor*adrenaline and serotonin. Despite the presence of brain *nor*adrenaline in the free form, it does not decline for an hour. Again, it has been shown (307) that the monoamine oxidase is distributed throughout the whole length of the adrenergic nerves. Thus it is possible that, in adrenergic elements, the levels of amine may be rigorously controlled by the action of monoamine oxidase on free amines, when either the amine has been released, or the stored depots have reached a limit of saturation. This aspect has been borne out by a study (308), which has conclusively pointed to the importance of *intra*cellular shifts in distribution of the amines (in shifts between the particulate and cytoplasmic components). It is quite obvious that careful and quantitative enzyme-kinetic studies using isotopically labelled materials are indicated in this field, and that nothing further will be gained by speculation, or by experiments using relatively crude sampling or fractionation techniques, and relatively simple behavioral measures.

5. Drugs Interfering with the Storage and Release of the Catecholamines and Serotonin: Reserpine and Related Compounds

The interaction between drugs and neurohumoral substances within the brain has been especially examined in regard to the possible action of reserpine and LSD-25. It was shown in 1955 (309) that reserpine potentiates the hypnotic effects of hexo-barbital and ethanol in mice, and in this respect resembles the effects of large doses of serotonin. Both effects were found to be antagonized by LSD-25 (310), which, by itself, did not antagonize barbiturate hypnosis. Pursuing this observation, it was also shown that reserpine led to the release of a large amount of serotonin from depots such as the brain and the small intestine (by far the largest storehouse of serotonin), and an increase in the excretion of 5-hydroxy-indole acetic acid (5-HIAA), a metabolite of serotonin. Moreover the time-course of the sedative effects paralleled, in a general ways the reduction of concentration of serotonin; in fact, the sedative effects persisted after reserpine had disappeared from the brain. That the effects of reserpine were exerted on the "binding", rather than the synthesis of serotonin was made likely by the observation that the urinary excretion of 5-hydroxy-indole acetic acid returned to normal levels if reserpine continued to be administered. Also, a "liberation" of serotonin from platelets (without change in bleeding time) was reported following reserpine. The effects of iproniazid were in keeping with the general view that free serotonin was susceptible to amine oxidase. If this reaction is inhibited by pre-treatment with iproniazid, prior to reserpine administration, the serotonin concentration in brain does not change appreciable after administration of reserpine. In this circumstance, however, (as was mentioned earlier), reserpine no longer exerts its tranquilizing powers. The effect, in fact, is the reverse; there being motor excitement, dilation of pupil, and tachypnoea (311). Moreover iproniazid does not only block the tranquilizing effects of reserpine, but also prevents its potentiating effects on barbiturate narcosis. It has, in fact, been suggested that whereas serotonin itself may act as a stimulant, the aldehyde formed by the oxidation via amino oxidase may act as a depressant. The combination of reserpine and iproniazid according to this view would increase rather than diminish the level of free serotonin; whereas, presumably, reserpine alone would increase the formation of the aldehyde (312). This theory bears some resemblance to that put forward some time ago concerning the possible pharmacological role of oxidation of amines to aldehydes, and referred to above (304). It is important to stress that the impairment of serotonin storage just described appears to be confined to reserpine, rescinnamine and some allied compounds.

The complexity of the matter, however, is illustrated by a number of further observations. First, reserpine not only depletes serotonin, but also lowers the level of noradrenaline in the brain (313), a property it shares with a number of drugs, in which a similar effect had been observed earlier (314). Secondly, Dopamine, a precursor of adrenaline, also disappears from the brain following treatment with reserpine (308). Thirdly when considered quantitatively, there is, in contrast to other catecholamine depleting drugs, no parallelism in the case of reserpine between the central sympathetic activity as judged by adrenal medullary catecholamine depletion, and the loss of catecholamines from the brain (315). Lastly, the striking reduction of brain catecholamines by reserpine does not, in keeping with the above findings, result in a reduction of the electrical activity of the sympathetic outflow of the preganglionic fibers, despite a marked reduction of excitability of postganglionic fibers in the sympathetic chain. This would rather tend to suggest that a low residue of catecholamines, or of serotonin is not necessarily related to a loss of central sympathetic activity. Furthermore, animals sedated by reserpine can be aroused by a number of drugs, such as morphine, amphetamine and LSD-25 (315).

The above discrepancies serve to emphasize the multiple nature of the effects of reserpine at central and peripheral sites, and the distinction which has to be borne in mind in regard to its effect on catecholamines and serotonin storage at these sites. For any given dose. as was mentioned earlier, the drug not only causes the liberation of stored *nor*adrenaline and serotonin, but apparently renders the tissues incapable of taking up amines that continue to be produced. After the amine stores are released, the three amines that continue to be formed will not flow from their sites of synthesis "in a persistent stream". Whether or not these free amines will exert a physiological effect at a receptor site will depend on the concentration achieved at the receptor sites. If an amine is synthesized at a rate slow enough to allow metabolism by monoamine oxidase before appreciable amounts can reach the receptor sites, then, to all intents and purposes, reserpine "depletes" the hormone. On the other hand the amine may be synthesized rapidly enough to outweigh the oxidation by monoamine oxidase. It has in fact been suggested (298) that even after administration of reserpine, brain serotonin is manufactured at a more rapid rate than *nor*adrenaline. These differential rates if borne out, may be of the utmost importance in arriving at a balanced view of the action of the drug. The essential facts, however, can only be arrived at by suitable kinetic studies. Such studies are now proceeding in several laboratories (316).

The finding that reserpine releases catecholamines from peripheral, as well as intracerebral stores at least suggests that the hypotensive and sedative effects of the drug may depend on rather different mechanisms. Since the *nor*adrenaline is synthesized relatively slowly at peripheral nerve endings, the effect of reserpine at these sites may, in fact, be regarded as effective depletion and the peripheral sympatholytic effects of reserpine may well be due to this peripheral depletion of *nor*adrenaline. In an animal given large doses of reserpine sufficient to release peripheral *nor*adrenaline ganglionic stimulants fail to elicit the usual peripheral sympathetic effects (317, 318). On the other hand in small doses, reserpine exerts much less effect on brain *nor*adrenaline and serotonin. The hypotensive effects of small doses of reserpine thus may well have a strong peripheral component. The central effect on the brain, on the other hand, may be due to its effect on serotonin rather than *nor*adrenaline. Evidence to support this suggestion comes from the examination of the effects of Compound SU 5171 (a semisynthetic reserpine analogue) (319). This compound at a dose of 0.5 mg/kg depletes brain *nor*adrenaline by about 85%, but has little effect on brain serotonin. Animals thus treated show little retardation despite a lowering of brain *nor*adrenaline by about 50%. With higher (2 mg/kg) dose of the drug there is 65% depletion of brain serotonin, the animals now showing definite sedation. The effects on behavior of the animals are short lasting, and largely disappear within six hours. During this time the serotonin level in the brain rises and returns to about 65% normal. In contrast, the *nor*adrenaline level remains the same throughout the period, perhaps because of a slower biosynthesis of *nor*adrenaline compared with that of serotonin. After six hours the animals show almost complete recovery, despite an almost complete depletion of *nor*adrenaline.

The superimposition of stress in the above experiment led to an extension of these findings. It had been shown in a different study (320), that exposure of rats to stress of cold (0°) or warm (37°) environment prevented the release of serotonin by reserpine. It also prevented sedation by the drug. In a similar series (319), where the experiments were repeated, and the brain *nor*adrenaline as well as serotonin were followed, it could be shown that *nor*adrenaline (though not serotonin), was markedly lowered by the procedure. Again, thus, the brain catecholamine level bore less relation to the effect (or lack of effect) of reserpine than the level of serotonin.

It is discrepancies such as these which suggest that one may be dealing with rather *local* and *relative* shifts, at intra-cellular level. Some experiments are in keeping with this view.

In these studies (308) the intra-cellular distribution of adrenaline, *nor*adrenaline and hydroxy tyramine (Dopamine) was examined in terms of a partition between mitochondria and cytoplasm of the substances concerned. The brain stem of the rabbit was used. The normal distribution was compared with that following reserpine and the effect of the administration of Dopa was also studied. It was found that in the untreated animal, adrenaline, *nor*adrenaline and Dopamine were present in the ratio of 1 : 4 : 5 and that each was distributed approximately equally between the particulate fraction (consisting mainly of mitochondria) and the cell sap. Reserpine was used in doses, which brought about the disappearance of approximately 50% of the catecholamines within four hours. It was found that the rate of disappearance of all three amines was similar. However, the cytoplasmic fraction was depleted more rapidly then the particulate fraction; and this depletion was maintained irrespective of whether amine oxidase had been inhibited by prior injection of iproniazid. The intravenous injection of DOPA in the reserpinized animal was found to restore the concentration of adrenaline and *nor*adrenaline to normal levels within an hour. Interestingly enough, however, the level of Dopamine was increased far beyond the control level. The concentration of amines was raised in both cellular fractions, suggesting that reserpine did not prevent the uptake of amines by the particulate component. The effect of DOPA on brain catecholamines in the untreated animal was similar. It, too, caused a striking rise in Dopamine; though adrenaline and *nor*adrenaline were not raised above their normal level. This suggested that the brain stem tissue was capable of rapid synthesis of adrenaline, provided DOPA was supplied; and that normal concentrations were close to saturation level. The above study did not examine the effect of similar procedures on the intra-cellular distribution of serotonin, which, presumably because of its greater susceptibility to monoamine oxidase, might have shown a rather different pattern. However, there is some evidence that, following reserpine, serotonin (in contrast to other catecholamines) disappears more rapidly from the particulate than the soluble fraction. This would not be out of keeping with the original suggestion that the action of reserpine depends on free serotonin. There, as elsewhere, more accurate estimates of the *rates* of synthesis, storage, release and disposition must be awaited. Until they are available on the basis of isotopically labelled material, and systematically related to drug response curves over a wide dose range, the evidence must of necessity remain inferential.

6. Drugs Presumed to Exert a Central Adrenergic Effect

Amphetamine and Mescaline have already been mentioned elsewhere. The electrophysiological effects of amphetamine are briefly reviewed below.

It is uncertain whether methylphenidate or pipradrol should be classed in this group. There are, however, two synthetic amphetamine derivatives, Methylenedioxyamphetamine (MDA) and Trimethoxyamphetamine (TMA) with marked psychoactive powers. MDA, taken in divided doses (up to 0.4 mg/kg) leads to mental changes, not unlike those seen with moderate doses of mescaline. Elevation of blood pressure, dilation of pupils, sweating, and other sympathomimetic effects are regularly noted. TMA produces rather similar effect, though there is apparently less change in blood pressure. The doses are about four to five times less than those of Mescaline.

7. The Ambiguous Position of LSD-25

The suggestive chemical relationship between serotonin and LSD-25 led to studies of possible antagonism between the two compounds, based on the hypothesis of possible competition between them for the same receptors (322). Serotonin exerts contractile effects on a number of smooth muscle preparations, such as the rat uterus, the bronchial tree of the cat and guinea pig, the vessels of the perfused rabbit ear, and the hind limb of the cat and dog. These effects can be tested for serotonin specificity by comparison with other spasmogenic agents such as carbaminoyl choline, acetylcholine, oxytocin and adrenaline. It could be shown that a number of ergot alkaloids and their synthetic derivatives did, indeed, antagonize the effects of serotonin as tested in the rat uterus, and the rabbit ear. Of these LSD-25 was found to be the most powerful and most highly specific agent, a concentration as low as 0.3 of µg per liter inhibiting a concentration of 16 µg/l of serotonin (323). The antagonism was less marked when the guinea pig ileum was used. Dibenamine, an antagonist of adrenaline, exerted a powerful and specific. antiserotonin effect in the rat uterus, but such actions were less marked and less specific when tested on the rabbit ear and guinea pig ileum preparation. A number of other substances, like some antihistamines, hexamethonium and yohimbine either had no antagonistic effect, or were nonspecific. Mescaline had no effect when so tested. The authors tersely observed "our most active antagonist produces temporary madness in very small doses. It may be possible to find an antagonist without this effect on the brain. On the other hand it is possible that 5-HT in our brain plays an essential part in keeping us sane" (324).

In an independent, study proceeding in another laboratory (325, 326), the effects of LSD-25, harmine, yohimbine and a number of other compounds was examined; against the contractile effects of serotonin on the sheep carotid artery ring. Again LSD-25 was found to be a powerful inhibitor of these effects. In a speculative leap it was proposed that these pharmacological findings "indicate that serotonin has an important role to play in mental process and that the suppression of its action may result in mental disorder. In other words, it is the lack of serotonin, which is the cause of the disorder. If now a deficiency of serotonin in the central nervous system were to result from metabolic rather than pharmacologically induced disturbance, the same mental operation would be expected to become manifest. Perhaps such a deficiency is responsible for the natural occurrence for the disease" (327). It was further suggested by these authors that the action of : serotonin might be linked to its contractile effects upon oligodendroglia in tissue culture, the effect of serotonin being envisioned as promoting a stirring of the extracellular fluids by oligendroglia and thus affecting the nutrition of the brain.

The intellectual history of suggestions such as these reminds one of the early history of the universal role of acetylcholine in central humoral mediation, a suggestion which had to be modified with time. Similarly, there is now a steady accumulation of facts, which make a direct linear relationship between serotonin blockade and psychosomimetic action unlikely. A number of controversial facts have to be accounted for; only a few of these will be quoted.

1. Whereas, as stated above, doses of the order of 1 μg/liter of LSD-25 inhibited the action of serotonin on the rat uterus, lower concentration (of the order of 0.05 to 2 μg/l sensitized the preparation) (328). Some Tranquillizers, Chlorpromazine, Reserpine, Azacyclonol, inhibit the serotonin effect.

2. Low concentration of LSD-25 may mimic, rather than antagonize the effect of serotonin in the isolated heart preparation of the clam (Venus Mercenaria) (329).

3. High doses of LSD-25 (of the order of 1 mg/kg) may lead to excitement (330) and symptoms not unlike those seen following iproniazid or 5-hydroxytryptophane (both of which are known to raise the serotonin level).

4. The hyperpyretic effects of LSD-25 can also be seen with 5-hydroxytryptophane, where, again, the brain serotonin level is presumably raised (331).

5. The depressant effect of serotonin on the transcallosal monosynaptic pathway (332) is mimicked, rather than antagonized, by LSD-25. This effect, though seen markedly with serotonin, lacks specificity for serotonin. It is also seen with epinephrine, gamma amino butyric acid and bufotenin.

6. More pertinent than any above findings however is the fact that the analogue of LSD-25, 2-Brom-n lysergic acid diethylamide (BOL 148) although a powerful antagonist of serotonin (333) exerts little effect on mental function in man (334). BOL 148 has been administered in very high doses to patients suffering from carcinoid tumor; again no mental effect were observed (334).

7. Similarly, BOL 148 while having no effect on hexobarbital sleeping time in mice and rats nevertheless antagonized the potentiation of hexobarbital sleeping time effected by either serotonin or reserpine (335). Since, in this respect, the non-psychosomimetic agent BOL 148 acts not unlike its psychosomimetic congener, LSD-25, it would seen unlikely that the anti-serotonin properties of LSD-25 were solely related to its psychosomimetic properties.

8. As an extension of the above studies, the psychosomimetic potencies of 13 congeners of LSD-25 (which included Stereoisomer Variants with substitution in the amine group, substitution in the ring system, and substitution in rings as well as variation in the amid-group) were compared. In these studies (339) it was found that, with exception of the acetylation of the indole nitrogen, all changes made in the LSD-molecule reduced, rather than increased, the psychomimetic potency of the drug, bromination at the 2-carbon causing the greatest inactivation. Tested in isolated muscle preparations, the high potency as a serotonin antagonist was not correlated with high potency as a psychosomimetic compound. The authors concluded that the data "did not support but did not disapprove the 'serotonin deficiency' hypothesis of the LSD-psychosis".

9. Despite the lack of relation between LSD-25 and BOL 148 in regard to their psychosomimetic effects some cross tolerance between BOL 148 and LSD-25 could be established. It had been noted that though no decrease of subjective effects of LSD-25 could be seen, when BOL 148 (in doses of 0.5 to 1 mg) was administered intravenously at the height of LSD-intoxication; the administration of 2–3 mg during 24 hours prior to their administration of LSD-25 resulted in a partial attenuation of mental reaction caused by LSD-25 (337). A more extensive study of cross tolerance has also established the phenomenon between LSD-25 and Psilocybin (338).

10. It has been pointed out (339) that LSD-25 and its two congeners leading to mental effects, namely Lysergic acid, Monoethylamine and Acetyl LSD, also caused central autonomic

effects. A thorough study in the rabbit has shown that LSD-25 elicits these responses in doses as small as those which cause mental changes in man. The autonomic effects include a rise in body temperature (with a threshold of 0.5 µg/kg), hyperglycemia, mydriasis, piloerection, tachycardia, leukocytosis and changes in EEG which are characterized by the disappearance of spindle burst and absence of slow activity. All these effects suggested to the authors, stimulation of mesencephalic and diencephalic structures and all have pronounced sympathotonic character. The effects are suppressed by ganglion blocking agents, (such as hexamethonium compounds) and by the hydrogenated alkaloids of the ergotoxin group, particularly by Hydergine. BOL 148, did not cause this central stimulation of the sympathetic system. This syndrome of sympathetic excitation may be considered a "counterpart of the syndrome of central sympathetic depression produced by reserpine which is characterized by predominance of vagal function and such symptoms as fall of body temperature, bradycardia, miosis and sedation". It is of interest that a more recent systematic survey of pharmacological properties again emphasises a redistribution of the central and peripheral sympathetic and parasympathetic effects among a number of LSD-congeners (340).

11. To add to an already confused issue, LSD-25 has been shown to be a powerful inhibitor of the non-specific cholinesterases of human brain and serum (see above, ref. 87). BOL 148, equally, is such an inhibitor. On the other hand a number of non-psychosomimetic drugs (including chlorpromazine) share this cholinesterase inhibitory property with LSD-25. Significantly neither LSD-25 nor BOL 148 fit into any of the three classes of the inhibitors defined for the anticholinesterases.

The findings so far would thus suggest that although LSD-25 possesses powerful antiserotonin properties, its psychotomimetic effects cannot be unequivocally linked to this attribute alone; that, furthermore, the possibility of a sympathomimetic or central adrenergic mechanism (as manifested by autonomic response) must also be borne in mind; and that, in addition, an imbalance in the turnover of a choline ester cannot be altogether excluded.

Perhaps it would be well to pause at this point, and consider, very briefly, the implications of the polyvalent effects, so common among psychotropic drugs (see Section II), and exemplified in this instance by LSD-25. The antiadrenaline actions of some of the antihistamines, or the antiacetylcholine properties of some of the tranquillizers could be equally cited. The suggestive facts in this area indeed are bound merely to confuse an already tangled issue; and by their own accumulation point to the urgency of enquiries of rather a different kind. It is regrettable that though many excellent studies have centered on interaction of drugs with single substances, and single neurohumoral systems, very few studies have so far considered the effects of graded doses of the same drug on the *relative* concentration of suspected key substances (or the activity of their associated enzyme systems) in discrete areas of the brain; or attempted to quantify the possible interaction between substances in relation to chemically induced behavioral states or chemically induced electrophysiological change. Yet it may well be the *relative* ratio of one substance to another, the ratio, say of a choline ester, a catechol amine or an indole amine in a particular place at a particular time, which may profoundly affect the net effect of a drug within a complex cell assembly. *Change* in concentration would thus seem to be of more moment than absolute amount; and the rate of reaction may be at least as cogent as the kind of reaction one is considering. It may in fact, be the *relative inter*action (i. e. the overlap of reactions proceeding at different rates) which may affect the anchoring or release of a particular substance from its subcellular binding site; and thus modulate a particular gating mechanism within e particular neural net.

That such relative shifts in concentration may, in fact, decisively influence the physiological action of neuro-effector agents at a particular site is illustrated by an early set of experiments (341, 342). It was shown that small amounts of adrenaline applied in experiments, which made possible the separate perfusion of the spinal cord, could profoundly affect the response to a given dose of acetylcholine applied to the perfusate. Small doses of adrenaline steadied the response to acetylcholine; large doses increased the (patellar) reflex; and very large doses led to a prolonged diminution of responsiveness. In related experiments the interaction between acetylcholine and adrenaline was further examined, using the superior cervical ganglion preparation (343). In both studies, the balance of evidence suggested that whereas adrenaline had relatively little effect when used by itself, it was indeed capable of profoundly modifying the response to a given dose of acetylcholine. Small doses usually led to facilitation, larger doses to inhibition. The pattern of responses elicited varied; yet interaction between these two groups of agents, and the very wide repertoire of responses produces by this interaction was equally worthy of note. It would appear that adrenaline can profoundly modulate a given response to acetylcholine (344), and that the net result of this interaction may depend upon the relative proportions of a particular substance at a particular site at a particular time. A comparable study of such interactions in the brain stem is timely, and urgent.

8. The Possible Interaction between Drugs and Hormones

In a previous section reference was made to the possible effect of drugs on the storage and release mechanisms of neurohumoral substances at subcellular sites. Little is known at present of the physiological (rather than pharmacological) factors which govern such mechanisms One would naturally suspect ionic shifts, though the evidence in this respect so far is very circumstantial. Equally, the role of hormones in these transactions is at present hardly more than suggestive.

There is a sizeable body of evidence, recently reviewed (345), to suggest a close physiological interaction between the cortical steroids and the catecholamines. The two groups of hormones would appear to operate physiologically as one functional unit. The steroids maintain the integrity and responsiveness of tissues to the adrenalines. Many actions of the physiologically present catecholamines cannot be elicited in the absence of the steroids. Equally, and perhaps of more moment, is the evidence to suggest that many actions of the steroids may, in fact, more properly be ascribed to the adrenalines. Of more immediate concern to the subject under discussion, are the early indications of the effects of hormones on levels of neuro-effector substances in the brain itself. Adrenalectomy, for example leads to a rise in brain serotonin (346). Exposure of rats to the stress of both a cold (0°C) and a warm (37°C) environment prevents the release of serotonin by reserpine (320); it also prevents sedation by this substance.

In other studies (347) it could be shown that a marked depletion of *nor*adrenaline (though not serotonin) could be obtained in rats after exposure to cold stress. A differential response of this kind is of great interest, and may point to an, as yet, unexplored dependence of drug effects on hormonal equilibria within the brain itself. It will indeed be advisable to examine in a consistent and systematic fashion the effects of graded doses of hormones, on both responsiveness, and on the effects of drugs on the binding of amines at their subcellular anchoring sites. This problem can be approached both at a strictly local as well as systemic level. Thus, for example, it can be shown that very small stereotactically placed implants of a hormone (stilboestrol dibutyrate) in the posterior hypothalamus will release a stereotype form of behavior, (namely sexual behavior) in the cat (348). The effect shows some specificity both for hormone and the placement of the hormone. Our present state of knowledge does not permit speculation as to the precise neuronal mechanisms governing this release of a well organized and coded behavioral pattern by a locally acting hormone. Earlier studies, however, would make one suspect a participation of the neuro-effector substances in the ultimate mediation of pituitary responses (349); and it is conceivable that, in the above experiments also, a *local* interaction between the hormone and elements in the immediate vicinity of the implant may lead to significant changes in the net balance (i. e., the relative rates of synthesis, storage, release and disposition) of neuro-effector substances at a strictly regional level. Noted also should be the effects of chlorpromazine on other endocrine functions. Both glycosuria, and breast changes have been reported following its administration.

Only little can be gained at present from the clinical data available in this pharmaco-endocrine field. The indications are suggestive. There is, for example a significant and linear relationship between an increase in anxiety and anger and plasma hydrocortisone levels (350). Moreover, and perhaps less expected, it has also been shown that severe depression is accompanied by elevated plasma-hydrocortisone level, and that deeply retarded patients show hormone levels higher than the less depressed group (351). Depression would thus appear to be an active stress response; and the retarded, tearless state a final phase in an active, adaptive process. This phase, of course, is largely inhibitory as against the excitatory components commonly seen in the so-called agitated depressive syndromes. Systematic studies of the effects of antidepressants on plasma hydroxycorticoid levels are called for.

It would be improper to speculate at present as to the possible effect of the various degrees of pituitary adreno-cortical mobilization on the binding and release of neuro-effector substances in nodal or trigger areas of the brain. It may even be that the reverse is true, and that differential proportions of catechol amines within the brain may affect the degree of adreno-cortical mobilization. There is some suggestive evidence for the influence of purely situational factors on the relative proportions of noradrenaline and adrenaline in plasma (352). Tested in monkeys, it was found that situations, which allow possible flight or escape from a stressful situation lead to a mobilization of *nor*adrenaline. Situations, on the other hand, structured as to bar the "way out", and favoring acceptance and inhibition as the response carrying the highest adaptive value lead to a rise of adrenaline. Mobility or "underactivity"; "freedom of choice" of "escape" or "acceptance" appear to have some correlates in the levels of plasma *nor*adrenaline or adrenaline. It is suggested that these humoral correlates be sought in the brain, as well as in the plasma. To date the data are scanty; and many more will be needed before testable hypotheses to account for these various states can be put forward.

d) On the Need for a Study of Regional Chemical Process within the Brain

The findings cited above and many others, omitted in the present context, serve to emphasize the role of a strictly regional or local economy within the brain in its function as a detector, and organizer of spatio-temporal change in the course of adaptive behavior. The topographical and cytological sub-organization of even quite small areas of, the brain has been mentioned. It is reflected in sharp regional differences in the chemical constitution at cellular, and, quite possibly, sub-cellular levels. Nor would one be justified in assuming that local, and, in some areas, rather specific chemical properties are not reflected in differences in local permeability of the blood brain barrier; or in strictly local changes in small vessel tone. There are, in fact, indications that the converse may be true; and that in some areas, for example, the hypothalamus may be differentially permeable to some metabolites and that change in local function may be related to change in local blood flow. The principle of shielding, and of metabolic autonomy, so strikingly reflected in the rigorous selectiveness of the blood/brain barrier, may well have deeper meaning, and have to be carried into the chemical architecture of the brain itself. For all one knows, there may be pericellular barriers in some areas, and local vascular shunts may well meet varying local needs. It may no longer be sufficient to look for differences in enzyme constitution between gross cell masses to account for a differential susceptibility of the nervous system to neuroleptic agents. Such differences must be sought at a more discrete level. Like no other organ in the body the brain has evolved as an aggregate of sub-organs resulting in, if one may so put it, an assembly of chemically mediated homeostats. The chemical traces of this evolution are becoming evident with time. A principle of metabolic compartmentalization (353) is emerging, of which the highly localized synthesis, storage, release and disposition of neuro-effector substances at sub-cellular sites is merely an instance. The convergence and overlap of a few interlocking chemical reactions may profoundly affect the excitability thresholds at particular sites at a particular time. The nodal midline areas concerned with some of the basic steering mechanisms of behavior appear to be peculiarly susceptible to such chemical shifts. Only overall data are so far available on the nature of these shifts; they do however, bear some resemblance to mechanism employed in neurohormonal mediation elsewhere.

It has been felt by the writer for some time (354) that these and cognate interactions may depend upon the presence and the uneven distribution in the central nervous system of small *families* of compounds derived from neuro-effector substances long familiar for their peripheral effects, yet possessed of special properties in the central nervous system, not shared in peripheral autonomic nets. Acetylcholine, adrenaline and serotonin may be prototype molecules of this kind; but one need only compare the effects of acetylcholine with succinyl choline, *nor*adrenaline with its methylated congener to see how profound the effect of even slight changes in molecular configuration may be. The astonishing chemical evolution undergone by the steroids is an example of the same economy. It is therefore not surprising that behind the "true" and "specific" acetylcholinesterase in the brain there now stand the so-called non-specific cholinesterase. Behind adrenaline there is dopamine, which has a high distribution in areas not necessarily rich in *nor*adrenaline. Behind serotonin there is melanotonin (5-methoxy-N-acetyltryptamine), a substance found in especially high concentrations in the pineal gland (355). It is evident that hypotheses solely linked to one or other of the old-established agents have not stood the test of time. It is upon *distribution gradients* of closely related substances, and appropriate coenzyme systems that some of the modulating and gating mechanisms in the enzyme and central nervous system may well depend.

It is therefore encouraging that methods for the analysis of regional transaction within the brain are now becoming available. The quantitative histochemistry of some enzyme systems in relation to cell populations is becoming a feasible undertaking (356), and is bound, sooner or later, to be related to the action of drugs at subcellular sites. Equally, the effect of drugs (357) and hormones (358) applied to discrete areas of the brain is now being studied in relation to behavior; and through the interpretation of such local effects is an admittedly difficult, and indeed forbidding, task it is bound to become more feasible and discrete with growing experience of the field. Furthermore, the electrophysiological correlates of these procedures are bound to be explored, and to be increasingly related to the electrophysiological correlates of conditioning viewed in terms of the coding and transformation of signals within the brain (359) It is this interaction between the regional neurochemistry, (both in its broad topographical as well as subcellular implications), electrophysiology, mathematics, and behavior, which holds out the highest promise for or a coherent science of behavioral pharmacology of the future.

D. Electrophysiological Evidence

a) The Effect of Some Drugs on the Activity of Single Units within the Central Nervous System

The recently developed techniques for peri and intra-cellular recording from single units (including the use of single and multi barrelled micropipettes) (360, 361) has made possible the analysis of phenomena at a level of organization of the central nervous system hitherto beyond the reach of direct enquiry. These methods of recording have two great advantages. In the first place, they make it possible to influence the synaptic sites directly by the electrophoretic application of chemical substances to the immediate milieu of the neurone. This effectively bypasses some problems of access which include (as has been mentioned above) the blood brain barrier (and possible pericellular barriers). Secondly the introduction of an intracellular electrode makes it possible to study the condition of the neural membrane itself, and thus to relate the excitatory post-synaptic potential to the events across the membrane.

It has been shown that the transmission across synapses occurs not by the spread of electrical currents, but through the liberation of specific chemical substances liberated from the pre-synaptic membrane (362). These substances alter the ionic permeability of the subsynaptic membrane, and consequently initiate specific ionic fluxes across the membrane. These fluxes in turn initiate the post-synaptic currents that cause the transient depolarization and hyperpolarization of the post-synaptic membrane which are produced respectively by synaptic excitatory or inhibitory action. Acetylcholine is regarded as a transmitter substance of a few types of central synapses though by no means as the universal transmitter. There is evidence that the excitatory transmitter substances act by making the sub-synaptic membrane more permeable to small ions (363) just as is the case at the neuromuscular junction (364). Extensive experimental investigation has led to the conclusion that "post-activation potentiation is attributable to two events localized in the immediate region of the pre-synaptic membrane: A mobilization there of relatively small amount of synaptic transmitter substance, there being thus increased amounts available for immediate release; and an increased size of pre-synaptic impulse" (365). Impulses, however, "can also be generated in a nerve cell by another method that is of particular value in relation to the problem of locating the site at which impulses arise in nerve cells. When the axon of nerve cells is stimulated, an impulse travels antidromically up to the nerve cells and usually invades it, generating an antidromic spike potential. When thus recorded by microelectrode in the soma, the antidromic spike potential has two main components. Evidence from intensive studies (362, 366, 367) suggests that the initial small spike is generated by the impulse in the initial segment of the neurone, (the axon hillock plus non-medullated axon) while the later (large) spikes are produced when the impulse enters the somato-dendritic membrane. The two spikes have been referred to as I.S. (initial spike) and (S.D.) (soma dendritic spike) respectively. With normal motor neurones the level of depolarization is higher for the somatic dendritic membrane than for the initial spike membrane. Yet the S.D. threshold is never less than twice the I.S. threshold. Several others types of neurones of the central nervous system significantly also show differences between the I. S. and the S.D. membranes. For example, in neurones in Clarke's column, the I.S.–S.D. separation is much more prominent than in the neurone of a cutaneous ascending pathway.

Apposed to the concept of central excitation there is the concept of inhibition This term signifies the depression of neuronal excitability which occurs independently of any conditioning excitatory synaptic activity on that neurone, and also independently of any depression of the excitatory synaptic bombardment that is employed in testing for the suspected inhibition. It can be shown "that the inhibitory action of motor neurones may be explained satisfactorily by the transient increases which are produced in their membrane potentials and which have been designated as inhibitory post-synaptic potentials (IPSP). A comparative synaptic inhibitory action has also been observed in crustacean stretch receptors and has also been recorded in neurones of Clarke's column (365).

By investigating the effects of varying the membrane potential by current applied through the microelectrode, it can be shown that the IPSP is produced by a process of ionic diffusion across the sub-synaptic membrane that has an equilibrium potential of about 10 mv more hyperpolarized than the resting membrane potential (i. e. about –80 mv). It can also be shown by an ionophoretic injection through the microelectrode, that this ionic diffusion is satisfactorily explained by the hypothesis that inhibitory synaptic transmitter *increases* the permeability of the sub-synaptic membrane to ions below a critical size (i. e. potassium chloride), though not to the somewhat larger ions, like sodium. This type of ionic mechanism appears to occur with all types of central inhibition so far investigated with regard to an effect on inhibition. Strychnine has been found to have a rapid depressing action on inhibitory synaptic action (368). More recently, a series of amino acids has been examined in this respect (using the multibarrel micropipette techniques) with special reference to Gamma amino acid (361). The results cast doubt on a specific (synaptic) as against a more general (membrane) effect of some of these amino acids.

Several aspects should be noted in the context of the above. First, the electrophysiological evidence suggests possible structural differences in terms of submicroscopic organization between the axon hillock and the soma surface. Here there are even some crude structural correlates. The Nissl substance is much finer in the area of the axon hillock, which thus appears clearer; nor is the density of synaptic knobs in this area as high as elsewhere (365). Secondly, the precise chemical milieu in the immediate vicinity of the neurone (and thus, the glial glyco or lipoproteins) may determine the electrochemical events on these special submicroscopic patches of the unit. Though some evidence in this regard is available for the spinal cord, the evidence stemming from the reticular formation and the cerebral cortex remains fragmentary to date.

A systematic microelectrode analysis of the activity of individual reticular neurones (369) has furnished convincing evidence of the existence of convergence in these neurones. Some reticular neurones possess enormous tactile receptor fields; and can for example, be activated by the movement of a few hairs on any limb, trunk, whiskers or by auditory stimulation. It is this convergence which makes for the term "reticular mixing pool", and which makes an analysis of these closely packed inhomogeneous cell masses so inordinately difficult.

Particular interest attaches to an analysis of the temporal patterns of discharge of units within the reticular formation. Such an analysis has been attempted (370). It was shown that the temporal characteristics of discharge patterns differed. The median latencies of discharge were used to construct a spatio-temporal diagram of response of the reticular network to such peripheral stimulation. It was found, furthermore, that responses to stimulation at mere threshold intensity varied more in their timing than did responses to stimulation at many times threshold intensity. Moreover, interaction between volleys from spatially separated afferent sources was found to be either inhibitory or occlusive. It was argued that reticular neurones with a wide receptor field, which respond similarly to different afferent sources, may be related to the generalized function of the reticular formation. However, those, which respond with different *temporal* patterns of discharge to stimulation of different afferent sources, may be related to local behavioral responses or to local signs of perception. A given discharge of a particular neuron may even contribute to both localized and generalized function, depending on the connections of the neuron with other neurones.

This study is mentioned in some detail because it brings into focus an area which, in the view of the writer, is of high potential yield in an analysis of drug effects on elements in the reticular formation, and indeed elsewhere. The spacial-temporal topology must be judged as the nearest approximation to the coding of "meaning" within the nervous system; and the influence of chemicals on those patterns of discharge may be very relevant. Only beginnings in this complex field are evident so far. Thus, for example, the patterns of discharge of respiratory neurones have been recently examined in detail; and a provocative hypothesis on the nature of the rhythmic discharge from these units has been put forward (371). Significantly, though, the exquisite susceptibility of the units to CO_2 remains a mystery.

An attempt has also been made to examine the effect of a few drugs on units within the reticular formation using a floating type microelectrode, (which, in that preparation, has the great advantage of "riding" with the cell). The effect of chlorpromazine was also studied, blood pressure being recorded simultaneously to control for vasomotor effect (372, 373). The units selected for observation were classified as reticular in character from the fact that they showed convergent responses, and from the effects observed by stimulation with microelectrodes after recordings had been completed. Observation was also made on a number of units belonging to the specific sensory projection systems, such as, for example, units situated in the mesencephalic nucleus of the fifth nerve, or the superior colliculus. The drugs were administered intravenously and by the intra-carotid route.

The studies concerned primarily the effects of adrenaline, acetylcholine and chlorpromazine, and it is for this reason that they are mentioned here. With adrenaline, variable effects were observed. The activity of units were either unaffected or showed an increase or decrease in the rate of discharge. Following intravenous injection, effects were usually seen only during a rise in blood pressure but following intracarotid injections of (1–5 µg), the effects were similar, though no change in blood pressure could be observed. The effects of acetylcholine (which was applied in doses of 0.2–1 µg by the intracarotid route) were somewhat different. These responses were of two kinds: first, a primary increase or decrease in discharge starting within a few seconds of injection and lasting only a few seconds; and secondly, a response of much longer latency. This latter response appeared more constant, and was observed in every unit tested, whereas the primary effect was not always seen. The secondary effect was invariably accompanied by a slight fall in blood pressure, though no change in blood pressure was observed during the primary effect. These effects were still present after bilateral denervation of the carotid sinus, and also following the injection of a paralyzing dose of tubocurarine. The units, therefore, were capable of either being facilitated or inhibited following the intracarotid administration of these drugs. It was of interest, also, that units belonging to the specific sensory systems of the brain stem were not affected by the injection of adrenaline. This difference in susceptibility is in keeping with more recent findings with other specific sensory systems; and it may well be that the interaction-in time between specific and non-specific projection systems may depend to a significant degree upon the convergence and temporal apposition of patterns of discharge along there two pathways in relation to *local* chemical states.

Chlorpromazine, when applied in doses of 24 mg, led to a marked decrease in the frequency of the spontaneous activity of the units. Moreover, the units became much less responsive to peripheral stimuli. Thus, a unit "which previously responded to light stabbing or stroking of one of the legs with a burst of 9 to 10 spikes, consistently produced only two or three spikes in response to a similar stimulus after chlorpromazine had been injected". This effect was observed with doses of 2 to 4 mg intravenously, an admittedly high dose. Further increase in this dose did not increase the effect; and even with the largest dose, some response to the tapping of the legs was always obtained. If pentobarbital or sodium pentothal were administered after chlorpromazine, all spontaneous activity disappeared, and no responses from the unit could be obtained. The activity reappeared within 20 to 30 minutes after injection, and eventually recovered fully when the effects of the barbiturates had worn off. The effect was not observed with barbiturate alone. It was suggested there was a synergism between chlorpromazine and barbiturates.

A further site at which unit activity has been recently studied is the cerebral cortex. In clear and convincing experiments (374) it was shown that single cells in the cortex could be activated by the electrophoretic application of acetylcholine to such units. In the writer's laboratory, multibarrelled micropipette studies are now being pursued in various parts of the brain stem and the archepallium (374a). Precise studies such as these hold out high promise and may, in time, illuminate the chemistry of synaptic transmission at high central level. They may also be relevant to microelectrode studies in the conscious animal where the relation of patterned inhibition to the process of attention is worthy of note. Diminished firing of some cortical units upon arousal, and the inhibition of unit discharge in the motor cortex upon stimulation of the thalamic reticular formation has been shown (375). Furthermore, there are indications that the excitability of cortical elements is *increased,* rather than diminished, during sleep (376). Such findings employ direct lead microelectrodes. The recent introduction of a "non-wired" device for the study of single unit activity in the unrestrained animal (using a miniature transmitter) is of particular promise here (377).

Despite their evident success, findings such as the above leave one curiously dissatisfied, for there is one parameter not usually represented in such experiments. None take into account the over-all, and relatively slow, shifts in Direct Current (D.C.) potential which have been recorded in the cortex, using suitable electrodes. It is evident that the change in D.C. polarization could either attenuate or enhance cortical potential. The periodic fluctuations in the normal electroencephalogram have, in fact, been ascribed to oscillation of two oppositely directed electrotonic D.C. components (378). That drugs are capable of influencing these D.C. potentials has been shown in the case of veratrine, strychnine and novocain (379). Veratrine leads to a negative shift of the cortical D.C. potentials; Strychnine, on the other hand, produced little or no change. Novocain led, without changes in D.C. potential, first to an enhancement and then to an attenuation of the positive phase of the evoked potential. The state of polarization of the cortex was stressed by these authors; and the role of subcortical influences from the higher thalamo reticular system could be conceived as influencing the D.C. changes in the cortex itself. The activation of subcortical elements by catecholamines and related agents may thus at least be conceived as leading to such D.C. shifts.

More recently, in the writer's laboratory, an attempt has been successfully made to record D.C. potentials in the conscious unanesthetized animal using a specially adapted small calomel electrode, which could be directly applied to the dura (380). Using this technique, changes with auditory stimulation have been noted. Its use in pharmacological studies must await further experiments.

b) The Effects of Some Drugs on Central Synaptic Transmission

A brief review of the subject will have to suffice. For reasons already mentioned the subject is still controversial, arguments being based more often on inference, than on evidence. Until these are resolved by the application of suitable microelectrodes techniques, speculation is bound to continue.

The effect of LSD-25 has been studied in the so-called transcallosal system, in which the cortical response in one hemisphere is recorded following the stimulation of the correspond ing cortical area of the contralateral hemisphere (381, 382). It was found that following the intracarotid administration of LSD-25 in a pentobarbital anaesthetized cat, there was a reduction of the post-synaptic component of this transcallosal response. Similar results were obtained in the unanaesthetized cat. The specificity of this inhibitory effect, however, is not very great since it is also observed with adrenaline and *nor*adrenaline. A rank ordering of these inhibitory effects has been attempted. Mescalin and adrenolutin, adrenochrome and *nor*adrenaline are classified as exerting a "low" inhibitory effect on this preparation; γ-amino butyric acid adrenalin and LSD-25, a "medium" effect; serotonin and bufotonin, a "high" effect. To convey a range of the rank order, the ratio of effectiveness of bufotenin as compared to mescalin is set as 10,000 to 1. An attempt has been made to relate this rank order to clinical effectiveness. It has in fact, been argued by the same authors that excessive synaptic inhibition might be related to the occurrence of hallucinations (383).

The controversial nature of the field, however, is illustrated by a further finding in another laboratory. Studied for its effect on the evoked potentials in the auditory and visual systems, it was found that LSD-25 caused facilitation of the primary cortical responses to auditory(click) and visual (photic) stimulation in cats rendered immobile by succinyl choline (384). Also, even relatively low doses of LSD-25 (4 μg per kg) altered the recovery cycles in these two systems. This alteration consisted of a bi-phasic response: there being first a shortened initial recovery phase, followed by a prolonged phase of supernormality. Higher doses of LSD-25 (40–60 μg/kg) depressed the auditory evoked potential while still facilitating evolved potential in the visual system. The facilitation was not observed when pentobarbital anaesthesia was used. The cortical response stimulation of the lateral geniculate radiation was also facilitated by LSD-25. When the effects of LSD-25 on the response of the visual cortex to simultaneous stimulation of the geniculate radiation fibres, and the homolateral suprasylvian gyrus was recorded, LSD-25 was found to cause inhibition to the suprasylvian stimulation, while simultaneously bringing about a stimulation of the striate response to geniculate radiation stimulation. On the other hand, the facilitatory effect of the suprasylvian stimulation on the response to subsequent geniculate radiation was blocked by 15 µg/kg doses of LSD-25. These findings led the author to conclude that LSD-25 may exert a differential effect on axodendritic as compared with axosomatic synapses. Thus, while inhibiting transmission across axo-dendritic sites, LSD-25 was suggested to cause facilitation of axosomatic transmission.

Three points emerge from the above data. The first is the lack of specificity of the so-called inhibitory responses for agents as different as the catecholamines and related substances, psychoactive indoles, antiserotonins, and membrane active amino acids. Secondly, with one agent, LSD-25, both facilitatory and inhibitory effects can apparently be obtained according to dose range. Thirdly, using high doses, differential effects in different systems can apparently be also obtained. The precise reasons for these differential effects remain far from clear. Whether synaptic membrane components, excitable chemically but not electrically, can produce either depolarizing or hyperpolarizing electrogenesis cannot be ascertained, until the effects of graded doses of the same agent applied to a synapse have been studied.

A further detailed study of the effects of LSD-25 on synaptic transmission has been made in the visual system of the cat (385). Under pentobarbital anaesthesia the intracarotid administration (30 µg/kg) of LSD-25 caused a mean decrease of 80% in the amplitude of the geniculate postsynaptic response to a single shock of the optic nerve. "Whereas geniculate transmission was blocked by LSD-25, transmission within the retina and between geniculate radiation fibres and cortical cells was extremely resistant to inhibition by LSD-25." The onset of the effect on geniculate transmission was rapid, occurring within 5–10 sec of the administration of LSD-25, with recovery following within 1 hour. With intravenous administration, a much greater amount of LSD-25 was required. Furthermore, pentobarbital sodium was found to sensitize the preparation to LSD-25. Thus in the conscious animal the amount required to block geniculate transmission was 5 times greater than that required in the acute, anaesthetized preparation. This block, once established, was associated with behavioral blindness, though the responsiveness to auditory stimuli was preserved. Repetition of the same experiment in monkeys required higher doses of LSD-25 still (of the order of 0.5 to 1 mg) which, taken weight for weight, is, indeed, a very large dose.

The effects of LSD-25 on thalamic recovery time have been studied in curarized cats using relatively high doses of LSD-25 (386). LSD-25 was found not to affect either the thalamic recovery cycle, nor the amplitude of recorded electrical activity. The differences between this finding and the finding cited above may be accounted for by differences in dosage and differences in technique.

In sum, then, little definitive information is available on the action of psychoactive drugs on synaptic transmission within the Central Nervous System. However, studies now in progress on their electrophysiological effects in elements of the *limbic* system hold high promise (386a).

c) The Effect of Some Drugs on Interneurones

Recent microelectrode studies have emphasised the role of interneurones in the maintenance of central inhibition within the spinal cord. The Renshaw cells (387) have been particularly examined in this regard. This cell has been found to fire repetitively to a single antidromic volley. It has also been shown that interneurones excited by the stimulation of dorsal roots have different firing patterns (388).

That such interneurones may indeed be affected by some drugs, is suggested by studies of the effects of drugs on the facilitatory and inhibitory stimulus response curves of the patellar reflex. Earlier studies on mephenesin showed that the facilitation of this reflex could be depressed by this drug without depression of the actual reflex (389). Pentobarbital and meprobamate in doses insufficient to cause overt ataxia, also depressed facilitation in a similar manner. Thus, without an appropriate choice of dose, mephenesin-like drugs could not be differentiated from barbiturates. In more recent studies by the same group (390) (using carefully adjusted doses and parameters of stimulation) higher doses of mephenesin were found to produce a profound depression of facilitation without affecting the patellar reflex. It was concluded that mephenesin selectively depressed direct central facilitation induced by stimulation of the contralateral sciatic nerve; these findings being consistent with a hypothesis that interneurones were involved in direct central facilitation, and that these interneurones may have pharmacological properties different from those of the Renshaw cell, and the motor neurone. The chemical relationship of mephenesin to meprobamate will be noted. Once again, the findings are suggestive, though hardly more.

d) The Effect of Some Drugs on Pathways Involving the Reticular Formation, and on the Arousal Response

The neural substrate of the reticular formation and its relation to the arousal response has been considered elsewhere in this volume. In view of the altered responsiveness engendered by some of the so-called neuroleptic agents in the normal subject and in various clinical states, an examination of drug effects on pathways involving the reticular formation and on the arousal response are particularly relevant; though it is well to bear in mind the inhomogeneity of the system and the limited inferences which can be drawn from any such experiments. To speak of the effects of a drug on the Reticular Activating System without specifying which of the many thresholds operating in the reticular system are referred to is an inappropriate use of the term. The organization of pathways feeding into the reticular formation from peripheral sensory receptors; the rich Reticulo fugal and Reticulopetal pathways connecting the reticular system with more rostrally situated cell groups; the existence of convergent units within the reticular formation; and the importance of inhibition in the organization of patterns within this closely knit neural feltwork all collude to make a *fractionation* (391) of responses of drug effects within this system inordinately difficult.

It was shown in 1953 (392) that pentobarbital inhibited responses in the reticular formation evoked by peripheral stimuli, and blocked the arousal response to stimulation of the reticular formation. Subsequent studies (393) showed a differential action of anaesthetics of interneuronal blocking agents on thresholds for the recruiting and the EEG response. In this context, however, a more recent report of the EEG arousal following the application of barbiturate into the circulation of the lower brain stem should be noted. In this study (394) the ingenious technical maneuver of clamping of the basilar artery (and adequate cannulation of the lingual and subclavian arteries) allowed the selective introduction of barbiturate into the vascular bed separately supplying the rostral pons, the midbrain and upper cerebrum, or the medulla and caudal pons. Here the intravertebral introduction of small amounts of barbiturates regularly elicited an *arousal* reaction, which was interpreted as being due to a transient inactivation of a synchronizing influence originating in the lower brain stem. Thus, even a barbiturate can elicit both kinds of effects, according to route of application and dose of application. This juxtaposition of findings well illustrates the paradoxes, which await the investigator in this field.

Using a combination of procedures which allowed for simultaneous measurement of the EEG arousal function of the reticular formation and also for the measurement of thresholds for a similar response following stimulation of the peripheral nerve and stimulation of the diffuse thalamic projection system, the effect of a number of drugs were examined in another series of studies (395). The drugs were selected with a view to eliminating those which altered blood pressure or body temperature. It was found that mephenesin did not affect EEG activation from reticular stimulation, but did block arousal from the diffuse projection system. Pentobarbital, on the other hand, blocked EEG arousal from stimulation of the reticular formation and of the thalamus. It also depressed responses in the reticular formation to sciatic stimulation and to intrareticular stimulation. The inhibitory effect of reticular formation stimulation on responses in the auditory system was also blocked by pentobarbital. Reserpine had no effect on EEG or behavioral arousal elicited from stimulation of either the reticular formation or the diffuse thalamic projection system. Chlorpromazine caused only slightly elevated EEG responses to stimulation of the reticular formation and the diffuse thalamic projection system and the behavioral responses to reticular formation stimuli, but markedly raised the threshold for behavioral arousal from the diffuse thalamic projection system. Responses in the reticular formation to evoked activity from peripheral nerve and to intrareticular stimulation were enhanced by chlorpromazine, as was the inhibitory effect of stimulation of the reticular formation on responses in the auditory system. It was concluded that chlorpromazine may act on the reticular formation in opposite manner from pentobarbital. Pentobarbital would appear to depress the elements in the reticular formation to the point at which attention and consciousness are disturbed. Chlorpromazine, on the other hand, increases reticular input and conduction and "enhances the controlling or filtering effect of the reticular formation on lateral sensory pathways with little effect on the reticular mechanisms of consciousness" (395).

In a parallel study in the author's former laboratory (396, 397), the effect of a number of drugs on arousal responses was examined. A distinction must be made between behavioral and electrocortical arousal; and, equally, between arousal produced by direct stimulation of elements in the reticular formation, and indirect stimulation by way of one of the sensory pathways. The *encéphale isolé* (398) is suitable for such studies. In this preparation, a waking state can be readily distinguished from the drowsy or "sleeping" state. The first state is accompanied by low voltage, fast activity not unlike that seen in the intact alert animal; the second, by slow waves at 1–4 cycles per second, or spindle activity at (6–12 cycles) per second. The correspondence between electrical activity and behavioral states in these preparations is maintained throughout, although individual variations in patterns of sleep activity can often be encountered. Furthermore, because of the intact cranial nerve connections, such a preparation is capable of arousal by tactile or auditory stimuli. It is, of course, also aroused by direct electrical stimulation of the brain stem reticular formation; here sharp behavioral arousal is reflected in a corresponding activation of the electrocorticogram.

In such experiments, the arousal thresholds can be determined by applying a stimulus (rectangular pulses of 1 m/sec duration at frequency of 300 cycles per second) for a fixed period (10 sec), and by gradually increasing the stimulus voltage to a point where behavioral and electrocortical arousal can be independently noted. Similarly, arousal thresholds to sensory (auditory) stimulation can (though somewhat crudely) be expressed in terms of the voltage which, when applied to a loudspeaker delivering a note of constant frequency, results in arousal. Responses to single clicks can also be determined at the auditory cortex in the same experiment.

A number of drugs were tested using this procedure. Amphetamine in doses of 0.01–1 mg/kg led to a progressive lowering of both the threshold for EEG arousal, and behavioral arousal in response to direct stimulation of the reticular formation; similarly, there was also a fall, at much the same rate, in the threshold for arousal by auditory stimulation, while the threshold for single click responses recorded at the cortex remained comparatively unchanged. In doses of 1 mg/kg, there was permanent alerting of the preparation, both in terms of electrical activity and behavior. LSD-25 on the other hand, while exerting (in doses of 1–20 μg/kg) relatively little effect on arousal to direct stimulation of the reticular formation, caused, a marked fall in the threshold for arousal by auditory stimulation. This could be seen in doses of the order of 1–2 μg/kg. Atropine (in doses of 02 to 4 mg/kg) led to the usual appearance of the characteristic slow wave activity in the electrocorticogram, but left the behavioral threshold (as judged by the criteria enumerated above), relatively unchanged. Although both tactile and auditory stimuli still produced behavioral alerting after atropine, they did not modify electrical activity. There thus appeared a wide divergence between the threshold for electrocortical arousal, and of arousal in terms of behavioral response.

Physostigmine produced effects opposite to those of atropine, leading to a fall of threshold for electrical activity, with relatively little change in behavioral threshold. If injected after atropine (in doses 0.01 to 0.8 mg/kg) this drug would lead to a progressive lowering of the EEG arousal threshold, as the slow activity induced by atropine gradually gave way to the low voltage fast activity seen with physostigmine. The behavioral threshold, however, was not markedly affected by this drug.

The above parameters were found useful in a subsequent examination of the effects of chlorpromazine and some ten other tranquillizing drugs on the arousal responses in the *encéphale* preparation (397). The drugs included Promazine, Acepromazine, Hydroxyzine, Benactyzine, Imipramine, Hyoscine, Reserpine, Rescinnamine, Deserpidine, Meprobamate and Azacyclonal. According to the responses observed, the drugs were found to fall into four groups. These were:

Group I. This included drugs which caused only slight diminution of the arousal responses to direct stimulation of the brain stem reticular formation, but a rise of threshold to arousal by indirect sensory (auditory) stimulation. Comprised in this group are Chlorpromazine, Promazine, Acepromazine and Hydroxyzine. It should be noted that the interaction between these drugs and amphetamine, atropine and physostigmine was in keeping with previous findings. Whereas chlorpromazine appeared to block the effects of amphetamine, the latter drug still produced some effects when given after promazine, acepromazine and hydroxyzine; though it never led to complete alerting. Atropine and physostigmine, on the other hand, when superimposed on chlorpromazine, produced their marked effect on electrical activity of the brain, but did not modify overt behavior. Most of the drugs in this group share anti-adrenalin properties, though some also show an action against 5-hydroxytryptamine, histamine, and acetylcholine.

Group II. Drugs in this group led to an increase in arousal thresholds, but, at the same time, produced a "dissociation" between electrical activity and behavior (see below). Comprised in this group are Benactyzine, Imipramine and Hyoscine. These drugs did not antagonize the alerting effects of amphetamine on behavior; moreover, they did not markedly affect thresholds for behavioral arousal, induced by sensory stimulation. It is well to remember that benactyzine and hyoscine are atropine analogues; and that imipramine, closely allied to promazine, also shares some anti-acetylcholine properties. Drugs in this group exert comparatively weak anti-epinephrine action and appear more effective in blocking the blood pressure and anti-spasmodic effects of acetylcholine than drugs in the other groups.

Group III. This group comprised drugs which had relatively little effect on arousal thresholds but which, in full doses, caused marked changes in the electrocorticogram towards the "activation" pattern. Included in this group are reserpine and two related compounds rescinnamine and dereserpidine. These drugs produced no changes in the threshold for arousal by stimulation of the brain stem, although they did, in high doses, lead to a change in the electrocorticogram towards a faster frequency. This, however, appeared unrelated to the behavioral state, the preparation usually showing little evidence of arousal. Drugs in this group, although possessing some anti-spasmodic activity against epinephrine, acetylcholine and histamine, share a depleting action on the stores of serotonin and of catecholamines in the brain.

Group IV. Drugs in this group could not be shown to exert any marked effect either on electrocortical activity or on the behavioral arousal threshold. Included in this group are meprobamate and azacyclonal. Meprobamate (in doses of 20–40 mg/kg) had no effect on threshold of arousal induced by direct stimulation of the reticular formation. Equally, the responses to afferent stimulation showed little change; and even with large doses, the electrocorticogram remained relatively unaltered. Somewhat similar effects were observed with azacyclonal.

The above studies give an indication of the broad and empirically crude nature of any grouping so far possible on the basic of neurophysiological evidence. It is obvious that the electrophysiological effects of the diverse tranquillizers are not necessarily related to their clinical effectiveness, and that such effects can, at best, only give a very inadequate indication as to their mode of action.

e) The Effect of Some Drugs on the Electrical Activity of the Brain and its Relation to Behavior

A number of studies have been carried out on the effect of drugs on the electrical activity of the brain in the conscious unanaesthetized animal, and in suitable acute preparations. Only a few can be quoted, and the reader is referred to the extensive source material (399). Studied in rabbits treated with Curare (400) it was found that small doses of LSD-25 (1 to 5 µg/kg) led to a decrease in amplitude and an increase in the frequency of the EEG, while higher doses of LSD-25 (10 µg/kg) caused a continuous "alert" pattern (i.e. low voltage fast activity). The effects were to some extent prevented by azacyclonol. The latter drug did not prevent the effects of DFP (a powerful anticholinesterase) and amphetamine.

Another series of studies previously reported by the author (396, 401–403) can only be briefly reviewed here. These concerned drugs interacting with acetylcholine (such as physostigmine atropine, hyoscyamine); some central sympathomimetic amines (dl-amphetamine, d and l-amphetamine); LSD-25; and chlorpromazine. The patterns of responses for each were established first; and the interaction between the various members subsequently examined.

Observed in the conscious cat preparation, carrying permanently implanted cortical and subcortical electrodes, the effects of the drugs were found to fall into two broad groups. Physostigmine (an anticholinesterase) used in relatively small doses (0.05–0.3 mg/kg ip.) led to low voltage fast activity closely resembling (though not entirely identical with) that seen in fully alert animals. However, provided the dose of the drugs was kept suitably low, no corresponding "alerting" of overt behavior could be detected, The animals appeared quiet, and resting, despite an incongruous low-voltage fast electrocorticogram. On the other hand atropine (1–2 mg(kg) and its isomer, l-Hyoscyamine (0.4–0.8 mg/kg) led to high voltage slow activity which, in some respects, resembled the activity seen in deep sleep. However, here again there was no correspondence between electrical activity and behavior. The animals were fully awake and, in some instances, showed motor excitement. It should be stressed, however, that in those early experiments no psychological test situations were employed; and that subtler deficits in performance may have therefore gone undetected. The discrepancy between electrical activity and overt behavior, however, was quite striking, and in the case of atropine, was in keeping with observations noted independently in the corticogram of the dog (404).

In contrast to the above three drugs (all related to the action of acetylcholine), amphetamine (1–5 mg/kg) both in its optically active, and inactive form regularly led to low voltage fast ("alert") activity in the conscious animal. This was accompanied by behavioral excitement. The effects of LSD-25 (in doses of 15 to 25 µg/kg) were less regular. At times they resembled those of amphetamine; at others they showed rhythmic activity (at about 15 cycles/sec). A striking feature of the effects of LSD-25 was the dependence of the patterns seen on the precise environmental setting of the experiment. For example, when carried out in a constant environment chamber placed in an open laboratory, (where, presumably, noises from other rooms could penetrate), the effects noted were the ones just described. However, if these experiments were carried out in a sound proof room, rhythmic activity at a rather slower rate (4–7 cycles/sec) was noted. This activity could be blocked by sensory stimuli. It thus appeared that one effect of LSD-25 was to sensitize the animal inordinately to its environment.

When considered in terms of the relationship of electrical activity to overt behavior, the drugs thus appeared to fall into two groups. The first comprised those drugs (physostigmine, atropine and l-hyoscyamine) which, within the crude framework of gross behavioral change, showed a lack of correlation between the effects on electrical activity, and on behavior. The second group covered drugs (the amphetamines, LSD-25 and to a lesser extent mescaline) where the correlation between the effect on electrical activity, and on behavior was much closer. Moreover, when the drugs were used in combination with each other, the gross behavior effects were always dominated by the second group (the amphetamines and LSD-25) whereas the effect on electrical activity was dominated by the first. The interaction, for example, between atropine and amphetamine showed this quite clearly.

The distinction between these two groups of drugs was borne out further by acute experiments, in which the effects of high spinal and mesencephalic section were studied. These experiments were carried out in the *encéphale* and *cerveau isolé*, preparations long found useful in enquiries concerned with the mechanisms subserving sleep and arousal. The *encéphale isolé* (severed at the level of the first cervical vertebra) receives afferent impulses from the cranial nerves only. It alternates (as mentioned above) both behaviorally and electrically, between periods of drowsiness and a limited form of alerting, (as shown by eye movement, retraction of the nictitating membrane, and movement of the vibrissae). The *cerveau isolé* is severed at the level of the midbrain. It shows drowsiness or sleep only, and responds to afferent stimuli in a much more limited way.

When examined in these preparations, physostigmine, atropine and 1-hyoscyamine, used in doses comparable to the conscious preparation led to effects closely resembling those seen in the conscious preparation; there being, again, marked effects on electrical activity, with relatively little effect on the admittedly limited behavior of the preparation. The effects were independent of the transient effects of the drugs on blood pressure. Effects on *local* cerebral vascular tone, however, were not excluded by these experiments.

In contrast to the above three drugs, the effects of amphetamine, although readily obtainable in the *encéphale isolé* preparation, could no longer be observed in the *cerveau isolé* preparation, even where relatively high doses of the drugs were used. LSD-25, on the other hand, produced no effects on either the electrical activity or the behavior of either of these acute preparations. Some effects in the monkey, however, were noted.

In the absence of evidence to the contrary it was assumed that the effects of physostigmine were related to its anticholinesterase activity, and presumably due to the endogenous accumulation of acetylcholine, or a related choline ester within the central nervous system. Similarly the effects of atropine and 1-hyoscyamine were thought to be due to a blockade of cholinergic sites. There are, of course, differences between the central and the peripheral effects of atropine and physostigmine, both in the terms of dosage, and reversibility of effects. Nevertheless, a cholinergic element may be presumed to be involved in these central effects. The lack of correlation between electrical activity and behavior, and the independence of the effects observed of mesencephalic and spinal connections, would, however, suggest a diffuse distribution of this element, and a possible representation of it at high subcortical and/or cortical, as well as mesencephalic, levels.

In this respect, amphetamine differed from the drugs just considered. In the case of this agent, there appeared closer a correlation between electrical activity and behavior; furthermore the effects on electrical activity and behavior were modified by mesencephalic (though not spinal) transection. In view of the striking part played by the tegmental reticular substance in behavioral and electrical arousal, it was suggested that the effect of this drug might be exerted on elements either intimately related to, or located in the brain stem reticular activating system. The presence of nor-adrenalin in this area of the brain; the extensive studies on sympathetic humoral influences in this area; and the albeit circumstantial evidence of the presence of adrenaline-sensitive elements in the brain stem (405, 406) are all in keeping with this suggested mode of action of this powerful centrally acting sympathomimetic amine.

The effects of LSD-25 were somewhat different, and in their susceptibility to, and dependence on afferent input suggested the involvement of an element particularly and peculiarly related to the afferent pathways. This element had to be distinguished from the element involved in the action of amphetamine. It was judged to play a key part in the organization of sensory experience; and to do so, primarily, by way of a discrete, highly patterned inhibitory mechanism, reciprocating with, and depending on afferent input. Whether this mechanism was linked to the natural turnover of an indole, possibly in elements in the limbic system (with which LSD-25 interfered) seemed uncertain at the time.

The grouping established for the above six drugs was found to obtain also when the study was extended to an examination of the interaction between them and chlorpromazine (396). Both chlorpromazine and methopromazine were administered, in divided doses, alone and in combination. Given alone, chlorpromazine led to striking behavioral changes, and effects on the electrical activity. Previously friendly and affectionate animals showed marked indifference to both environment and observer; and, on occasion, became slightly aggressive when disturbed. The electrical activity reflected these changes in behavior, the record usually being dominated by regular waves at 5–8 cycles/sec interspersed by slow waves at 2–4 cycles/sec. Neither behavioral nor electrical arousal response could be obtained in these animals. When chlorpromazine was given in combination with the drugs mentioned, it was noted that whereas both the behavioral and the EEG effects of amphetamine and LSD-25 (administered in full doses) could be blocked by premedication with chlorpromazine, the effects of atropine and physostigmine on the electrical activity of the brain persisted, in the presence, even, of high doses of chlorpromazine; nor did these latter drugs appreciably modify the behavior patterns attributable to chlorpromazine. When administered in small doses (0.2–1 mg/kg) in the *encéphale isolé*, chlorpromazine led, in some (though not all) experiment, to a transient blocking of the spindle and slow-wave activity often seen in this type of preparation. This effect usually passed within about two minutes. Larger doses, however, (1.5–4 mg/kg) produced an increase in the slow spindle activity in the preparation, and also made the preparation more difficult to rouse. Chlorpromazine had little effect on the *cerveau isolé* preparation; such effects as were found were associated with a fall in blood pressure, and could thus not be readily distinguished from the circulatory effects of the drug in this preparation.

f) The Importance of Peripheral Receptors in Determining Apparently Central Effects

The ambiguous effects of chlorpromazine are mentioned because they stress the care which has to be exercised in viewing what are apparently central effects as purely central effects. It is indeed most unlikely that any drug or any neurohumoral agent exerts a central effect only. The feedback between the brain stem, and peripheral baro
and chemoreceptors, such as the carotid sinus and the carotid body, and the play of proprioceptive activity upon the brain stem is much too close, and too constant to allow for any such artificial separation; and any analysis of an apparently central drug effect [such as, for example, the effects of reserpine) soon bares a peripheral component. The subject will not be gone into; it has been well considered by others (391). It is mentioned here merely to avoid emphasis where it does not belong.

IV. SOME DRUG EFFECTS ON ANIMAL BEHAVIOR

A. Effect on "Conflict" and the So-Called Experimental Neurosis

The principle of Pavlovian conditioning techniques and theory are referred to elsewhere in this volume, and have also been referred to in the present chapter. Pavlov conceived the cortex "as a grandiose mosaic upon which are distributed, at a given moment, a huge number of points of application of external excitations, now stimulating, now inhibiting the various activities of the organism. Since, however, these points are in a definite and reciprocal functional relationship, the cerebral hemispheres are, at any given moment, a system in a state of dynamic equilibrium which one might call stereo-type" (407). However as pointed out in an outstanding review (408), Pavlov was forced to conclude that constitution played an important part in determining the degree of stability of such a dynamic equilibrium since his experimental animals (dogs) displayed a different capacity for developing and retaining the so-called "positive" and "negative" conditioned responses. In describing these so-called constitutional types, Pavlov went as far as speaking of animals as being of an "Excitable", "Lively",

"Calm" and "Inhibitory" temperament. The emphasis on genetic and constitutional factors should be noted; there being, here, much less allowance than there is at present for sensitisation of the organism to particular stimulus constellations and social situation, during an early developmental period.

Early in the conditioning studies, however, it was observed that an extensive disruption of behavior could be produced in animals when they were required to make difficult differentiations between stimulus situations carrying a positive and negative connotation, such as the famous illuminated Circles and Ellipses. A similar disruption was seen following catastrophic occurrence. Under such circumstances all differentiations of even simple conditioned response were found to disappear. The animal manifested marked defense and escape reactions, or remarkable inactivity (inhibition); or varying proportions of both sets of phenomena. These Pavlov considered as being an experimentally induced neurotic reaction and explained it by the assumption that "under certain conditions the clashing of excitation with inhibition led to a profound disturbance of the usual balance between these two processes and, in greater or less degree, and for a longer or shorter time, to a pathological disturbance of the nervous system". These changes manifested not only in motor behavior but also in the area of autonomic function. Thus experimental neurosis in dogs lead to long lasting disturbances in respiratory rhythm and cardiac rhythms, excretory functions, sexual behavior, and social behavior (Gantt, 409). Similar observations were made in sheep (410).

In his characteristically vigorous way, Pavlov extended these concepts to the explanation of behavior in man, and putting forward the existence of "second signalling systems" associated with "the kinesthetic–motor–speech" areas and subserving the functions of language, of cognitive function, and of abstraction. Further, he distinguished between three levels of integration in man, the aforementioned "secondary signalling system" of language, the first signalling system's of "Conditioned Responses", and, of course, the system of "Unconditioned Responses". It should be noted that these theories were developed long before a detailed study of the subcortical system subserving arousal and focussed attention, and the visceral and neuroendocrine integration of affective responses, was recognized. The systems were supposed to function principally in the cortical areas; though in his later writings, no attempt was made on the part of Pavlov to localize the two signalling systems in a particular cortical area, but to regard them more as *functional* systems widely distributed about the cerebral cortex, carrying out the analysis and synthesis of signals originating at the sensory receptors. Furthermore, the nature of the temporary connections in the establishment of conditioned responses was never clearly specified, any point in the cerebral cortex being capable of developing such a conditioned connection. It is well to reflect here how well certain principles defined by Pavlov have stood the test of time. The first is the juxtaposition of excitation and inhibition in the function of the nervous system at whatever level examined, and the role, particularly of inhibition in the organization, coding and grouping of signals. The second is the steady departure from a topographical point of view of the organization of the nervous system, and the acceptance of a spatio-temporal topology of signals within cell assemblies. Thirdly, there is preliminary evidence, both at a behavioral and electrophysiological level, for the formation of temporary connections (411). It is, incidentally, of interest how the obvious inhibitory and delaying function of the secondarily signalling system (inasmuch as it replaces motor and behavioral discharge by symbolic verbal patterns) can be compared to the "Symbolic Barrier" proposed by Luria (412). This was conceived as being interposed between the so-called "receptors", and the "effector" discharge apparatus. That this inhibitory symbolic barrier can break down under "conflict" or "stress" was to some extent suggested by the effects of emotionally charged verbal material on voluntary and involuntary motor responses (413). More recent adaptations of this technique open an engaging area for experimental work, particularly in regard to the value of verbal and non-verbal cues in human conditioning. It is of course commonplace that affective states in man can be affected profoundly by purely verbal stimuli. Yet the effect of drugs on human conditioning responses, and particularly verbally conditioned responses, remain relatively unexplored.

The above considerations are mentioned to convey both the promise and the limitations of the purely conditioning approach in the single organism, which naturally (at least during the past) has lent itself more readily to adaptation to the animal than to the human experiment. In regard to the effect of drugs, the technique was particularly developed by Masserman (414) using instrumental conditioning procedures. In essence the procedure involved the apposition of reward and punishment situation in a manner so as to induce, with a high degree of predictability, motivational conflict within the animal. In the original experiment carried out in cats, animals starved for twenty-four hours to ensure a state of hunger, were trained to obtain a small pellet of fish by lifting the hinge lid of a box with their mouth. By keeping the lid firmly closed, except immediately after the administration of a light buzzer signal, the animals learned to approach the food box and obtain food only after these stimuli were presented. Further training could lead cats to learn to activate these signals themselves by pressing a platform switch in various ways. This pattern, once established was then altered by delivering a disconcerting stimulus (such as an air blast, or mild electric shock) just as the animal attempted to lift the lid covering the food box in a manner which it had learned to associate with reward. When these procedures were repeated, "kinetic tension, (anxiety) mounts, and behavior becomes hesitant, vaccilating, erratic, and poorly adaptive", regressive. Such cats show resistance to placement in the experimental cage, resistance to handling, and attempts to escape from the experimental cage; and significantly alternate between approach and avoidance to the food box. They may adopt peculiar postures, may show cleaning behavior, or varying patterns of purposeless excitation. Anyone who has alternatively petted and punished a dog may have observed similar situations in more homely surroundings. It is also known that the variety and intensity of such anxious and neurotic patterns can be increased by various manipulations designed to augment the drive or the punishment. The behavioral effect can be diminished by reducing the intensity of drive, (for example, force-feeding) or by showing encouragement and approbation of the animal (for example, petting). An attempt to quantify these changes has recently been made (415).

Studied in such situations of experimental neurosis or motivational conflict alcohol and barbiturates were found to exert marked effects. Thus, for example, in sixteen cats trained to obtain food by lifting the hinged cover of the box after activating a platform switch, the administration of alcohol led to a brief excitatory period which in turn, was followed by the abolition of learned responses in the order in which they had been acquired, concomitantly with development of ataxia and other motor signs of alcoholic intoxication. As the intoxicating effects of alcohol wore off, learned responses were said to appear in the reverse order. Smaller doses of alcohol reduced restiveness and phobic reactions markedly, the animals responding to the light-buzzer signals, and occasionally also activating the platform switch. "Submissive cats and also those which had surrendered their dominance while neurotic, once again, under alcohol, began to preempt the food from their partners, even though their mild disorientation and ataxia made them more vulnerable to competition and to repeated physical attacks."

These effects were seen about thirty minutes after alcohol, but could be observed up to three to eight hours later. Ten of the sixteen cats displayed a preference for milk containing 5% alcohol as long as they remained neurotic, and chose plain milk after they had been "cured" by non-pharmacological procedures. It was argued on the basis of this evidence that alcohol exerted "a selective action on more recently acquired complex neurotic patterns." Barbiturates were found to alleviate the signs of experimental neurosis and to restore dominance in cats which had lost this feature after the induction of motivational conflict. Here again it was argued that barbiturates "disorganized recently formed intricate and complexly motivated adaptive patterns into earlier and more direct perception-responses, and thereby temporarily mitigated experimentally induced neurotic behavior. Significantly, in a later account (416) morphine was found to exert effects not unlike those of barbiturates; reserpine, chlorpromazine and mepobromate produced comparatively less immediate relief from experimentally produced neurotic behavior in both cats and monkeys than did alcohol or barbiturates and a greater number of sympathetic and motor complications. Furthermore, no drug could prevent the effect of long continued adaptional conflict in any of the animals studied.

An attempt to quantify the above procedure was made (417) in testing the antiacetylcholine drug, benactyzine. Employing the method of Masserman for producing experimental neurosis in cats with modification designed to facilitate such quantification, these authors found that injection of relatively small doses of benactyzine (0.75 to 2.0 mg) one-half to four hours before testing, "normalized" behavior as indicated by a diminution of displacement activity, (like licking, rubbing, playing, sharpening claws and extra manipulation of the signal switch), and also led to a reduction in duration of a full feeding cycle which showed a tendency to become prolonged after the induction of motivational conflict. In this respect benactyzine was found to be superior to alcohol, which in relatively high doses (3–3.7 ml of absolute alcohol) shortened the duration of the feeding cycles, but had little effect on displacement activity. Significantly, another anti-acetylcholine drug, scopolamine, had little effect on the experimental neurosis induced in this manner. There was also confirmation of the lack of chlorpromazine on this effect.

Another method of studying the conditioned avoidance response was employed (418) in the initial studies on chlorpromazine. Here an auditory stimulus (the ringing of a bell for two seconds) was coupled with an electric shock delivered through the floor of the experimental cage; the animals being trained to avoid the shock by climbing a vertical rope stretched between the floor and a rest platform. In rats in which stable responses were established, chlorpromazine, in a dose of 1 mg per kg "definitely retarded the response to the auditory stimulus, as well as slowing down the speed of the reaction". At higher doses there was a total inhibition of the response. "In general, the rat treated with chlorpromazine becomes disinterested in the bell ringing, which no longer incites the flight from pain. As with untrained normal rats the subject moves curiously around the cage without paying attention to the auditory stimuli or to the vertical cord, although his interests can at any moment be awakened with some foreign excitation" (418). In a later study the same author reports the effect of chlorpromazine on the agitation of mice placed on a hot plate. In a development of the rope-climbing technique (419) an attempt was made to measure separately the conditioned avoidance vis ... vis the unconditioned escape reaction. As in the previous experiments, rats were trained to avoid an electric shock (the unconditioned stimulus) by associating it with a bell (conditioned stimulus). In early training, the rats would escape the electric shock on to the pole safety area. After approximately ten training trials, the rat would consistently climb the pole whenever the bell was rung. When this response was elicited by the bell alone, it was considered a conditioned response. When animals failed to exhibit a conditioned response after drug administration, the unconditioned stimulus (shock) was presented in order to determine if the unconditioned response could be elicited. The responses were classed into three groups. Normal trained animals, or animals treated with ineffective drugs showed both positive conditioned and unconditioned responses (Class I). Animals which had their conditioned responses affected by the drug, and still maintained an unconditioned responses, were considered to show a specific block of conditioned response (Class II). Animals which had both conditioned and unconditioned responses blocked were considered to show a non-specific block (Class III). Here again, findings suggested that chlorpromazine, reserpine and morphine produced a specific (Class II) block of the conditioned response. Alcohol, several barbiturates and meprobamate, on the other hand, produced non-specific blocks (Class III) of the conditioned response; and even these non-specific blocking effects were produced only at doses, which produced marked incapacitating effects. The rope climbing techniques have also been used in testing the effects of human serum fractions on behavior (420).

B. The Fractionation of Over-All Behavior

a) General Considerations: The Operant Conditioning Techniques

The above examples illustrate the difficulties inherent in drawing all too readily on over-all behavior for a paradigm of neurotic behavior. This matter has been mentioned earlier, where reference has been made to the need for assessing the relative contributive sensory cues; the relative strength and relation to each other of appetitive drives; the strength of the inhibitory mechanisms innate or acquired, which normally regulate the release of these drives; and the strength of the motor apparatus normally at their disposal to bring about their discharge. That apparently paradoxical results can be obtained if these factors are not allowed for is shown by several observations, of which two will be quoted. In self stimulation studies (see below) reported in 1957 (421) it could be shown that in rats carrying permanently implanted electrodes in the medial forebrain bundle just below the fornix, dual effects from stimulation via the same electrodes could be regularly observed. The animal would press a bar to turn on the stimulation and thus show initial reward effect. This, however, would be followed by the turning off of the stimulus (brought about by the turning of a wheel) and presumably signified an escape from a punishing effect as the stimulus continued. The sequence would be regularly repeated. It was suggested that it reflected a differential rate of recruitment of the patterns of reward and punishment behavior when the systems subserving them were stimulated simultaneously.

It was of interest in these experiments that drugs with so opposite an effect as methamphetamine (2 mg/kg) and chlorpromazine (4 mg/kg) produced roughly similar effects on the over-all rate of bar pressing. However, when the positive and negative components were measured separately, striking qualitative differences could be shown. Methamphetamine increased the average time to turn the stimulation off. Chlorpromazine, on the other hand, had its largest effect on the opposite measure, namely the time the animal waited before the stimulation was turned on. The time to turn the stimulation off was also increased, but to a much lesser extent. Thus an over-all measure (bar pressing) may in fact, obscure two measures related to different effects, possibly on different systems and this despite a single electrode placement, which may be, mistakenly, associated with a single effect.

That such compound effects are likely is also borne out by another study, where operant conditioning techniques (see below) were employed. It could for example, be shown both in the rat, and the monkey (422) that whereas pentobarbital exerted an early effect on avoidance behavior, i.e., reduced a number of responses which prevented the delivery of a shock to the animal, the same drug exerted relatively little effect on appetitive behavior (i.e., when the animal was lever-pressing for sugar pellet reward). Hyoscine, on the other hand, had the obverse effect. Even in small doses it led to an immediate depressant effect on reward behavior, leaving avoidance behavior relatively less affected.

The earlier techniques mentioned above employed visual methods, and the quantification of visually observed responses. In some respects, the method has tremendous advantages. It allows one access to cues and situations, which may well be missed by a purely instrumental approach. Yet it holds within it also certain limitations, most particularly a precise analysis of the temporal sequence of stimulus and response patterns, and the probability of interaction between such patterns. It is here that the operant conditioning techniques, introduced over the past twenty-five years by B. F. Skinner and his co-workers and pupils (423–427) become most relevant and fruitful. Essentially, the method is based upon "a simple principle, namely that the characteristic features of a particular form of behavior are to a large extent determined by the environmental events that have been consequent upon past occurrences of the behavior" (428). A rat, for example, in pressing a lever and obtaining food, operates upon the environment. As has been pointed out (428), reproducibility among subjects within a given species, has been enhanced by "selecting for measurement and manipulation a response whose topography is congenial to the organism and one that the organism can perform, and immediately be in a position to repeat; by selecting an environmental consequence or 'reinforcement' that is appropriate for a particular individual; by limiting the experimental environment; and utilizing motivational levels that are strong enough to override many experimental developed variables". For example, a food or water-deprived animal is placed in a chamber where a lever can be pressed to obtain an appropriate reward. The apparatus can be set automatically by an appropriate electronic device, to reward each depression of the lever, or it can be set, equally, to yield an intermittent reward in accordance with automatically controlled schedule which makes the reward available. If the animal makes a lever response, only after lapse of a constant or variable interval of time, this is referred to as the so-called fixed or "variable interval" reinforcement. Equally, it can be set so that the reward is available after the animal has made a specified number (constant or varied) of responses (the so-called "fixed or variable ratio reinforcement") or alternately as the animal holds down its output to some predetermined low level (the so-called "differential reinforcement of low rates"). In this situation, only responses are rewarded which followed the last preceding response by some pre-determined interval (say, 20 seconds). As the reward is continuously withheld, the animal eventually stops making lever responses. "By using electronic programming techniques of stimulus situations, various schedules of reinforcement can be made to produce characteristically different output curves, which are readily distinguishable. These different kinds of outputs can be placed under the control of the stimulus, by having the signal stimulus (for example, a light) present when one schedule is in force and, another signal (for example, sound) present when another schedule is in operation. Different schedules may thus be presented sequentially and all tested during a single run after the animal has been properly trained. The purpose of the technique is thus to place an arbitrary sample of behavior under experimental control, so that behavioral processes may be investigated as a function of the various operations."

b) The Measurement of the Strength of Appetitive Drives

It has already been pointed out above that fractionation of overall behavior in terms of individual components is necessary. The appetitive drives having survival value (like hunger and thirst) present an obviously relevant group. The measurement of consummatory or goal responses is one obvious way of quantifying these appetitive drives. Thus, the amount of water drunk or food eaten may be used as a measure of thirst or hunger. A so-called drinkometer (429) has been developed for measuring consumption of water or liquids. Curiosity can be measured by the number of objects investigated (430) and there are, of course, well developed methods for measuring the effect of androgens on the copulatory responses in rats (431). It should, however, be noted that while consummatory responses often agree with other measures of the drive, such agreement is by no means universal. It can, for example, be shown that although the volume of food consumed by a rat may not continue to increase with periods of deprivation longer than twenty-four hours, other measures, in fact, may continue to increase (432). Similarly, for instance bilateral lesions in the region of the ventro medial nucleus of the hypothalamus may cause a marked increase in eating, but can also cause a decrease in the rate at which the animal will work for food, or decrease the amount of quinine required to stop an animal from eating (433). A further measure of appetitive drive is the speed of approach to the object of the consummatory response. Thus, for example, male rats who copulate with the female run to the female faster than non-copulatory rats. A rather similar measure is strength with which an animal will pull when temporarily restrained on the way to a goal (434). This measure has been used in a study of the effect of alcohol and sodium amytal (435). A fourth index of strength of appetitive drive is the rate of operant behavior. As pointed out below, in this arrangement the animal operates a single device, which automatically delivers the goal object (food or drink). The device has the advantage of being operated by a relatively stereotype movement. The lever pressing (or pecking of keys) (436) can be used to study thirst, hunger fear and explorative drive, and the aversive and rewarding effects of electrical stimulation of the brain. Furthermore, there are the so-called preference tests (437). Here an animal is given a choice between two or more goal objects. This method has been useful in studies of specific hungers and palatability. Lastly, another way of measuring strength of drive is by inducing an animal to cross an electric grid on the way to the goal (438). This has also been used in self-stimulation techniques (see below).

c) The Effect of Some Drugs on Fear and Conflict

As was pointed out above, a procedure commonly employed in studying "anxiety" and "fear" in the experimental animal is the so-called avoidance conditioning technique. In this type of experiment, an animal is permitted to prevent delivery of an electrical shock by making appropriate responses. When this response is not made, the animal receives a shock ("punishment") which may or may not be preceded by a warning signal. It was pointed out in an important review (439) that few studies had adequately controlled for motor effects, sensory decrements and general malaise, any or all of which would produce depression of avoidance behavior independently of any specific emotional change. It can, for example, be shown that a dose of reserpine, which depresses avoidance behavior in the monkey (440) also completely depressed behavior maintained by food reinforcement. On the other hand, d-desoxyephedrine, which depressed food reinforcement, may produce an increase in avoidance responding. Avoidance behavior does not only depend on drugs, but also upon the behavioral variables involved in the avoidance situation. For example, on a schedule which delivers shock to rats every time they allowed 20 seconds to elapse without depressing a lever, a given dose of reserpine does not produce decrement in lever pressing. However, when the schedule was set so as to deliver it only on one-fifth of the occasions, on which they were "due", the same dose of reserpine produced a marked depression in the rate of avoidance responding (441). Chlorpromazine, on the other hand, decreased shock avoidance behavior in a more direct fashion. A further variant of this operant conditioning technique was the assessment of disruption of one form of behavior, by superimposing a parallel signal which ended in delivery of an electric shock. Animals were trained to give a stable level base line of behavior by reinforcing lever-pressing responses with food on a variable interval schedule. While the animals were lever-pressing a stimulus of several minutes duration was presented contiguously and terminated by delivery of an electric shock. It was found that after several such periods of stimulus and shock, the stimulus itself came to produce a complete disruption of the animal's ongoing behavior (442). Lever pressing ceased during the stimulus and was resumed only after the receipt of the unavoidable shock. This variant is of interest inasmuch as it approximates the anxiety situation consequent upon anticipation of an unpleasant stimulus and the disruption of ongoing behavior by this anticipatory set. Employing this conditioned suppression technique, some striking effect of amphetamine and reserpine could be shown (443). Disruption of ongoing behavior by the presence of a second stimulus could be relieved or cured by continued reserpine treatment. Amphetamine was found to exert an opposite effect, intensifying the degree of behavioral suppression.

It is also of interest that this technique provides ready control for non-specific effects, which are reflected by the *rate* of responding on the variable interval reinforcement schedule between stimulus presentations. Here again, some interesting differential effects were observed. Amphetamine, for example, while producing greater suppression of responding during the warning stimulus, actually *increased* the response output in the absence of the stimulus. Reserpine, while increasing the response rate during the warning stimulus, produced in fact a *lower* output between stimuli. Pure motor effects are thus unlikely to account for these effects.

There is one other aspect, which is only just beginning to be studied systematically. The effect of drugs on the natural extinction of conditioning emotional response is of obvious importance. In some of the early studies directed toward the elucidation of this problem (443A, 443, 444), the effects of chlorpromazine upon extinction of such a conditioned responses were investigated. Suppression of ongoing behavior was first established in the manner outlined above, by pairing a stimulus with a shock, until ongoing behavior was completely disrupted during the anticipatory signal. Extinction was then followed through, with or without the drug, by presenting the warning signal, but omitting the shock. It was of interest that whereas animals who had received the drug during the extinction procedure, still displayed the anticipatory disruption of behavior after the drug was discontinued, animals not receiving the drug showed no effect on the progress of extinction, which had its usual effect in eliminating the emotional response. Thus chlorpromazine, far from permitting the animal to unlearn its fear, actually prevented the normal extinction process from occurring.

d) Self-Stimulation Techniques

The evidence quoted above serves to emphasize several sources of error in experiments in this field. As has been pointed out, the effect of drugs on over-all behavior is composite, and has to be fractionated, as far as possible into components making up the total response. Also of moment is the *temporal topology* of one form of behavior in relation to another, which may proceed simultaneously. Thirdly, there are indications (as in the experiments quoted above) of the close juxtaposition of opposite (i. e. appetitive and aversive) forms of behavior, and a delicate balance between the two. It is perhaps in regard to the third that the pharmacological studies using self-stimulation techniques become most relevant. It was shown by Olds and Milner (445) that rats carrying electrodes, implanted into various parts of the brain and arranged in a circuit, so as to make it possible for the animal to deliver shock to himself by stepping on a pedal, exhibited two broad groups of effects. In certain electrode placements, which included the system centered on the hypothalamus and most of the rhinencephalon and projected into the thalamus and mid-brain, animals continued to self-stimulate themselves rapidly for long periods, usually "preferring this auto encephalic stimulation to all other pursuits". If, however, the electrodes were placed in a smaller area, which included the greater part of the reticular activating system and the dorsal posterior hypothalamus and extended forward between the mammillary thalamic tract and the fornix, the animals were found not to choose the stimulation and, in fact, avoided such stimulation. On such occasions, even an accidental tripping of the lever would result in an animal avoiding this lever again. There is also an area extending to the dorsal posterior hypothalamus, in which stimulation "always produced ambivalence effects." Presumably, it is this area, which also is involved in the experiment quoted above. A differentiation in the motivational effects can also be achieved from different parts of the positive system. Thus, for example, with the electrodes in the posterior hypothalamus, stimulation rates may be of the order of 5,000 times an hour. With the electrodes in the anterior hypothalamus, the rates may be much lower (of the order of 400 per 1,000 responses per hour). In the septal or amygdaloid region of the forebrain they average from 500 to 1,000 per hour. It can furthermore be shown that, using an obstruction rats will cross painful foot shock in order to get to the lever and to induce self-stimulation. Again, rats with very high response rate would cross a grid with strong shock in order to stimulate themselves. A rat with a very low response rate would be stopped by a relatively weak shock. It is suggested that differentiation within the positive response system may be related to the number of "positive motivational units excited". This concept is in need of further elucidation, as is the relation of the "negative" motivational system to the system subserving subjective *pain*.

Using these techniques, the effects of a number of drugs on the rate of self-stimulation with different electrodes in animals and with different electrode placement were examined (446, 447). It was shown that, with the electrode in the ventral posterior hypothalamus, chlorpromazine, for example, produced marked inhibition of self-stimulation. On the other hand, no effect was observed with the electrode in the middle hypothalamus. Meprobamate, pentobarbital and morphine, on the other hand, increased the very low rate of self-stimulation in the negative area. On the basis of these, and cognate findings, it was proposed that whereas " meprobamate, morphia and pentobarbital caused a very mild depression on the positive system, they caused also a major depression in the negative system. Amphetamine, on the other hand, was judged to bring about an augmentation in the positive system with, perhaps, a lesser augmentation of the negative system. Chlorpromazine was judged to cause a total depression of the positive system. The studies have also been extended to allow for the self-injection of drugs by an animal into its own brain down an implanted fine pipette. The effects of LSD-25 and monoamine oxidase inhibitors are suggestive, but must await further refinements of technique.

Though the above studies draw attention to the binary arrangement of the motivational system, it would be well to be aware of the limitation inherent in an all-too-exclusive approach to the problem in these terms. As pointed out above, the wide topographical distribution of these areas and their convergence and overlap within certain nodal regions in the brain, does not mean they can be in any way localized to these "areas". Nor would it be entirely correct to assume that the positive areas have predominately sympathetic autonomic response, whereas the negative areas are predominately parasympathetic in character. Inhomogeneity is the rule in the Central Nervous System. Parameters of electrical stimulation may be important in the mobilization of various elements. A mosaic of cell assemblies populated by elements of both cholinergic and non-cholinergic nature would seem more likely; and though the ultimate effector pathways do in fact effect predominantly sympathetic and parasympathetic discharge, a central intermingling of these elements need not necessarily be excluded by the predominant peripheral involvement of one system or another.

e) Non-Specific Drug Effects, and Some Special Responses

It will have been apparent from the foregoing how general are the methods so far employed in the analysis of drug effects on animal behavior, and how little can be said with confidence of specific effects of drugs on any particular system. This, however, does not imply unawareness on the part of experimenters of the possible overlap of specific effects by such general effects (for example, general excitatory or depressive effects on the motor system, or sensory deficit). One way of circumventing this danger obviously lies in the assessment of the *frequency* of occurrence of a particular drug effect on a particular form of behavior in various temporally structured stimulus response situations. Thus, for example, in studying the effect of drugs on pecking behavior of pigeons, it could be shown that pentobarbital may depress behavior in the fixed interval and fixed ratio schedules (see above). However, the dose response curves were found to be markedly different in two types of behavior (436). Fixed ratio performance (i. e., where the number of pecks to obtain reward was fixed) was shown to be more resistant to pentobarbital than it was to fixed interval performance (where the reward was forthcoming only after a fixed time). Furthermore, a relatively low dose of pentobarbitol which almost completely suppressed fixed interval behavior may actually *increase* the responses rate on a fixed ratio schedule. In evaluating the specificity of a drug effect therefore, a *family* of dose responses curves, taken over a wide range of time intervals following drug administration, would appear to be at least one sure method of preventing over-generalization and, in fact, attaching significance to the effect of a particular drug on a particular form of behavior. A technique for the study of the effects of drugs upon discriminative capacity may be quoted (447A). In these experiments, quoted above, pigeons were presented with two response keys, which they had to peck to obtain reward. The keys were separated by a vertical bar. The keys and bar could be independently illuminated and the birds were to discriminate to obtain the correct reward. Two measures were plotted: one was the total number of responses emitted by the bird and the other was percentage of responses, which were correct. It was found that LSD-25 soon after administration produced a decline in total responses but at the same time an *increase* in accuracy. Chlorpromazine, on the other hand, was found to decrease both accuracy and output. Pentobarbital decreased accuracy and increased output. Meperidine reduced both accuracy and output. Alcohol and sodium barbital were found to increase the total response output, while decreasing accuracy. It will be seen that, taken with the measures outlined above, it is possible to assess, albeit approximately, the contribution of any sensory deficit upon the total drug effect.

Special responses

A number of special responses have been described for psychoactive drugs the full significance of which must, for the present, remain obscure. One is the effect of LSD-25 and related compounds on spider web formation (438B). LSD-25 alters the spinning behavior of the spider, resulting in irregularities in the web (which, it may be noted, is exceedingly rich in adrenaline). The fighting habit, and indeed posture of siamese fighting fish is affected by LSD-25 (439B), as are the state of the operculum and of the snail (*Ambularia cuprina*). In mice receiving oral mescaline, an increase in scratching episodes may be observed (440B). The number of such paroxysms may be counted and used for the assay of the interaction between mescaline and a number of drugs. Many other such special forms of behavior are constantly turning up, particularly in pharmaceutical laboratories. Very few, however, have, as yet, been investigated in depth.

C. Drug Effects in Relation to Social Setting and Social Cues

The dependence of drug effects, on social setting has already been mentioned at the beginning of this chapter. Thus it was shown in 1940 (37) that grouped mice were more susceptible to the stimulant effects of amphetamine and allied compounds than single mice. The relation of the LD-50 of adrenaline, methyl amphetamine, ephedrine and amphetamine to various degrees of confinement was examined in a subsequent paper (38). It was found that, with the area kept constant and the number of mice increased from 1 to 10, the toxicity of adrenaline was doubled and that of amphetamine nearly increased tenfold. the increase in mortality by ephedrine and methedrine fell between these two extremes. It was also shown that a reduction of temperature markedly reduced the effects of aggregation on the toxicity of amphetamine, the toxicity of the drug falling almost to a figure comparable to that obtained in solitary mice under similar conditions. It was noted that the animals were almost inactive at 60°. In a subsequent paper (39), a number of other factors were further allowed for. These included weight of the animal; environmental noise; confinement of the area in which the animal was placed; and aggregation (that is, the presence of other animals). The latter factor was felt to exert the greatest effect under conditions normally employed in experimental laboratories. Intensity of illumination and the transparency of boundary walls appeared to have little effect on results. It was concluded on the basis of these findings, "that the essential feature of these amines is that unlike other Central Nervous stimulants they induce in a mouse a state of excitability rather than excitement. Lethal doses almost invariably killed the solitary mouse as the result of violent convulsion, which therefore may appear when excitation in the central nervous system has reached a critical level. Doses themselves not lethal may thus become so as the result of external factors raising the excitation to a critical level." A further careful examination of the influence of aggregation on amphetamine toxicity and interaction between amphetamine and chlorpromazine (41) showed that, in a single mouse, pentobarbitone and chlorpromazine exerted only a slight protective effect against the toxicity of amphetamine. In groups of mice, pentobarbitone had no effect on the LD-50. A marked protection, however, was achieved with phenobarbital at doses, which produced ataxia and sleepiness. With chlorpromazine a significant protective effect was observed in doses well below those producing impairment in consciousness. Reserpine and promazine were also found to be protective; the latter, however, less so than chlorpromazine.

In a subsequent paper (445B), the effect of aggregation (that is, number of mice) confinement, i. e. decrease of space and temperature were re-examined. The dose of amphetamine ranged between 10 and 200 mg per kg. Identical groups were kept at temperatures of 25° and in a cold room at 10° cg for periods of five hours. It was found that at room temperature, aggregation increased the toxic effects of amphetamine. Confinement, however, had less influence on mortality. Increasing the number of animals from three to five per container did not cause any significant difference in result. The influence of temperature on the toxicity of amphetamine was found to vary with exposure. For the first few hours, the temperature at 10°C. had a definite protective effect on grouped animals, and only a slight one on single animals. Later however, this protection was lost to varying degrees. On the other hand, temperatures lower than 10°C increased the toxicity of amphetamine. A short exposure of mice to 10° either before or after the injection of amphetamine, however, had a protective effect. Cold had a sedating and quieting effect on normal animals and counteracted the excitation caused by amphetamine. A promising variant of the above investigations has been reported in regard to the ability of adrenergic blocking agents to antagonize some of the central actions of dextroamphetamine in mice in different states of aggregation (446B). The agents included dibenzyline, phenylhomoveratryl piperazine, phentolamine and dibozane, and were compared for their effectiveness with chlorpromazine. It was found that these agents indeed did protect mice from lethal effects of dextroamphetamine; and that, as in the case of chlorpromazine and reserpine, this effect was most marked when the mice were observed in groups. It was also shown that the same adrenergic blocking agents reduced the motor activity induced by dextroamphetamine in mice. The protective action against dextroamphetamine however was not necessarily related to intrinsic sedative property of the adrenergic blocking agent. Dibenzylene was quite effective in protecting mice from the lethal effects of amphetamine, though having only a relatively slight effect in reducing amphetamine induced motor activity. Reserpine was found to protect against the lethal effect of dextroamphetamine at doses which did not cause sedation and below those required to reduce the motor activity of dextroamphetamine. It is however clear that in these experiments the central vis-…-vis the peripheral component of action, cannot be fairly apportioned, and further analysis is needed to distinguish between such central and peripheral effects.

That such interaction between social circumstance, doses and type of response is not confined to stimulant compounds is shown by an observation on barbiturates. It was noted that certain barbiturates actually increased rate of activity of groups of mice (447B) in spite of careful selection of adequate depressant doses determined in isolated animals. A scheme was devised to identify successive stages of activity induced by the CNS depressants. These studies demonstrated that the sequence of increasing depression was obscured by an incongruous phase of excitability produced by most barbiturates in animal groups. If, however, the hyperactivity was assigned its proper place in the scheme, the subsequent states of depression followed with a high degree of consistency from animal to animal and for all CNS depressants.

The depression level profile for each depressant appeared distinctive even to the point where a difference in metabolism between two shortacting barbiturates was suggested. Dose depressant profiles for the tranquilizers were shown to differ from those for the barbiturates in several ways. First, there was a wide dose range for producing depressant effects. Secondly, there was absence of a hyperactive phase. Thirdly, there was an inability to produce complete immobilisation and lastly, there was long duration of action, at low levels of motor activity. Comparison of the effects observed in mice isolated from each other with the effects observed in mice put together in groups showed another important difference between tranquilizers and barbiturates. Phenobarbitol used in doses which produced full hypnosis in mice isolated from each other "not only failed to depress mice grouped together, but actually caused marked increase in the rate of spontaneous activity"; and much higher doses were required for depressant effects to be noted in grouped mice. In complete contrast, neither the time nor the degree of depression induced by chlorpromazine and reserpine were influenced in the group situation. Such interaction between drug response and social setting are of obvious relevance, not only in the experimental, but also in the clinical field. They are briefly considered elsewhere.

D. Drug Induced Disturbances in Timing: Increments and Decrements of Adaptative Behavior

One may be permitted to return briefly to operant conditioning techniques because they make possible an accurate and quantitative analysis of temporal sequence in controlled stimulus (and response) situations, and thus are particularly suitable for the analysis of the effects of some drugs upon temporal orientation. That such effects may be of moment in the successful adaptive (including social) performance of animals is self-evident. "Good" adaptation implies an appropriate response at the appropriate time. The serial organization in time is thus essential for an appropriate response. The effect of drugs on temporal orientation has been examined in a number of laboratories. In one such procedure, rats were rewarded for lever pressing only when they spaced their responses at least 20 seconds *apart* (448). Rats learn rapidly to respond appropriately, as this is acquired in the test situation after relatively few trials. Amphetamine, in increasing doses, was found to shift the peak of distribution towards shorter values, indicating that the animals were responding too early. There was here an orderly shift of the temporal patterning of responses, suggesting that the effect of the drug was not simply an excitatory effect. Alcohol, sodium pentobarbital and reserpine, however, led to markedly different effects. Sodium pentobarbital unlike amphetamine "completely destroyed all evidence of timing". On the other hand, with reserpine the responding was eventually completely suppressed, the timing remained intact as long as there was enough residual behavior to provide an adequate measure (449).

Though not entirely comparable, another line of experiments suggests an effect of drugs, particularly LSD-25 on the capacity to serially organize information in time. This centers on the so-called delayed response and *delayed* alternation tasks, as observed in monkeys (450). In this experimental situation an animal (having responded appropriately by pressing a panel and obtaining a reward) is required to wait two seconds before pressing another panel (previously not associated with reward) in order to receive another reward. It can be shown that this delayed alternation task, is impaired by frontal lobe and basal ganglia lesions; but relatively unaffected by temporal lobe lesions. Experiments designed to test the effect of LSD-25 on the accuracy of performance of such delayed alternation task in doses as low as 5μg. per kg, showed impairment in performance of delayed alternation problems. The effect of the drug was reflected primarily in the accuracy of response, although increasingly large doses tended to depress the rate of performance. Tolerance to the effects of LSD-25, though falling off rapidly, persisted for several days. Unlike LSD-25, amphetamine, pentobarbital and chlorpromazine either did not produce changes in accuracy or, when they did, these changes were relatively small compared with the effects on the pressing rates. The effects of LSD-25 were not unlike those obtained following bi-frontal lesions in the monkey, though speculation in this regard is premature.

It is reactions such as these, which may in time lead one to a clearer definition and analysis of decrements in adaptive behavior induced by small doses to this drug. To date these decrements are most obviously seen in man and have indeed been studied recently (451). Moreover, cognate tests, going as they do beyond the mere effect of drugs on motivational systems, indirectly may lead also to a clearer analysis of the effects of drugs on the so-called "cognitive" functions; and thus contribute to the evolution of models much more suitable to the testing of the effects of drugs on intellectual impairment than has been possible so far. "Behavioral toxicity" is so far a term principally applied to man. It describes the various and subtle decrements of function seen with marginal doses of the drugs – showing slight errors in judgement, intellectual capacity and motor skill. So far, no real animal model to test for these subtle changes is available. Yet, the need for such models is urgent; and is more likely to be met in the study of delayed responses, than the effect of drugs on the affect systems alone.

V. SOME FACTORS AFFECTING DRUG RESPONSES IN MAN

A. Somatic and Metabolic Considerations

Even the most cursory acquaintance with psychotropic drug effects in man suggests striking differences in the individual reaction. The differential susceptibility to alcohol is well known and equally, a personal equation runs through most psychosomimetic drug-induced experiences. It is therefore surprising how little systematic knowledge is available in this area of work. Though the evidence is so far only very inadequate and circumstantial, it would be well to allow for such differences as being, in part, due to metabolic idiosyncrasy, We may absorb, metabolise and excrete drugs in slightly deviant ways. Roger Williams (452) has marshalled impressive evidence for the argument of biochemical individuality, and the so-called genotropic concept. He has summarized the genetic basis of anatomical variations, (including the observed variations between organs in similar species); of individuality in composition, (particularly in the blood proteins, blood and salivary amino acids and the gastric and intestinal juices); individual enzymatic patterns (including blood phosphatase, cholinesterase, amylase, and some other enzymes); individuality in endocrine function (including variation of thyroid parathyroid, insulin, estrogen, androgen, steroid and pituitary activity) and individuality in nutrition. It is self-evident that if, indeed, such individual biochemical variation exists, this may be of utmost moment in determining the final reaction pattern between a given dose of a drug and the biophysical soma with which it interacts.

Indeed, this interaction poses some well-known paradoxes in general pharmacology. It was noted by Clark (453) that dose responses relationships appear more direct when intact animals are used than when a specific tissue, (such as the epidermis) is employed as a test object. It was suggested by him that simplicity of the tissue response is more apparent than real, because, in the intact animal, the effect of a drug is indeed the summation of a larger number of variables; these, between them, contributing to the total response. The view could thus be posed (though not necessarily agreed to) that we may expect to find the most striking evidence for biochemical individuality when we look at detail rather than at such crude summation as the total adaptive statistical response of a complex organism. For example, although in man the inter-individual variation androsterone excretion may vary 35 fold, the excretion of total keto-steroids may vary much less (i.e. 3 fold) (454). The obverse, however, could also be argued. Namely, that in the metabolic interplay between interrelated organ systems and the scanning function of the nervous system (and of its viscero-endocrine-motor projections) would make for a wide range of variation of the same organism to standard metabolic and pharmacological loads over *time*. A genetically determined chemical individuality would thus appear to be too crude and rigid a model; and in any metabolic considerations, biochemical *reaction* patterns acquired during maturation, and susceptible to self-limiting fluctuations must be equally taken into account. To loading studies designed to elucidate inter-individual biochemical differences from a purely genetic view, (such, as a study for example, responses of twins to a standard biochemical or pharmacological load), one must, therefore, add studies of the reactivity patterns of individuals to drugs *over time;* and do so in precisely defined social situations. The two approaches, far from being mutually exclusive, are, in fact, complementary.

A simple substance known for its different effect in different individuals is ethyl alcohol. Even early studies showed that the degree of sobriety was not necessarily related to blood alcohol levels (455). Metabolic and enzymic adaptation with a sustained supply of substrate is a well-known biological phenomenon; and its role in the possible production of addiction is considered elsewhere. Again, the problem of sensitivity to drugs and of side reactions should be noted. Such reactions may be seen upon first administration or following continued use. They may be observed in drugs as diverse as antibiotics, antihistaminics and psycholeptics. Thus, for example, in an early study in which 50,000 units of penicillin were administered over two and a half days to 28 normal individuals; 7 showed severe side reactions. More relevant the blood levels of penicillin may be maintained in some individuals for longer periods than in others. A similar state obtains in the case of phenylbutazone (Butazolidin). Studied in 60 subjects, blood levels range as widely as 60 to 150 mg per liter. Significantly, though it may show a day-to-day constancy in the individual suggesting that the rate at which the drug is metabolized may vary (between 17 and 35%) in different individuals. In fact, this inter-individual variation in the metabolism of phenylbutazone is even more widely scattered in different species; its biological "half-life" being three hours for rabbits, six hours for dogs and rats, and seventy-two hours for man. In this context a very remarkable tolerance of rabbits to atropine should be noted (456). The ability to hydrolyze atropine in this species is related to the presence of an atropine esterase, an inherited enzyme characteristic (457). Furthermore, the enzyme does not appear in the blood until two months after birth. On the other hand, human infants and unweaned animals may tolerate a relatively large dose of atropine.

The above findings emphasize the need for systematic loading studies of the effects of drugs and metabolites in different groups of normal controls, in selected clinical syndromes, and in the families of both. In the field of the chemotherapies of infectious diseases where the degree of systemic bacteriostasis is obviously related to the maintenance of adequate blood drug levels, the exigencies of the problem have forced the development of adequate chemical methods. Strangely enough, however, in the chemotherapies of the nervous system, and of the behavior disorders, the need for comparable tools and techniques is only just beginning to be realized. The needs in this area, to be sure, arc both more complex and more challenging. For not only is it necessary to obtain data on the absorption, blood level metabolism, and clearance of a particular drug; but also, to relate these to the levels of hormones (such as for example, the 17-Hydroxy-corticoids and blood catecholamine level) inasmuch as they may be affected by the drugs.

As an example of inter-individual variation in drug reactivity patterns, one study of vascular response variability may be quoted. A series of early studies by Funkenstein and his colleagues (458), have suggested s relationship between blood pressure responses to injected epinephrine and methacholine and the clinical course in various groups of psychiatric patients. The subject has been reviewed (459) and will not therefore be commented in in any detail. What was relevant in this imaginative approach was the attempt to establish drug reactivity patterns in individual patients in terms of a somatic response, and to relate these patterns to patient category, and to prognosis. Although the many variations in technique, the lack of an adequate recording system and of adequate sampling, (particularly in regard to age and initial blood pressure) make the original claims doubtful, the approach must stand as a useful and early example of a type of study which is in urgent need of extension and elaboration in carefully selected groups.

In a later development of the same approach it was shown that the excretion rate for *nor*adrenaline was higher in aggressive and hostile patients than in patients showing timidity and fear. The latter showed a higher excretion of adrenaline. There was also evidence that when subjects were given mecholyl, the degree of hypotensive responses was related to the *nor*adrenaline level; the greater the hypotensive response, the lower the *nor*adrenaline level. It was further noted that the infusion of adrenaline and noradrenaline during the mecholyl test caused an increase in the hypotensive response when adrenaline was used and a decrease when *nor*adrenaline was employed.

Such trends are suggestive, though care must be exercised in accepting these findings at their full value. In the first place, as already mentioned, the clearance patterns for the catecholamines are only now becoming established, and the increased output of one component against another need not necessarily reflect corresponding blood levels. It may equally signify the retention or active metabolism of the component whose presence in the urine is reduced. Secondly, adrenaline and noradrenaline only represent a *small* fraction (about 7%) of the total metabolic products excreted in the urine; a full metabolic balance sheet of catecholamines in man is, now, however, a real possibility and clear and definitive evidence in this regard is now coming forward (460–462). Lastly, neither plasma nor urine levels can, at present, be related with any confidence to highly localized intracerebral changes; though here in estimation of blood hormone levels may be more relevant than an estimation of urine levels. It is in this context that the studies of hormone levels in anxiety and depression are timely. Two groups of studies are urgently needed in this area. In the first place, much more detailed information is required of the levels, turnover and excretion patterns of hormones in the individual human subject in various affective states, both natural and experimentally induced (such as stress states, states of sleep deprivation, and states of sensory isolation and in a number of pathological syndromes). Particular attention should be paid in such studies to longitudinal follow-through in the same subject, and the inner consistency or variability of such patterns *over time.* The mere occurrence of diurnal variations in the excretion patterns of hormones strongly suggests the need for such studies. Secondly, systematic metabolic loading studies, using amino acids and the precursors and products of substances known to play a part in the regulation of the central and autonomic nervous system must assume their place in long-term investigations of the chemical topology of mental disorder. Such studies should be extended to or combined with drug loading studies of the kind mentioned above, where the availability of compounds possessing an overriding property (such as the anticholinesterases, the serotonin antagonists, the acetylcholine adrenaline and ganglion blocking agents) may play a very useful part. Lastly, there is an equally urgent need for the study of the excretion patterns of some commonly used phrenotropic drugs, such as the phenothiazines, in individual patients over time. The remarkable lag in excretion patterns in the phenothiazines should be noted. Moreover, as mentioned above, there are few isolated instances (463) where there is evidence of the conversion of a substance into a more, rather than less active substance in the body. Such studies as indeed all others mentioned above, should be linked to genetic studies, extended to twins, and normal siblings. This may be particularly profitable in an area such as the biochemical study of schizophrenia, where the indications for a genetic background are strongly suggestive.

B. The So-Called Individual (Inter Subject) Variation

The above remarks may serve to emphasize the manner in which an individual biochemical pattern, be it genetically determined or acquired in later life by a process of exposure ("sensitisation"), may affect the pharmacological response to a particular drug. Yet it is evident that in the complex transaction between the ingestion of a drug and the output of a particular form of behavior other factors may be pre-eminently important. It is commonplace knowledge that different personality patterns may react to a drug in very different ways (463A) and that even in the same individual, the retrospective or anticipatory set in a particular situation may lead to very different results with the same drug, (even in the same dose) according to the circumstances which precede, or accompany, or follow a particular medication. Some studies are now beginning to define this complex field. (464, 464A) though, again one encounters a situation all too familiar; namely, the inadequacy of the tools of investigation to the purpose of the investigation. For the problem is essentially a treble one; namely the definition of the dimension of the personality; the accurate recording of drug induced mental change and the correlation of one group of data with the other. Various psychometric scales can serve in some measure to assess the personality of the subjects and a battery of suitable projective sensory-motor tests, as well as an inventory questionnaire can be used to describe (and, if possible, measure) drug-induced change. Thus, two suggestive early papers (465, 466) have examined the correlation between the psychoasthenia (Pt) and Depression (D) scales of the MMPI (Minnesota Multiphasic Personality Inventory) performance on a number of psychological tests and the subjective effects of two-dose levels of LSD-25, Secobarbital, Chlorpromazine, Meperidine and, also, placebo. The tests included speed of addition tests, modified digit symbol tests, pursuit rotor, tachystoscopic discrimination of circle size, and tactual threshold determination. A 46-item symptom questionnaire was also administered to the subjects.

The results did not suggest a significant correlation between the objective (i. e. performance) and subjective psychological effects of a given drug. The drugs, which produced greater mean objective effects however, also produced greater mean subjective effects. All drugs, in the doses given, impaired performance on the psychological tests. It was incidentally noted that Meperidine hydrochloride (in 50 and 100 mg doses) did not impair performance of the same psychological tests. Also in this series, it was found that, whereas LSD-25 exerted significant effects on intellectual and perceptual tasks, it caused relatively little impairment of motor tasks. Chlorpromazine and secobarbitol, on the other hand affected motor tasks, but did not cause significant impairment of performance on simple intellectual and perceptual tasks.

That these patterns, however, could in no way be regarded as specific for the drugs was shown by a comparison of the subjective effects with the Psychoasthenia (Pt) and Depression (D) scales of the MMPI. Here a significant, or almost significant, relationship to the subjective effects of 200 mg of secobarbitol, 200 mg of chlorpromazine and a 50 μg dose of LSD-25 was noted. The more deviant the subject on these two MMPI scales, the greater were the subjective effects of these drugs. That this correlation however was sensitive to dose was shown by the lack of relationship between subjective effects and the MMPI when a higher dose (100 μg) of LSD-25 was used. Here the subjective LSD experience was noted irrespective of deviation on the MMPI scale. Thus, whereas some effects of the drug may be more related to personality patterns others are more related to the drug itself. As pointed out earlier it may well be that delicate neurohumoral shifts may partake in the patterns of interaction between the total person and the environment. It could be proposed that although some such patterns ("Depression", "Anxiety", "Hysteria") may be "learnt" in early infancy the thresholds of their release in subsequent life may depend upon delicate shifts in balance between interacting systems within the brain and the peripheral autonomic nets. It is therefore not surprising that it is particularly *low* doses of the drug which correlate with psychological personality traits. These doses may be expected to shift the thresholds of compensatory mechanisms and bring about the emergence of stored patterns of behavior of less adaptive value. Higher doses, on the other hand, may lead to disruption of far greater magnitude, and exert effects, which are more characteristic of the drug than of the personality with which it interacts. Mentioned in this context may be the studies of barbiturates on language and the subjective denial of illness (467), which may be seen in brain damaged patients in these circumstances. It is, in fact, felt that the study of language in various drug induced states (and particular in relation to low drug doses) may offer an unusually fertile field for the classification and grouping of those drug induced phenomena which, in the most personal of all idioms may be regarded as unique, or, at any rate individual. It is here that psychopharmacology could interact with linguistics, with communication theory and with psychoanalysis.

C. The Placebo Response

Implicit in the foregoing is the concept of the Placebo, and (by implication) of the Placebo Reactor. This familiar principle, long embedded in clinical usage (and particularly in the ancient world) has been well described as the "only single action which, all drugs have in common" (468). Literally translated it signifies "I shall please." It is the effect attributable to a particular medication or procedure, where the symbolic transaction accompanying a particular medication or procedure assumes the significance of the procedure itself. In view of the profound influence of verbal and non-verbal cues on human behavior and the profound therapeutic effect of such cues, it would hardly be surprising if behavior, or subjective experience, were not influenced by what, in Pavlovian language, may be termed "secondary (symbolic) situations". The subject has been well reviewed (469–471).

The conditioning of visceral responses by purely symbolic cues had in fact received extensive study in the Pavlovian laboratory and that of his pupils (472) and the effect on heart rate, respiration, sudomotor activity of purely verbal stimuli in man is well known. Factors such as gastric motility can be influenced by purely verbal stimuli. Equally, placebos can lower blood pressure (when compared with reserpine (473) or bring relief in cases of arthritis (474). They may even lead to side reactions, such as stuffiness of nose (in the case of reserpine), and headaches, and disturbances of sleep. These effects, far from being minimal, are very real to the patient. Significantly, they are particularly apparent in stress states (475). It is a sardonic commentary on the bias and complacency of the medical sciences that so powerful a factor in the therapeutic transaction should have been singled out only recently for methodical scrutiny.

An important question is presented by the so-called Placebo Reactor. There is however no consensus of opinion about the characteristics of the reactor. He has been described as a recognisable entity, but only in the sense that interview and psychologic testing can differentiate him from a nonreactor. Different distributions of scores for reactors from non-reactors have been claimed by some. Others, on the other hand, were unable to isolate features sufficiently characteristic. In fact, the lack of predictability to placebo response has been singled out as one of it characteristics (470). This may be due to a lack of cognisance of the total setting in given experimental situations.

There is a further factor which should be borne in mind. Usually, the patient is referred to as placebo reactor; the "reactor" among the observer staff being conveniently ignored. Yet suggestibility knows no such distinction; it must be inquired into, and allowed for, wherever it is met. Another feature is the usually negative attitude assumed in the face of a placebo response. This, again, is difficult to understand. For the subjective relief afforded by placebo in what is essentially a subjective disorder may be very real, and in excess even of that produced by a more active preparation. Rather, therefore, than treat the placebo merely as a source of error in an all-too-cleanly designed investigation, it would be appropriate, and rewarding, to investigate positive placebo responses in much the same way as any drug responses. The interaction of the personality traits of the subject with those of the observer, and with the total social situation, will be as relevant here as in any other study, and should reveal and define synergisms generally suspected only on clinical grounds.

The aspects touched on above reflect the false sense of security, which the inclusion of a placebo in a drug trial may lull one into. It is extremely difficult to maintain inert placebo medication for any length of time. Taste, or texture, or solubility may give it away; the side effects of the active preparation may show themselves clearly and unmistakably; and the staff may attempt to break the code by devious routes. In part, such difficulties may be met by a long period of placebo medication, preferably based on an "inactive placebo" followed by an "active placebo" period. The active placebo should be designed to mimic the side effects of the drug under test, or possess some striking peripheral property. The complete unawareness of the patient of any change in terms of both medication and attention is essential throughout a trial; as is the early detection of placebo reactors amongst those making up the *observer* team. In an early controlled trial of chlorpromazine by C. Elkes (476) it was found that minor improvements were reported daily during the first weeks of the trial, irrespective of whether the patients were receiving the drug or inert placebo. It was found also, that there were differences between observers in this regard. Only after this enthusiasm had waned, and a mood of healthy indifference (and even boredom) had supervened in the ward, could the effects of the active preparation be more clearly discerned. These effects, once established, showed a high relapse rate upon substitution of the active preparation by placebo.

D. Other Factors: Attitude of Investigator: Physical and Social Setting: Subject Observer Interaction

There are a number of other factors entering into the drug response in the individual human subject. Some of these have been considered recently by several authors (464, 477), and the reader is referred to these papers for more detailed guidance.

It is the experience of those working in the field that not only does the investigator's attitude influence his own observations, but that these attitudes may overtly, or covertly be transmitted both to the subject and to colleagues partaking in a study. The "double blind" and "triple blind" design (whereby the observer is not aware of the research design) mitigate against this tendency. Yet it is well to realize how the subject/observer interaction may, in fact, form the very core of the phenomena induced by psychoactive drugs, and equally, may manifest in terms of therapeutic yield. Far too little is known of such factors: we are, as yet, in no position to precisely weigh the role of verbal, and, above all, nonverbal cues in the observer/subject transaction during a drug induced state. Yet so important is this transmission of attitudes judged to be in terms of therapeutic efficacy that some centers have deliberately decided against using the double-blind technique in a clinical setting. It can, however, be shown that interactions between attitudes and drug effects can be studied within a double blind design without sacrifice of either accuracy, or a substantial loss of therapeutic efficacy.

Similarly the physical setting of a drug study may be of great moment. This does not only imply size and physical appearance of room, noise or isolation crowding or solitariness, but also such rather unexpected factors, as climate (and even weather conditions). Similarly the degree of individual isolation, the group interaction between subject and the setting, and values of the group in which the individual finds himself or, for that matter, of the institutional setting to which he belongs and the expectations of such institution, may profoundly affect the ultimate response to a particular procedure or medication. These, again, have received study without being especially related to the pharmacotherapies. Such an attempt, however, has recently been made (478).

VI. THE RELATION OF DRUG-INDUCED MENTAL CHANGES TO PSYCHODYNAMIC PROCESS

In one of his last essays Freud wrote, "We are here concerned with therapy only in so far as it works by psychological methods, and for the time being we have no other. The future may teach us how to exercise a direct influence, by means of particular chemical substances upon the amounts of energy and their distribution in the apparatus of the mind" (479). It is timely (479A) that thought in this direction be resumed, and an attempt made to relate the concepts and entities defined and postulated by psychoanalytic theory to the ordered and sequential display of endopsychic phenomena induced by the psychotropic drugs. As has been mentioned earlier, these changes bear some resemblance to other phenomena which, although transient and relatively rare, form part and parcel of normal subjective human experience. The existence and overlap of these two groups of phenomena serve to emphasize the inadequacy of this binary approach which, even at this stage, continues to distinguish between a so-called, "organic" and a "functional" or "psychodynamic" orientation. Even the briefest reflection would suggest that these viewpoints are more representative of the relative positions of the observers than of the phenomena themselves. The sharing of common elements between drug-induced states and other states encountered in the absence of drugs suggests common denominators between the physiology of the so-called normal mental life and its alteration by known chemical variables. Equally, the theories of personality structure, and an understanding of the nature of the cohesive forces entering into its organization, may be refined and gain in depth by a systematic study of drug-induced changes in man. A more consistent and careful preoccupation with such matters may contribute to an understanding of the element making for the unique effects of n particular drug in a particular clinical situation; and thus for more discrimination in their use. A careful paper by Lindemann (480) has considered some of these aspects; what follows is largely based on views expressed in this paper.

Psychoanalytic studies are concerned with the detailed analysis of conscious content, and of behavior in terms of its meaning to the individual who maintains, or is attempting to maintain, an equilibrium between inner drives, with their unconscious and preconscious aspects, and the demands of environment in an ever-changing continuum. Both normal and abnormal behavior can be seen as parts of a comprehensive action pattern of a goal-directed organism. The personality system may be regarded as the determining integrative instrument of such goal-directed behaviours, usually relating inner experience to outer perceptual cues, and relating past experience to the anticipation of future events in a way which makes the plan of action relatively satisfying, or safe. Both normal and abnormal behaviour may be viewed as attempts to maintain an optimal equilibrium compatible with particular circumstances. Such evidence as is available strongly suggests that action patterns may be profoundly influenced by patterns acquired and "learned" during an early developmental period. Equally however, behaviour at any given time is profoundly affected by the attitudes, goals, norms and aspiration of members making up the social setting of an individual. A compromise between what is innate, and past, and learnt, and what is actual and "present", is thus being struck constantly by the operation of a highly organized and continuous homeostatic adaptive process. It is this system of integrative processes which comprises the so-called Ego functions postulated by psychoanalytic theory.

It is, as yet, difficult to be certain of the precise nature of the process, which is constantly at work at various functional levels, balancing perceptual or associative cues against executive functions. In a sense it represents a continuous effort of problem solving by rehearsing anticipated situations and making choices between various possible and future actions. These symbolic duplicate models for real situations (481), which presumably are of the essence of "thought", may represent a conscious outline or mapping of an anticipated program of action. They may also show themselves in a variety of sets of imagery manifesting less in terms of a clear and anticipated action than of the emergence of a preformed and affectively charged pattern representing a compensatory fulfilment or satisfaction in situations when reality precludes appropriate action. The degree of cohesion and strength of this integrative system determines the appropriateness of the action vis-a-vis the ever-changing demands of outer reality. The functions concerned in this Ego system can operate at levels of perception, recall, anticipation, and action. They mature with growth, although even in the normal and mature individual they may falter physiologically in such instances as dreams or the experience of hypnagogic imagery. It is here that earlier and more infantile modes of thought and functioning emerge.

It is the cardinal contribution of psychoanalytic theory to regard these phenomena as part and parcel of normal human adaptive behaviour, and to view their persistent or recurrent appearance in mental disturbances, be it of a psychoneurotic or psychotic character as the emergence of highly organized compensatory mechanisms not dissimilar in character from the compensatory nature of symptoms in other clinical entities. The neurophysiological basis of these delicate and highly organized integrative processes is yet completely unexplored though one would hope that animal ethology, neurophysiology, neurochemistry and, ultimately, information theory may contribute to their understanding. To some extent these mechanisms would appear to depend on sensory input; reduction of input, as in sensory isolation experiments (482), strikingly alters levels of awareness and of consciousness, and the ordered exceedingly rapid processes which makes for appropriate action in terms of the "here and now". Some aspects of these dysfunctions of the brain as an organ of information in relation to schizophrenic disorder have been considered by the author elsewhere (483).

In a more limited sense, a not dissimilar course is observed in the process of free association during personal analysis. As is common knowledge, this is arranged to facilitate the influx into consciousness of material previously stored at preconscious or unconscious levels. Those experienced in the technique know how material, which at first may look confused and lacking in pattern, does in fact arrange itself in an ordered and meaningful way, and how emotional attachments to incidents, figures, and objects in the patient's early environment are later transferred to the therapist. This transference situation is accompanied by a reliving and rehandling of a previous situation not possible during the original adaptive process. It is this "working-through" on the part of the patient in the face of a challenge posed by previous unresolved conflicts which is reputed to make ultimately for therapeutic success. Equally, it is possible that during these intensely charged states the executive functions of the ego may be so overwhelmed by a return of the affect originally attached to older events that an "acting-out" of the original experience is now possible, or likely. It is this "acting-out" which poses serious problems in the management of severe neurotic disturbances, and in the psychotic states in which the integrative functions of the ego are most seriously disturbed.

In the light of the above considerations, it may now be relevant briefly to examine the possible effects of organic variables (including drugs) on these integrative functions. To be sure accurate information in this regard is only slowly becoming available, and such knowledge as has been attained comes from the study of organic brain injury, deliria, and, to a lesser extent, sensory isolation. Drug effects while having certain elements in common with other nonpharmacological challenges differ from them in certain important respects. In terms of chemistry, dosage and interaction, drugs can be discriminate, delicate, and capable of varied manipulation. It is, however already apparent that, although certain special features may attach to special drugs, it may be a gross over-simplification to speak of drug-specific reactivity patterns. On the contrary, experience suggests that *the same drug, in the same dose, in the same subject may produce very different effects according to the precise interpersonal and motivational situation in which it is given.* In the integrative functions with which it interferes, and in the "set" which it alters, environment both past present, and anticipated, plays a dominant part. Such factors must be constantly taken into account in a study of the integration and disintegration of ego functions. On the other hand, the perceptual and cognitive modalities may very definitely play a part in this process. It is, for example, known that full doses of some drugs such as mescalin, LSD-25 or marihuana may lead to a marked distortion of perception which is likely to be due to a disorganisation, at a high central level, of the coding of information coming from the sense or ans. Again, ego rupture may show itself by a disturbance of the critical appraisal of perceptual cues, and s reduction in the caution with which plans of action are usually integrated with percept; or again, by a striking reduction of involvement on the part of the subject in the phenomena which he may be witnessing, often accompanied by a striking motor inactivity seen in such subjects. The range of of phenomena indeed is wide. The intense and dramatic quality of perceptual distortion and dream imagery should not detract from the equally relevant changes in other areas. It is perhaps significant that most of these changes have been observed with relatively large doses. The discriminate and systematic study of small, graded doses in individual subjects has so far received far too little attention.

With such considerations in mind, it may be appropriate to review briefly the implications of the psychotropic drugs for individual psychotherapy. Drugs for example, can be used to facilitate the influx of material into consciousness, their so-called psycho-exploratory or abreactive use. This can be accomplished by small doses of sedatives such as amylobarbital. The light induction stage of ether anaesthesia (484) has been used to obtain a similar effect. Again, some so-called stimulant drugs, such as amphetamine and methylamphetamine, have been used for the same purpose (485). More recently LSD-25 (486, 487) in varying doses, or mescalin (488) have also been employed. The use of these drugs demands the most careful case selection, and thorough familiarly with individual psychopathology of the particular patient. The main indication for LSD-25 therapy so far have been severe and crippling neuroses, particularly of the obsessional kind, neurotic reaction forms related to a known psychological trauma, and certain character disorders. The known contra-indications are the appearance of severe conversion symptoms, anxiety states, depressive or suicidal states developing after the first three or four treatments. The dangers have been recently reviewed (489) The use of the psychosomimetic drugs as part of a deliberate therapeutic process must, for the present, be regarded as purely exploratory and experimental; though the theoretical yield in this field could, indeed, be very great.

The role of the tranquillizers, both major and minor, in psychotherapy is strictly limited, their use being essentially symptomatic. These drugs can serve in the management of those phases of s psychotherapeutic process where anxiety may be severe and overwhelming enough to lead to an "acting-out" on the part of the patient with consequences likely to be unacceptable or dangerous to the patient or those around him. The greatest care and judgement is required in the use of these drugs in this therapeutic setting; for it must be clear that an affective blunting, induced by full doses of tranquillisers, is essentially incompatible with a relearning, which is at the very core of successful psychotherapy. The indiscriminate use of such drugs is likely to confirm the very infirmities it is wished to relieve. Anxiety quantities, which operate as signals for the presense of alarming and challenging situations, are important items to be mastered by the personality in the course of its development and normal function. If they are reduced, their contribution to personality growth in terms of increasing anxiety-tolerance or frustration-tolerance is hampered. This is illustrated in certain common situations, such as grief states, where early confrontation and acceptance of severe mental pain leads ultimately to their successful resolution. Symptoms can be evidence of constructive psychological work as much as of defect. The indiscriminate use of tranquillizers in such states is likely to lead to an unresolved, extended state, resulting in obtunding, depression, and a continuing pathological process.

VII. SOME IMPLICATIONS OF THE FUTURE USE OF THE PSYCHOTROPIC DRUGS: THEIR EFFECTS ON HOSPITAL MILIEU, AND THE GENERAL FUNCTIONAL PATTERN OF THE MENTAL HOSPITAL

In an age of revolutions, one is apt to get used to revolutions. In considering the impact of the pharmacotherapies on the management of the psychoses in a mental hospital, one is apt to be reminded of the violent changes brought about in the past by the introduction of other somatic therapies, such as deep insulin coma, electroshock and the lobotomies. Each of these has wielded changes, based essentially upon relatively short-term results; only in recent years could these be viewed against the perspectives of long-term follow-up studies. The changes in management, and the attendant changes in attitude, however, have stayed and become cumulative. It is quite possible that a similar fate may befall the pharmacotherapies of mental disorders, though three important differences distinguish them from earlier treatment and encourage a more hopeful view. The first is the fact that these therapies can be graded and made individual in a way, which was quite impossible with the less variable and massive procedures used in the past. Secondly, they can be used on a scale far larger than the earlier therapies. Thirdly, whereas in the past systematic studies of mode of action followed essentially empirical findings and measures, the empirical findings of the pharmacotherapies are being increasingly related to a growing body of modern theoretical neuropharmacology and neurochemistry. Theories are thus likely to keep abreast of clinical findings in a way never before witnessed in psychiatry; and are likely to make these ever more precise, discriminate and long-term.

The impact of the drug therapies on mental hospital population is essentially threefold. They have altered the immediate management and treatment of certain types of acutely disturbed psychotic patients; they have mobilised large chronic populations hitherto excluded in the continued-treatment units of the average mental hospital; and, in individual cases, have made possible measures of rehabilitation which would have been very difficult to achieve in their absence. Lastly, they have increased and made more urgent the contacts between the mental hospital and the community. In terms of all these effects the drugs are wielding profound changes in staff attitudes at all professional levels. The precise pattern of these changes at present is far from dear, and for the moment can only be discussed in the broadest terms.

Effect on Staff Attitudes and the Demand for Fresh Skills

There seems little doubt, on the evidence so far available, that the drugs have confronted the staff with a challenge unlike any challenge experienced during similar periods of transition in the past. The more ready management of the overtly disturbed patients has already been referred to; yet, as any sensitive observer will have noted, this may merely reflect the manifest shell of a state of mind in which the patient, perhaps for the first time may be accessible to individual and group influences from which a defensive pathological process has shielded him hitherto. The patient's environment (of which his physician, or ward personnel, or other patients, or family, or friends are an inseparable part) becomes more meaningful, for good or ill. It is significant that staff attitudes to this change are by no means uniform, and may reflect long-standing idiosyncrasies. Some may welcome this change; others may lapse into a significant denial that any change has occurred at all. In sum, some take up the challenge; while others transfer their own responsibilities to the chemicals, which they are now happy to employ. There is little doubt, even in the light of relatively short clinical experience that the increased accessibility of patients seen in some forms of pharmacotherapy (for example in the so-called overactive or turbulent phase of reserpine therapy or the state following treatment by some stimulant compounds, such as amphetamine, iproniazid, or LSD-25) offers novel and yet totally unexplored opportunities in terms of both individual and group psychotherapy. The modulating effect of the group, be it composed of patient, nurses or attendants, and their varying interaction with each other, can profoundly affect norms of individual behavior within the group. Equally, the play of transference and counter-transference situations within the group of s ward community can be used to great effect, and, incidentally, supply the social psychiatrists and sociologists with a wealth of material for research. Thus, the acquisition of elementary skills in group process, and the management of the acute and fluctuating changes seen in these processes may be forced by pharmacotherapies in a measure quite unforeseen at their inception. It is usual to think of such skills in terms of medical personnel only. It is submitted that this is an error. Anyone working in this field cannot fail to be impressed by the high stores of ability and skills to be found in nurses, aides and attendants in meeting the day-to-day needs of patients for intimate human relationship. Quite apart from any other consideration, the degree and continuity of the patients' exposure to ward personnel ensures their central position in any therapeutic or rehabilitative programme. Formation of ward clubs, for example, under the (passive) leadership of a charge nurse or senior aide, or even patient, may go a long way towards changing the day-to day milieu of the ward in which the individual patient functions. Properly considered and balanced, such measures may contribute greatly towards distributing therapeutic skills, and making the most of the scarce medical skills that are available.

It is important in this context that early and thorough thought be given to a definition of the skills needed to carry the pharmacotherapies to their full yield. A good deal of initial consideration has also to be given to the types of investigators who are likely to contribute maximally to a definition of these situations and skills. It is the writer's impression that only rarely can observers with a purely academic training in one of the social or behavioral sciences be taught the relevant action cues to a therapeutic transaction, (be it individual or social), unless they have worked in the mental hospital themselves. On the other hand, these very skills can often be found in a native state in relatively untrained personnel though their definition and analysis may be beyond their power. It is suggested that on the one hand, research nurses, research attendants, and research ward administrators be selected from the most promising professional personnel working at an operational level, and that they be joined by investigators of more formal training who could serve in the formulation and communication of the operation.

Changing Patient Needs: Effect on Layout of Future Treatment Units and of Extramural Treatment Facilities

There is a further area in which the evolution of the pharmacotherapies may bear upon the functional pattern of the mental hospital. The emergence of new categories of patients is becoming increasingly apparent and may powerfully influence the layout and architecture of the future treatment unit. A commensurate grouping of patients according to changing therapeutic needs is clearly necessary: yet it is far from definite what these changing needs are, since no adequate quantitative data in this regard are at present available. Empirical findings suggest that a small proportion of chronic patients may be capable of family placement. Again some patients, though disagreeable, are unsuitable for rehabilitation without disrupting family structure, and require sheltered work, or a hostel type of accommodation in a type of institution only sparsely available, yet quite distinct from a mental hospital, or a geriatric ward, or the average industrial rehabilitation center. With some patients the family, though able to accept them, is unwilling to do so. Others may require a minimum of general medical and psychiatric care and may be better left in a setting such as a mental hospital from which they may pursue daily extramural work. The patients may thus require varying degrees of general medical skill and nursing care; of social or individual psychiatric care; of extramural vis-...-vis intramural employment; of contact with, or avoidance of, their families; of re-education or industrial training; or of continued chronic institutional isolation. The pattern is changing constantly. No accurate figures in this respect are available, and systematic surveys in representative sample populations will have to be undertaken before any valid conclusions in this respect can be drawn.

These considerations are bound to affect the layout of the mental hospital itself, and of the extramural facilities with which it is connected. Within the hospital, more Day Space will be needed and the bay-type ward (giving privacy with a maximum of open space) may well gain support. More intramural workshop and light-industrial space will also be required, as will more club space and perhaps even residential family accommodation for the occasional problem family. Equally, more space will be needed for group meetings and for contacts with professional and non-professional personnel within the community, such as the general practitioner and the visiting nurse and health worker. Furthermore, a totally new type of institution may be required for those patients who no longer belong to the mental hospital proper, are employable, need a minimum of nursing care, yet cannot be returned to their families without disrupting the family structure. Yet other institutions may be needed for patients who may require high degrees of care and even security measures.

It is quite impossible to predict the precise proportion of these various services (or their precise location in relation to other treatment units) without first thoroughly surveying the needs in different cultural settings. It would, however, be prudent not to be misled by the initial discharge figures, which may boomerang into high readmission figures with the passage of time. It is, nevertheless, clear that the pharmacotherapies are likely to affect these figures both ways (490); but not the pharmacotherapies alone. The concept of a therapeutic community is emerging not only from within the mental hospitals themselves, but also from a consideration of the relationship of the mental hospital services to general hospital services. In as far as can be judged at present, one is inclined to envisage relatively small mental treatment units geographically close to general hospitals; a wide zone of out-patient and social rehabilitative services subserving both general and mental services; mobile extramural teams centered on these services; and central research and statistical services, guiding the work of both.

The Use of Psychotropic Drugs in the Community: Behavioral Toxicity and the Problem of Self-Medication

Mild sedation, mild stimulation, or a combination of both has been an ever-present feature of treatment in general practice and in the outpatient setting. It is therefore not surprising that with the increasing incidence of mild stress disorders, and the initial high promise held out by the psychotropic drugs in the psychoses, enthusiasm should have been high for their possible us in the neuroses also. The last five years have seen an enormous increase in the consumption of these drugs within the open community. No doubt massive commercial pressures and suggestibility have played their part. There are, however encouraging signs that the many ignorances which led to this regrettable and dangerous state of affairs are being recognized and faced. The dust is settling and the limitations of these drugs in general practice and in the open community are emerging slowly and unmistakeably.

There are several false assumptions, which lie at the bottom of the use of these drugs in outpatient practice. The first is that their usefulness in the psychoses implies a role in the neuroses also. This view does not take into account the profound differences in drug reactivity between the fully established psychotic patient and the neurotic reaction type, or the normal. Dose range alone suggests these differences to be very real. Secondly, it is often thought that a chemical splinting of a disturbed pattern of adaptive behaviour in which the symptoms are part of a highly reactive fluctuating process could lead to a resolution of the disorder; it does nothing of the kind, and may in fact impair the very adaptive powers upon which recovery depends. Thirdly the illusion of the nontoxicity of this group of drugs is essentially based on the old concept of somatic aide effects and somatic toxicity. It is, however, becoming quite clear that a totally new type of toxicity, taking into account slight and subtle decrement in mental functioning and deficits in behaviour, is needed to describe the phenomena most commonly observed in the abuse of these drugs. The problem of psychological drug-dependence, and of addiction (491) also arises. In these areas no adequate data are available.

The problem of self-medication and of effectiveness of the minor tranquillisers has been touched on a number of occasions (491–493). One such paper (494) has examined its impact upon a large number of patients presenting principally symptoms of anxiety. One-third of the patients reported ill-effects, many of them quite serious. Another (495) compared in controlled trial the effects of benactizyne and placebo. The trial periods and numbers here were regrettably short, but within the limits of this particular trial, patients were found to react more favourably to amylobarbital and placebo than any of the tranquillizers used in the study. Whatever differences may have been missed, they cannot obviously have been very great. Many more instances of this kind could be quoted.

It is suggested that no accurate information on the subject will be available until several distinct aspects of the problem are covered by suitably planned inquiries. The first is a systematic survey, in the light of data available from manufacturers, the distributive trade and responsible public bodies, of the scale and the pattern of consumption of drugs obtainable without prescription, as well as the drugs prescribed in representative samples of out-patient services and of general practice. Secondly, the minimal safe doses must be defined not merely in terms of somatic side effects such as skin eruption, agranulocytosis, jaundice, Parkinsonism, purpura, tremor, but also in terms of the subjective reduction of well-being and objective behavioural deficits (such as reduction of motor skill, sluggishness, recklessness, or lack of judgement). Marked mental side effects such as undue depression (relatively common in, for example, out-patient use of reserpine in hypertensives) must also be allowed for. Thirdly, an inquiry into the factors making for self-medication in different samples of the population in relation to social class and cultural background is needed. Equally, a complementary inquiry into the motives of the general practitioner making for particular idiosyncrasies of choice must be inquired into. It is only upon the basis of such information that any recommendations can become more than well intentioned empirical measures. It is clear that here as in every other area of mental health, psychopharmacology interacts powerfully with sociology and so-cial psychiatry. In the area of the psychoses the pharmacotherapies may decisively prepare the ground for the long and highly skilled task of individual and social rehabilitation. In the field of the neuroses the obverse may well be true; as psychotherapeutic skills become more wide-spread and the fundamental principles of human adaptive behaviour freed of theoretical en-cumbrances, become increasingly part of the body of general medical education and medical practice, the out-patient use of the psychotropic drugs will shrink to small and reasonable pro-portions. Public reactions (both medical and lay) indicate that this day may not be too distant.

VIII. MEASUREMENT IN THE CLINICAL SETTING: THE NEED FOR METHODOLOGICAL TOOLS

It will have become apparent from the foregoing how manifold are the methodological dif-ficulties which beset the field under discussion (496, 464). To attribute these specifically to the pharmacotherapies would be misleading; rather would it seem that these therapies are forcing many issues which have lain dormant in psychiatry (and, indeed, in the human behav-ioral sciences) for some time. These issues are likely to be encountered in any setting, where psychotropic drugs are used. They may be seen at the level of the normal volunteer, the indi-vidual patient, the clinical trial in small or large groups, within a hospitals, or in the commu-nity at large. They impinge upon such problems as the individual variation and the placebo re-sponses, the careful use of descriptive terms, and the selection and training of observers. Only a few aspects will be touched upon by way of closing.

The Calibration of Linguistic Tools: The Assessment of the Non-Verbal Element

It may be justifiably argued that, for the present, clinical observation and judgement remain the moat sensitive research tool in any large-scale study of psychotropic agents. Yet several major sources of error pervade it. The first is the time sampling of the clinical interview or clinical "impression". This interview usually takes place in the physician's office, in s setting totally different from the patient s usual ward environment; it represents a special sample of the patient's total 24-hour cycle; and may, in part, be actually influenced by the interview situ-ation. Whatever its merits, it certainly is not a sample of "free" behaviour. Secondly the inter-view, unless carefully (though imperceptibly) structured, may omit facets which, though un-important in the immediate context, may turn out to have important bearing upon an aspect of later research. Thirdly, the method usually employed for recording is descriptive and anec-dotal. According to the skills of a particular interviewer the picture ultimately given may be more, or less, accurate or complete. Fourthly, whatever the picture, it does not, as a rule, take account of the observations of persons other than the interviewer – thus again reflecting the re-striction of the time-sample of the average clinical examination.

It is the third of the questions raised above which is perhaps the most pertinent; for it is ob-vious that unless the phenomena seen are described and grouped in a way which conveys them accurately and reliably to others, they can hardly be more than personal impressions. For that reason, the calibration of terms which would minimise descriptive overlap and ambiguity, must be at the very core of any research in this peculiarly clinical field. Various research docu-ments have been and are being developed to do justice to the problem, and to measure im-provement and deterioration in the individual patient (497). Some employ glossaries, some checklists, some three or five point scales: all of them, however, attempt to describe the clinical change in terms likely to minimise semantic error. It is only fair to say that, in any calibration of a scale or document by several independent observers (through an "identity-parade" type of presentation of selected patients), the observers are usually drawn from the same hospital or group of hospitals. In fact, having defined their terms, physicians learn to use them, and begin to work as a group. It is a totally different matter to know how other professional groups would receive the same scale. Such inter-hospital comparisons are now in progress. It would indeed be most instructive to determine the frequency with which different terms were being used to describe different phenomena. The most appropriate terms may thus, in time, be encouraged to survive, and others to lapse by disuse. The same problem applies with even more force to assessment of behavioural change by non-medical personnel; the day nurse, the night nurse, the aide, the psychiatric social worker, even the patient's relatives on visiting day (or when the patient is out visiting) see the patient for much longer periods than the physician, and may thus (if properly selected) become most valuable to members of the observers' team. Yet unless they agree to use particular terms to describe particular phenomena, it is difficult to form a firm opinion of a particular clinical state. Here, too, then, semantic problems become paramount in document design. It is suggested that, in this area, problems will be more readily solved if the terms finally agreed are based upon terms used most frequently by the more intelligent and senior non-medical staff, and that solution will only be delayed by the imposition of new words of essentially medical connotation; the terms should be simple, direct and unambiguous, and unencumbered by technical jargon.

Another aspect concerns the assessment of the non-verbal element. It has been claimed that the language of gesture if properly used is the most economical form of communication available (498). Little is known of the precise organization of these patterns of expression: In any psychoanalytic work, one is certainly impressed by the information contained in all aspects of non-verbal behaviour. These clues are more familiar to those who think intuitively than to those with a strongly deductive bent of mind; to artists rather than scientists. An analysis of the phenomena, however, is possible.

Essentially, again, the problem is one of method; a fully developed clinical sense pays much attention to averbal clues. But for more precise information two aspects come to mind. The first is the documentation of a total situation, which includes both verbal and non-verbal elements, and the separate and independent analysis of these two aspects. The second is the correlation between what is expressed averbally and what, in fact, is perceived by the observer. The first is made possible by the sound-film technique, and by separate analysis of the sound track, the silent film, and the various aspects of mime in such a film record of an ordinary experimental session. The second, by the independent scoring (in terms of rank order) by subject and observer of items of importance at any particular time throughout a session, and a comparison of these rank orders in terms of coincidence, or lack of correlation. It is quite obvious that such a process is not only laborious but expensive; yet if a clearer understanding of non-verbal communication (499) is to be reached, it will, sooner or later, have to be undertaken in some such way. The writer has examined the problems of subjective and objective observation in psychiatry elsewhere (500).

A further aspect, which has already been touched upon, is the lack of any agreed language to describe the unusual drug-induced subjective states. Here, again, familiarity with these phenomena will no doubt create new semantic tools. These however, will have to be used with the greatest care and discrimination until the unusual qualities which they describe have, in fact, been thoroughly and adequately explored..

The Selection of Observers, and Some Requirements of Trial Design

The foregoing remarks serve to bring into focus dependence of any interpretation of the effects of psychotropic drugs in man on the quality of the observers taking part in an investigation, particularly since the observation of total behaviour may depend much more upon non-medical than medical personnel. It has been found repeatedly in trials conducted in mental hospitals, or in out-patient clinics, that even one biased and unreliable observer can undo the work of a carefully organized group. The selection of observers, therefore, lies at the very core of any drug trial.

A procedure which has been found useful by the writer, is to select a small group of staff, both medical and non-medical, irrespective of rank, and to submit them to a "trial of a trial" procedure. This essentially consists in allowing them to observe a small group of patients intensively over a fixed (say four week) period, and determining the skill with which they note and describe change in terms previously agreed. It is remarkable and rewarding to note how many competent observers can be found in the non-dominant as well as the dominant strata of a particular professional group. A small group having been selected, discussion meetings are arranged in which methodology of a particular trial (be it in-patients or out-patients) is gone into, the semantic criteria finally agreed, and suitable documents carefully considered and accepted. A two-phase placebo trial (comprising an "active" and an "inactive" placebo) is then begun and the correlation between the different observers again noted. It is this period which has been found particularly important; for it is then that the research instrument, in the shape of a *group* of people, is beginning to form, and a common and agreed language is found to emerge by trial and error. In an early trial on chlorpromazine (476) it was found that the nurses and aides gradually became the most valuable members of the research team, and it was upon the retrospective examination of their completed documents that an assessment could most reliably be based. It was also found that the attitude of the staff changed perceptibly as the trial proceeded, and that new recruits for the observer teams were continuously brought forward. Some of these had to be rejected because of over-enthusiasm and suggestibility; others stayed to be trained further.

It is a debatable point whether at this stage it is advisable to convey to the observers, in the course of their training, more than the elements of psychopharmacology. Too detailed a discussion and, most particularly, too detailed a description of symptoms and changes, may merely result in the appearance of these symptoms in subsequent records. It is best to maintain a friendly but neutral attitude; to answer specific questions, and to keep interest alive, without, if possible, biasing the subject in any way.

A great deal could be said of the desiderata of trial design, which have been considered at previous meetings (496) and only the briefest summary is in place here. A trial should be *long,* that is, long enough for the spontaneous fluctuations in the clinical picture (and in the long-term effects of any drug) to manifest unequivocally; but not too long to offset its own advantages by loss of initiative on the part of personnel. 12 to 16 weeks would seem a suitable period. It should be *blind,* the code being, unknown to anyone concerned with the conduct of the trial. It should be both *inter-group controlled* and *self-controlled,* that is, the patient (in the latter case) acting as his own control, and the drug (in different doses, and with placebo to match these different doses) being administered alternately over repeated periods. It should be *documented* by keeping a round-the clock record of behaviour thus necessitating observations on the part of non-medical as well as medical personnel (day nurse, night nurse, aides, psychiatric social worker, general practitioner, the patient's relatives, and the patient himself). It should be *statistically validated* both in design and in assessment; and finally it should be based on the retrospective and blind examination of documents, and only subsequently matched against the code of the trial. Some of these conditions – long-term planning, observer training and blind design – could be met in almost any hospital community. Equally, it is obvious that the amount of the information obtained from a trial will depend entirely on the scope of the questions, which are being posed. These will vary with the character of the hospital or community in which the investigation is being planned, and it is most desirable that they be specified in the fullest possible detail. Thus psychopharmacology, by the very questions it poses in the clinical field, furthers the tools of social psychiatry; and it is upon the interaction of these two areas and their relation to developmental process in man, that the growth of Clinical Psychiatry within the next decade may well depend.

The author gratefully acknowledges the help of his secretary, Mrs. Edna Van Lill, and Mrs. Jeanette Pearce (Librarian, The Adolf Meyer Library, Phipps Clinic) in checking the references.

REFERENCES[*]

1. Kety, S. S. (Ed.): The Pharmacology of Psychotomimetic and Psychotherapeutic Drugs. N. Y. Acad. Sci. 66 (1957).
2. Wikler, A.: The Relation of Psychiatry to Pharmacology. Baltimore: Williams and Wilkins 1957.
3. Garattini, S. and V. Ghetti (Eds.): Psychotropic Drugs. Amsterdam: Elsevier Publ. Co. 1957.
4. Cole, J. O., and R. W. Gerard (Eds.): Psychopharmacology Problems in Evaluation. National Academy of Sciences, National Research Council. Washington 1959.
5. Kline, N. S. (Ed.): Psychopharmacology Frontiers. Boston: Little, Brown Co. 1959.
6. Bradley, P. B., P. Deniker, C. Raduoco-Thomas (Ed.): Neuropsychopharmacology. Amsterdam: Elsevier 1959.
7. Lewin, L.: Phantastica, Narcotic and Stimulating Drugs – Their Use and Abuse. New York: Cutton 1931.
8. Stoll W. A.: Lysergs"ure-diethylamid – ein Phantastikum aus der Mutterkorngruppe. Schweiz. Arch. Neurol. Psychiat. 60. 279-323 (1947).
9. Beringer, K.: Der Meskalinrausch. Berlin 1927.
10. Mayer-Gross W. and H. Stein: šber einige Ab"nderungen der Sinnest"tigkeit im Meskalinrausch. Z. ges. Neurol. Psychiat. 101, 354 (1926).
11. Galton, F.: The Visions of Sane Persons. Pop. Sci. Month. New York 29, 519-531 (1881).
12. Galton, F.: Statistics of Mental Imagery. Mind 5 301-318 (1880).
13. James, W.: The Varieties of Religious Experience. A Study in Human Nature (Gifford Lectures on Natural Religion 1901/02). New York: Longmans 1928.
14. Müller, J. v.: Physiology of the Senses, Voice and Muscular Motion (Müller's Elements of Physiology and Supplement). London: Taylor, Walton & Maberly 1848.
15. Leaning, F. E.: Proc. Soc. Psychic Res.35 (1925).
16. Ladd G. T.: Contributions to the Psychology of Visual Dreams. Mind (new series) (London) 1, 299-304 (1892).
17. Mitchell S. W.: Remarks on the Effects of Anhelonium Lewinii (The Mescal Button). Brit. Med. J. 1896 II, 1625-1629.
18. Ellis, H.: The World of Dreams. London 1911.
19. Klüver, H.: Mescal, the "Divine" plant and its psychological effects. London 1928.
20. Klüver H.: Mechanisms of Hallucinations. p. 175. In: Q. McMemar and M. A. Merrill, L (Eds.): Studies in Personality, New York 1942.
21. Hilgard E. R. L., S. Kubie, and E. Pumpian-Mindlin (Eds.) Psychoanalysis as Science. Stanford Univ. Press 1952.
22. Stewart, C. C.: Variations in Daily Activity Produced by Alcohol and by Changes in Barometric Pressure and Diet. With a Description of Recording Methods. Amer. J. Physiol. 1, 40 (1898).
23. Pavlov, I. P.: Conditioned Reflexes. London 1927.
24. Gantt, W. H.: Physiological Bases of Psychiatry. Springfield. Chaa. C. Thomas 1958.
25. Massermann, T.: Behavioral Pharmacology in Animals. In: Neuropyschopharmacology, p. 97, Bradley P. B. et al. (Eds.). Amsterdam: Elsevier 1959.
26. Miller, N. E.: Objective Techniques for Studying Motivational Effects of Drugs on Animals. In: Psychotropic Drugs, p. 83, Garattini, S., and V. Ghetti (Eds.). Amsterdam: Elsevier 1957.
27. Brady, J. V.: Procedures, Problems and Perspectives in Animal Behavioral Studies of Drug Activity. In: Psychopharmacology, Problems in Evaluation, p. 255. Cole, J C. and R. W. Gerard (Eds.). National Academy of Sciences, National Research Council, Washington 1959.
28. Rosvold, H. E.: Evaluation of the Effects of Pharmacological Agents on Social Behavior. In: Psychopharmacology, Problems in Evaluation. Loc. cit. p. 244, 1959.

---

[*] The references in the present article end in 1961. In a subject advancing as rapidly as Psychopharmacology this may mark the paper as one more concerned with a "Psychopharmakologie der Vergangenheit" than "der Gegenwart." The author however is less intent to keep up to date than to outline, however broadly, the constants of the subject, as they appear to him.

29. Beach F. A.: A Review of Physiological and Psychological Studies of Sexual Behavior in Mammals. Physiol. Rev. 27, 240 (1947).
30. Sequard, J. P.: Genetic Differences in Hoarding. J. comp. physiol. Psychol. 47, 157 (1954).
31. Carpenter, C. R.: Societies of Monkeys and Apes. Biol. Sympos. 8, 177 (1942).
32. Lorenz, K. Z.: The Comparative Method in Studying Innate Behavior Patterns. In: Physiological Mechanisms in Animal Behavior Patterns, pp. 221-288. London: Cambridge University Press 1950.
33. Tinbergen, N.: The Hierarchical Organization of the Nervous Mechanisms underlying Instinctive Behavior. In: Physiological Mechanisms in Animal Behavior Patterns, pp. 305-312. London: Cambridge University Press 1950.
34. Waelsch, H. (Ed.): Biochemistry of the Developing Nervous System. New York: Academic Press 1955.
35. Hess, E. H.: Effects of Meprobamate on Imprinting in Waterfowl. Ann. N. Y. Acad. Sci. 67, 724-732 (1957).
36. Elkes J., J. T. Eayrs, and A. Todrick: On the Effect, and Lack of Effect of Some Drugs on Postnatal Development in the Rat. In:. Waelsch, H. (Ed.). Biochemistry of the Developing Nervous System, N.Y.: Academic Press 1955.
37. Gunn, J. A., and M. R. Gurd: Action of Some Amines Related to Adrenaline. Cyclohexylalkylamines. J. Physiol. (Lond.) 97, 453 (1940).
38. Chance M. R. A.: Aggression as Factor Influencing Toxicity of Sympathomimetic Amines in Mice. J. Pharmacol. exp. Ther. 87, 214 (1946).
39. Chance, M. R. A.: Factors Influencing Toxicity of Sympathomimetic Amines to Solitary Mice. J. Pharmacol. exp. Ther. 89, 289 (1947).
40. Chance, M. R. A.: Personal Communication.
41. Lasagna, L. and W. P. McCann: Effect of Tranquilizing Drugs on Amphetamine Toxicity in Aggregated Mice. Science 125, 1241 (1957).
42. Evarts, E. Y.: A Discussion of the Relevance of Effects on Animal Behavior to the Possible Effects of Drugs on Psychopathological Process in Man. In: Psychopharmacology, Problems in Evaluation. Cole, J. C., and R. W. Gerard (Eds.). National Academy of Sciences National Research Council, p. 284. Washington 1959.
43. Schmitt, F. O.: The Structure and Properties of Nerve Membranes. In: Richter, D. (Ed.). Metabolism of the Nervous System, p. 35. London. Pergamon Press 1957.
44. Elkes, J., and J. B. Finean: The Effect of Drying upon the Structure of Myelin in the Sciatic Nerve of the Frog. Diac. Faraday Soc. 6, 134 (1949).
45. Elkes, J., and J. B. Finean: Effects of Solvents on the Structure of Myelin in the Sciatic Nerve of the Frog. Exp. Cell. Res. 4, 32 (1953).
46. Pope A.: The Relationship of Neurochemistry to the Microscopic Anatomy of the Nervous System, p. 341. In: Waelsch, H. (Ed.). Biochemistry of the Developing Nervous System. New York: Academic Press 1955.
47. Lowry, O. H.: A Study of the Nervous System with Quantitative Histochemical Methods. In: Waelsch, H. (Ed.). loc. cit. p. 350.
48. Jasper, H. H., et al. (Eds.). The Reticular Formation of the Brain. Henry Ford Hospital International Symposium. Boston: Little, Brown and Co. 1958.
49. MacLean, P. D.: The Limbic System ("Visceral Brain") in Relation to Central Gray and Reticulum of the Brain Stem. Psychocom. Med.17, 355 (1955).
50. Olds, J.: Selective Effects of Drives and Drugs on "Reward" Systems of the Brain. In: Neurological Basis of Behaviour, p.124. Wolstenholme, G. E. W., and C. M. O'Connor (Eds.). London: J. A. Churchill 1958.
51. Ingram W. R., F. L. Hannet, and S.W. Ranson. The Topography of the Nuclei of the Diencephalon of the Cat. J. comp. Neurol. 55, 333 (l932).
52. Ingram, W. R.: Nuclear Organization and Chief Connections of the Primate Hypothalamus. Ass. Res. nerv. ment. Dis. 20, 195 (1940).
53. Olszewski, J.: The Cytoarchitecture of the Human Reticular Formation. In: Brain Mechanisms and Consciousness, p. 54. Delafresnaye, J. F. (Ed.). Oxford: Blackwell 1954.
54. Adey, R. W. Organization of the Rhinencephalon. In: The Reticular Formation of the Brain. Loc. cit. p. 621.
55. Nauta, W. J.: Hippocampal Projections and Related Neural Pathways to the Mid-brain in the Cat. Brain 81, 319 (1958).
56. French, J. D.: Corticofugal Connections with the Reticular Formation. In: The Reticular Formation of the Brain, p. 491. Jasper, H. H., et al. (Eds.). Boston: Little, Brown and Co.1958.
57. Brobeck, J. R.: Neural Regulation of Food Intake. Ann. N. Y. Acad. Sci. 63, 44 (1955).
58. Anderson, B., P. A. Jewell, and S. Larsson. In: Neurological Basis of Behaviour. Wolstenholme, G. E. W., and C. M. O'Connor (Eds.). Loc. cit. p. 76, 1958.
59. Sawyer, C. H.: The Reticular Formation of the Brain; loc. cit. pp. 223-229.
60. Vogt, M.: The Concentration of Sympathin in Different Parts of the Central Nervous System Under Normal Conditions and After the Administration of Drugs. J. Physiol. (London) 123, 451 (1954).
61. Twarog B. M., and I. H. Page: Serotonin Content of Some Mammalian Tissues and Urine and a Method for its Determination. Amer. J. Physiol.175, 157-161 (1953).
62. Roberts, E., P. J. Harman, and S. Frankel: Gamma Aminobutyric Acid Content and Glutamic Decarboxylase Activity in Developing Mouse Brain. Proc. Soc. esp. Biol. N. Y. 78, 799 (1951).
63. Elkes J.: Effects of Psychosomimetic Drugs in Animal and Man. In: Neuropharmacology, pp. 205-295: Trans action of the 3rd Conf.. Josiah Macy, jr., Found. Abramson, H. A. (Ed.). Madison, N. J.: Madison Printing .1957.
64. Dell, P. G.: Humoral Effects on the Brain Stem Reticular Formations. In: The Reticular Formation of the Brain; loc. cit. pp. 365-379 1958.
65. Bradley, P.B., J. Elkes: The Effects of Some Drugs on the Electrical Activity of the Brain. Brain 80, 77-117 (1957).
66. Elkes J.: Drugs Effects in Relation to Receptor Specificity within the Brain. Some Evidence and Provisional Formulation. In: Ciba Foundation Symposium on the Neurological Basis of Behavior, p. 303. Wolstenholme, G. E. W., and C. M. O'Connor (Eds.). London: J. A. Churchill 1958.

67. Elkes, J.: Drugs Influencing Affect and Behaviour. Proceedings of Kaiser Hospital Symposium on The Physiology of Emotions. Featherstone, R. M., and A. Simon (Eds.) Springfield Ill.: C. C. Thomas 1961.
68. McCullogh, W. S., and W. Pitts: A Logical Calculus of Ideas Immanent in Nervous Activity. Bull. Math. Biophys. 5, 115-133 (1943).
69. Uttley, A. M.: The Classification of Signals in the Nervous System. EEG Clin. Neurophysiol. 6, 479-494 (1954).
70. MacKay, D. M.: The Nomenclature of Information Theory. Symposium on Information Theory, London, pp. 194-195 1950.
71. Sholl. D. A.: A Dendritic Organization in Neurons of Visual and Motor Cortices of the Cat. J. Anat. (London) 87, 387 (1953).
72. Galambos, R., and H. Davis: The Responses of Single Auditory Nerve Fibres to Acoustic Stimulation. J. Neurophysiol 6 39-57 (1943).
73. Allanson, J. T. and I. C. Whitfield: The Cochlear Nucleus and its Relation to Theories of Hearing. Third London Symposium on Information Theory, p. 269. Cherry, C. (Ed.). London: Butterworth 1956.
74. Kuffler, S. W.: Neurones in the Retina: Organization, Inhibition and Excitation Problems. Cold Spr. Harb. Symp. quant. Biol.17, 281-292 (1952).
75. Whitfield, I. C.: The Physiology of Hearing. Progr. Biophys. 8, 1-47 (1957).
76. Isbell, H., E. J. Miner and C. R. Logan: Cross Tolerance Between D-2-Brom Lysergic Acid Diethylamide (Bol-148) and d-Diethylamide of Lysergic Acid (LSD-25). Psychopharmacologia 1 102-116 (1959).
77. Hoagland, H.: A Review of the Biochemical Changes induced "in vivo" by Lysergic Acid Diethylamide and similar Drugs. Ann. N. Y. Acad. Sci. 66 445-458 (1957).
78. Bain, J. A.: A Review of the Biochemical Effects "in vitro" of Certain Psychotomimetic Agents. Ann. N. Y. Acad. Sci. 66, 459-467 (1957).
79. Bain, J. A.: Biochemical and Neuroenzymological Considerations in the Study of Neuropharmacological Drugs. In: Psychopharmacology, Problems in Evaluation. Cole, J. C. and R. W. Gerard (Eds.); loc. cit. pp.199-206 (1959).
80. Lewis, J. L., and H. McIlwain: Action of Some Ergot Derivatives, Mescaline, and Dibenamine on Metabolism of Separated Mammalian Cerebral Tissues. Biochem. J. 57, 80 (1954).
81. Berger, M., H. J. Strecker, and H. Waelsch: Biochemical Effects of Psychotherapeutic Drugs. Ann. N. Y. Acad. Sci. 66, 806-811 (1957).
82. Axelrod, J., R. O. Brady, B. Witkop, and E. Y. Evarts: The Distribution and Metabolism of Lysergic Acid Diethylamide. Ann. N. Y. Acad. Sci. 66, 435-444 (1957).
83. Szara, S.: Dimethyltryptamine: Its Metabolism in Man; the Relation to its Psychotic Effect to Serotonin Metabolism. Experientia (Basel) 12, 441 (1956).
84. Salzman T. P., and B. B. Brodie: Physiological Disposition and Fate of Chlorpromazine and a Method for its Estimation in Biological Material. J. Pharmacol. exp. Ther. 118, 46 (1956).
84A. Lin, T. H., L. W. Reynolds, I. M. Rondish, and E. J. van Loon. Isolation and Characterization of Glucuronic Acid Conjugates of Chlorpromazine in Human Urine. Proc. Soc. esp. Biol. (N. Y.) 102, 602 (1959).
85. Posner, H. S.: Metabolism of the Phenothiazine Tranquillisers in Humans. Proc. Am. Chem. Soc. Abstr., 81, 1959.
85A. Huang, C. L., and A. A. Kurland:. A Quantitative Study of Chlorpromazine and its Sulfoxides in the Urine of Psychotic Patients. Amer. J. Psychiat.118, 428 (1961).
86. Szara, S., and E. Hearst: (in press).
87. Thompson, R. H. S., A. Tickner, and G. R. Webster: Action of Lysergic Acid Diethylamide on Mammalian Cholinesterases. Brit. J. Pharmacol. exp. Ther. 10, 61 (1955).
88. Rothlin, E.: Lysergic Acid Diethylamide and Related Substances Ann. N. Y. Acad. Sci. 66, 668-676 (1957).
89. Trendelenburg, P.: Physiologische und pharmakologische Versuche über die Dünndarmperistaltik. Naunyn Schmiedeberg's Arch. exp. Path. Pharmak. 81, 55 (1917).
90. Ginzel, K. H.: The Effect of Lysergic Acid Diethylamide on Some Autonomic Reflex Patterns. In: Psychotropic Drugs, pp. 48-54. Garattini, S. and V. Ghetti (Eds.). Amsterdam: Elsevier 1957.
91. Paton, W. D. M.: The Action of Morphine and Related Substances on Contraction and on Acetylcholine Output of Coaxially stimulated Guinea-pig Ileum. J. Pharmacol. 12, 119 (1957).
92. Cerletti, A.: Discussion of Comparison of Abnormal Behavioral States Induced by Psychotropic Drugs in Animals and Man. Discussion. In: Neuro-Psyohopharmacology, p. 117. Bradley, P. B., P. Deniker, and C. Radouco-Thomas (Eds.). Amsterdam: Elsevier 1959.
93. Ginzel K. H.: Personal Communication.
94. Ginzel K. H.: Some Central Effects of Lysergic Acid Diethylamide on Vasomotor Responses. J. Physiol. (Lond.) 129, 61 (1955).
95. Marrazzi, A. S., and E. R. Hart: Relationship of Hallucinogens to Adrenergic Cerebral Neurohumore. Science 121, 365 (1955).
96. Killam, K. F., and E. K. Killam: A Comparison of the Effects of Reserpine and Chlorpromazine to those of Barbiturates on Central Afferent Systems in the Cat. J. Pharmacol. exp Ther.116, 35 (1956).
97. Evarts, E., V. Landau, W. Freygang jr., and W. H. Marshall: Some Effects of Lysergic Acid Diethylamide and Bufotenine on Electrical Activity in the Cat's Visual System. Amer. J. Physiol. 182, 594-598 (1955).
98. Bradley, P. B., and A. J. Hance: The Effect of Chlorpromazine and Methopromazine on the Electrical Activity of the Brain in the Cat. EEG Clin. Neurophysiol. 9 191 (1957).
99. Bradley, P. B. and B. J. Key: A Comparative Study of the Effects of Drugs on the Arousal System of the Brain. Brit. J. Pharmacol. 14, 340-349 (1959).
100. Bradley, P. B., A. Mollica: The Effect of Adrenalin and Acetylcholine on Single Unit Activity in the Reticular Formation of the Decerebrate Cat. Arch. ital. Biol. 94, 168 (1958).
101. Delay, J.: Discussion of Pharmacologic Treatment of Schizophrenics. In: Psychopharmacology Frontiers, p. 426. Kline, N. S. (Ed.). Boston: Little, Brown & Co.1959.

102. A. M. A., Council on Drugs, J. Amer. Med. Ass. 166, 1040 (1958). Psychotherapeutic Drugs.
102A. Freyhan, F. A.: On Classifying Psychotropic Pharmacology. Comprehens. Psychiat. 2, 241 (1961).
103. Jacobsen, E.: In Ataractic and Hallucinogenic Drugs in Psychiatry. WHO Technical Report No. 152 WHO, Geneva. pp. 22-29, 1958.
104. Jacobsen, E.: The Comparative Pharmacology of Some Psychotropic Drugs. Bull. WHO. 21 411-413. (1959).
105. Burke, J. C., G. L. Hassest jr. and J. P. High: The Tranquilizing Activity of 10-(3-dimethylaminopropyl) 2-(trifluoromethyl)-phenothiazine Hydrochloride (MC 4703) and Related Phenothiazines in Animals. J. Pharmacol. exp. Ther. 119, 136 (1957).
106. Kinross-Wright, V.J.:. Phenothiazines in treatment. In: Psychopharmacology Frontiers, p. 428. Kline, N. S. (Ed.), Boston: Little, Brown & Co 1959.
107. Freyhan, F. A.: Clinical and Investigative Aspects. In: Psychopharmacology Frontiers; Kline, Boston, p. 7. 1959.
108. Grebe, R. M: Chlopromazine Hydrocloride: Handbook of Toxicology. (Ed.). Vol, IV. Tranquilizers, pp .14-17. Nat. Acad. of Sciences. Nat Res. Council. Philadelphia and London: W. B. Saunders, 1959.
109. Bein, H. J.: The Pharmacology of Rauwolfia. Pharmacol. Rev. 8 435 (1956).
110. Grebe, R. M.: Reserpine: Handbook of Toxicology. (Ed.). Vol. IV. Tranquillizer, pp. 90-94. Philadelphia: W. B. Saunders Co. 1959.
111. Ataractic and Hallucinogenic Drugs in Psychiatry. WHO Technical Report, No. 152 1958, p. 31.
112. Grebe, R.M.: Hydroxyzine: Handbook of Toxicology. (Ed.). loc. cit. p. 27.
113. Fabing, H. D: New Blocking Agent against the Development of LSD-25 Psychosis. Science 121, 208 (1955).
114. Grebe, E R. M.: Meprobamate. Handbook of Toxicology. (Ed.). loc. cit. p. 42-47 1959.
115. Zeller, E. A. and J. Barsky: "In vivo" Inhibiton of Liver and Brain Monoamine Oxidase by l-Isonicotinyl-2 Isopropyl Hydrazine. Proc. Soc. exp. Biol. (N. Y.) 81, 459 (1952).
116. Benson, V. A., P. L. Stefko and M. D. Roe: Pharmacologic and Toxicologic Observations on Hydrazine Derivatives of Isonicotinic Acid. Amer. Rev. Tuberc. 65, 376 (1952).
117. Grebe, R. M.: Iproniazid: Handbook of Toxicology. (Ed.). loc. cit. pp. 30-38 1959.
118. McGill University Conference on Depression and Allied States. Canadian Psychiatric Association Journal. Vol. 4, Special Supplement 1959.
119. Sigg, E. B.: Pharmacological Studies with Tofranil. In: McGill University Conference on Depression and Allied States. Loc. cit. p. 75, 1959.
120. Barger, G., H. Dale: Chemical Structure and Sympathomimetic Action of Amines. J. Physiol. (Lond.) 41 19 (1910).
121. Chen, K. K. and C. F. Schmidt: Ephedrine and Related Substances. Medicine 9, 1 (1 930).
122. Alles, G. A.: The Comparative Physiological Actions of dl-β-Phenylisopropylamines. J. Pharmacol. exp. Ther. 47, 339 (1933).
123. Pfeiffer, C. E. Jenney, W. Gallagher, R. P. Smith, W. Bevan, K. F. Killam, E. K. Killam, W. Blackmore: Stimulant Effect of 2-Dimethylaminoethanol – Possible Precursor of Brain Acetylocholine. Science 126, 610 (1957).
124. Killam, E. K., H. Gangloff, B. Konigsmark and K. F. Killam: The Action of Pharmacologic Agents on Evoked Cortical Activity. In: Biological Psychiatry p. 53. Masserman, J. H. (Ed.). New York: Grune & Stratton 1959.
125. Connel, P. H.: Amphetamine Psychosis. Maudsley Monographs. The Institute of Psychiatry. London: Chapman & Hall 1958.
126. Wikler, A.: Loc. cit. pp. 204-205, 261-262.
127. Schwarz, B. E., R. H. Bickford and H. P. Rose: Reversibility of Induced Psychosis with Chlorpromazine. Proc. Mayo Clin. 30 407 (1955)
128. Cerletti, A.: In Neuropsychopharmacology, p. 291. Bradley, P. B., P. Deniker and C. Raduoco-Thomas (Eds.) Amsterdam: Elsevier 1959.
129. Erspamer, V.: Pharmacology of indole-alkylamines. Pharmacol. Rev. 6, 425 (1954).
130. Evarts, E. Y.: Some Effects of Bufotenine and Lysergic Acid Diethylamide on the Monkey. Arch. Neurol. Psyciat. (Chic.) 75, 49 (1956).
131. Fabing, H. D. and J. R. Hawkins: Intravenous bufotine injection in the human being. Science 123, 886 (1956).
132. Böszörményi, Z. and S. Szara: Dimethyltryptamine. Experiments with Psychotics. J. ment. Sci. 104, 445 (1958).
133. Szara, S.: The Comparison of the Psychotic Effect of Tryptamine Derivates with the Effects of Mescaline and LSD-25 in Self-Experiments. In: Psychotropic Drugs. Garattini, S., V. Ghetti (Eds.). Amsterdam. Elsevier 1958.
134. Bratgard, S. O., T. Lindquist: Demonstration of 82 BR in Nerve Cells. J. Neurol. Neurosurg., Psychiat. 17, 11 (1954).
135. Cade, J. F. J.: Lithium Salts in the Treatment of Psychotic Excitement. Med. J. Aust. 36, 349 (1949).
136. Schou, M.: Biology and Pharmacology of the Lithium Ion. Pharmacol. Rev. 9 17 (1957).
137. Schou, M.: Lithium in Psychiatric Therapy. Stock taking after ten years. Psychopharm. (Berl.) 1, 65 (1959).
137A. Cleghorn, R. A. (Ed.): Proc. 3rd World Congress of Psychiatry. Montreal 1961. Univ. of Toronto Press 1962.
138. Harris, G. W.: Neural Control of the Pituitary Gland. London 1955.
139. Mason, J. W.: Visceral Functions of the Nervous System. Ann. Rev. Physiol. 21 353 (1959).
140. The Reticular Formation of the Brain. Henry Ford Hospital International Symposium. Jasper, H. H. et al. (Eds.). Boston, Little Brown & Co. 1958.
141. Himwich, W. H., W. G. VanMeter, and H. Avens: Drugs used in the Treatment of the Depressions. In: Biological Psychiatry, p. 27. Masserman, J. H. (Ed.). New York: Grune & Stratton 1959.
142. Morruzzi, G., and H. W. Magoun: Brain Stem Reticular Formation and Activation of the EEG. Electroenceph. Clin. Neurophysiol. 1 455 (1949).
143. Nauta, W. J. H., and H. G. J. M. Kuypers: Some Ascending Pathways in the Brain Stem Reticular Formation. In: Reticular Formation of the Brain, p. 3. Jasper, H. H. (Ed.). Boston: Little Brown & Co.1958.
144. Nauta, W. J. H.: Hippocampal Projections and Related Neural Pathways to the Mid-Brain in the Cat. Brain 81, 319 (1958).

144A. Pribram, K. H., and L. Kruger: Functions of the "Olfactory Brain". Ann. N. Y. Acad. Sci. 58, 109 (1954).
145 French, J. D.: Corticifugal Connection with the Reticular Formation. In: Reticular Formation of the Brain. Loc. cit. p. 491 1958.
146. Papez, J. W. A.: A proposed Mechanism of Emotion. Arch. Neurol. Psychiat. (Chic.) 38,725 (1937).
147. Brady. J. V.: The Paleocortex and Behavioral Motivation. In: Biological and Biochemical Bases of Behavior, p. 192. Harlow, H. F., and C. N. Woolsey (Eds.). University of Wisconsin Press 1958.
148. Nauta, W. J. H.: Hippocampal Projections and Related Neural Pathways to the Mid-Brain in the Cat. Loc. cit. p. 339, 1958.
149. In:gram, W. R.: Nuclear Organization and Chief Connections of the Primate Hypothalamus. Ass. Res nerv. ment. Dis. Proc. 20, 195. (1940).
150. Olszewski, J.: The Cytoarchitecture of the Human Reticular Formation. In: Brain Mechanism and Consciousneas. p. 54. Delafresnays, J. F. (Ed.) Oxford: Blackwell Scientific Publications. 1954.
151. Brobeck, J. R.: Neural Regulation of Food Intake. Ann. N. Y. Acad. Sci. 63 44 (1955).
152. Hess W. R.: Das Zwischenhirn. Basel: Schwabe 1949.
153. Hare, K., and W. A. Gellhorn: Influence of Frequency of Stimulus Upon the Response to Hypothalamic Stimulation J. Neurophisiol. 4,266. (1941).
154. Olds, J.: Studies of Neuropharmacologicals by Electrical and Chemical Manipulation of the Brain in Animals with Chronically Implanted Electrodes. In: Neuropsychopharmacology, p. 20. In: Bradley, P. D., P. Deniker, and C. Raduoco-Thomas (Ed.). Amsterdam: Elsevier 1959.
155. Sokoloff, L.: The Action of Drugs on the Cerebral Circulation. Pharmacol. Rev. 11, 1 (1959).
156. Kety, S. S.: The Effects of Circulation and Energy Metabolism of the Brain. In: A Pharmacologic Approach to the Study of the Mind, p. 3. Featherstone, R. M. and A. Simon (Eds.). Springfield: C. C. Thomas 1959.
157. Kety, S. S. and C. F. Schmidt: Determination of Cerebral Blood Flow in Man by Use of Nitrous oxide in Low Concentrations. Amer. J. Physiol.143, 53 (1945).
158. Kety, S. S., W. M. Landau, W. Freygang jr., L. P. Rowland and L. Sokoloff: Estimation of Regional Circulation in the Brain by the Uptake of an Inert Gas. Fed. Proc. 14, 85 (1955).
159. Kety, S. S.: Loc cit. p. 5.
160. Jayne, H.W., P. Scheinberg, M. Rich and M. S. Belle: Effect of intravenous papavernine hydrocloride on cerebral circulation. J. Clin. Invest. 31 111 (1952).
161. Battey, L. L., A. Heyman and J. L. Patterson: Effects of Ethyl Alcohol on Cerebral Blood Flow and Metabolism. J. Amer. Med. Ass. 152 6 1953.
162. Moyer, J. H., A. B. Tashner, S. J. Miller, H. Snyder and R. O. Bowman: Effect of Theophylline with Ethylenediamine (aminophylline) and Caffeine on Cerebral Hemodynamics and Cerebrospinal Fluid Pressure in Patients with Hypertensive Headaches. Amer. J. Med. Sci. 224, 377 (1952).
163. Crumpton,, C. W., W. C. Klingensmith, N. J. Keffer and J. H. Hafkenschiel: Effects of Protoveratrine on Cerebral Hemodynamincs and Oxygen Metabolism in Hypertensive Subjects. Fed. Proc. 10, 32 (1951).
164. Hafkenschiel, J H., and C. K. Friedland: Effects of l-hydrazino phthalazine on cerebral blood flow, vascular resistance oxygen uptake and jugular oxygen tension in hypertensive subjects. J. Clin. Invest. 32, 655 (1953).
165. Hafkenschiel, J. H., C. W. Crumpton, J. H. Moyer, and W. A. Jeffers: Effects of dihydroergocornine on cerebral circulation of patients with essential hypertension. J Clin. Invest. 29, 408 (1950).
166. Hafkenschiel, J. H., A. M. Sellers, G. A. King, and M. W Thorner: Preliminary observations on the effects of parenteral reserpine on cerebral blood flow, oxygen and glucose metabolism, and electroencephalograms of patients with essential hypertension. Ann. N. Y. Acad. Sci. 61, 78 (1955).
167. King, B. D., L. Sokoloff and R. L. Wechsler: Effects of l-Epinephrine and l-nor-Epinephrine Upon Cerebral Circulation and Metabolism in Man. J. Clin. Invest. 31, 273 (1952).
168. Abreu, B. E., G. W. Lidle, A. L. Burks, L. Sutherland, H. W. Elliott, A. Simon, and L. Margolis: Influence of Amphetamins Sulfate on Cerebral Metabolism and Blood Flow in Man. J. Amer. Pharm. Ass. 38, 186 (1949).
169. Ecker, P. G., B. D. Polis. Naval Air Development Center Report No. NADC, MA-5507. Johnsville, Pa. 1955.
170. Sokoloff, L., S. Perlin C. Kornetsky and S. S. Kety: The Effects of n-Lysergic Acid Diethylamide on Cerebral Circulation and Over-all Metabolism. N. Y. Acad. Sci. 66, 468 (1957).
171. Aizawa, T., Y. Goto, Y. Tazaki, S. Hamaya, and K. Makino: The Effects of Chlorpromazine on Cerebral Circulation and Metabolism. Keio J. Med. 2, 205 (1956).
172. Kleh, J., and J. F. Fazekas: Use of Reserpine in Hypertensive Arteriosclerotic Syndrome. Amer. J. Med. Sci. 228 560 (1954).
173. Scheinberg, P.: Cerebral Circulation and Metabolism in Hyperthyroidism. J. Clin. Invest. 29 1010 (1950).
174. Craigie, E. H.: On the Relative Vascularity of Various Parts of the Central Nervous System of the Albino Rat. J. comp. Neurol. 31, 429 (1920).
175. Craigie, E. H.: The Comparative Anatomy and Embryology of the Capillary Bed of the Central Nervous System. Res. Publ. Ass. Nerv. Ment. Dis. 18, 3 (1938).
176. Wolff, H. G.: The Cerebral Blood Vessels – Anatomical Principles. Res. Publ. Ass. Nerv. Ment. Dis. 18 29 (1937).
177. Brierle, J. B.: The Blood-Brain Barrier. In: Richter, D. (Ed.). Metabolism of the Nervous System, p. 132. London: Pergamon Press 1957.
178. Sokoloff, L.: Local Blood Flow in Neural Tissue. In: Windle, W. F. (Ed.). New Research Techniques in Neuroanatomy, p. 51. Springfield Illinois: Charles C. Thomas 1957.
179. Kety, S. S. and J. Elkes (Eds.): Regional Neurochemistry. The Regional Chemistry Physiology and Pharmacology of the Nervous System. Oxford and New York: The Pergamon Press 1961.
180. Stern, L. and R. Gautier: Recherches sur le liquide céphalorachidien. Les rapports entre le liquide céphalo rachidien et la circulation sanguine. Arch. int. Physiol. 17, 138 (1921).
181. Obersteiner, H.: The Anatomy of the Central Nervous Organs in Health and Disease. London: Ch. Griffin 1890.

182. Hess A.: Ground Substance of the Developing Central Nervous System. J. comp. Neurol. 102 65 (1955).
183. Pappenheimer, J. R.: Passage of Molecules through Cappillary Walls. Physiol. Rev. 33, 387 (1953).
184. Krogh, A.: Active and Passive Exchanges of Inorganic Ions Through the Surface of Living Cells and Through Living Membranes Generally. Proc. Roy. Soc. Med. B 133 140 (1946).
185. Bering, J. A.: Water Exchange of Central Nervous System and Cerebrospinal Fluid. J. Neurosurg. 9, 275 (1952).
186. Hahn, L. and G. Hevesy: Rate of Penetration of Ions Through Capillary Walls. Acta physiol. scand. 1, 347 (1941).
187. Noonan, T. R., W. O. Fenn and L. F. Haege: Effects of Denervation and of Stimulation on Exchange of Radioactive Potassium in Muscle. Amer. J. Physiol. 132, 612 (1941).
188. Dobbing, J.: The Blood-Brain Barrier. Physiol. Rev. 41, 130 (1961).
189. Brodie, B. B.: Report to American Heart Association, 1959.
190. Fleischauer, K.: Regional Differences in the Structure of the Ependyma and Subependymal Layers of the Cerebral Ventricles of the Cat. In: Kety, S. S. and J. Elkes (Eds.). Regional Neurocliemistry p. 279. Oxford and New York. The Pergamon Press 1961.
191. Weil-Malherbe, H., L. G. Whitby and J. Axelrod: The Blood-Brain Barrier for Catecholamine in Different Regions of the Brain. In: Kety, S. S., and J. Elkes (Eds.). Regional Neurochemistry, p. 284. Oxford and New York. The Pergamon Press 1961.
191A. Quadbeck, G.: On the Possibility of Altering the Exchange of Material Between the Blood and CNS for Therapeutic Purposes. Act. neurochir. (Wien). Suppl. VII, 152 (1961).
192. Folkow, B., and U. S. von Euler: Selective Activation of Noradrenaline and Adrenaline Producing Cells in the Cat's Adrenal Gland by Hypothalamic Stimulation. Circulat. Res. 2, 191 (1954).
193. Feldberg, W., and S. L. Sherwood: Injections of Drugs into the Lateral Ventricle of the Cat. J. Physiol. (Lond.) 128, 148 (1954).
194. Haley, T. J. and R. W. Dickinson: Pharmacological Effects Produced by Intracerebral Injection of Drugs in the Conscious Mouse. J. Amer. Pharm. Ass. Sci. Ed. 4, 432 (1956).
195. HLEx T. J., and W. G. McCoR3rsex: Pharmacological Effects Produced in Intracerebral Injection of Drugs in the Conscious Mouse. J. Pharmacol.12 12 (1957).
195A. Grundfest, H.: Functional Specifications for Membranes in Excitable Cells. In: Kety S. S. and J. Elkes (Eds.): Regional Neurochemistry, p. 378. Oxford and New York: The Pergamon Press 1961.
196. DeRobertis, E.: Morphological Bases of Synaptic Processes and Neurosecretion. In: Kety, S. S., and J. Elkes (Eds.). Regional Neurochemistry, pp. 248-258. Oxford and New York. The Pergamon Press 1961.
197. Quastel, J. H. and A. H. M. Wheatley: Effects of Amines on Oxidation of the Brain. Biochem. J. 27. 1609 (1933).
198. Block, W., K. Block and B. Patzig: Zur Physiologie C 14-radioaktiven Mescaline im Tierversuch. Hoppe-Seyler's Z. physiol. Chem. 291, 119 (1952).
199. Schueler, F. W.: Effects of Succinate in Mescaline Hallucinations. J. Lab. Clin. Med. 33 1297 (1948).
200. Schueler, F. W.: Effect of Succinate in Mescaline Hallucinations. J. Lab. Clin. Med. 33, 1301 (1948).
201. Block, W., K. Block and B. Patzig: Zur Physiologie des C 14-radioaktiven Mescalins im Tierversuch. Hoppe Seyler's Z. physiol. Chem. 290, 160 (1952).
202. Clark, L. C., R. P. Fox, F. Benington, and R. Morin: Effect of Mescaline, Lysergic Acid, and Related Compounds on Respiratory Enzyme Activities of the Brain. Fed. Proc. 13, 27 (1954).
203. Bain J. A.: A Review of the Biochemical Effects "in vitro" of Certain Psychotomimetic Agents. Ann. N. Y.Acad. Sci. 66, 461 (1957).
204. Leis, J. L., and H. McIlwain: Action of Some Ergot Derivatives Mescaline and Dibenamine on Metabolism of Separated Mammalian Cerebral Tissues. Biochem. J. 57, 680 (1954).
205. Bain, J. A.: A Review of Biochemical Effects "in vitro" of Certain Psychotomimetic Agents. Ann. N. Y. Acad. Sci. 66, 463 (1957).
206. Poloni, A. and G. Malfezzoni: Le Variazioni dell'Attivita Colinergica del Tessuto Cerebrale per Effetto della Bulbocapnina della Mescalina, E. della Dietilamide dell'Acido Lisergico. Sist. nerv. 4, 578 (1952).
207. Thompson, R. H. S., A. Tickner, and G. R. Webster: Action of lysergic acid diethylamide on Mammalian Cholinesterases. J. Pharmacol. 10, 61 (1955).
208. Evans, F. T.: The Effect of Several Psychotomimetic Drugs on Human Serum Cholinesterase. Psychophar macologia (Berl.) 1, 231 (1960).
209. Evans F. T.: The Effect of Several Psychotomimetic Drugs on Human Serum Cholinesterase. Psychophar macologia (Berl.) l, 237 (1960).
210. Collier, H. B. and G. M. Allenby: Enzyme Inhibition by Derivatives of Phenothiazine. IV. Inhibition of Succinoxidase Activity of Rat Liver Mitochondria. Canad. J. Med. Sci. 30 443 (1952).
211. Wase, A., W. J. Christensen and E Polley: The Accumulation of S 35-Chlorpromazine. Arch. Neurol. Psychiat. (Chic.) 73, 54 (1955).
212. Grenell, R. G., J. Mendelson and W. D. McElroy: Effects of Chlorpromazine on Metabolism in Central Nervous System. Arch. Neurol. Psychiat. (Chic.) 73, 347 (1955).
213. Berger, M., H. J. Strecker, and H. Waelsch: Biochemical Effects of Psychotherapeutic Drugs. Ann. N. Y. Acad. Sci. 66, 808 (1957).
214. Berger, M., H. J. Strecker, and H. Waelsch: The Biochemical Effects of Psychotherapeutic Drugs. Ann. N. Y. Acad. Sci. 66 808 (1957).
215. Hesselbach, M. L., and H. G. DuBuy: Localization of Glycolytic and Respiratory Enzyme Systems on Isolated Mouse Brain Mitochondria. Proc. Soc. exp. Biol. N. Y. 83, 62 (1953).
216. Brodie, B. B. and C. A. M. Hogben: Some Physico-chemical Factors in Drug Action. J. Pharmacol. 9, 345 (1957).
217. Williams, R. T.: Detoxication Mechanisms. New York: John Wiley & Sons 1959.
218. Salzman, N. P. and B. B. Brodie: Physiological Disposition and Fate of Chlorpromazine and a Method for its Estimation in Biological Material. J. Pharmacol. exp. Ther. 118, 46 (1956).

219. Fishman, V. and H. Goldenberg: Metabolism of Chlorpromazine Organic-Extractable Fraction from Human Urine. Proc. Soc. exp. Biol. N. Y. 104, 99 (1960).
220. Posner, H.: (Personal Communication).
221. Lin, T. H. L. W. Reynolds, I. M. Rondish, and E. J. van Loon: Isolation and Characterization of Glucuronic Acid Conjugates of Chlocpromazine in Human Urine. Proc. Soc. exp. Biol. (N. Y.) 102 602 (1959).
222. Posner, H.: (loc. cit.).
223. Fishman, V., A. Heaton, and H. Goldenberg: Metabolism of Chlorpromazine. III. Isolation and Identification of Clorpromazine-N-Oxide. Proc. Soc. exp. Biol. (N. Y.) 109, 548 (1962).
224. Posner, H. S., E. Hearst, W. L. Taylor and G. J. Cosmides: Model Metabolites of Chlorpromazine and Promazine Relative Activities in Some Pharmacological and Behavioral Tests.J. Pharmacol. exp. Ther 131, 84 (1962).
225. Cochin,.J. L., A. Woods and M. H. Seevers: The Absorption and Urinary Excretion of Mescaline in the Dog. J. Pharmacol. exp. Ther. 101, 205 (1951).
226. Slotta, K. H., and J. Mueller: šber den Abbau Mescalins und mescalin"nlicher Stoffe im Organismus. Hoppe Seyler's Z. physiol. Chem. 238, 14 (1936).
227. Harley Mason, J., A. H. Laird and J. R. Smythies: The metabolism of mescalin in the human; delayed clinical re-actions to mescalin. Confin. neurol. (Basel) 18, 152 (1958).
228. Mokrash, L. C. and L. Stevenson: The Metabolism of Mescaline with a Note on Correlations Between Metabolism and Psychological Effects. J. nerv. ment. Dis. 129, 177 (1959).
229. Szara S., E. Hearst, and F. Putney: Metabolism and Behavioural Action of Tryptamine Derivatives. Int. J. Neuropharm. 1, 111 (1962).
230. Szara S.: Hallucinogenic Effects and Metabolism of Tryptamine Derivatives in Man. Fed. Proc. 20, 88 (1961).
231. Axelrod, J., R. O. Brady, B., B. Witkop, and E. V. Ewarts: The Distribution and Metabolism of Lysergic Acid Diethylamide. Ann. N. Y. Acad. Sci. 66, 435 (1957).
232. Axelrod, J., R. O. Brady, B. Witkop, and E. V. Evarts: The Distribution and Metabolism of Lysergic Acid Diethylamide. Ann. N. Y. Acad. Sci. 66 447 (1957).
233. Elkes, J.: Discussion. In: T.M. Tanner (ed.) Prospects in Psychiatric Research, pp. 126-135. Oxford, Blackwell Publications (1957)
234. Richter, D., and J. Crossland: Variation in Acetylcholine Content of Brain with Physiological State. Amer. J. Physiol. L59, 247 (1949).
235. Tobias, J. M., M. A. Lipton, and A. A. Lepinat: Effect of Anesthetics and Convulsante on Brain Acetylcholine Content. Proc. Soc. exp. Biol. (N. Y.) 61, 51 (1946).
236. Feldberg, W., and M. Vogt: Acetylcholine Synthesis in Different Regions of Central Nervous System. J. Physiol. (Lond.) 107, 372 (1948).
237. Ord, M. G., and R. H. S. Thomson: Pseudo-cholinesterase Activity in Central Nervous System. Biochem. J. 51 245 (1952).
238. Elkes, J., and A. Todrick: On the Development of the Cholinesterase in the Rat Brain. In: Waelsch, H. (Ed.). Biochemistry of the Developing Nervous System, p. 309. New York, N. Y.: Academic Press 1955.
239. Bayliss, B., and A. Todrick: The Use of a Selective Acetylcholinesterase Inhibitor in the Estimation of Pseudocholinesterase Activity in Rat Brain. Biochem. J. 62, 62 (1956).
240. Elkes, J., J. T. Eayrs, and A. Todrick: On the Effect and the Lack of Effect of Some Drugs on Postnatal Development in the Rat. In: Waelsch, H. (Ed.). Biochemistry of the Developing Nervous System, p. 499. New York, N. Y. Academic Press (1955).
241. Rosenzweig, M. R., D. Krech, and E. L. Bennett: Brain Enzymes and Adaptive Behavior. In: Wolstenholme, G. E. W. and C. M. O'Connor (Eds.). The Neurological Basis of Behaviour, p. 337. London: J. & A. Churchill 1958.
242. Desmedt, J. E. and G. Lagrutta: Control of Brain Potentials by Pseudocholinesterase. J. Physiol. (Lond.), 129, 466 (1955).
243. Lembeck, F. Zur Frage der zentralen šbertragung afferenter Impulse. III. Das Vorkommen und die Bedeutung der Substanz P in den dorsalen Wurzeln des Rückenmarks. Naunyn-Schmiedebergs Arch. exp. Path. Pharmak. 219, 197 (1953).
244. Stürmer, E., and J. Franz: šber pharmakologische Eigenschaften hochgereinigter Substanz P aus Pferdedarm. Med. Exp. 5, 37 (1961).
255. Holton, F. A., and P. Holton: The Possibility that ATP is a Transmitter at the Sensory Nerve Endings. J. Physiol. (Lond.) 119, 50 P (1953).
256. Vogt, M.: The Concentration of Sympathin in Different Parts of the Central Nervous System under Normal Conditions and after the Administration of Drugs. J. Physiol. (Lond.) 123 451 (1954).
257. Amin, A. H. B. B. Crawford, and J. H. Gaddum: The Distribution of Substance P and 5-hydroxy-tryptamine in the Central Nervous System of the Dog. J. Physiol. (Lond.) 126, 596 (1954).
257A. Weil-Malherbe, H., and A. D. Bone: Intracellular Distribution of Catecholamines in the Brain. Nature (Lond.) 180, 1050 (1957).
258. Carlson, A.: The Occurrence, Distribution and Physiological Role of Catecholamines in the Nervous System. Pharmacol. Rev. 11, 490 (1959).
259. Lerner, A. B., J. D. Case, Y. Takahashi, T. H. Lee, and W. Mori: Isolation of Melatonin, the Pineal Gland Factor that Lightens Melanocytes. J. Amer. Chem. Soc. 80, 2587 (1958).
260. Holtz, P.: Role of L-Dopa Decarbosylase in the Biosynthesis of Catecholamines in Nervous Tissue and the Adrenal Medulla. Pharmacol. Rev. 11, 327 (1959).
261. Purpura, D. P., M. Girado, T. G. Smith, D. A. Callan, and H. Grundfest: Structure Activity Determinants of Pharmacological Effects of Amino Acide and Related Compounds on Central Synapase. J. Neurochem. 3, 238 (1959).
262. Roberts, E. P. J. Harman and S. Frankel: Gamma Aminobutyric Acid Content and Glutamic Decarboxylase Activity in Developing Mouse Brain. Proc. Soc. exp. Biol. (N. Y.) 78 799 (1951).
263. Roberts, E.: Formation and Utilization of Gamma-aminobutyric Acid in Brain. Progr. Neurobiol. 1 11 (1956).
264. Roberts, E.: The Biochemistry of Gamma Aminobutyric Acid in the Central Nervous System. Proc. West. Pharmacol. Soc. l, 29 (1958).

265. Roberts, E. (Ed.): Inhibition in the Nervous System, and γ–Amino Butyric Acid. New York and Oxford. Pergamon Press (1960).
266. Salvador, R. A., and R. W. Alberts: The Distribution of Glutamic Gamma Aminobutyric Transaminase in the Nervous System of the Rhesus Monkey. J. biol. Chem. 234, 922 (1959).
267. Killam, K. F.: Convulsant Hydrazides. II. Comparison of Electrical Changes and Enzyme Inhibition Induced by Administration of Thiosemicarbazide.J. Pharmacol. exp. Therap.119, 263 (1957).
268. Dasgupta, S. R., E. K. Killam, and K. F. Killam: Drug Action on Rhinencephalic Seizure Activity in the Cat. J. Pharmacol. exp. Ther. 122, 16 A (1958).
269. Eidelberg, E., C. F. Baxter, E. Roberts, C. A. Saldias, and J. D. French: In Roberts, E. (Ed.), loc. cit. p. 365.
270. Florey, E. and H. McLennen: Effects on an Inhibitory Factor (factor 1) from Brain on Central Synaptic Transmission.:T. Physiol. (Lond.) 130, 446 (1955).
271. Waelsch, H.: Metabolism of Proteins and Amino Acids. In: Richter, D. (Ed.): Metabolism of the Nervous System, p. 431. Oxford and New York: Pergamon Press 1957.
272. Waelsch, H.: Compartmentalized Biosynthetic Reactions in the Central Nervous System. In: Kety, S. S., and J. Elkes (Eds.). Regional Neurochemistry, p. 57. Oxford and New York: Pergamon Press 1961.
273. Ambache, N.: The Use and Limitations of Atropine for Pharmacological Studies on Autonomic Effectors. Pharmacol. Rev. 7, 467 (1955).
274. Sawin, P. B., and D. Glick: Atropinesterase, Genetically Determined Enzyme in Rabbit. Proc. Nat. Acad. Sci. (Wash.) 29 55 (1943).
275. Gray, G. W.: and J. Seevers: "In vivo" Observations on the Nature of Atropine Tachyphylaxia exhibited by Intestinal Smooth Muscles. J. Pharmacol. exp. Ther. 113 319 (1955).
276. Cushny, A. R.: Die Atropingruppe. Handbuch der experimentellen Pharmakologie. Berlin: Springer 1924.
277. Ostfeld, A. M.: Dose Response Data for Autonomic and Mental Effects of Atropine and Hyoscine. Fed. Proc. 18, 44. (1959).
278. Jacobsen, E, and Y. Skaarup: Experimental Induction of Conflict Behaviour in Cats. Its Use in Pharmacological Investigation. Acta pharmacol. (Kbh.) 11, 117. (1955).
279. Berger, F. M., C. D. Hendley, and T. E. Lynes: Pharmacology of a Psychotherapeutic Drug: Benactyzine (β-diethylamino-ethyl benzilate HCl). Proc. Soc. Exp. Biol. (N. Y.) 92, 563 (1956).
280. Bradley, P. B., J. Elkes: The Effects of Some Drugs on the Electrical Activity of the Brain. Brain 80, 11 (1957).
281. Jacobsen, E. and E. Sonne: Effect of Benzilic Acid Diethylamoethyl Ester, HCl (Benactyzine) on Stress Induced Behavior in Rat. Acta pharmacol. (Kbh.) 11, 135 (1955).
282. Hargreaves, G. R., M. Hamilton and J. M. Roberts: Benactyzine as an Aid in Treatment of Anxiety States. Brit. Med. J. 1957 I. 306.
283. Abood, L. G., J. H. Biel and A. M. Ostfield: The Psychotogenetic Effects of some N substituted Piperidyl Benzilates. In: Bradley, P. B., P. Deniker and C. Raduoco-Thomas (Eds.): Neuropsychopharmacology, p. 433. Amsterdam: Elsevier 1959.
284. Lebovits, B. K., M. Visotky, and A. M. Ostfeld: LSD-and JB 318: A Comparison of two Hallucinogens. Arch. Gen. Psychiat. 2, 390 (1960).
285. Nickerson, M.: Blockade of the Actions of Adrenaline and Noradrenaline. Pharmacol. Rev. 11, 43 (1959).
286. Tripod, J.: Beeinflussung der zentralerregenden Wirkung von Weckaminen durch Pharmaka mit spezifisher Wirkung auf das autonome Nervensystem. Helv. Physiol. Pharmacol. Acta 10, 403 (1952).
287. Nickerson, M.: Blockade of the Actions of Adrenaline and Noradrenaline. Pharmacol. Rev. 11, 455 (1959).
288. Nickerson, M. and L. S. Goodman: Pharmacological Properties of New Arenergic Blocking Agent, N,N-dybenzyl β-chlorothylamine. J. Pharmacol. Exp. Ther. 89, 167 (1947).
289. Slater, I. H. and G. T. Jones: Pharmacologic Properties of Ethoxybutamoxane and related Compounds. J. Pharmacol. Exp. Ther. 122, 69 A (1958).
290. Ohler, E. A. and R. W. Sevy: Inhibition of Stress Induced Adrenal Ascorbic Acid Depletion by Morphyne, Dibenzyline and Adrenal Cortex Extract. Endocrinology 59, 347 (1956).
291. Tepperman, J. and J. S. Bogardus: Attempts at Pharmacologic Blockade of the Secretion of Adrenocorticotrophin. Endocrinology. 43, 448 (1948).
292. Markee, J. E., J. W. Everett: The Regulation of the Sex Cycle. Recent. Hormone Res. 7, 139 (1952).
293. Sawyer, C. H., J. E. Markee and J. W. Everett: Further Experiments on Blocking Pituitary Activation in the Rabbit and the Rat. J. exp. Biol. 113, 659 (1950).
294. Redish, W., E. C. Texter, R. M. Howard, p. H. Stillman, J. M. Steele: Action of SKF 88 A (phenoxyethyl derivative of Dibenamine) upon Certain Functions of Sympathetic Nervous System in Man. Circulation 6, 352 (1952).
295. Rockwell, F. V.: Dibenamine Therapy in Certain Psychopathologic Syndrones. Psychosom. Med. 10, 230 (1948).
296. Rosenblueth, A., W. B. Cannon: Some Circulatory Phenomena Disclosed by Ergotoxine. Amer. J. Physiol. 105, 373 (1933).
297. Konzett, H. and E. Rothlin: Investigations on Hypotensive Effect of Hydrogenated Ergot Alkaloids. J. Pharmacol. (Lond.) 8, 201 (1953).
298. Brodie,B. B., S. Spector and P. A. Shore: Interaction of Drugs with Norepinephirine in the Brain. Pharmacol. Rev. 11, 552 (1959).
298A. Brodie, B. B., S. Spector and P. A. Shore: Interaction of Drugs with Norepinephrine in the Brain. Pharmacol. Rev. 11, 548 (1959).
299. Bosworth, D. M., J.W. Fielding: Chemotherapy in Certain Forms of Juvenile Tuberculosis. N. Y. Med. J. 54, 2327 (1954).
300. Crane, G. E.: Iproniazid (marsilid) Phosphate, a Therapeutic Agent for Mental Disorders and Debilitating Diseases. Psychiat. Res. Rep. Amer. Psychiat. Ass. 8, 142 (1958).
301. Delay, J., B. Laine et J. F. Buisson: Note concernant l'action de l'isonicotinyl-hydrazide utilisé dans le traitement des états depressifs. Ann. Méd. Psychol. 2, 689 (1952).
302. Zeller, E. A., J. Barsky and E. R. Berman: Amine Oxidases; inhibition of monoamine oxidase by l-isonicotinyl 2-ispropylhydrazine. J. biol. Chem. 214, 267 (1955).

303. Zeller, E. A.: The Role of Amine Oxidases in the Destruction of Chathecolamines. Pharm. Rev. 11, 387 (1959).
304. Mann, P. J. G., and J. H. Quastel: Benzedrine (β-Phenylisopropylamine) and Brain Metabolism. Biochem. J. 34, 414 (1940).
305. Horita, A.: Comparative Clinical Pharmacology of a Monoamine Oxidase Inhibitor (JB 516) and Related Compounds. In: Featherstone, R. M. and A. Simon (Eds.): Pharmacology Approach to the Study of the Mind, p. 271. Springfield: Charles C. Thomas 1959.
306. Axelrod, J.: Presence, Formation and Metabolism of Normetanephrine. Science 127, 754 (1958).
307. Koella, G. B. and A. De T. Valk: Physiological Implications of Histochemical Localization of Monoamine Oxidase. J. Physiol. (Lond.) 126, 434 (1954).
308. Weil-Malherbe, H. and A: D. Bone: The Effect of Reserpine on the Intracellular Distribution of Chatecholamines in the Brain Stem of Rabbit. J. Neurochem. 4, 251 (1959).
309. Brodie, B. B., A. Pletscher and P. A. Shore: Evidence that Serotonin has a Role in Brain Function. Science. 122, 968 (1955).
310. Shore, P. A., S. L. Silver and B. B. Brodie: Interaction of Reserpine, Serotonin and Lysergic Acid Diethylamide in Brain. Science 122, 284 (1955).
311. Brodie, B. B., A. Pletscher and P. A. Shore: Possible Role of Serotonin in Brain Function and in Reserpine Action J. Pharmacol. 116, 9 (1956).
312. Holtz, P., H. Balzer, E. Westerman and E. Wezler: Beeinflussung der Evipannarkose durch Reserpin, Iproniazid und biogene Amine. (Effect of Reserpine, Iproniazid and Biogenic Amines on Evipan Narcosis.) Arch. exp. Path. Pharmakol. 231, 333 (1957).
313. Holzbauer, M. and M. Vogt: Depression by Reserpine of the Noradrenaline Concentration in the Hypothalamus of the Cat. J. Neurochem. 1, 8 (1956).
314. Vogt, M.: The Concentration of Sympathin in Different Parts of the Central Nervous System under Normal Conditions and after the Administration of Drugs. J. Physiol. (Lond.) 123, 451 (1954).
315. Vogt, M.: Catecholamines in Brain. Pharmacol. Rev. 11, 483 (1959).
316. Axelrod, J.: In preparation.
317. Carlsson, A., M. Lindquist and F. Magnusson: 3,4-Dihydroxy-phenylamine and 5-Hydroxytrytophan as Reserpine Antagonists. Nature (Lond.) 180, 1200 (1957).
318. Muscholl, E. and M. Vogt.: The Action of Reserpine on the Peripheral Sympathetic System. J. Physiol. (Lond.) 141, 132 (1958).
319. Brodie, B. B.: (personal communication).
320. Garattini, S., L. Valzelli: Researches on the Mechanism of Reserpine Sedative Action. Science 128, 1278 (1958).
321. Alles, G. A.: Subjective Reactions to Phenethylamine Hallucinogens. In: Featherstone, R. M. and A. Simon (Eds.): A pharmacologic approach to the study of the mind, p. 238. Springfield, Ill. Charles C. Thomas 1959.
322. Gaddum, J. H.: Antagonism between Lysergic Acid Dyethylamide and 5-Hydroxytryptamine. J. Physiol. (Lond.) 121, 15P (1953).
323. Gaddum, J. H., K. A. Hameed: Drugs which Antagonize and 5-Hydroxytryptamine. J. Pharmacol. 9, 240 (1954)
324. Gaddum, J. H. In: Ciba Symposium on Hypertension. Boston: Little, Brown & o. 203, 69 (1953).
326. Wooley, D. W. and E. Shaw: A Biochemical and Pharmacological Suggestion About Certain Mental Disorders. Science 119, 587 (1954).
327. Wooley, D. W. and E. Shaw: A Biochemical Pharmacological Suggestion About Certain Mental Disorders. Proc. nat. Acad. Sci. (Wash.) 40, 228 (1954).
328. Costa, E.: Effects of Hallucinogenic and Tranquilizing Drugs on Serotonin Evoked Uterine Contractions. Proc. Soc. Exp. Biol. (N. Y.) 91, 39 (1956).
329. Shaw, E., D. W. Wooley: Some Serotonin-like Activities of Lysergic Acid Diethylamide. Science 124, 121 (1956).
330. Evarts, E. V.: Some Effects of Bufotine and Lysergic Acid Diethylamide on the Monkey. Arch. Neurol. Psychiat. (Chic.) 75, 49 (1956).
331. Horita, A. and J. H. Gogerty: The Pyretogenetic Effect of 5-Hydroxytryptophan and its Comparison with that of LSD-J. Pharmacol. exp. Ther. 122, 195 (1958).
332. Marrazzi, A. S. and E. R. Hart: Relationship of Hallucinogens to Adrenergic Cerebral Neurohumors. Science 121, 365 (1955).
333. Cerletti, A. and E. Rothlin: Role of 5-Hydroxytryptamine in Mental Diseases and its Antagonism to Lysergic Acid Derivatives. Nature (Lond.) 176, 785 (1955).
334. Schneckloth, R., T. H. Page, F. Del Greco and A. C. Corcoban: Effects of Serotonin Antagonists in Normal Subjects and Patients with Carcinoid Tumors. Circulation 16, 523 (1957).
335. Salmoiraghi, G. C., I. Sollero and I. H. Page.: Blockade by Bromo lysergic-acid-diethylamide (BOL) of Potentiating Action of Serotonin and Reserpine on Hexobarbital Hypnosis. J. Pharmacol. 117, 166 (1956).
337. Ginzel, K. H. and W. Mayer-Gross: Prevention of Psychological Effects of D-lysergic Acid Diethylamide (LSD 25) by its 2-brom Derivative (BOL 148). Nature (Lond.) 178, 210 (1956).
338. Isbell, H., A. B. Wolbach, A. Wikler and E. J. Miner: Cross Tolerance between LSD-and Psilocybin. Psycho pharmacologia (Berl.) 2, 147 (1961).
339. Rothlin, E.: Lysergic Acid Diethylamide and Related Substances. Ann. N. Y. Acad. Sci. 66, 668 (1957).
340. Cerletti, A.: Discussion of "Comparison of Abnormal Behavioural States Induced by Psychotropic Drugs in Animals and Man." Neuropsychopharmacology, p. 117. Bradley, P.B., P. Deniker and C. Raduoco-Thomas (Eds.) Amsterdam: Elsevier & Co. 1959.
341. Schweitzer, A. and S. Wright: The Action of Adrenaline on Transmission in the Sympathetic Ganglia, which May Play a Part in Shock. J. Physiol. (Lond.) 88, 476 (1937).
342. Bülbring, E. and J. H. Burn: Observations Bearing on Synoptic Transmission by Acetylcholine in the Spinal Cord. J. Physiol. (Lond.) 100, 337. (1941).
343. Bülbring, E.: The Action of Adrenaline on Transmission in the Superior Cervical Ganglion. J. Physiol. (Lond.) 103, 55 (1944).
344. Burn, J. H. The Relation of Adrenaline to Acethylcholine in Nervous System. Physiol. Rev. 37, 377 (1945).

345. Ramey, E. R. and M. S. Goldstein: The Adrenal Cortex and the Sympathetic Nervous System. Physiol. Rev. 37, 115 (1957).
346. De Maio, D.: Influence of Adrenalectomy and Hypophysectomy on Cerebral Serotonin. Science 129, 1678 (1959).
347. Brodie, B. B., K. F. Finger F. B. Orlans, G. P. Quinn and F. Sulser: (in press).
348. Harris, G. W., R. P. Michael and P. P. Scott: Neurological Basis of Behavior, p. 236. London: Churchill, 1958.
349. Sawyer, C. H.: Activation and Blockade of the Release of Pituitary Gonadotropin as Influenced by the Reticular Formation. In: Reticular Formation of the Brain. Henry Ford Hosp. Internat. Symposium, p. 233. Boston: Little, Brown & Co. 1958.
350. Persky, H. D. A. Hamburg, H. Basowitz, R. R. Grinker, M. Sabshin, S. J. Korchin, M. Herz, F. A. Board and H. A. Heath: Relation of Emotional Responses and Changes in Plasma Hydrocortisone Level After Stressful Interview. Arch. Neurol. Psychiat. (Chic.) 79, 434 (1958).
351. Board, F., R. Wadeson and H. Persky: Depressive Affect and Endocrine Functions. Arch. Neurol. Psychiat. (Chic.) 78 612 (1957).
352. Mason, J. W.: Personal communication.
353. Waelsch, H.: Compartmentalized Biosynthetic Reactions in the Central Nervous System. In: Kety, S. S. and J. Elkes (Eds.). Regional Neurochemistry, p. 57. Oxford and New York. Pergamon Press 1961.
354. Elkes J.: Ignorances in Biochemistry Endocrinology and Pharmacology. In: J. M. Tanner (Ed.). Prospects in Psychiatric Research, p. 126. Oxford. Blackwell Scientific Publications 1953.
355. Lerner, A. B. J. D. Case, Y. Takahashi, T. H. Lee, and W. Mori: Isolation of Melanotonin, the Pineal Gland Factor that Lightens Melanocytes. J. Amer. Chem. Soc. 80, 2588 (1958).
356. Pope, A., A. A. Hess and J. N. Allen: Quantitative Histochemistry of Proteolytic and Oxidative Enzymes in Human Cerebral Cortex and Brain Tumors. Progr. Neurobiol. 2, 182 (1957).
357. Olds, J., and M. E. Olds: Positive Reinforcement Produced by Stimulating Hypothalamus with Iproniazid and other Compounds. Science 127, 1175 (1958).
358. Michael, R.: An Investigation of the Sensitivity of Circumscribed Neurological Areas to Hormonal Stimulation by Means of the Application of Oestrogens Directly to the Brain of the Cat. Regional Neurochemistry, p. 465. Oxford: Pergamon Press 1961.
359. John, E. R. and K. F. Killam: Electrophysiological Correlates of Avoidance Conditioning in the Cat. J. Pharmacol. exp. Ther. 125 252 (1959).
360. Curtis, D. R. and R. M. Eccles: The Effect of Diffusional Barriers Upon the Pharmacology of Cells within the Central Nervous System. J. Physiol. (Lond.) 141 446 (1958).
361. Curtis, D. R.: The Effects of Drugs and Amino Acids upon Neurons. In: Kety, S. S., and J. Elkes (Eds.): Regional Neurochemistry, p. 403. Oxford: Pergamon Press 1961.
362. Fatt, P.: Biophysics of Junctional Transmission. Physiol. Rev. 34, 674 (1954).
363. Coombs, J. S., J. C. Eccles, and P. Fatt: Electrical Properties of Motoneurone Membrane. J. Physiol. (Lond.) 130, 291 (1955).
364. del Castillo, J., B. Katz: Biophysical Aspects of Neuro-Muscular Transmission. Progr. Biophys. 6, 121 (1956).
365. Eccles, J.: The Behaviour of Nerve Cells. In: Ciba Symposium on Neurological Basis of Behaviour, pp. 29, 34, 35. London. Churchill 1958.
366. Araki, T. and T. Otani: Response of Single Motoneurons to Direct Stimulation in Toad's Spinal Cord. J. Neurophysiol. 18, 472 (1955).
367. Fatt, P.: Sequence of events in synaptic activation of a motoneurone. J. Neurophysiol. 20, 61 (1957).
368. Bradley, K., D. M. Easton and J. C. Eccles: An Investigation of Primary or Direct Inhibition. J. Physiol. (Lond.) 122, 474 (1953).
369. Moruzzi, G.: The Physiological Properties of the Brain Stem Reticular System. In: CIOMS Symposium on Brain Mechanisms an Consciousness, p. 21. Oxford: Blackwell Scientific Publications 1954.
370. Amassian, V. E.: Spatiotemporal Patterns of Activity in Individual Reticular Neurons. In: Reticular Formation of the Brain. Henry Ford Internat. Symposium, p. 69. Boston: Little Brown & Co. 1958.
371. Salmoiraghi, G. C., and D. B. Burns: Notes on Mechanism of Rhythmic Respiration. Neurophysiol. 23, 14 (1960).
372. Bradley, P. B.: Microelectrode Approach to the Neuropharmacology of the Reticular Formation. In: Garrattini, S. and V. Ghetti (Eds.). Psychotropic Drugs, p. 201. Amsterdam: Elsevier 1957.
373. Bradley, P. B., A. Mollica: The Effect of Adrenaline and Acetylcholine on Single Unit Activity in the Reticular Formation of the Decerebrate Cat. Arch. ital. Biol. 94, 168 (1958).
374. Gr"sser, O. J., G. Saur, U. Cornelis: Neuropharmakologie: Zentrale Wirkungsmechanismen chemischer Substanzen. Klin. Wschr. 36, 1157 (1958).
374A. Salmoiraghi, G. C.: In preparation.
375. Whitlock, D. C., A. Arduini and G. Moruzzi: Microelectrode Analysis of Pyramidal System During Transition from Sleep to Wakefulness. J. Neurophysiol. 16, 414 (1953).
376. Fleming, T. C., P. R. Huttenlochner and E. V. Evarts: Effects of Sleep and Arousal on the Cortical Response to Lateral Geniculate Stimulation. Fed. Proc. 18, 46 (1959).
377. Malcolm, J. L.: The Electrical Activity of Cortical Neurons in Relation to Behaviour, as Studied with Micro electrodes in Unrestrained Cats. In: Ciba Symposium on Neurological Basis of Behaviour, p. 295. London: J. & A. Churchill 1958.
378. Jung, R.: Neuronal Discharge. Electroenceph. Clin. Neurophysiol. Suppl. 4. 57 (1953).
379. Goldring, S., and J. L. O'Leary: Correlation Between Steady Transcortical Potential and Evoked Response. 1. Alterations in Somatic Recieving Area Induced by Veratrine, Strychnine KCl and Novocaine. Electroenceph. Clin. Neurophysiol. 6, 189 (1954).
380. Gumnit, R. J., D. C. Potential Changes from Auditory Cortex of Cat. J. Neurophysiol. 23, 667 (1960).
381. Marrazzi, A. S., and E. R. Hart: Relationship of Hallucinogens to Adrenergic Cerebral Neurohumors. Science 121, 365 (1955).
382. Marrazzi, A. S.: The Effect of Drugs on Neurons and Synapses. In: Fields, W. S. (Ed.): Brain Mechanisms and Drug Actions, pp. 45, 325. Springfield, Ill.: Charles C. Thomas 1957.

383. Marrazzi, A. S.: Pharmacodynamics of Hallucination. In: West, L. J. (Ed.): Hallucinations, p. 36. New York. Grune & Stratton 1962.
384. Purpura, D. P.: Electrophysiological Analysis of Psychotogenic Drug Action. Arch. Neurol. Psychiat. (Chic.) 75, 122 (1956).
385. Evarts, E. V. W. Landau, W. Freygang jr., and W. H. Marschall: Some Effects of Lysergic Acid Diethylamide and Bufotenine on Electrical Activity in Cat's Visual System. Amer. J. Physiol. 182, 594 (1956).
386. Killam, K. F. and E. K. Killam: A Comparison of the Effects of Reserpine and Chlorpromazine to those of Barbituates on Central Afferent Systems in the Cat. J. Pharmacol. exp. Ther. 116, 35 (1956).
386A. Brücke, F. G. Gogolak, C. L. Stumpf: Die Wirkung von LSD-auf die Makro und Mikrot"tigkeit des Hippocampus. Naunyn-Schmiedeberg's Arch. exp. Path. Pharmak. 240, 461 (1961).
387. Eccles, J. C., P. Fatt and K. Koketsu: Cholinergic and Inhibitory Synapses in Pathway from Motor-Axon Collaterals to Motoneurones. J. Physiol. (Lond.) 126, 524 (1954).
388. Frank, K. and M. G. F. Fuortes: Unitary Activity of Spinal Interneurones of Cats. J. Physiol. (Lond.) 131, 424 (1956).
389. Henneman, E., A. Kaplan, and K. R. Unna: Neuropharmacological Study on Effect of Myanesin (Tolserol) on Motor Systems. J. Pharmacol. exp. Ther. 97, 331 (1949).
390. Abdulian, D. G., W. R. Martin and K. R. Unna: The Effect of Pharmacologic Agents on the Nervous System ARNMD Symposia, Vol. 37, p. 72. Baltimore: Williams & Wilkins 1958.
391. Koella, W. P.: Physiological Fractionation of the Effect of Serotonin on Evoked Potentials. In: Neuropharmacology, p. 199. Transaction of 5th Conference. New York. Josiah Macy Jr. Foundation 1959.
392. French, J. D. M. Verzeano and H. Magoun: Neural Basis of Anesthetic State. Arch. Neurol. Psychint. (Chic.) 69, 519 (1953).
393. King, E. E.: Differential Action of Anesthetica and Interneuron Depressants upon EEG Arousal and Recruitment Responses. J. Phacmacol. exp. Ther. 116 404 (1956).
394. Magni, F., G. Moruzzi, G. F. Rossi e A. Zanchetti: EEG Arousal Following Inactivation of the Lower Brain Stem by Selective Injection of Barbiturate into the Vertebral Circulation. Arch. ital. Biol. 97, 33 (1959).
395. Killam, K. F., and E. K. Killam: Drug Action on Pathways Involving the Reticular Formation. In: Reticular formation of the brain, p. 111. Henry Ford Hosp. Internat. Sympos. Boston: Little, Brown & Co. 1958.
396. Bradley, P. B. and A. J. Hance: The Effect of Chlorpromazine and Methopromazine on the Electrical Activity of the Brain in the Cat. Electroenceph. Clin. Neurophysiol. 9, 191 (1957).
397. Bradley, P. B., and B. J. Key: A Comparative Study of the Effects of Drugs on the Arousal System of the Brain. J. Pharmacol. 14, 340 (1959).
398. Bremert, F.: Cerveau isolé et physiologie du sommeil. C. R. Soc. Biol. (Paris) 118, 1235 (1935).
399. Evarts E. V.: A Review of the Neurophysiological Effects of Lysergic Acid Diethylamide (LSD) and other Psychotomimetic Agents. Ann. N. Y. Acad. Sci. 66, 479 (1957).
400. Rinaldi, F., and H. E. Himwich: Drugs Affecting Psychotic Behavior and the Function of the Mesodiencephalic Activating System. Dis. Nerv. Syst. 16, 133 (1955).
401. Bradley, P. B., J. Elkes: The Effects of Some Drugs on the Electrical Activity of the Brain. Brain 80, 77 (1957).
402. Elkes, J.: Effects of Psychosomimetic Drugs in Animals and Man. In: Neuropharmacology, p. 205. Transactions of the Third Conference. Josiah Macy Jr. Foundation 1957.
403. Elkes, J.: Drug Effects in Relation to Receptor Specificity within the Brain. Some Evidence and Provisional Formulation. In: Ciba Found. Symposium on Neurological Basis of Behaviour, p. 303. London: Churchill 1958.
404. Wikler, A.: Pharmacologic Dissociation of Behavior and EEG "Sleep Patterns" in Dogs: Morphine, N-allylnor morphine and Atropine. Proc. Soc. exp. Biol. (N. Y) 79, 261 (1952).
405. Rothballer, A. B.: The Effects of Catecholamines on the Central Nervous System. Pharmacol. Rev. 11, 494 (1959).
406. Salmoiraghi, G. C.: Personal Communication.
407. Pavlov, I. P.: Conditioned reflexes and psychiatry. New York: International Publishers 1941.
408. Wikler, A.: The Relation of Psychiatry to Pharmacology. Baltimore. Williams & Wilkins 1957.
409. Gantt, W. H.: Experimental Basis for Neurotic Behavior. New York: Paul B. Hoeber 1944.
410. Anderson, 0. D., and R. Parmenter: Psychosom. Med. Monogr. Suppl. 2, 1 (1941).
411. Morrell, F.: Some Electrical Events Involved in the Formation of Temporary Connections. In: Reticular Formation of the Brain. p. 545. Henry Ford International Symposia. Boston: Little Brown & Co. 1958.
412. Luria, A. R.: The Nature of Human Conflicts. New York: Liveright Co. 1932.
413. Huston, P. E. D. Shakow and M. H. Erickson: A Study of Hypnotically Induced Complexes by means of the Luria Technique. J. Gen. Psychol. 11, 65 (1934).
414. Masserman, J. H.: Behavior and Neurosis. Chicago: Univ. of Chicago Press 1943.
415. Jacobsen, E. and Y. Skaarup: Experimental Induction of Conflict-Behaviour in Cats: Its Use in Pharmacological Investigation. Acta pharmacol. (Kbh.) 11, 117 (1955).
416. Masserman, J. H.: Behavioral Pharmacology in Animals. In: Bradley, P. B., P. Deniker, and, C. Raduoco-Thomas (Eds.): Neuropsychopharmacology, p. 97. Amsterdam: Elsevier 1959.
417. Jacobsen, E. and E. Sonne: Effect of Benzilic Acid Diethylaminoethyl Ester HCL (benactyzine) on Stress Induced Behavior in Rat. Acta pharmacol. (Kbh.) 11, 135 (1955).
418. Courvoisier, S.: International Symposium on Clorpromazine, Pharmacodynamic Basis for Use of Chlor promazine in Psychiatry. J. Clin. Psychopath. 17, 25 (1956).
419. Cook, L.: In Bradley, P. B., P. Deniker and C. Raduoco-Thomas (Eds.): Neuropsychopharmacology, p. 123. Amsterdam: Elsevier 1959.
420. Winter, C. A., L. Flataker, W. P. Boger, E. V. C. Smith and B. E. Sanders: The Effects of Blood Serum and of Serum Fractions from Schizophrenic Donors Upon the Performance of Trained Rats. In: Chemical Pathology of the Nervous System, p. 641. Jordi Folch-Pi. (Ed.). Oxford: Pergamon Press 1961.
421. Miller, N. E.: Objective Techniques for Studying Motivational Effects of Drugs on Animals. In: Garattini, S., and V. Ghetti (Eds.). Psychotropic Drugs, p. 83 Amsterdam: Elsevier 1957.
422. Brady, J. V.: In Bradley, P. B., P. Deniker, and C. Raduoco-Thomas (Eds.). Neuropsychopharmacology, p. 275. Amsterdam. Elsevier 1959.

423. Skinner, B. F.: The Behavior of Organisms. New York: Appleton-Century, Crofts 1938.
424. Keller, F. S.: Light-aversion in the white Rat. Psychol. Rec. 4, 235 (1941).
425. Sidman, M.: Avoidance Conditioning with Brief Shock and no Exteroceptive Warning Signal. Science 118, 157 (1953).
426. Brady, J. V. and H. F. Hunt: An Experimental Approach to the Analysis of Emotional Behavior. J. Psychol. 40, 313 (1955).
427. Dews, B.: Studies on Behavior. I. Differential Sensitivity to Pentobarbital of Pecking Performance in Pigeons Depending on the Schedule of Reward. J. Pharmacol. exp. Ther. 113, 393 (1955).
428. Sidman, M. Behavioral Pharmacology. Psychopharmacologia. (Berl.) 1, 1 (1959).
429. Hill, J. H., and E. Stellar: An Electronic Drinkometer. Science 114, 43 (1951).
430. Berlyne, D. E.: Novelty and Curiosity as Determinants of Exploratory Behaviour. Brit. J. Psychol. 41, 68 (1958).
431. Beach, F. A., and A. M. Holz-Tucker: Effects of Different Concentrations of Androgen Upon Sexual Behavior in Castrated Male Rats. J. comp. physiol. Psychol. 42, 433 (1949).
432. Miller, N. E.: Effects of Drugs on Motivation; the Value of Using a Variety of Measures. Ann. N. Y. Acad. Sci. 65, 318 (1956).
433. Miller, N. E.: In R. W. Gerard (Ed.): Methods in Medical Research. Vol. III, p. 216. N.Y. Year Book Publ. 1950.
434. Brown, J. S.: Gradients of Approach and Avoidance Responses and Their Relation to Level of Motivation. J. comp. physiol. Psychol. 41, 450 (1948).
435. Bailey, C. J., and N. E. Miller: J. exp. Psychol. 45, 205 (1952).
436. Dews, P B.: Modification by Drugs of Performance on Simple Schedules of Positive Reinforcements. Ann. N. Y. Acad. Sci. 65, 268 (1956).
437. Young, P. T.: Motivation of Animal Behavior. In: C. P. Stone: Comparative Psychol. 3rd edition, p. 62. New York: Prentice-Hall 1951.
438. Jenkins, T. N., L. H. Warner, and C. J. Warden: Standard Apparatus for the Study of Animal Motivation. J. comp. Psychol. 6, 361 (1926).
438B. Witt, P. N.: D-Lysergs"ure Diethylamid (LSD 25) im Spinnentest. Experientia (Basel) 7, 310 (1951).
439. Brady, J L: A Comparative Approach to the Evaluation of Drug Effects Upon Behavior. In: W. S. Fields (Ed.). Brain Mechanisms and Drug Actions. Springfield, Ill.: Charles C. Thomas 1957.
439 B. Abramson, H. A.: Blocking of the LSD-25 Reaction in Siamese Fighting Fish. In: Neuropharmacology, p. 9. Transaction of Third Conference. New York: Josiah Macy Jr. Foundation 1958.
440. Weiskrantz, L., and W. A. Wilson jr.: The Effects of Reserpine on Emotional Behavior of Normal and Brain-operated Monkeys. Ann. N. Y. Acad. Sci. 61, 36 (1955).
440B. Cook, L. In: Bradley, P. B., P. Deniker. and C. Raduoco-Thomas (Eds.): Neuropsychopharmacology, p. 125. Amsterdam: Elsevier 1959.
441. Sidman, M.: Drug Behavior Interaction. Ann. N. Y. Acad. Sci. 65, 282 (1956).
442. Estes, W. K., and B. F. Skinner: Some Quantitative Properties of Anxiety. J. exp. Psychol. 29, 390 (1941).
443. Brady, J. V.: Assessment of Drug Effects on Emotional Behavior. Science 123, 1033 (1956).
443A. Hunt, H. F.: Some Effects of Drugs on Classical Type Conditioning. Ann. N. Y. Acad. Sci. 65, 258 (1956).
444. Hunt, H. F.: Effects of Drugs on Emotional Responses and Abnormal Behavior in Animals: In Cole, J. O., and R. W. Gerard (Eds.): Psychopharmacology, p. 268. Washington: Nat. Acad. Sciences, Nat. Res. Council 1959.
445. Olds, J., and P. Milner: Positive Reinforcement Produced by Electrical Stimulation of Septal Area and other Regions of Rat Brain. J. comp. physiol. Psychol. 47 419 (1954).
445B. Höhn, R., L. Lasagna: Effects of Aggregation and Temperature on Amphetamine Toxicity in Mice. Psychopharmacologia (Berl.) 1, 210 (1960).
446. Olds, J.: Selective Effects of Drives and Drugs on "Reward" Systems of the Brain. In: Ciba Symposium on Neurological Basis of Behavior, p. 124. London: J. & A. Churchill 1958.
446B. Maxwell, D. R.: In Bradley, P. B., P. Deeniker, and C. Raduoco-Thomas (Eds.): Neuropsychopharmacology, p. 365. Amsterdam: Elsevier 1959.
447. Olds, J.: Studies of Neuropharmacologicals by Electrical and Chemical Manipulation of the Brain in Animals with Chronically Implanted Electrodes. In: Bradley, P. B., P. Deniker, and C. Raduoco-Thomas (Eds.): Neuro psychopharmacology, p. 20. Amsterdam: Elsevier 1959.
447A. Blough, D. S.: Ann. N. Y. Acad. Sci. 66, 733 (1957).
447B. Brown, B.: Behavioral Effects of Drugs Derivable from Observation of Intact Normal Animals. In: Cole, J. O., and R. W. Gerard (Eds.). Psychopharmacology, p. 236. Washington National Acad. of Science and National Research Council 1959.
448. Sidman, M.: Technique for Assessing the Effects of Drugs on Timing Behavior. Science 122, 925 (1955).
449. Sidman, M.: Drug Behavior Interaction. Ann. N. Y. Acad. Sci. 65, 282 (1956).
450. Jarvik, M. F., and L. Uhr: Impairment by Lysergic Acid Diethylamide of Accuracy in Performance of a Delayed Alternation Test in Monkeys. In: Uhr, L., and J. G. Miller (Eds.): Drugs and Behavior, p. 326. New York: John Wiley & Sons 1960.
451. Miller, J. G., and L. Uhr: Behavioral toxicity as measured by tests of simulated driving and of vision: drugs and behavior, p. 326. New York. John Wiley & Sons 1960.
452. Williams, R. J.: Biochemical Individuality. New York: John Wiley & Sons 1956.
453. Clark, A. J.: The mode of action of drugs in cells. Baltimore: Williams & Wilkins 1933.
454. Williams, R. J.: Loc. cit. p. 89.
455. Williams, R. J.: Etiology of Alcoholism; Working Hypothesis Involving Interplay of Hereditary and Environ mental Factors. Quart. J. Stud. Alcohol. 7, 567 (1947).
456. Ellis, S.: Benzoylcholine and Atropine Esterases. J. Pharmacol. exp. Ther. 91, 370 (1947).
457. Sawin, P. B., and D. Glick: Atropinesterase Genetically Determined Enzyme in Rabbit. Proc. Nat. Acad. Sci. (Wash.) 29, 55-59 (1943).
458. Funkenstein, D. H., M. Greenblatt, and H. C. Solomon: Autonomic Nervous System Changes Following Electric Shock Treatment. J. Nerv. Ment. Dis. 108, 409 (1948).
459. Feinberg, I.: Current Status of the Funkenstein Test. Arch. Neurol. Psychiat. (Chic.) 80, 488 (1958).

460. Labrosse, E. H., J. Axelrod, I. J. Kopin, and S. S. Kety: J. Clin. Invest. 40, 253 (1961).
461. Labrosse, E. H., J. D. Mann, and S. S. Kety: The Physiological and Psychological Effects of Intravenously Administered Epinephrine, and its Metabolism in Normal and Schizophrenic Men. III. Metabolism of 7-H 3 epinephrine as Determined in Studies on Blood and Urine. J. Psychiat. Res. 1, 68 (1961).
462. Weil-Malherbe, H.: The Fluorimetric Estimation of Catechol Compounds by the Ethylenediamine Condensation Method. Pharmacol. Rev. 11, 278 (1959).
463. Szara, S.: 6-Hydroxylation: An Important Metabolic Route for α-Methyltryptamine. Experientia (Basel) 17, 76 (1961).
463A. Eysenck, H. J.: Drugs and Personality. 1. Theory and Methodology. J. Ment. Sci. 103, 119 (1957).
464. Uhr, L., and J. G. Miller: Drugs and Behavior. New York. John Wiley & Sons 1960.
464A. Lindemann, E., u. J. M. v. Felsinger: Drug Effects and Personality Theory. Psychopharm (Berl.) 2, 69 (1961).
465. Kornetsky, C., and O. Humphries: Relationship between Effects of a Number of Gentrally Acting Drugs and Personality. Arch. Neurol. Psychiat. (Chic.) 77, 325 (1957).
466. Kornetsky, C., O. Humphries and E. V. Evarts: Comparison of Psychological Effects on Certain Centrally Acting Drugs in Man. Arch. Neurol. Psychiat. (Chic.) 77, 318 (1957).
467. Weinstein, E. A., and R. L. Kahn: Denial of Illness. Springfield, Ill.: Charles C. Thomas 1955.
468. Modell, W.: The relief of symptoms, Chapter 4. Philadelphia: W. B. Saunders & Co.1955.
469. Lasagna, L., F. Mosteller, J. M. v. Felsinger, and H. K. Beecher: Study of Placebo Response. Amer. J. Med. 16, 770 (1954).
470. Wolf, S.: The Pharmacology of Placebos. Pharmacol. Rev. 11 689 (1959).
471. Beecher, H. K.: The Measurement of Subjective Responses. New York: Oxford University Press 1959.
472. Gantt, W. H.: Physiological Bases of Psychiatry. Springfield, Ill.: Charles C. Thomas 1958.
473. Palmer, R. S.: Hypotensive Action of Rauwolfia Serpentina and Reserpine: Double Hidden Placebo Study of Ambulatory Patients with Hypertension. Amer. Practit. 6, 1323 (1955).
474. Taut, E. F., and E. W. Passarelli: Placebos in the Treatment of Rheumatoid Arthritie and other Rheumatic Conditions. Ann. rheum. Dis. 16, 18 (1957).
475. Beecher, H. K.: Evidence for Increased Effectiveness of Placebos with Increased Stress. Amer. J. Physiol. 187, 163 (1956).
476. Elkes J. and C. Elkes: Effects of Chlorpromazine on the Behavior of Chronically Overactive Psychotic Patients. Brit. Med. J. 1954 II, 560.
477. Rinkel, M. (Ed.). Symposium on Specific and Non-Specific Factors in Psychopharmacology. New York. Philosophical Library (1962).
478. Cooperative Multihospital Study. Psychopharmacology Service Center. Washington: D. C. (in preparation).
479. Freud, S.: An Outline of Psychoanalysis. New York: W. W. Norton & Co.1949.
479A. Kubie, L. S.: A Psychoanalytic Approach to the Pharmacology of Psychological Processes. In: Uhr, L., and J. G. Miller (Eds.). Drugs and Behavior, p. 209. New York. John Wiley & Sons 1960.
480. Lindemann, E.: Working Paper. WHO/AHP 10. Study Group on Ataractic Agents. Geneva: WH0 1958.
481. Craik, K. J. W.: The Nature of Explanation. New York: Cambridge Univ. Press 1943.
482. Bexton, W. H., W. Heron, and T. H. Scott: Effects of Decreased Variation in the Sensory Environment. Canad. J. Psychol. 8, 70 (1954).
483. Elkes, J.: Schizophrenic Disorder in Relation to Neural Organization: The Need for some Conceptual Points of Reference. In: Folch-Pi, J. (Ed.): Chemical Pathol. of the Nerv. System, p. 648. Oxford: Pergamon Press 1961.
484. Sargant, W., and H. J. Shorvon: Acute War Neurosis. Special Reference to Pavlov's Experimental Observations and the Mechanism of Abreaction. Arch. Neurol. Psychat. (Chic.) 54, 231 (1945).
485. Delay, J., P. Pichot, P. Romaniet et R. Genest: L'emploi de methedrine en psychiatrie, l'exploration des mutismes. Ann. méd.-psychol. 105, 50 (1947).
486. Sandison, R. A., A. M. Spencer, and J. D. A. Whitelaw: Therapeutic Value of Lysergic Acid Diethylamide in Mental Illness. J. ment. Sci. 100, 491 (1954).
487. Abramson, H. A. (Ed.): The use of LSD-in psychotherapy. New York: Josiah Macy Jr. Foundation 1960.
488. Denber, H.C.B., S. Merlis: Studies on Mescaline Action in Schizophrenic Patients. Psychiat. Quart. 29, 421 (1955).
489. Cohen, S.: Lysergic Acid Diethylamide Side Effects and Complications. J. Nerv. Ment. Dis. 130, 30 (1960).
490. Kramer, M.: Publ. Health Monograph, No. 41. Washington: D.C. U.S. Govt. Printing Office 1956.
491. Hazards of Tranquillity (Annotation). Brit. Med. J. 1957 II 92.
492. A. M. A. Council on Drugs: Potential Hazards of Meprobamate. J. Amer. Med. Ass. 164, 1332 (1957).
493. Dickel, H.A., H.Dixon: Inherent Dangers in Use of Tranquilizing Drugs in Anxiety States. JAMA 163, 422 (1957).
494. Raymond, M. J., C. J. Lucas et al.: A Trial of five Tranquilizing Drugs in Psychoneurosis. BMJ 1957 II, 63.
495. Hargreaves, G. R., M. Hamilton and J. M. Roberts: Benactyzine as an Aid in Treatment of Anxiety States; Preliminary Report. Brit. Med. J. 1957 I, 306.
496. Psychopharmacology, Problems in Evaluation. Cole, J. O., and R. Y. Gerard (Eds.). National Acad. of Science, National Research Council, pp. 393-432: Washington, D. C., 1959.
497. Lorr, M.: Rating Scales, Behavior Iventories, and Drugs. In: Uhr, L., and J. G. Miller (Eds.): Drugs and Behavior, p. 519. New York: John Wiley & Sons 1960.
498. Critchley, M.: The language of gesture. London: Arnold 1939.
499. Ruesch, J., and W. Kees: Non Verbal Communication. Berkeley University of California Press 1956.
500. Elkes, J.: Subjective and Objective Observation in Psychiatry. The Harvey Lectures Series 57, p. 63. New York: Academic Press 1962.

Part Five

SCHIZOPHRENIC DISORDER AS A DISORDER OF CHEMICALLY MEDIATED INFORMATION PROCESSING IN THE BRAIN

PAPER

16. Joel Elkes: *Schizophrenic disorder in relation to levels of neural organization: The need for some conceptual points of reference.*
Reprinted with the agreement of Elsevier Science from J. Folch-Pi (ed.) *The Chemical Pathology of the Nervous System* (pp. 648-665). London, Pergamon Press, 1961

ARGUMENT

Paper 16 examines disturbances of cognitive function as a central feature of schizophrenic disorder, and compares drug induced changes in perception, affect, and behavior to the phenomenology of the schizophrenias. It finds the similarities partial and unconvincing. The author argues that schizophrenic disorder represents a decompensation or failure of a fundamental organizing process in the brain concerned with the processing of information at perceptual, affective and cognitive levels. The central feature of this process is chemically mediated discriminate inhibition involving several levels of functioning simultaneously. Attention, vigilance and serial ordering of information in time are seen as attributes of this process.

The paper suggests that this process involves cell ensembles in subcortical areas reciprocally governing cortical functions. The thalamus, lenticular, pulvinar, globus pallidus and caudate nuclei as well the amygdala and the hippocampal areas should be considered. A plea is made for studying regional chemical topology of the brain in relation to the relative distribution, balance and inter-relation of regionally distributed families of neurotransmitters, such as norepinephrine, serotonin, GABA, and dopamine. Dopamine is singled out because of its (at the time) recently discovered presence in the caudate and lentiform nuclei. Drugs could be used a discriminate probes in the study of the chemical pathology of schizophrenic disorder.

PAPER 16

SCHIZOPHRENIC DISORDER IN RELATION TO LEVELS OF NEURAL ORGANIZATION: THE NEED FOR SOME CONCEPTUAL POINTS OF REFERENCE[*]

Joel Elkes

Clinical Neuropharmacology Research Center, National Institute of Mental Health, and Saint Elizabeth Hospital Washington, D.C.

It is important, as has been pointed out in an adjoining review (1) , not to misuse quantitative biochemical techniques in inadequate controlled clinical material. Therein, no doubt, lies a major source of error. Yet, though the most immediate, and without doubt, the most pertinent et present, it is not the only source. There are others, which, though less pressing, merit consideration at this stage, inasmuch as they bear upon the phenomenology of schizophrenic disorders, and their possible neurophysiological correlates. It is the purpose of this communication briefly to examine some of these sources; and to attempt, in a tentative and very preliminary way, to relate them to some conceptual points of reference, which, in the view of the writer, should be borne in mind in investigations in this field.

For the past few decades research in human neuropharmacology, and in schizophrenia, has been pervaded by three attitudes which are in danger of hardening into tacit assumptions, despite an oft-avowed awareness to the contrary. The first of these is the view that the overt and florid behavioral symptoms of schizophrenic illness (hallucinations, delusion, disturbances of affect, and of motor behavior) are representative and characteristic of schizophrenic illness; the second that psychotropic drugs, by the mimicry or relief of overt symptoms of the psychoses, may be used to furnish one with reliable scale models of the schizophrenias; and the third that peripheral biochemical indicators in body fluids can be related to what may well be essentially localized intracerebral biochemical events. It is these assumptions, and their unfortunate collusion with each other, which one would like to question. They make for a conceptual matrix which is hybrid and unsatisfactory; and though little can be done to improve it at the present stage, it may perhaps be well at least to define some components which, at this, or any stage, have no business in it.

1. DISTURBANCE OF COGNITIVE FUNCTION AS A CENTRAL FEATURE OF SCHIZOPHRENIC DISORDER

In the first place it would be well not to be misled by what is manifest in the schizophrenias. The florid clinical symptoms of the acute attack and the varied manifestations of the illness as

---

[*] Reprinted with the agreement of Elsevier Science from J. Folch-Pi (ed.) *The Chemical Pathology of the Nervous System* (pp. 648-665). London, Pergamon Press, 1961

it takes its course may merely obscure a more malignant and behaviorally silent process, which, in an established case, proceeds relentlessly, irrespective of the outer shell of symptoms, and their ebb and flow during remission and relapse. Thus, for example, depersonalization and derealization (the feeling of unreality, strangeness, and foreignness of a person either about himself, or in relation to his environment) though seen in early schizophrenia may be observed equally in the hysterical reaction (2), the depressive depersonalization syndrome, and in organic brain disease (2). It is also seen in Mescal (3) and LSD-25 (4) intoxication. The violent affective changes are seen in the manic-depressive psychoses. Illusions and hallucinations are well known in the organic syndromes, such as alcoholic encephalopathy; they can also be evoked by temporal lobe stimulation (5). Equally delusion of the most extravagant kind are encountered in organic brain disorders (for example, syphilitic encephalopathy) or in the affective psychoses; latent delusional material may be activated in drug induced states(6). These few spurious examples could be enlarged; they are merely cited to emphasize the lack of specificity of these phenomena for schizophrenic process. Yet if we are to relate physiological of biochemical findings to the schizophrenias with any prospect of theoretical yield, we must, even at this early stage, be much more rigorous and specific about the description of the phenomena we are studying, and look to cognate phenomena elsewhere.

These phenomena need not strike on at first behaviorally at all. But anyone who has engaged a quiet schizophrenic in conversation, or read in schizophrenic's letter, will instantly know what one means. Its is the quality defined by Bleuler (7, 8) as disconnectedness (Zerfahrenheit) a lack, or loosening, or fragmentation of association; an inability to order an relate stimulus situations to each other or to stored memory traces, an inability to "abstract" common denominators from related situations, and to organize these into a coherent, sequential, cognitive process. There is in the schizophrenic a reduction of the capacity to categorize and group phenomena on the basis of common or shared properties, or, at times, a paradoxical inversion of the frame of reference usually employed for such grouping. A phrase such as, "The air is still here, the air between the things in the room; but the things are not there any more" (9), conveys this aspect. The language of the schizophrenic thus no longer functions as an adaptive instrument in the commerce between the patient and his environment.

This inability to generalize and abstract is directly related to another property namely the excessively concrete quality of schizophrenic thinking (10) which, as well as being apparent clinically, may also show in psychological tests (11). It is very difficult for a schizophrenic patient to grasp the make-believe of any fictitious situation, such as story, or a proverb (12) read to him; and his actions towards it although at times of an inner consistency, may, in fact, be totally inappropriate because of the false assumptions which underlie it. A word when used by schizophrenic appears as part of an object or a situation, not a representative of it (13). Such changes however, are on occasion encountered in patients with irreversible organic brain damage (13).

These disturbances are related to a third type of dysfunction seen in the schizophrenic, namely lability, incongruousness and exaggeration of affective responses at the beginning of the illness followed at a later stage by a "flattening" of affect and an incapacity to modulate or grade the response: "Affective rigidity", as Bleuler put it (14), "is on of the surest signs of the disease." This, however, must be clearly distinguished from a inability to make such a response (14). The touching of a particular constellation of ideas in a schizophrenic may, very often, provoke a violent response, even in an apparently indifferent patient; and in the dereistic and autistic preoccupations of a withdrawn chronic schizophrenic one finds the extravagant fulfillment of active endeavors, wishes and fears. These permeate the delusional material, and dye deep the thought process of the schizophrenic. The affective apparatus is therefore capable of functioning. Its threshold, and smoothness of operation however are very different from normal, and it responds to cues very different from the normal.

The above three properties – disturbance and fragmentation of association, an excessive concretization of thinking, a lack of appropriateness and of modulation of the affective response – are linked to a fourth consistent finding in the schizophrenias, which forms an outstanding an measurable characteristic of the disease process. This is the inabilitiy of a schizophrenic to consistently maintain, for any length of time, a state of *readiness* to incoming stimuli in an experimental situation which demands response to such stimuli (15) . The disturbance is most clearly shown in comparing the reaction time of normals with that of schizophrenics, the most marked differences between the two groups appearing in relation to the so-called preparatory interval (that is the interval between a warning signal, and a stimulus to which the subject is instructed to respond). This preparatory interval is related to what is commonly known as attention, and to the older, and very valuable concept of vigilance (16). It can, however, in this instance be reduced to a measure which, of all the scores so far available, clearly differentiates normal from schizophrenic subjects without any overlap (17). This measure, termed „Set Index" (18) thus forms a valuable anchor for quantitative studies of a pharmacological and biochemical kind. It is mentioned again below in a different context.

2. THE SUPERFICIAL RESEMBLANCE OF DRUG-INDUCED MENTAL DISTURBANCES TO SCHIZOPHRENICS PROCESS

The above consideration may serve to sharpen the relation of drug included mental changes to the phenomenology of established schizophrenia, and point to similarities as well as to possible differences. The similarities have indeed been obvious since the turn of the century (19, 20) but, for reasons considered elsewhere (21), did not interact with the neurological and behavioral sciences until the last few decades. Yet the term psychosomimetic, though drawing attention to similarities between the two sets of phenomena which may be real enough,, tends to obscure certain differences which are equally real. The changes in affect (lability, or flattening, or incongrousness, inappropriateness, and exaggeration of response) are seen in both LSD-25 and Mescal intoxication, and particularly in early schizophrenia; however, as pointed out above, they lack specificity for the schizophrenic. Similarly, disturbances of body image, and the disturbances of feeling of identity covered by the terms depersonalization and derealization, are seen in both sets of conditions; but not in them alone (21).

Disturbances of perception, although often quoted as a common, denominator, in fact show marked differences between the two sets of conditions. In the Mescal or LSD-25 induced states, visual symptoms predominate, and auditory, tactile and gustatory modalities are involved much less frequently. On the other hand, auditory symptoms predominate in schizophrenia. Furthermore, the visual illusions and hallucinations seen in LSD-and Mescal intoxication are characterized by the appearance of the so-called entoptic phenomena or "form constants" (22). These include faintly moving geometrical figures (lattice, chessboard, tapestry, cobwebs, tunnels); an alteration in number (polyopia), size (dysmegalopsia) and shape (dysmorphopsia), of the objects perceived, and a change of visual perspective. Such changes, however as pointed out in a most pertinent critique (22), are not confined to Mescal intoxication. They are seen equally in such diverse conditions as hypoglycaemia, nitrous oxide or carbon dioxide inhalation, in states of dehydration, and in non-specific or toxic deliria. More pertinent, visual changes such as described above are only seen rarely in established schizophrenia; when they occur, they may be associated either with the onset, or an acute exacerbation of the disease. Form constants are very rarely encountered, and apparent movement of objects is distinctly uncommon. Such visual hallucinations as may appear are much more organized and personally meaningful to the schizophrenic patient. They may represent either an activated memory trace, or the fusion of a memory, or a wish, or a fear, with a misidentified, and ambiguous object in the patient's environment (such as any of us are apt to do in dim light). They are used a bizarre props in a visually projected play of the patient's imagination.

Attention is draw to these differences both in the incidence and character of the visual manifestations for two quite separate reasons. In the first place, it is casually assumed that the sensory disorganization in the drug induced states can be equated with corresponding changes in schizophrenia. Plainly, it cannot. Secondly, even if visual disorganization is manifest in both states, the level of disorganization induced by either Mescal or LSD-would appear to be of a rather different order from that seen in schizophrenia. The disturbance of color vision and the appearance of form constant and of fine apparent movement in Mescal intoxication would suggest a disturbance of the perceptual processes at a more discrete level of organization, than the emergence, or the creation-by-fusion of imagery which, whether an illusion based on a misidentification of sensory cues, or a condensation of such cues with an emergent stored memory trace, is well formed, animated and real to the patient in his own personal idiom. The administration of Mescal to schizophrenics leads to the appearance of new sets of symptoms (23). Thus, even if we were to assume a basically similar mechanism to account for both sets of changes (which, at this stage, would be precarious assumption), we would have to grant that the same process did rather different things at different levels of organization. The visual changes may or may not be related to electrophysiological data suggesting the involvement of elements in the lateral geniculate body (24), and the retina (25, 26) in LSD-intoxication. The role of retroretinal structures (27), as giving rise to persistent after-images has also to be borne in mind, as has the possibility of interference with fine eye movement, and the physiological fine nystagmus which makes for definition of the visual image (28). Whatever the level of interference, it is clear that the coding and successive transformation of information along the visual pathway, including its central projections, may be disturbed sufficiently in drug intoxication to interfere with normal perception of color size, shape, distance, position and texture of objects. This is a rather different matter from a disturbance manifesting, for example, in the appearance of a patient's mother dressed in the clothes of his wife, whispering affectionate greetings to him as he is on his way to supper in a dimly lit hall. A very much larger and more highly organized preformed and stored aggregate of information is released in accordance with needs of the patient at the time.

The affective connotation of illusional or hallucinatory material is borne out even more markedly in the auditory symptoms which, though rarely seen in drug intoxication, are common in schizophrenic illness. Sometimes these manifest as simple noises, such as blowing, raring, rattling, shouting; more often, as emotionally charged sounds, such as of repeated short sentences implying a wish, actual or repressed, a fear, or a command. Somehow, there is, here too, emergence of stored information, polarized strongly in terms of its affective meaning. As Bleuler put it (29), "hallucinations do not express sensory material but thoughts, feelings and drives". They may use sensory cues, and even sensory illusions. But the form they ultimately assume draws heavily upon performed and repressed memory traces carrying a strong affective charge. The predominance of auditory over visual disorders of perception in established schizophrenia may be due to the constant variation of visual vis-a-vis the relatively invariant auditory input during day-to-day life; this may make for more ready corrections in the visual than the auditory field. Furthermore, inasmuch as the process of conceptual thinking is closely related to the evolution of the signaling system of spoken language, it may not be unexpected for this system to become increasingly affected by the thought disorder so characteristic of the illness; though the difference between aphasia and this type of disturbance will no doubt be noted

3. SCHIZOPHRENIC DISORDER AS A DISTURBANCE OF INFORMATION PROCESSING BY THE BRAIN

Thus we are left with relatively few features which, with any confidence, can be related to the syndrome of the schizophrenias. At the somatic level, which has been recently reviewed elsewhere (30) and will therefore not be touched upon here, there is indication of autonomic imbalance, with some indication of sympathetic predominance, and significant deviation from the normal responses in stress situations (31). At the phenomenological level of clinical observations there is a striking lack of "play" and modulation of the affective apparatus; yet, at the same time, a strong affective coloring of all ideational material, despite its inappropriate and bizarre nature. Equally, there are occasional perceptual disturbances, more common in the auditory than in the visual area; a disturbance of cognitive functioning showing as an inability to abstract common elements from related situations, an undue concretization of thinking, and a dependence on verbal stimuli as they are presented; and a corresponding disturbance of language as an instrument of communication. At a psychometric level there is the consistent finding of disturbance of preparatory set, or a state of readiness in anticipation of events in the future (15).

It is suggested that these findings are not unconnected, and that they represent the decompensation or failure of a quite fundamental organizing process in the brain which, during wakefulness in the normal, and at tremendous speed, registers, transforms, codes, matches and correlates new against stored information, and, in a succession of such transactions, computes the probabilities which are of optimum service to the adaptive needs of the organism. It is furthermore suggested that these transformations proceed simultaneously at different, yet closely interrelated neural level, that they employ shifting reciprocal, and highly discriminate inhibitory mechanism in a successive elimination of redundant information; and that the final product – be it percept, or a motor act, or an "idea" – represents a condensed symbolic model of succession of operation which, whether stereotype or unique, comprise traces and elements of its various phases in a temporally coded pattern. The ability to organize rapidly changing and fluctuating inputs by a process of convergence and occlusion into a temporal topology of high information content would thus seem to be an outstanding characteristic of higher nervous nets. This is most clearly seen in the process of perception (32), where evidence suggests an early, selective, and highly discriminate adjustment or "gating" of thresholds along the sensory pathway.

It is, by now, reasonably that perceptual definition and invariance requires variable stimulation of receptors over time. This, for example, appears true in the case of the retina, where a mirror arrangement to keep an image constant on the retina despite fine eye tremor leads to the disappearance of the image (33). A scanning operation (34), a sort of "fingering over" (35), of the visual field by the spherically arranged array of receptors must be assumed to make for sharpness and detail of image. Furthermore, it can be equally shown that both in the visual (36) and the auditory pathway (37) the pattern, transmitted from the receptor to the first cell relay involves in each and every instance, a highly patterned, inhibitory process, the inhibition reciprocating with excitation in a sort of miniature Sherringtonian rule. The information leaving the receptors is thus already condensed and coded; and undergoes further transformation along its upward path by the operation of further inhibitory processes which, unlike the graded responses to stimulus situations, increasingly emphasize its on/off characteristics (38), That this information, relayed by way of sensory nuclei, is nevertheless profoundly stimulus influenced is brought out by two sets of experiments, each involving the auditory pathway. In the first (39), the evoked potentials in the cochlear nucleus were recorded in response to a click, and followed through, by a process of repetition, to the point of extinction. The click was then paired with an electric shock, and conditioning reestablished; it was then allowed to fade again. It was noted that during extinction there was a marked reduction in the evoked electrical activity in the cochlear nucleus, the caudate nucleus and the auditory cortex. However, when the click signified impending shock, the responses were considerably higher.

The second experiment (40) involved the presentation of visual (mouse) or olfactory (fish smell) stimulus in the conscious cat while evoked potentials from the cochlear nucleus were being recorded in response to auditory stimulation. Again, there was a marked reduction of such response while the animal was attending to these competing stimuli. It was suggested by the authors that this attenuation of discharges was brought by inhibitory influences emanating from the midbrain reticular system.

Phenomena such as these suggest a much more active participation of the attention and affect systems in the selective organization of sense data than is generally assumed; a participation which in man becomes more evident as sense data become ambiguous, or reduced. In these circumstances (as in a presentation of ambiguous figures (41) or an attenuation of sensory input) the interaction between sensory information and stored, and affectively charged memory traces becomes more obvious. It is, as if there were a first-order monitoring or preliminary grouping of sensory stimuli in terms of their appetitive-positive-pleasurable or aversive-negative-painful connotation; the process resulting either in the suppression or distortion of what is perceived, or the emergence of an associated memory trace which carries an affective meaning very different from that of the presenting stimulus. The wish may thus become not only father to the thought, but also to the image. In dim light, for example, the aggressive, destructive, orally preoccupied schizophrenic will mistake his visiting wife for his much hated mother and viciously attack her; or savor blood in the roses which she brings him. In view of the promptness of these affective responses the various stages of the operation must take place at very high speed. The fast, rich and direct cable system connecting the various levels of the limbic system to each other (42-45); the relative closure of this system; and its efferent connections both upward into the basal ganglia and downward into the brain stem (45) make this system, which embodies much that is clearly appetitive or aversive, a possible neural substrate for this preliminary grouping of information. The intimate anatomical relationship of this system to the hypothalamus and the brain stem nuclei should be particularly noted. It is presumably these connections which provide the efferent loops ultimately leading to the discharge of the repertoire of motor responses known as "innate" or "instinctual" behavior. Three qualities of these responses may be mentioned the present context. First, they are limited and stereotype in range; second, they are related to functions and processes which have survival value (hunger, thirst, combat, sex): and third, other things being equal, they are normally acted out with relatively little delay. The fast computation of sensory cues thus comes up with a limited but prompt and normally appropriate motor answer, using a programming which has been laid down at a genetic or early developmental level. The firmness and specificity of these inborn motor patterns, or the sensory cues which elicit them (46) is a remarkable degree and comparable to the specificity of the physical attributes of a species. It must therefore be presumed to be carried at the gene level.

4. DELAYING MECHANISMS, AND THE SERIAL ORDERING OF INFORMATION IN TIME

Attention has been drawn in the preceding section to the promptness of discharge of the affective patterns of behavior. Yet, it is evident that in normal waking life in man the full range of these patterns is only sparingly used; and usually used under stress. Equally, however, as was indicated earlier, the whole context of symbolic thought and language is profoundly guided by the affect systems, which continuously compel choices and compromises between mutually occlusive responses. It is evident that the far-reaching modifications of this immediate responsiveness of the higher nervous system is related to the evolution of delaying systems which discriminately block the immediate response; and that it is associated with an increasing power to substitute condensed symbols and secondary signals of objects and events for objects and events, or for the sensory cues by which they are normally represented. In the motor field, the increasing condensation of the normal range of motor activity to high-information content responses – such as gesture, speech and writing – are examples of the same economy. Somehow, then the higher nervous system has developed an ability to relate new sets of cues to stored memory traces. And to "abstract" or group new information in terms of categories, rather than isolated items. It is these functions which, as mentioned earlier, are characteristically disturbed in the schizophrenias. In the organic disturbances of language, aphasia or agraphia, there are neurological correlates. To date no comparable correlates have become evident in schizophrenia.

This disturbance of cognitive function may not be unrelated to another disturbance evident in the fully developed schizophrenic patient. Such patients show a diminished ability to order information serially in time (47), or to recognize the mutual occlusiveness of different sets of responses, which cannot coexist in the same segment of time, and remain appropriate responses. There is furthermore (though this, of necessity, is not regularly seen) a diminished ability to recognize past, present, and future sequentially. A schizophrenic may condense in one brief sentence temporally separated elements, and present them as a subjectively coherent, but objectively paradoxical whole. He will introduce long-standing memory traces into conversation as if they ware actual events, and thus be both illogical and doubly oriented. Yet, orientation and logic and, for that matter, the structure of language, require a rigorous regulation of the amount of information allowed within a time span; and serial order is implicit in the concept of causality where one event is, by definition, preceded by another. Appropriate response to a situation implies the retrospective validation and matching of new against stored information, a reduction of randomness, and an increase in probability in the correct assessment of outcome over a given bit of time. Time is thus the main axis around which the waking brain constructs its models of reality; and the success of the higher nervous system in its evolution may well be related to an increasing ability for inhibition and delay of initial responses and for accurate appraisal responses of probabilities over time.

It is therefore of moment to any view seeks neurophysiological correlates in schizophrenic process that the very properties which have been singled out as characteristic of this process are also shared by two other groups of phenomena, both of which are rapidly becoming accessible to controlled investigation. The first of these is the reduction in sensory input (the so-called "sensory isolation") where in normal human subjects, profound disturbances of thinking have been observed as a result of systematic cutting off of visual, auditory and tactile stimuli for extended periods (48, 49). The second is represented by the dream process, which occurs physiologically during light sleep, and which, because of the electrophysiological accompaniments of dreaming (50), can now be followed sequentially in suitably instructed volunteers. The early, and inordinately penetrating description of the natural history of dreams (51) singles out four characteristics of this physiological type of thought disorder. First, the material has a strong affective coloring: The fusion of wish or a fear with an image or event is regularly seen. Second, the dream material is not bound by the logic of waking life; arbitrary and mutually occlusive elements may coexist in the same scene. Third, there is a fusion of memory with percept, a memory actually appearing as a well organized hallucination. Lastly, there is a striking disregard of considerations of time. As in schizophrenic thought disorder, temporally separated elements coexist and a stimulus applied to the sleeper during dreaming may be projected both backward and forward in time.

That such profound changes in the processing in information should in fact occur physiologically without any extraneous chemical intervention gives pause for thought. It poses the question as to whether the process seen overtly in dreaming may not represent an early phase in a continuum of information-processing by the brain which, by way of related stages ultimately leads to the highly condensed, appropriate and logical responses of normal, waking adaptive behavior. Stated in a more definitive way (as indeed in suggested by psychologists from a phenomenological point of view), we are consciously aware of only a small and ever changing portion of the total input and store of information being carried by the brain, this portion being the end product of a complex and exceedingly fast succession of processes which furnish us with finished patterns of adaptive value. At the present state of knowledge the so-called "primary" process of psychologists (51) would appear to involve a continuous taking in of information, possibly subliminally (41), without actual participation by awareness; and a clustering, massing, grouping and polarization of this information against genetically coded patterns. These patterns have a strong appetitive or aversive connotation, and have little sense for delay, or of time in terms of a current stimulus situations. This first phase of preliminary analysis, however, may be used, and quite selectively used, by another process proceeding simultaneously. This process (which has been called "secondary") arrives by a succession of increasingly accurate computations and the "abstraction" of common cues from related situation, at responses carrying the highest adaptive values in terms of the "Here" and the "Now". It allows for the separation of, and serial ordering of events in time. In anticipating the future, it takes account of the experience of the past. It is capable of recognizing similarities on the basis of relatively few cues, and of rigorous suppression of material which is irrelevant. It is thus, a process capable of discrimination, appropriateness, and logic.

It is not irrelevant in the context of the above that, whereas the first kind of process is physiologically seen in relaxed-day-dreaming, in light sleep, or in sensory isolation, a second process implies not only wakefulness, but also attention and a anticipatory set with regard to new incoming information. For, by its very nature, the power to discriminate, to abstract, and to think categorically, i.e., in terms of a category, implies having functionally available frames of reference comprizing similar cues from the past; it also implies the rigorous and reciprocal suppression of cues which are irrelevant in regard to the particular operation in hand. The attending and waking brain may thus be as specialized a state of activity as the sleeping or unconscious, or anaesthesized brain; and it is in the study of the transitional states, and the disturbances of the attention process, that we may look to the most ready models of schizophrenic thought disorder.

5. ATTENTION, "SET" AND VIGILANCE: THEIR POSSIBLE RELATION TO INTERNAL INHIBITION AND TO SCHIZOPHRENIC DISORDER

Reference has already been made to the inability of the schizophrenic to maintain a state of readiness or set to incoming stimuli, and an inability to smoothly move from the anticipation of one set of stimuli to the anticipation of another. Is has also been pointed out that there is some similarity between the dream process and schizophrenic thought disorder. To say that the schizophrenic merely regresses to an older form of functioning is really begging the question. The child-like and dream-like behavior of the schizophrenic is, in fact, distinct from either. The schizophrenic uses the most delicate instrument of adult communication, namely language, in the service of processes for which language is not normally intended. He uses mechanisms normally seen as manifestations of light sleep in situations which, in terms of muscle tone, movement, respiration, and other somatic correlates, are certainly not those of light sleep. Any formulation, however crude, must take these two groups of facts into account.

It is, therefore, particularly encouraging that the last decade has seen far-reaching advances in the exploration of the electrophysiological equivalents of states of arousal and attention, which, it is submitted, may be very relevant to any future experimental approach to schizophrenic thought disorders. The findings in these fields to date have received extensive review (52, 53) and only a few aspects may be mentioned here. First, a distinction must be made between arousal (i.e., wakefulness), and general alerting on the one hand, and specific alerting or focussed attention on the other. Whereas the former may be related to a "grosser and more tonically operating component in the lower brain stem, subserving global alterations in excitability" (54), the latter may rest in "a more cephalic, thalamic component with greater capacities for fractioned, shifting influence upon focal region of the brain" (54). Again, it has been shown that descending reticular systems are capable of influencing the excitability of afferent relays both in the spinal cord (55) and in the upper brain stem (56). A mounting body of evidence, recently comprehensively reviewed (57), suggests a marked central control of sensory transmission systems. For example, a shift of attention from one stimulus (sound) to another (sight) in an attending animal is capable of inhibiting electrical discharges from relay centers (to cochlear nucleus) evoked by the stimulus initially presented (40). Lastly, and perhaps more pertinent to the present argument, there is increasing evidence pointing to the relation to the attention process, whether general or discriminate, to a patterned *inhibition of activity* of cortical neurons. This is reflected in the so-called cortical excitability cycle, and its relation to the α rhythm (58). It is seen, at a more discrete level, in *diminished* firing of some cortical units upon arousal, or the inhibition of unit discharge in the motor cortex upon stimulation of the thalamic reticular formation (59). Furthermore, there are preliminary indications that the excitability of cortical elements is *increased* during sleep (60). Yet a number of investigations, both at the level of sensory relay nuclei or of cortical elements point to the relation of patterned inhibition to the discriminate coding of information. This appears equally true in the visual (36), in the auditory (39, 61), the olfactory (62), and the somatic sensory area (63) pathways. The power of the higher brain stem nuclei in bringing about discrimination of function may thus well rest in their ability to apprehend and block redundant information, and so to increase the information content of the patterns which ultimately result, The diminished excitability of some neurones in thalamic cortical nets during attention may thus be as significant as the increased excitability of such neurones during sleep. It is at least conceivable that whereas the first approximation qualitative computation of stimulus in terms of affective connotation is carried through by elements in the limbic system, and its most immediate projections, the more discriminate and delayed responses are dependent for their analyses on information fed simultaneously into thalamo cortical nets. Presumably, these interrelated processes are normally in equilibrium. Increasing attention and improved "set" would, in this view, be related to a state of increased, rather than diminished inhibition. In sum, the higher nervous system is more remarkable for its ability to ignore, than its ability to perform.

It has been suggested earlier(64) that this finely set inhibitory process may in some way, yet ill understood, be defective in schizophrenia. In the normal, the process falters strikingly with the reduction of sensory input, and apparently in sleep. It would thus appear to be locked to moderate sensory input, and to be diminished during sleep, Since schizophrenia is not associated with sleep and some symptoms of it are at least temporally alleviated by barbiturates (65) one would almost be tempted to suggest a disassociation, or imbalance between the sleep-wakefulness mechanisms, and the mechanisms subserving discriminate and specific attention. The latter could conceivably include elements in the upper brain stem (such as the Lenticular, Pulvinar, Globus Pallidus and Caudate nuclei), and any areas serving as relay systems in transcortical transactions. Yet such a crude anatomical localization would be functionally unjustified. It would not allow for the interdependence of the various cellular masses of the brain in its smooth operation. What may look like overinhibition in the cortex may, in fact, reflect overactivity of sub-cortical centers, and what may be seen as underactivity in the hypothalamic pituitary systems (in electrophysiological or hormonal terms) may, in fact, be due to an imbalance between the hippocampal and amygdalar elements of the Limbic system (66). The brain, more than any other organ in the body, is structurally, functionally, chemically an inhomogeneous organ. The role of steep chemical gradients within it, and of the possible role chemical fields (65, 67) has yet to be explored in neurophysiological and functional terms. The recent great advances in the chemical topology of the brain and particularly those in regard to the differential synthesis, storage and release, breakdown and distribution of catecholamines, 5-hydroxytryptamine and γ-aminobutyric acid now demand a careful and systematic scrutiny of the *inter*relationship of these substances an their derivatives in chemical, electrophysiological behavioral terms in various regions of the brain. For if, indeed, reciprocal relationships between various brain areas are part and parcel of its functioning, the relative *ratios* of substance to each other, and their rate of turnover and change in concentration may be much more important than the absolute amount of any particular substance at a particular place at a particular time. This may apply equally to areas of the brain with which neurohumoral processes have been associated, as to strictly cellular or peri-cellular levels. The concept of metabolic pools (68) and the role of subunits of the neurone in maintaining these pools may be relevant here.

It was suggested some time ago (64, 65, 67, 69) that rather than thinking in unitary terms it might be useful to consider the possible selection by chemical evolution of families of compounds which, while related to neuroeffector agents familiar to us at the periphery, were possessed of a differential distribution throughout the Central Nervous System. The titre of one or other of these substance in key areas of the brain stem was envisaged as capable of profoundly modulating the activities of large neurone pools at a distance (65, 67). It was further suggested that the *inter*action between these substances could well determine the states of excitation or inhibition within a particular neural net. There is reasonable evidence now to support the association of epinephrine with the brain stem arousal mechanism (70). Epinephrine sensitive areas have been located in the midbrain reticular formation by direct application of epinephrine (71). Microelectrode studies also suggest the existence of such epinephrine "sensitive units" (72). It is, however, well to remember that epinephrine, applied in larger doses intracisternally leads to somnolence rather than wakefulness (73); and that, in a number of experimental situations, the response to acetylcholine can be profoundly modified by varying concentrations of epinephrine (74). Thus, relative ratios of particular substances, their precursors and products may be much more important than absolute amounts. It is of interest in the context of the above that Dopamine, as well as epinephrine, have now been identified in the higher brain stem structures (such as the caudate and lentiform nuclei – 75); and that is this respect, at any rate, these higher cell masses differ significantly from other areas hitherto examined. Such differences may well become more apparent with increasing experience in the field, and may have their place in a chemical pathology of thought disorder.

It is in problems such as these that the discriminate use of drugs possessing one or other overriding property, or of specific antimetabolites, can be of great theoretical yield. It will, however, only contribute to an understanding of schizophrenia, insofar as the models used in these investigations are clearly related to the phenomena of the group disorders known as the schizophrenias. As was pointed out in a pertinent paper (76), the animal behavioral model has to take into account those attributes (such as delayed response, serial ordering of information in time, and ability to abstract) which are most closely related to corresponding dysfunction in man. The local application of drugs and metabolites to discrete brain areas in the conscious primate may gradually enhance our knowledge of the kind and distribution of the chemical processes concerned with the adequate discharge of these functions. Furthermore, much more attention should be paid to the electrophysiological, biochemical and hormonal changes attending the intermediate state separating wakefulness from sleep, or the states following sensory isolation or prolonged deprivation of natural sleep. In the schizophrenic the qualitative effect of drugs on overt behavior may be grossly misleading and, as has been pointed out, leave the nuclear psychotic process untouched (77). On the other hand, data on the effect of drugs on set and attention in the schizophrenic are conflicting (78, 79), and pose many more questions than they answer. Yet the use of graded doses of drugs, singly and combination, in such studies may contribute pharmacological, and quite possibly biochemical points of reference in areas which may be related to the central dysfunction of the schizophrenic. This will particularly apply to studies of perception, attention, set and the capacity of handling information over time. Any clear indication of an interaction between chemical variables, and those dysfunctions my be useful in providing psychological frames of reference for future work in this field.

It may well be asked why a communication such as this should be submitted to a Symposium dedicated to the Chemical Pathology of the Nervous System. The writer's only excuse for this transgression in his feeling that care has to be exercised in the use of the term "schizophrenia", the over-inclusiveness of which may hide a number of quite different meanings; that the models employed for the study of schizophrenia are defective in several important respects; that any chemical variables in schizophrenia which the present or the future may reveal, demand interpretation in terms of their effects on brain mechanisms and, particularly, their effect on inhibitory process within the brain; and that pharmacological interventions in schizophrenia in appropriate experimental settings offer an unusual opportunity for the study of the human brain as a chemically mediated and, quite possibly, regionally organized organ of information.

SUMMARY

1. The clinical phenomena of schizophrenic illness are briefly considered, and their specificity for schizophrenic disorder examined. A number of symptoms seen in the schizophrenias are shared by other mental and neurological disorders. Disturbance of cognitive function, however, with its attendant loosening and fragmentation of association, is held a central feature of schizophrenic disorder. It appears to be related to a disturbance of the attention process, and to an inability to consistently maintain a state of readiness to incoming stimuli over time.

2. The manifestations of schizophrenic illness are briefly compared to the mental changes induced by the so-called psychosomimetic drugs. The resemblance between the two sets of phenomena is held to be superficial. The sensory disturbances seen in Mescal and LSD-25 intoxication are different from those reported in schizophrenia. True thought disorder is rarely seen in drug induced states, except after prolonged exposure.

3. A preliminary attempt is made to examine schizophrenic thought disorder in terms of a disturbance of information processing by the brain. Attention is drawn to evidence suggesting an active participation of the systems subserving in the processes of attention and motivation in the selective organization of sense data. The interaction between sensory information and stored, affectively charged memory traces is held to be more overt in the schizophrenic than in the normal. The possible role of the limbic system in a first order monitoring or preliminary grouping of sensory data in terms of their pleasurable or aversive connotation is considered. The stereotype nature and prompt discharge of instinctual patterns of behavior is stressed.

4. Attention is drawn to the existence of delaying systems in the higher neuraxis, which discriminately block immediate response, and make possible the serial organization of information in time. It is suggested that these delaying and inhibitory mechanism are related to an increasing power of the higher nervous system to substitute condensed symbols of high information-content for initial responses, and its power to abstract shared qualities, or universals, from isolated items. The diminished ability of the schizophrenic to order information serially in time is noted.

5. Attention is drawn to the psychological thought disturbance seen in the dream process, four features of which are stressed. It is suggested that the process seen overtly in dreaming may represent a psychological and early phase in a continuum of information-processing by

the brain. This, by way of related stage, ultimately leads to the highly condensed, appropriate and logical responses of normal, waking adaptive behavior. Two phases of the process are arbitrarily distinguished. The first of these would appear to involve a continuous taking in of information, possibility subliminally, without actual participation by awareness, and a clustering, massing, grouping and polarization of this information against genetically coded, affectively charged patterns of response. The second phase, which presumably proceeds simultaneously, may comprise a succession of increasingly accurate computations and "abstractions" of common cues from related situations, resulting ultimately in common denominators carrying the highest values in terms of waking, conscious adaptive behavior. This process allows for the separation of, a serial ordering of events in time. It requires both sensory input, and a preparatory set towards incoming stimuli. It is this process which falters during reduction of sensory input, and in sleep. It may be defective in schizophrenia.

6. The distinction between mere arousal and wakefulness and specific alerting and focussed attention is stressed. The evidence pointing towards the role of patterned and shifting inhibition in relation to the process of attention is briefly reviewed. Improved "set" appears to be related to a state of increased, rather than diminished, inhibition; this inhibition may emanate from higher brain stem nuclei, whereas arousal and wakefulness may be more related to mechanisms located at mesencephalic level.

7. It is suggested that this highly discriminate inhibitory process, concerned with specific attention, may in some way be defective in schizophrenia. The possibility of an imbalance between the sleep-wakefulness mechanism, and the mechanisms subserving discriminate attention is considered.

8. It is stressed that any biochemical or pharmacological approach to schizophrenia must clearly account for biochemical variables, not only in terms of their effect on the general manifestations of the illness, but more specifically, on those properties which are regularly, and measurably, related to the central schizophrenic disturbance. Such findings will ultimately demand interpretation in terms of brain mechanisms. The effect of chemical variables upon the role of inhibitory process within high thalamic or striatocortical nets may be particularly relevant to biochemical theory of the schizophrenias.

9. The regional chemical suborganization and inhomogeneity of the brain are briefly considered with special reference to the differential distribution of closely related substances within various areas of the brain. The relative ratio, and interaction between these substances may be more important than absolute amounts in determining the relative patterns of excitation and inhibition within higher neural nets.

10. It is suggested that pharmacological intervention in schizophrenia in appropriate experimental settings offers an unusual opportunity for the study of the human brain as a chemically mediated organ of information.

REFERENCES

1. Kety, S. S. (1960) An Examination of Current Biochemical Theories of Schizophrenia. This volume, p.684.
2. Ackner, B. (1954) J. Ment. Sci. 100, 838.
3. Lewin, L. (1931) Phantastica, Narcotic and Stimulating Drugs. Their Use and Abuse. Cutton, New York
4. Stoll, W. A. (1947) Arch. Neurol. Psych. 60, 279.
5. Penfield, W. (1958) The Role of the Temporal Cortex in Recall of Past Experience and Interpretation of the Present. In: Wostenholme, G.E.W. and O'Connor, C.M., Editors, Neurological Basis of Behavior. London J. & A. Churchill, 149.
6. Sandison, R. A. (1957) Personal communication.

7. Bleuler, E. (1951) Textbook of Psychiatry. Dover Publications.
8. Bleuler, E. (1950) Dementia Praecox. New York, International Universities Press.
9. Fischer, F. (1930) Zeitsch. f. ges. Neurol. u. Psychiat. 124, 246.
10. Goldstein, K. (1941) Methodological Approach to the Study of Schizophrenic Thought Disorder. In: Kasanin, J.S. Editor, Language and Thought in Schizophrenia. Univ. of California Press. p. 17.
11. Vigotsky, L. (1934) Arch. Neurol. and Psychiat. 31, 1063.
12. Benjamin, J. D. (1944) A Method of Distinguishing and Evaluating Formal Thinking Disorder in Schziophrenia. In: Kasanin, J.D. loc. cit. p.65.
13. Goldstein, L. (1944) loc. cit. p. 27.
14. Bleuler, E. (1950) Dementia Praecox. New York, International University Press. p. 47.
15. Huston, P. E., Shakow, D. and Riggs, L. A. (1937) J. Genet. Pychol. 16. 39.
16. Head, H. (1926) Aphasia and Kindred Disorders of Speech. Cambridge University Press.
17. Hunt, J., and Cofer, C. N. (1944) Psychological Deficit. In: J. McV Hhunt, Editor, Personality and the Behavior Disorders. New York, Ronald Press, p. 971.
18. Rodnick, E. H. and Shakow, D. (1940) Amer. J. Psychiat. 97, 214.
19. Kluver, H. (1928) Mescal. London.
20. Mitchell, S. W. (1896) Brit. Med. J. 2, 1625
21. Elkes, J. (1957) Psychotropic Drugs: Observations on Current Uses and Future Problems. Working Paper No. 1. World Health Organization Study Group on Ataractic Agents, WHO, Geneva.
22. Kluver, H. (1942) Mechanisms of Hallucinations. In: Studies in Personality. New York, McGraw Hill, P. 175.
23. Zucker, L. (1930) Z. Ges. Neurol. Psychiat. 127, 108.
24. Evarts, E. V. (1957) Ann. N. Y. Acad. Sci. 66, 479 .
25. Apter, J. T. and Pfeiffer, C. C. (1957) The Effect of the Hallucinogenic Drugs LSD-25 and Mescalin on the Electroretinogram Ibid. p. 508.
26. Zadur, J. (1930) Z. Ges. Neurol. 127, 30.
27. Marshall, E. R: (1937) J. Neurol. Psychopat. 17, 129.
28. Riggs, L. A. (1951) Science, 114, 17.
29. Bleuler, E. (1950) Dementia Praecox. New York, International University Press, p. 388.
30. Richter, D. (Ed.) (1957) Schizophrenia, Somatic Aspects. New York, The MacMillan Co.
31. Pincus, G. and HOAGLAND H. (1950) Amer. J. Psychiat. 106, 641.
32. Bruner, J. S. (1958) Res. Public Assoc. For. Res. Nerv. and Ment. Disease. 36, 118.
33. Ditchburn, R.W. (1958) In: Bruner, J. S. loc. cit. p. 134.
34. Graik, K. (1952) The Nature of Explanation. Cambridge University Press, Cambridge, England.
35. Bruner, J. S. (1958) loc. cit. p. 133.
36. Kuffler, S.W. (1952) Neurones in the Retina: Organization, Inhibition and Excitation Problems. Cold Spring Harbor Symp. 17, 281.
37. Whitfield, I. C. (1957) Progress in Biophysics and Biophysical Chemistry. London, Pergamon Press, 8, 1.
38. Whitfield, I. C. (1959) Sensory Mechnism and Sensation. Symp. On the Mechanisation of Thought Process. London, H. M. Stationary Office, In press.
39. Galambos, R., SCHEATZ, G. and VERNER, V. G. (1956) Science, 123, 376.
40. Hernandez-peon, R., Scherrer, H. and Jouvet, M. (1956) Science 123, 331.
41. Klein, G. S., Soence, D. P., Holt, R, R., and Gourevitch S. (1959) J. Abnorm. Soc. Psychol. In press.
42. Maclean, P. D. (1949) Psychosom. Med. 11, 338.
43. Pribram, K. H. and Kruger, L. (1954) Ann. N.Y. Acad. Sci. 58, 109.
44. Nauta, W. J. H. (1956) J. Comp. Neurol. 104, 247.
45. Brady, J. V. (1958) The Paleocortex and Behavioral Motivation. In: Harlow, H.F. & Woolsey, C.N. Ed.: Biological and Biochemical Bases of Behavior University of Wisconsin Press, p. 193.
46. Tinbergen, N. (1950) The Hierarchical Organization of Nervous Mechanism underlying Instinctive Behavior. In: Psychological Mechanisms in Animal Behavior. Cambridge University Press. p. 305.
47. Bleuler, E. (1951) loc. cit.
48. Benton, W. H. (1953) Some Effects of Perceptual Isolation in Human Subjects. Dissertation, Aug. 1953.
49. Benton, W. H., Heron, W., and Scott, T. H. (1954) Canad. J. Pychol. 8, 70.
50. Dement W. and Kleitman, N. (1957) EEG Clin. Neurophysiol. 9, 673.
51. Freud, S. (1900) The Interpretation of Dreams. Basic Writings of S. Freud; Modern Library N. Y., p. 183.
52. Jasper, H. H., Proctor, K. D., Knighton, R. S. Noshay, W. C. and Costello, R. T. (Eds) (1958): The Reticular Formation of the Brain. Boston, Little Brown & Co. p. 513.
53. Magoun, H. W. (1958) The Waking Brain. Springfield, Charles C. Thomas

54. Magoun, H. W. loc. cit. p. 116.

55. Hagbarth, K. E. and Kerr, D. I. B. (1954) J. Neurophysiol. 17, 295.

56. King, E. E., Naquet, R. and Magoun, H. W. (1957) J. Pharm. Exp. Therap. 119, 48.

57. Livingston, R. B. Central Control of Sensory Receptors and Sensory Transmission Systems. In: Handbook of Psychology, vol I. John Field, Editor, Amer. Psychol. Soc. In press.

58. Lindsley, D. B. (1958) The Reticular system and Perceptual Discrimination. In: Jasper et al. Editors, The Reticular Formation of the Brain; Boston, Little Brown & Co. p. 513.

59. Whitlock, D. C., Arduini, A. and MoruZZI, G. (1953) Neuropsychol. 16, 414.

60. Fleming, T. C. Huttenlocker, P. R. and EvartS, E. V. (1959) Fed. Proc. 18, 46.

61. Galambos, R. and Davis, H. (1943) J. Neurophysiol. 6, 39.

62. Adrian, E. D. (1954) Psychological Basis of Perception. In: Brain Mechanism and Consciousness. Adrian, E. D. et al. Editors, Blackwell, Oxford.

63. Mountcastle, V. B. (1957) J. Neurophysiol. 20, 408.

64. Elkes, J. (1958) Drug Effects in Relation to Receptor Specificity within the Brain: Some Evidence and Provisional Formulation. In: Wolstenholme, G.E.W. and O'Connor, C.M. Editors, Neurological Basis of Behavior. London, J. & A. Churchill, p. 303.

65. Elkes, J. (1957) Effect of Psychosomimetic Drugs in Animals and in Man. In: Abramson, H. A. (Ed.) Neuropharmacology Transactions. Third Conference of Josiah Macy Jr. Foundation, N. Y. p. 205.

66. Mason, J. W. (1958) The Central Nervous System Regulation of ACTH Secretion. In: Jasper, H.H. et al. Editors, Reticular Formation of the Brain. Boston, Brown Little & Co., p. 645.

67. Bradley, P. B. And Elkes, J. (1957) Brain, 80, 77.

68. Waelsch, H. W. (1960) New Aspects of Amine Metabolism. This volume, p. 576.

69. Elkes, J. (1953) In: Prospects in Psychiatric Research, Tanner, J.M. Editor, Oxford, Blackwell Scientific Publications, p. 126.

70. Dell, P., Bonvallet, M. and Hugelin, A. (1954) EEG Clin. Neurophysiol. 6, 599.

71. Rothballer, A. B. (1956) EEG Clin. Neurophysiol. 8, 603.

72. Bradley, P. B. and MollicA, A. (1958) Arch. Ital. Biol. 96, 168.

73. Leimdorfer, A. and Metzner, W. R. T. (1949) Amer. J. Psychol. 157, 116.

74. Burn, J. H. (1945) Physiol. Rev. 25, 377.

75. Carlson, A. (1959) Pharmacol. Rev, 11, 490.

76. Evarts, E. V. (1959) A Discussion of the Relevance of Effects on Animal Behavior to the Possible Effects of Drugs on Psychopathological Processes in Man. In: Psychopharmacology Problems in Evaluation. Cole, J. and Gerard. R.W. Editors, Washington, National Acad. of Sciences, p. 284.

77. Elkes, J. and Elkes, C. (1954) Brit. Med. J. 2, 560.

78. Huston P. E. and Singer, M. M. (1945) Arch. Neurol. Psychiat. 53, 365.

79. Huston, P. E. and Senf, R. (1952) Amer. J. Psychiat. 109, 131.

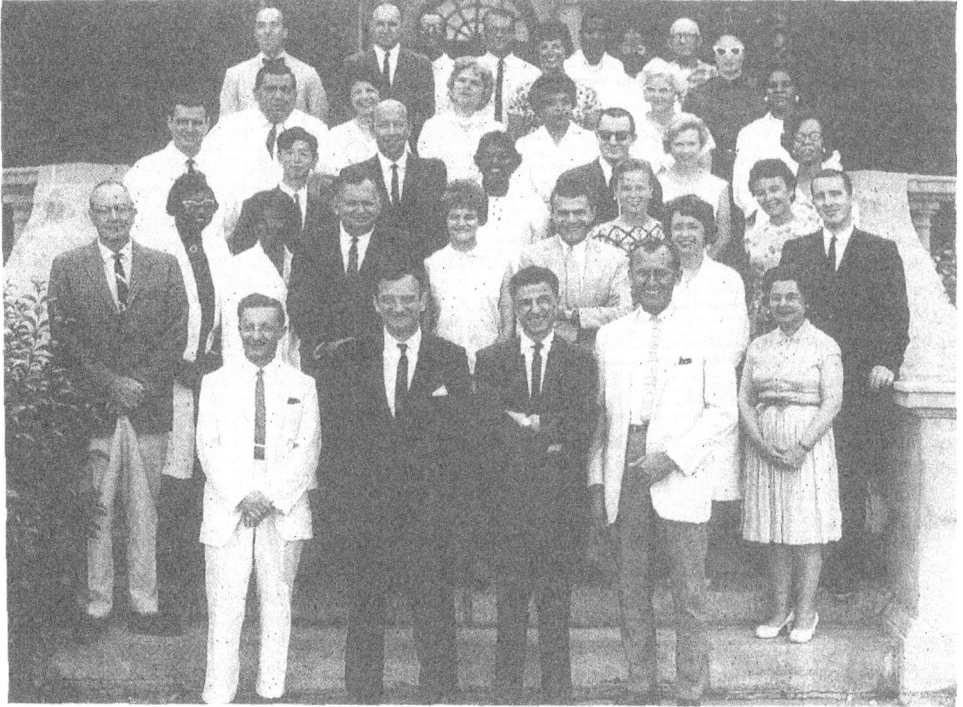

At St. Elizabeth's, 1961. Front row: H. Weil-Malherbe, J. Elkes, G. C. Salmoraghi, S. Szara

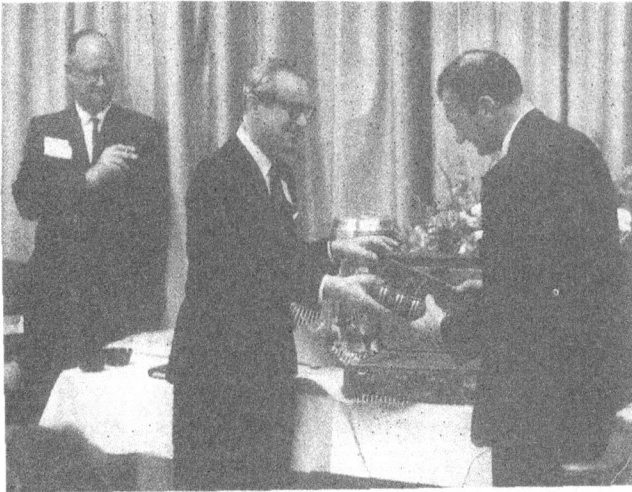

Farewell, St. Elizabeth's! Fritz Freyhan handing Joel Elkes a bound copy
of collected papers by staff.

Part Six

A PERSPECTIVE (1978)

PAPER

17. Joel Elkes: *Epilogue and foreglimpse. Letter to a young collegue considering a career in psychopharmacology.*
Reprinted with the kind permission of Academic Press from W.G. Clark and J. del Giudice (eds.) *Principles in Psychopharmacology* (Chapter 43, pp. 741–753). New York, Academic Press, 1978

CONTEXT

Paper 17 is the closing chapter to a textbook in psychopharmacology. It is written as a letter to an aspiring young colleague. The paper deals with chemical mapping and neurochemical specificities in the brain; the promise and drawback of metabolic loading studies; the promise of discriminate use of drugs in a taxonomy of mental disorders; the chemical correlates of coping, and well-being; and the possible chemical extension of physiological boundaries. It ends with the author's perennial plea for new mathematical languages for the description of the nonlinear stochastic phenomena, which are the business of much of a future psychopharmacology.

PAPER 17

EPILOGUE AND FOREGLIMPSE
Letter to a Young Colleague Considering a Career in Psychopharmacology

Joel Elkes

Reprinted with the kind permission of Academic Press from W. G. Clark and T. Del Gindice (Eds.) *Principles of Psychopharmacology* (Chapter 43, pp. 741–755) New York, Academic Press, 1978

Dear Jean:

Thank you for your letter. I was interested to learn of your wish to specialize in Psychopharmacology. You ask, a little despondently, "Where does the subject begin, and where does it end?", "What are its main trends at the present time?", "Where is it going in the future?" In answering, I am at some disadvantage. For I do not know where you come from. You do not say whether your background is in medicine, or psychiatry, or physics, -or biochemistry, or biology, or psychology, or the social sciences, or by way of several of these disciplines. Nor do you mention whether you might prefer clinical or basic psychopharmacology, or both. So perhaps I can be useful to you by giving you a little background, and suggest some directions where Psychopharmacology may be going in the next few years. The view will, of necessity, be a rather personal and parochial view, which I would like you to take with a hearty pinch of salt. Put what I say alongside your own training, reading, and conversations; and decide, after most thorough and careful reflection, whether there is enough joy and reward in it to make it worth your while.

In this year of 1977, with large national and international bodies representing psychopharmacology, with major journals (see Appendices 3 and 4, this text) devoted to its findings, and huge industries invested in its inventions, it is hard to realize that the field is barely a quarter of a century old. The discoveries of the early 1950's of LSD-25, of Chlorpromazine, and the Antidepressants coincided with rapid advances in cognate areas lying at the interface between "Brain" and "Behaviour". I remember one such occasion very well. Some 20 years ago in April, 1954, there was convened at Magdalen College, Oxford, the 1st International Neurochemical Symposium; Drs. Seymour Kety, Jordi Folch-Pi, the late Heinrich Waelsch and Louis Flexner were the American partners of the Committee. In Britain, there were Drs. Derek Richter, the late Geoffrey Harris, and myself (who acted as organizing secretary). The field was sparse in those days; yet we located 69 colleagues from 9 countries to attend what proved to be a most useful exchange.

Writing in the introduction to the Proceedings, we put our purpose this way:

We agreed that from the start it would be well to consider the brain as a biological entity in all its complexity of morphology and function, rather than as a homogenate, or an engineering problem. For that reason, we felt that the most useful contribution of a Symposium of this kind would be an attempt to reintegrate biochemical process with structure and function particularly with respect to the chemical topography of the brain, which. to us, seemed of greatest moment in an understanding of function. The program thus not only represents the framework of a conference, but also expresses an attitude. We feel that this approach may be helpful in slowly building the foundations for a rational therapy of disorders of the nervous system. (Waelsch, 1955)

We seem to be still at it; but it is significant that, as you mention in your letter, a little island on the horizon in 1954-what we called the CNS "Sympathins" (now called the catecholamines)-now has enlarged to a whole continent. The forces which brought us to this point are, in part, accidental and empirical, and in part, deliberate. It required the boot of empiricism (the discovery of the psychoactive drugs) to give us new facts of great clinical relevance. The Dialectic began when new facts began to hunt for explanations; and there it is the evolution of new *methods* which brought us to the position we are in today.

These methods were, in part, Anatomical and Physiological, in part Chemical, in part Behavioral and in part Clinical. In this respect, our field brooks no compromise, and compels conversation between various approaches like no other. It was a combination of Anatomy, Physiology, and Behavior which slowly bared the mosaic of the subsystems governing Sleep, Arousal, and focused Attention. It gave us an anatomical scaffolding for an understanding of the control of Hunger, Thirst, Sexuality, Social play, and Predatory Attack. It was the same combination, coupled with microphysiological approaches which led to an understanding of the role of convergence, filtering and funneling of signals in peripheral sense organs (such as Retina and Olfactory Bulb), integration at high central level (such as the Cerebellum) or the assignment of significance and value in what we call Affective terms in the pathways and structures of the Limbic System. It is here, too, that the organizing power of the Reward and Punishment systems emerged; with still another field (the sequential organization of motor performance, including Speech) being related to the striatum and the dominant hemispheres.

If all this sounds like the language of the 19th century cerebral "localizers" it both is, and isn't. The brain, to be sure, seemed and still does seem, an assembly of suborgans, a system of systems, a mosaic of biased homeostats. It has its nodal areas, its cables, and connections; and presumably in certain genetic respects, was "wired" for a purpose. But the "wiring", and the "control" centers, should not mislead. For equally clear, and emerging in the light of recent experimental evidence, were diffuse and generalized effects on large areas of the brain, or in the brain as a whole; phenomena of modulation, gating, and slow potential drifts. It is these which were related to the now established fact of differential cell populations in even small areas of the brain ; and the influence, by way of widespread a projections of some nodal midline areas (such as the locus coeruleus, the raphe nuclei, and the substantia nigra), over large areas.

Chemical Mapping and Neurochemical Specificities

While these developments were proceeding, a chemical map was being quietly superimposed upon functional anatomical findings. It started with painstaking dissection of gross areas of the brain and bioassay. (I still remember the excitement of reading the great paper of Feldberg and Vogt, 1948.) It proceeded to the sampling of ever smaller areas, by the application of the Linderstrom–Lang techniques to the analysis of single cells. The use of radioisotopes added to this dimension, and further elucidated the regional chemical organization within the CNS; but it did more. For by taking down the regional process to the organization of subcellular components, by showing up the astonishing precision and economy of the processes governing release, reuptake, and storage of chemicals – it related *spatial* subcellular organization to their turnover *in time*. It added the concept of quantal discharge of transmitters by differential synaptosomal populations, thus introducing a much needed statistical, probabilistic element into our thinking. It also made much more real the concept of heterogeneous cell populations, surmised by some of us early on. This proposition was literally illuminated by the advent of the pathbreaking cytofluorescent and immunocytofluorescent techniques developed in recent years by Falck, Hillarp, Fuxe, Goldstein, and others (see Chap. 4). We speak these days of adrenergic, noradrenergic, serotoninergic, dopaminergic, gabergic, histaminergic, and peptidergic neuronal pathways; others are emerging. All this is true, but with a reservation. For many of these neuronal populations overlap; they clearly interact. Nearly 20 yr ago one spoke of families of neuroregulatory substances, "whose number probably is quite small but whose influence upon the integrative action of higher nervous activity may be profound" (Bradley and Elkes, 1957). One thought of the operations of chemical fields in nodal areas of the brain and envisaged the basic states of consciousness as being determined by variation in local concentrations of these agents (Elkes, 1958). Thanks to modern methods the picture now is much clearer. We know something of the chemistry of the Medial Forebrain Bundle, the Locus Coeruleus, the Raphe System and the Nucleus Accumbens. We are just beginning to explore the detailed cytochemistry of those huge and mysterious masses of the Caudate, and Striatum, and the Globus Pallidus, and their relation to both the Limbic and the Frontoparietal system. How far modern methods have carried us in this regard! Like the Cloud Chamber in Physics, we have now a number of inferential approaches which allow us to draw conclusions of the likely chemical events at unit level. These are the subcellular fractionation and radioactive uptake techniques, using synaptosomes, mitochondria and ribosomes, giving one a fairly precise picture of intra- and pericellular kinetics; the radioimmunofluorescent approaches, allowing cytochemical localization of components at different specific neuronal sites; the combination of radioisotope techniques with electron microscopy; the microelectrode and micropipette studies (coming, among others, from our own laboratories at NIMH, St. Elizabeths; Salmoiraghi and Bloom, 1964) and allowing for the sequential application of drugs to single cells, thus making possible a mapping of chemical susceptibilities in different cell populations.

These methods have yielded a rich harvest. They have clearly confirmed that the principles of regional chemical economy within the CNS can be carried into the chemical specificities of the individual cell itself. They have linked certain enzymes with certain components. They also have made possible a detailed step-by-step analysis of the informational flow (the "feedback") between product and the enzymatic machinery governing production; between release and "uptake"; between storage, release, and disposition. When such findings are applied to neurons exerting scanning, filtering, condensing, and integrating functions, our analysis of that rather vague term modulation becomes possible in neurophysiological as well as chemical terms. What is even more exciting is that, by placing single-cell monitoring devices judiciously along a particular pathway in the learning animal, a monitoring of electrochemical events *preceding* actual behavior becomes possible. Attention, and even intention, are thus not beyond physiological scrutiny; as, of course, are the sequelae of learning.

The picture which is emerging in terms of chemical control systems already exceeds our early naive assumptions. Behind the old families of the Choline Esters, the Catecholamines and Indoles, there are the Membrane-active Amino Acids (such as GABA and Glycine), or

Substance P, exerting mainly an inhibitory function; there is Histamine; there are the ubiquitous Secondary Transmitters such as the Prostaglandins and Cyclic AMP, and now, the third generation (oligopeptides such as the hypothalamic morphinomimetic peptides, the Enkephalins or Endorphins) (Snyder 1975, and others). Moreover, the Catecholamines have clear effects on energy transfer systems, like adenyl cyclase, and thus could influence specificity in protein (or lipo- or glycoprotein) synthesis. There is the old and well known interaction between the catecholamines and the steroids; between both, and the neuroactive ions; and between simple oligopeptides (some of them fragments of such pituitary hormonal peptides such as ACTH) and ions (peptides, as you know, influence learning) (DeWied et al. 1975). Add to this studies which suggest that the mucopolysaccharides at the cell surface may in some "Signpost" fashion (Bogoch 1975), be related to specific encoding? (by way of glucosamines, as in bacteria), and you have an idea how complex a term "neuronal specificity" really has become. It cries out for a Systems Approach. There must clearly be both genetic and acquired labeling of the neurons surface and interface; and the incorporation of specific recognizers, and transponders into the cell surface. It is possible that in some way, still ill-understood, the amines, and other small molecules may provide letters in an alphabet in the building up of such small, informed cell ensembles. One does not need many letters. In fact, I have found a crude partitioning into three kinds of transactions (if I may so put it, three kinds of chemical languages), useful to myself. The first is the All-or-None discharge of the ionic battery which we know as nerve action potentials; the second is the play of stochastic neurohumoral interactive inhibitory influences which, at subthreshold, and in very specific ways, influence cell excitability; and the third, the actual transfer of materials from cell to cell, possibly by neurotubules. The time scale for the first (a sort of final "Yes" or "No" event) is short: a matter of milliseconds; for the third, it may be quite long (a matter of minutes to hours). It is well to reflect at this point that the CNS processes events in time, and detects and encodes coincidences and relations of events in time. It used *inhibition* as its agent of structure; and time as the axis along which it constructs its models of reality. It performs by banking "irrelevant" information; by, as we say, "ignoring". It is this stupendous capacity to selectively ignore which makes performances in the Here and Now possible. We do not precisely know the chemical correlates of this key selective inhibitory process. but it is, to my mind, a Key Question in psychopharmacology. We must ask whether the hemispheres function differently in this regard? Whether certain selected cell groups in certain metabolically very active nodal older areas of the brain (which always partake in this encoding process) are indeed functioning as first-approximation "germinal" model makers, building units which are then transferred to other cells; and whether, indeed, the brain uses a thermodynamic mode of information storage and transfer with which (with our standard neurophysiological models) we are still totally unfamiliar. In this context the holographic model (Pribram 1971) is very helpful, and one hopes that it will find wider acceptance in Psychopharmacology.

Whatever the idea, I hope I have conveyed to you that, if there be specificity in neuron populations, the old Monistic view is simple and naive in the extreme. Stochastic *inter*action would appear to be the language of the brain; an interaction which need no longer remain a matter of speculation. We have better tools now; and will have ever better tools later. There are the depleters, the enzyme inhibitors of synthesis and destruction; the false transmitters; the various fragments of behaviorally active oligopeptides; the corticoids, the electrolytes; the inhibitors of protein synthesis such as the puromycins, to be used either singly or in combination-especially in combination. It may seem a long road, but it should be a rewarding one. Just remember what the specific Cholinesterase Inhibitors (like DFP and TEPP) did for the whole field of Acetylcholine. We have come some way in defining the chemical specificities and specific release mechanisms operating in those deeply ingrained programs we know as innate behavior. Sexual activity, Aggression, and Predatory Attack are examples of such programs. Above all, thanks to our late and beloved Jim Olds and his colleagues, we know a good deal about both the anatomy, as well as the physiology and chemistry of the systems subserving Reward and Punishment (Olds 1976). There are also faint silhouettes forming around the chemistry of the Circadian rhythm, and the role of the β-receptors in them (Axelrod 1975), and the Chemical Parameters of Sleep and Wakefulness. Programs serving Survival, and basic states of Consciousness appear to have a counterpart in the chemistry of the neuro-regulatory centers of the Brainstem. But again and again a monistic concept does not suffice; and the *inter*action between the so-called Neurotransmitters, Hormones, and more lately the so-called Neuromodulators and membrane-active amino acids, remain to be worked out in greater detail. Here again you encounter one of the most compelling characteristics of Psychopharmacology.

While individual methods (be they physiological, chemical, or behavioral) are used in their own right, they become Psychopharmacology only if used in combination. We have already briefly mentioned the combination of microelectrophysiology with cytochemistry, and cellular pharmacokinetics in relation to behavior. At a somewhat more molar level, we can combine remote electrical and chemical stimulation with Telemetry, the recording of evoked potential, and computerized frequency analysis. The Electroencephalograph (EEG) has become a sensitive and discriminate technique for the study of drug threshold effects in man (in the organic brain disorders it can now be combined with Computerized X-ray Tomography). Three areas invite early inquiry. One is the effect of psychoactive drugs on Cortical polarity, and slow DC shifts within the . cortical mantle in relation to subcortical centers; a second, the effect of drugs on the short but enormously significant electrical events *preceding* a voluntary act (a sort of pharmacology of intention, or selective attention); and a third, the slow interhemispheric shifts, and interhemispheric synchrony bearing upon a complementarity of function between the 2 hemispheres, and on the nature of possible subcortical selectors linking the hemispheres into a smoothly functioning whole. It is here that the recently described Biofeedback techniques, and various nondrug procedures for inducing Alternate States of Consciousness may have particular value. These techniques are designed to develop selective Inward Attention. Their autonomic effects suggest functional shifts in cell populations concerned with autonomic control. Drugs, possessing perhaps an overriding property, used in small graded doses, could conceivably prove powerful analytic tools for study of the chemistry of these processes. Such drugs could affect thresholds, and used discriminately, conceivably enhance the efficacy of these procedures. Again one wonders about the midline structures and the place of the enkephalins in these phenomena. Already, there are reports of striking changes in the Respiratory Center during inter trance states. In any event the field lies fallow and awaits inquiry.

Peripheral Indicators of Central Events. Metabolic Loading, Psychobiological Response Patterns and the Taxonomy of Mental Disorder

But what, you will say, of the relation between central events and peripheral indicators of such events? Administering a drug is one thing; drawing inferences from the assay of ions or metabolites in fluctuating psychological and behavioral states is a more hazardous procedure. Such fluctuation may only palely reflect Central Events, involving highly localized, formidably shielded cell groups. Fortunately, however, the field looks less forbidding than even a decade ago. For one thing, there are metabolites like MHPG which reflect central, rather than peripheral turnover. There is also the possibility of using stable-isotope labeled materials in man. Quite possibly, also, we may come upon peripheral enzyme systems (such as MAO and COMT in blood elements) which may serve not only as indicators of a behavioral state, but as genetic markers in the patients' families. If alongside one were to put the wide range of specific loading materials (precursors, specific inhibitors and the like), one obtains an idea of how useful these methods could eventually be in defining specific psychophysiological patterns of reactivity. Already in the study of the Affective Disorders, or the Schizophrenias (and, even, potentially in disorders of the senium), there are indications of metabolic imbalances which may distinguish subgroups within a given syndrome in terms of individual reaction patterns to a chemical load. If one were to begin to combine such a metabolic study with systematic studies of Stress Responsiveness, and Graded Performance, one could, while monitoring physiological responses, also establish quantitative threshold responses to particular drugs. The interaction between the phenothiazines and prolactin secretion is a case in point. Slowly, thus, one is beginning to approach what one might call Psychochemical diagnostic procedures. A Space-Age Technology awaits to be used; and in your lifetime such psychochemical screening procedures may well become a Routine Admission procedure for patients, and provide a rational basis for Diagnosis, Therapy and even New Drug Design. Let me venture another aside in this context. You will have seen from perusing this volume how, already, cleavage planes are appearing in conventional Diagnostic Nosologics. They will go on appearing until we find that we have to look at mental disorder in a way very different from the way present labels suggest. In terms of functional states, and states of performance, our new grouping may well run across older categories. I find the subcategories of a mental status examination in a sense more useful than cozy diagnostic labels. Quantification should be possible: Attention, Intention and Vigilance; Sensory Discrimination, Autonomic Lability, Motor Coordination and Motor Performance, Access to Memory Stores, and Verbal Associative Structure, Imagery and Phantasy all reflect. various states of integration of the states we know as Consciousness. Thus, I believe that we may be standing on the threshold of a new Taxonomy of Mental Disorders, drawing upon a deeper biological understanding of both function and dysfunction. We also should be able to identify at-risk populations much more readily.

How much nearer such considerations will bring us to understanding of the genetics of mental disorder remains to be seen; but here again, I, for one, am quite hopeful. The operation of Genetic Factors in the etiology of both affective disorders and the schizophrenias now is reasonably established and, while still a long way from Garrod's true, inborn errors of metabolism (for example, Phenylketonuria), we have some hope in the use of enzymes as genetic markers. Perhaps the most engaging parts of the emerging story of psychogenetics and pharmacogenetics are the ways in which loading doses of drugs can bring out interspecies difference in the induction of certain enzyme systems in the brain; and the behavioral correlates of such differences in response to early environmental cues. It is for that reason that metabolic loading studies in pure strains may well elucidate some of the fundamental rules by which structural genes are evoked, or kept in abeyance, by early environmental influences. At the extreme end, the rigidly coded behavior patterns of insects offer opportunity for fundamental work. These studies are aided by rapid propagation, and relatively easy harvesting of actual genetic material. Mammalian species, such as the rodents, cats, and dogs (all subject to well documented genetically determined patterns of behavior), may provide other opportunities. It is here, too, that the study of chemical corollaries of early environmental influences (such as exploration, play, socialization, learning through modeling and the hierarchical structure of groups) may be of special moment. I have consistently felt for a long time that the techniques of Ethology have a place in the laboratory of behavioral pharmacology. There is a complementarity between this approa.ch, and the classical Skinnerian paradigm. Whereas the former can teach one a great deal about the development of social responsiveness and communication, and the internalization of early social cues in neurochemical and enzymatic terms, the latter makes possible a fine grain analysis of behavior in the single animal to a degree, and with a precision and reproducibility which make a metabolic experiment thoroughly rewarding. It is even possible these days, to study mutual reinforcement, socialization and altruism in groups of animals engaged in a mutually reinforcing learning task.

The excitement, however, really begins when one looks at the induction of enzyme systems as a result of early intervention, and the responsiveness of hormone levels in both brain and blood to early social experiences. I say Brain and Blood because the brain as you know is regarded by some of us as a formidable organ of internal secretion, trafficking both within itself, into the cerebrospinal fluid, and the blood stream. The oligopeptides are here to stay. Not only do they influence Pain and Pleasure and Reward and Punishment, but they clearly are also concerned with Activity, Behavior, and Learning (DeWied et al. 1975). The ability to cope is learned early; there are, so to speak, Chemical Correlates of these early rehearsals of infancy and early life which prepare the organisms for adult adaptation. Social Reinforcement is chemically transcribed. There would appear to be a chemistry of Separation and Loss, and of Coping and Not Coping, as there is chemistry of Competence and Mastery. Hans Selye speaks of Stress, Distress and Eu-stress (Selye 1974). In a decade from now I venture to think we may be able to put a chemical name and number alongside such concepts. Bear in mind, also, the tools we already have to affect storage sites, reuptake mechanisms, and processes of synthesis and destruction, and you will get an idea of the incredible opportunity which awaits you in the laboratory to define the chemical outlines of Competence and of Coping. I used to think that animal models had only Limited Value in relation to human psychopharmacology. Now I am more hopeful. The reason is that very gradually Psychopharmacology is edging toward its mother-source of Physiology; the blunderbuss chemical hammer is giving way to discriminately used specific probes. We used to intervene, and then speculate and infer. The fit now is closer; for, in a few lucky instances, we have indicators of the physiological processes predominantly affected. You are familiar with the Catecholamine Hypothesis of Depression, the Dopamine Hypothesis of Schizophrenia and the relation of anticholinergie effects to extrapyramidal symptoms. Let's face it; most drugs that we have still are the result of the serendipitous visitations of an idea, or an observation, upon a Prepared Mind. But now one can hope for more precision. This is also aided by studying the conformational properties of compounds in relation to Receptor Configuration. Remember that many of the psychoactive compounds are active charge transfer compounds; no wonder that electron orbital calculations now figure heavily in the design of psychoactive drugs. Please also recall that in the design of such drugs we may be looking, in some respects, for the very opposite characteristics we look for in our precision tools of neurochemical investigation. Whereas, in the latter we seek an overriding and highly specific property, the psychoactive drugs are more likely *sharers* of several properties. Many of them combine anticholinergic, antiserotonergic, antigabergic, antiadrenergic, and antihistaminic properties in varying proportions; and these are very early days yet. Whatever the inferred biology of a defective central process [be it an enzyme deficiency, receptor deficiency or overactivity of an enzyme, site occupation by a false transmitter, lack of cofactors (such as ions, or hormones, or modulatory secondary transmitters) or local curare-like blockade or hypersensitivity] it should, in time, be possible to design drugs counteracting a physiological deficit presumably related to a particular disorder. This process will be helped enormously by the study of the Metabolic Kinetics of drugs in the body, and the monitoring of effective drug levels or of metabolites in relation to Therapeutic Effectiveness. The routine determination of Lithium Levels presages things to come; though even now – 27 years after its discovery – the restitutive and prophylactic action of this simple salt remains quite obscure.

Coping, Self Regulation, and Well-Being

Beyond the field of the Functional Psychosis lies the whole field of successful Adaptation, and the enhancement of Coping by chemical means. Here the line between what is pleasurable and what is desirable becomes thin and precarious. For whereas one would wholly subscribe to a true physiology of well-being, one would hesitate to further its pharmacology unless it is physiologically rooted. The effects of prednisone on cortisol secretion have made one cautious in the use of this compound. There is a justifiable reaction against the chronic use of anxiolytics and mild antidepressants, both at the hands of the practitioner, and by way of self-medication. Drugs loosely intended to help one cope over the short run, all too often result in a sharp reduction in coping-capacity. Dependence travels in subtle guises. Also, if one has used psychoactive drugs discriminately, one cannot but be impressed by the inordinate interaction between the interpersonal and social setting, and the response to a particular drug. The same drug, in the same dose, in the same person will lead to very different responses according to the antecedents and circumstances attending medication. Expectation is a powerful factor, and the Placebo a most powerful remedy. They can even be addictive! Do not brush the Placebo effect aside; but rather go after it, and try to understand the neurobiology of its inordinate effectiveness. We are capable, apparently, of exerting much more control and self-regulation than we are ready to admit; Attention Set, and Intention (especially Intention maintained over time) matter a great deal. Inner Awareness is at least as important as outer Attention and Vigilance. Awareness is the gate to choice; and we would appear to have much more choice than we are ready to admit. In a Thing-polluted and Word-polluted world, it would appear a matter of individual survival to cultivate Awareness and Choice, above all else. You will see that I abhor the idea of a Happiness Pill. Yet I cannot but hope that the physiology and biochemistry of successful Coping and Well-Being (into Maturity and Old Age) will be taken as seriously in our research, as the psychobiology of the Depressive Disorders and of the Schizophrenias. What, precisely are the hormonal and neurohormonal consequences of adequate work, and fulfillment? of rest, recreation, play? and, above all, of simple, quiet, well-being? What is the biology of a Good Day? What are the hormonal differences between the compulsively taken vacation, and truly and deeply taking "Time Out", to reassess Priorities and Values and, perhaps, rearrange one's life? How do the parents of children of healthy families differ biochemically from families notoriously under stress? Why, among the older, do some stay young and others wither early? You will note that studies such as these will require the evolution of research methods carried deeply into daily life. Only by making the consumer the sharer, and partner both of information, and the benefits of such shared information, can one hope to develop the kind of open and cooperative partnership between researcher and consumer, which would give such work the Social Significance it potentially holds. There is a profound difference between Questionnaires administered by strangers and Self-Monitoring devices which help one through one's day; between "data collection" and participatory feedback to the client. You will see that here Applied Research merges gently with Health Education, and that it extends to Self-Help, Self-Care and Self-Regulation, growing out of informed knowledge on the part of the Consumer. You will also note that the tools of social psychology, and of educational psychology, (and particularly methods of self-monitoring and awareness training) can be of significance in such development. It is out of such studies (coupled, as always, with the good luck of a serendipitous discovery) that physiologically based restitutive compounds may perhaps emerge. After all, Vitamin and Megavitamin tablets have been on the average breakfast table for some time. Who knows what FDA-approved additives Junior will take a decade or two hence?

The Chemical Extension of Physiological Boundaries

Will, you ask, such discoveries be capable of extending physiological boundaries by pharmacological means? Here, I confess I resist speculation. Recent symposia (e.g., Evans and Kline 1971), have examined the implications of the psychochemical revolution, probable or otherwise ; clearly drugs are already at hand which affect fertility, sexual desire and performance, hunger and physical pain. The Circadian Clock could conceivably be manipulated to a 48-hr day, and possibly to prolonged chemically induced periods of hibernation. The counterpart of prolonged feats of physical endurance also can be envisaged. Thoughts on the chemical enhancement of retention, recall, learning ability and overall intelligence also must be taken seriously in view of the evidence already available on neuronal growth, the relation of protein synthesis to the consolidation of the memory trace. The implications for the mounting geriatric population were examined at a recent international symposium (Lehmann and Joulou 1977).

The so-called psychedelics form a chapter unto themselves. There has been, in recent years, a most welcome turning away from their mass use to responsible use by serious investigators, in a few well-equipped laboratories. These tools are very powerful, and dangerous. They can be used in the study of preconscious experience, and the induction of transpersonal states which give one an idea of the organization of the realms of the human unconscious (see Grof 1975). Meticulous preparation is essential in the conduct of any such experiments. The drugs have been used in the terminally ill. The emergence of very early memories, and of imagery and thought-forms described independently by cultural anthropologists, raises profound questions as to the racial, ethnic and transcultural attributes of the memory traces we carry within us. The dangers of these drug-induced states are self-evident; yet probably, we have so far only seen the forerunners of such compounds. While many have global effects, others will become (or already are) available, capable of affecting, in highly discriminative ways, the qualities of Selective Attention, which collectively comprise the universe of outer vigilance or inward awareness. Here again, comparison with non-drug-induced, physiological states – such as Concentration, Meditation, Yoga, Akido, Biofeedback and the like – is inviting. The drug "trip" is giving way to the concept of the non-drug journey. "Journey" involves purpose, effort, discipline, and an honest self-accounting. Clearly these states cannot be treated lightly: that they should have been sanctified by great religions suggests both their potency, and their danger; and their potential usefulness to Culture. There is no rule here except the rule of respect.

It is significant that our "Future–Shock"-prone age, should, by way of homeostatic adaptation, emphasize these intensely personal nondrug "centering" procedures: procedures demanding self-discipline, and making for self sufficiency and competence in the face of huge social and political upheaval. The transformation of cultures leads to the strange conversations. One cannot also help observing, in passing, how many of these developments have so far developed outside conventional Academia. This should surprise no one. At the turn of the century William James drew much from Benjamin Blood's Ether Dreams (Blood 1894), and his essays on the "Stream of Thought", "The Varieties of Religious Experience and Pluristic Mystic" were hardly in keeping with the spirit of the times. As he says (James 1890):

> What must be admitted is that the definite images of traditional psychology form but the smallest part of our minds as they actually live. The traditional psychology talks like one who should say a river consists of nothing but pailsful, spoonsful, quartpotsful, barrelsful and other molded forms of water. Even were the pails and pots all actually standing in the stream, still between them the free water would continue to flow. It is just this free water of consciousness that psychologists resolutely overlook. Every image in the mind is steeped and dyed in the free water that flows round it. With it goes the sense of its relations, near and remote, the dying echo whence it came to us, and the dawning sense whither it is to lead.

It is hard to tell how far these "Echoes" and this "Dawning Sense of Knowing" will lead one. But the study of non-druginduced intuitive states of concentration may well lead one to a study of the phenomena of the creative process. My physicist friends tell me that their best mathematical work often is done in a peculiar withdrawn state of almost mystic concentration. It would appear that the intuitive perception of space-time configurations is deeply readied in the unconscious; its clumsy read-out in ordinary language barely represents the tremendous condensation of symbols going into such a successful transaction. Elsewhere 1 have examined the role of language in psychopharmacology, and in science, with a special reference to physical sciences (Elkes 1963, 1970a,b); here I would simply plead for the study of transformation of language in alternate states of awareness. As Whorf (1956) and Chomsky (1972) and others have shown, there are deep organizational rules in the very nature of language ; and these rules extend deep into the unconscious. Our habitual linear way of ordering our lives only uses sparingly the creative power of the instrument we carry in our skull. Again we come up against the respective roles of the right and left hemisphere, and the linear and parallel analogs of the computer. By their own admission, the physicists appear to use these inner space devices more than some of us. However, they have one advantage: they have created accurate mathematical languages to describe relationships which defy the rules of conventional logic. Properties such as Complementarity, Noninclusiveness, and Coexistence appear in their relativistic mode to present a much more accurate picture of reality than the conventional metric rules by which we live. The timing of these concepts, also is interesting. Maxwell (1856), published his equations on Faraday's Lines of Force in the year of Freud's birth; and George Boole (1854), the father of Boolean Algebra, aimed in his "Investigation of the Laws of Thought" to test the ability of symbols to express logical proposition, "the laws of whose combination should be founded upon the laws of mental processes which they represent." I have argued elsewhere for the establishment, with serious long-term funding, of "Inner Space Laboratories" (Elkes 1970b), engaged in the training of selected "Intronauts", capable of navigating in Inner Space as seasoned travellers do in strange territory. It certainly would be much less expensive than putting a man on the moon, and, in terms of social yield, at least as useful. Isn't it curious, incidentally, that some of the extraordinary well-organized and competent men who did engage in Outer Space exploration, have turned inward and regard a knowledge of Inner Space as a legitimate enterprise?

The Need for Mathematical Languages

This brings me to one last point. The ability to recognize relationships, and particularly relationships in time, is the essential function of mathematics; and if mathematics and information theory have hesitated on the edge of the behavioral and the physiological sciences for so long, it is perhaps because, with certain notable exceptions, they have never really been tempered against the precise requirements of the physiological experiment at the bench level. The intellectual history of such distance and alienation is common enough; yet the history of physics suggests, in some measure, that sooner or later such isolation is broken; and that as experiments become more precise, their conceptual, mathematical models become more feasible, possible, and productive. Cybernetic theory, although drawing more heavily on biological models, has not returned to the parent science what it drew from it.

The climate, however, is now changing slowly and unmistakably. The time vector, and the probability of events in time, are invading theories of perception and of learning, just as they did the physical sciences of a century ago. Moreover, the essentially random nature of much of the assembly of units making up our information carrying system, is receiving steadily increasing recognition. The "wiring" theories of old are giving place to less rigid, more statistical and, yet apparently, more flexible and correct models. Information Theory has so far only tenuously interacted with genetics or immunochemistry, where its implications are obvious. In the CNS it has proved particularly valuable in the understanding of the coding process along sensory pathways, and very gradually the theoretical framework is being expanded to accept and manipulate data in other areas, such as the process of recognition of universals in language, and cognate secondary signaling systems. It would, therefore, seem advisable to give early thought to the bringing of mathematical talent into the physiological and neurochemical, as well as the psychological laboratory; and to exposing individuals so endowed to data at the laboratory level. It perhaps may be not too much to hope that concepts only partly and inadequately covered by the languages now employed will find their precise and compact mathematical expression through such a process of mutual exposure. The concept of the CNS as a chemically mediated organ of information may thus be made a little more real. For unless we understand the code and cipher in which the brain constructs and stores, silently and with uncanny speed, its models of reality, and the distortion of this coding, by controlled chemical means, we will, whatever language we choose to employ, and whatever chemical aspect we wish to follow, be standing outside the phenomena: our language will be descriptive, and do justice merely to some properties of the process, rather than the process itself. Yet a careful contemplation of clinical phenomena plainly makes demands higher than this; and whether we like it or not, we shall be faced with these demands in the light of the very experiments which clinical observations compel.

Closing

This has been a rambling letter; but like the Talmud, one cannot, so to speak, speak of Psychopharmacology standing on one leg. You will agree that it is a Large Country or, to change the metaphor, a City of Many Gates. I do not know by which door you propose to enter; but I would ask you please to scrutinize your particular door very carefully. You can clearly come to Psychopharmacology by way of Physics and Biophysics; from Biochemistry or Neurobiology ; from Experimental, Clinical or Social Psychology ; from Medicine, Psychiatry or from Anthropology. If you come from Physics, or Mathematics, or Systems Theory I can only say, for my personal part, that we need you, and I hope that you will be made welcome.

There are three requirements which will be necessary for you to enjoy the field. One is true expertise and craftsmanship in your own branches of science; a second, a working knowledge or the areas upon which your particular approach borders, and impinges and third, a *place of work* where there is true conversation extending through the length and breadth of the discipline. Thus, choose your approach carefully and align it with your own abilities. Choose your intellectual company (the literature is huge and varied); and choose your place of work. For Psychopharmacology is not only a body of knowledge, but represents an Attitude. It is a Transdisciplinary Discipline; and true cooperation and sharing is a condition for its continued growth. By and large, we live by barter and exchange among ourselves; and favor Win/Win rather than Win/Lose solutions.

This volume, with its rich appendices carries a very full bibliography, and also Appendix 6 makes a beginning to list places all over the world where active teaching and training is available. There should be no shortage of places to choose from: the Universities, Government, Industry and the Scientific Organizations of many Nations and International bodies, including UNESCO, NATO and WHO, support collaborative work, Fellowships, and Study plans in this new discipline. We have an International College of Neuropsychopharmacology and several international Journals. It was not always so. One recent meeting, for example (Ayd and Blackwell 1970), gave us occasion to recall how some of us began; there weren't many of us then. Indeed, it was a small and intimate group. In this context I also recall the proverbial smoke-filled room in which some of us, 6 years ago, planned the creation of the American College of Neuropsychopharmacology. There is no reward in my life that I value more than serving as its first President. As I said at the time:

> It is not uncommon for any one of us to be told that Psychopharmacology is not a science, and that it would do well to emulate the precision of older and more established disciplines. Such statements betray a lack of understanding for the special demands made by Psychopharmacology upon the fields which compound it. For my own part, I draw comfort and firm conviction from the history of our subject, and the history of our group. For I know of no other branch of science which, like a good plough on a spring day. has tilled as many areas in Neurobiology. To have, in a mere decade, questioned the concepts of synaptic transmission in the central nervous system; to have emphasized compartmentalization and regionalization of chemical process in the unit cell and in the brain; to have focussed on the interaction of hormone and chemical process within the brain; to have given us tools for the study of the chemical basis of learning and temporary connection formation; to have emphasized the dependence of pharmacological response on its situational and social setting; to have compelled a hard look at the semantics of psychiatric diagnosis, description and communication; to have resuscitated that oldest of old remedies. the placebo response, for

careful scrutiny; to have provided potential methods for the study of language in relation to the functional state of the brain; and to have encouraged the Biochemist, Physiologist, Psychologist, Clinician, and the Mathematician and Communication Engineer to join forces at bench level, is no mean achievement for a young science. That a chemical text should carry the imprint of experience, and partake in its growth. in no way invalidates study of symbols, and the rules among symbols, which keep us going. changing, evolving, and human. Thus, though moving cautiously, psychopharmacology is still protesting; yet, in so doing it is, for the first time, compelling the physical and chemical sciences to look hehavior in the face, and thus enriching both these sciences an d behavior. If there be discomfiture in this encounter, it is hardly surprising; for it is in this discomfiture that there may well lie the germ of a new science. (Elkes 1963)

That this field poses the ethical dilemma of sciences at its most poignant will not have escaped you. The specter of a Drug-polluted or Drugged society is here to stay, until faced responsibly through a process of education, and gradual permeation by an enlightened regulatory process. This must be based on evidence, and anchored in the consent of an informed public. As a member of the fraternity you will have a tremendous educational job on your hands. Do not be carried away by your own enthusiasm, and preoccupations, however satisfying they may be to you at a particular moment. The public is apt to misunderstand, unless you take the time to explain and put it in context. I personally believe, as I stated earlier, that the value of Pharmacology lies in leading us to its Source, to Physiology in our field; drugs may well illuminate the awesome restitutive powers which our bodies possess. unaided by chemical prostheses. It may well be that as our society becomes more tolerant, more cooperative and kindly, more rewarding in work, and more joyful in play, we may need less drugs, and not more. For the axis of it all, I suppose, is having a Good Day; which, now, I wish you, wherever you are.

Sincerely yours,

Joel Elkes

REFERENCES

Axelrod, J. (1975). The pineal gland: A guide to study the regulation of the adrenergic receptor. In: The Nervous System (D.B. Tower, ed.), Vol. 1, pp. 395-400. Raven, New York.

Ayd, F. J., and Blackwell, B. (eds.) (1970). Discoveries in Biological Psychiatry. Lippincott, Philadelphia, Pennsylvania.

Blood, B. P. (1874). The Anaesthetic Revelation and the Gist of Philosophy. New York and Amsterdam.

Bogoch, S. (1975). The "sign-post" function of brain glycoproteins: Order and disorder in the nervous system. In: The Nervous System (D. B. Tower, ed.), Vol. 1, pp. 591-600. Raven, New York.

Boole, G. (1854). An Investigation of the Laws of Thought. Walton & Maberly, London.

Bradley, P. B., and Elkes, J. (1957). The effects of some drugs on the electrical activity of the brain. Brain 80, 77-111.

Chomsky, N. (1972). Language and Mind. Harcourt, New York.

De Wied, D., Bohus, B., Urban, I., van Wimersma-Greidanus, B., and Cispen, W. H. (1975). Pituitary peptides and memory. In: Peptides: Chemistry, Structure, and Biology (R. Walter and J. Meienhofer, eds.), pp. 635-643. Ann Arbor Sci. Publ., Ann Arbor, Michigan.

Elkes,J. (1958). Drug effects in relation to receptor specificity within the brain: Some evidence and provisional formulations. Neurol. Ciba Found. Symp., 1957. pp. 303-332.

Elkes, J. (1963). The American College of Neuropsychopharmacology. A note on its history, and hopes for the future. Bull. Am. Coll. Neuropsychopharmacol. 1, 2-3.

Elkes, J. (1970a). Word fallout, or, On the hazards of explanation (Presidential Address). In: The Psychopathology of Adolescence (J. Zabin and A. M. Freedman, eds.), pp.118-137. Grune & Stratton, New York.

Elkes, J. (1970b). Psychopharmacology: On beginning in a new science. In: Discoveries in Biological Psychiatry (F.J. Ayd and B. Blackwell, eds.) pp. 30-52. Lippincott, Philadelphia, Pennsylvania.

Evans, W. O., and Kline, N. S. (eds.) (1971). Psychotropic Drugs in the Year 2000. Thomas, Springfield, Illinois.

Feldberg, W., and Vogt, M. (1948). Acetylcholine synthesis in different regions of the nervous system. J. Physiol. (London) 107, 372-381.

Grof, S. (1915). Realms of the Human Unconscious. Viking, New York

James, W. (1890). Principles of Psychology. Holt, New York. (Reprinted in 1950 by Dover, New York. Vol. 1. pp. 689)

Lehmann, H. E., and Joulou, L. (chairmen) (1977). Symposium on Geriatric Psychopharmacology. Proc. 10th Congr. Coll. Int. Neuropsychopharmacol. (CINP) (in press).

Maxwell, J. C. (1856) On Faraday's lines of force. In: Scientific Papers of J.C. Maxwell (W. D. Niven, ed.). Vol.1, pp.155-229. Cambridge Univ. Press, London and New York.

Olds, J. (1976) Behavioral studies of hypothalamic functions, drives and reinforcements. In: Biological Foundations of Psychiatry (R.G. Grenell and S. Gabay, eds.), Vol. II, pp. 321-448. Raven, New York.

Pribram, K. H. (1971) Languages of the Brain. Prentice-Hall, Englewood Cliffs, New Jersey.

Salmoiraghi, G. C., and Bloom, F. E. (1964) Pharmacology of individual neurons. Science 144, 493-499.

Selye, H. (1974) Stress Without Distress. Lippincott, Philadelphia, Pennsylvania.

Snyder, S. H. (1975) Opiate receptor in normal and drug altered brain function. Nature (London) 257, 185-189.

Waelsch, H. (ed.) (1955) Biochemistry of the Developing Nervous System. Academic Press, New York.

Whorf, B. J. (1956) Language, Thought and Reality. MIT Press, Cambridge, Massachusetts.

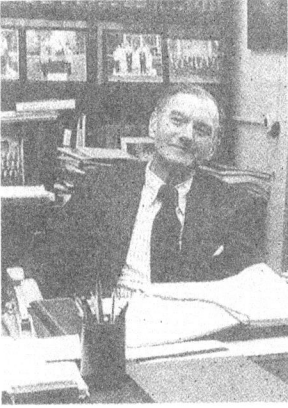

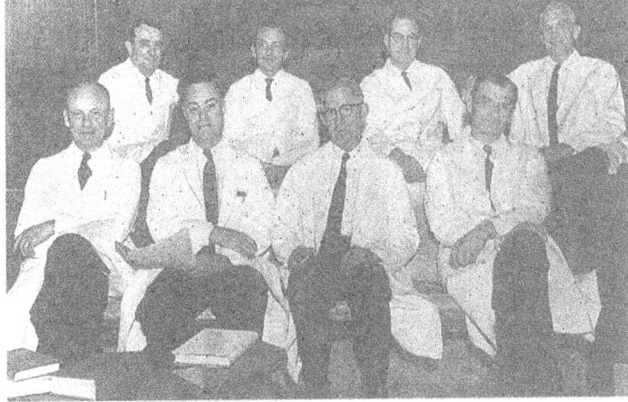

With residents

The Clinical Chiefs at John Hopkins, cca 1968
Front row, left to right: A. Barnes, R. Morgan, A. Blalock, J. Elkes.
Back row, from left: McGehee Harvey, I. Bennett, E. Maumenee, R.
Cooke.

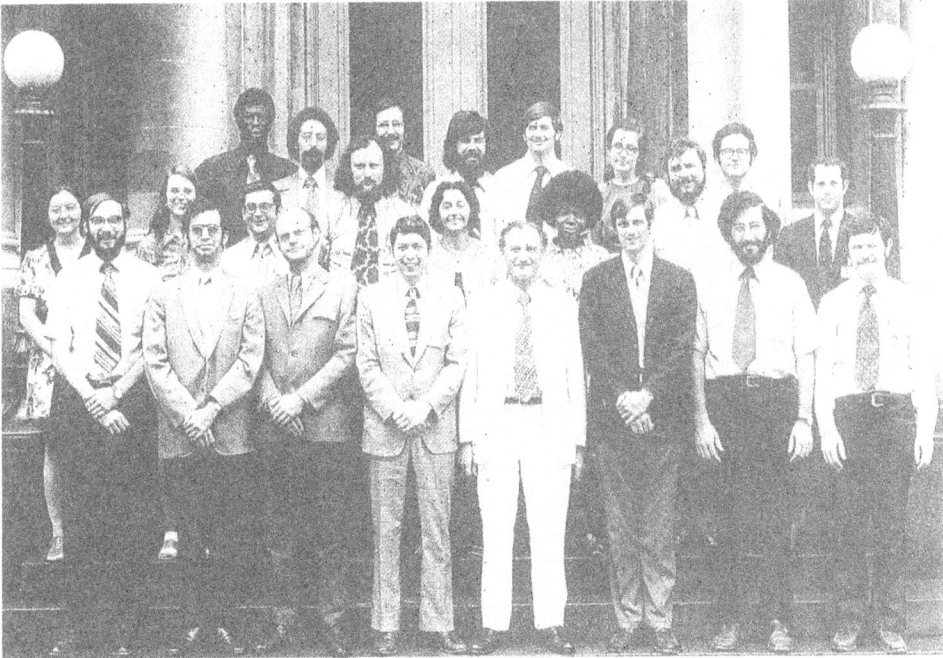

At Hopkins, 1969

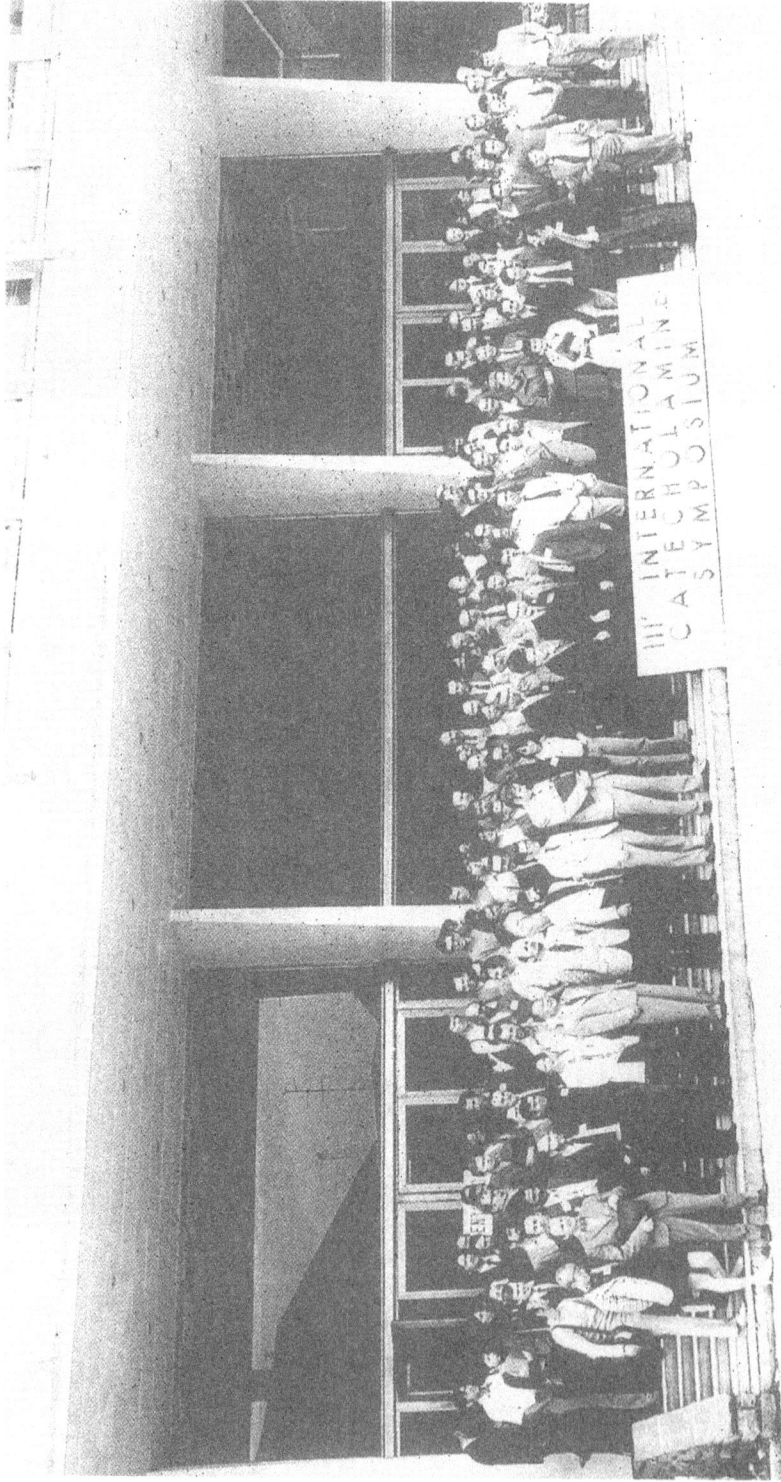

The Third International Catecholamine Symposium
Strassbourg, 1972

Part Seven

HUMANIZING THE EDUCATION OF PHYSICIANS – THE BEHAVIORAL SCIENCES IN THE SERVICE OF MEDICINE

PAPERS

18. J. Elkes: *Memorandum to the search committee for the Henry Phipps Chair of Psychiatry, at Johns Hopkins, 1963.*
    Reprinted with the kind permission of Slack Inc. from J. Elkes *Behavioral medicine: The early beginnings*. Psychiatric Annals 11: 27, 1963
19. J. Elkes: *On meeting psychiatry: A note on the student's first year.*
    Reprinted with the kind permission of the American Psychiatric Association from The American Journal of Psychiatry 122: 121-128, 1965, and with the kind permission of W.B. Saunders from Comprehensive Psychiatry 8: 236-245, 1965
20. L. Dickstein and J. Elkes: *Health awareness and the medical student: A preliminary experiment.*
    Reprinted with the kind permission of the Fetzer Institute from Advances (Institute for Advancement of Health) 4: 12-23, 1987
21. R.R. Rubin, J. Elkes, R.W. Maris, and P.E. Dietz: *Medicine and the Behavioral Sciences: The Johns Hopkins M.D.–Ph.D. Program.*
    Reprinted with the kind permission of The Johns Hopkins University Press from The Johns Hopkins Medical Journal 136: 268-270, 1975

ARGUMENT

Before accepting the Henry Phipps Chair at Johns Hopkins University in Baltimore (USA), Joel Elkes wrote a memorandum to the Search Committee (Paper 18). In this, he outlined his ideas how given an opportunity – modern psychiatry could "relate and translate the growing points of modern biology to the behavioral sciences, and the behavioral sciences to the body of clinical medicine." He emphasized the crucial role of transdisciplinary communication, and the need for the evolution of common language through joint work.

The name of the Department was changed from Psychiatry" to Psychiatry and Behavioral Sciences" in 1964. Many schools adopted a cognate change of name during the coming years.

At Hopkins, with the help of committed colleagues, Elkes introduced a course in the Behavioral Sciences during the students' first year. One of the important objectives of this course was to convey the message to the students early in their career that the "Behavioral Sciences has something to offer to medicine as a whole." At the beginning, no curriculum time could be found for this course during the week; it was therefore relegated to Saturday mornings. However, it was very well attended, and well received by the student body. Three departmental chairmen (of Pediatrics, Gynecology and Obstetrics, and Psychiatry), and several other senior members from other departments participated. An outline of this course is given in Paper 19.

To make the point further an M.D.-Ph. D. program in the Behavioral Sciences was put into operation between 1973 and 1975. (Paper 21). It was a cooperative effort between six departments of the University.

Throughout his career as a teacher, Joel Elkes has continued to be impressed by the excessive pressures put on students during their time in medical school, and the need for enhancing awareness of their own health needs, and honing their coping skills early in their career. The opportunity to do so arose when he was invited to a post-retirement post in the Department of Psychiatry and Behavioral Sciences in the University of Louisville (Kentucky, USA – Head of Department, Dr. John Schwab). In Louisville, Elkes met Dr. Leah Dickstein, at that time the Dean of Students, who shared his concerns. Together they developed what was to become known as the "Louisville Experiment," a four and a half day Workshop on Health Awareness offered annually to medical students during the week before official enrollment, on an entirely *voluntary* basis. Over some fifteen years 90 to 95% of every class have attended this workshop.

The workshop used both a didactic and experiential mode, by combining large presentations with small group exercises. Topics covered included Mode of Life as a factor in illness and disability; the psychobiology of human adaptation, stress, and the stress response; the physiology of nutrition, exercise, and relaxation; the psychology of time management and study skills; listening, and the give-and take of relationships; substance abuse and the impaired physician; and an introduction to the ethics of medical practice and of the place of Belief in Healing. There was an attempt to maintain a balance between presentations of scientific evidence and a participatory experiential "fun" approach to learning. A web of social support was created for students before they actually began their course work.

The message that "the behavioral sciences have something to offer to medicine as a whole" was also developed in Paper 21.

PAPER 18

MEMORANDUM TO THE SEARCH COMMITTEE
For the Henry Phipps Chair of Psychiatry, at Johns Hopkins, 1963[*]

Joel Elkes

Clinical Neuropharmacology Research Center,
National Institute of Mental Health, Washington, D.C.

The part played by psychiatry in modern medical education, medical practice and the growth of the biomedical sciences will in large measure depend on its ability to relate (and translate) the growing points of modern biology to the behavioral sciences and the behavioral sciences to the body of clinical medicine. The lag in the evolution of the subject reflects neither on its quality as a body of empirical knowledge, nor on its future as a clinical science.

Like other specialties, psychiatry is rooted in the natural history of the phenomena which are its business; like the other specialties, also, its growth as a science depends on the development of those areas of fundamental knowledge most directly related to an understanding of clinical states. Medicine, in its own evolution has leaned heavily on the growth of physiology; and Genetics owes some of their most fundamental advances to recent strides in the fields of Molecular Biology and Biophysics.

The sciences of normal and aberrant behavior of human communication and miscommunication of necessity depend on the growth of cognate disciplines. These are to be found in the recent developments in neurobiology (including neurophysics, neurochemistry, neuroendocrinology, neuropharmacology and neurocommunication) as in the psychological sciences, the social sciences and the sciences of communication. It is the task of psychiatry to mediate between the various areas by making them relevant to problems of aberrant human behavior, and in so doing to transform natural history into the beginnings of a clinical science.

As yet interaction is tenuous: the languages and frames of reference are too diverse to permit effective exchange. Yet it could be one of the major functions of a "Department of Psychiatry and Behavioral Sciences" in a modern School of Medicine to provide a setting for precisely this kind of dialogue and to do so at working as well as a discursive level. Common languages evolve out of common purpose. Common purpose is best pursued in a common setting.

The wide scatter of the areas impinging upon clinical psychiatry; their varying investigate approaches (which are in part experimental and in part historical in nature) and their representation both within and without the Medical School proper have so far often colluded in a conspiracy of silence: by and large, psychiatry has remained as isolated from the disciplines related to it, as these have from psychiatry. It is up to psychiatry to break the deadlock of isolation and it is up to related sciences to avail themselves of the opportunity offered by an ad-

---

[*]   Reprinted with the kind permission of Slack Inc. from J. Elkes *Behavioral medicine: The early beginnings.* Psychiatric Annals 11: 27, 1963

vancing and far-reaching clinical field. The growth of psychopharmacology (which has successfully engaged in inquiries ranging from the role of social field and personality structure to the neutral substrate of drug action) suggests that such in an interaction is, indeed, possible.

To fulfil these various functions, the Department of Psychiatry and Behavioral Sciences must be firmly rooted in the high quality of its Clinical Services and of its Clinical Teaching. This should be furnished by its own hospital facilities (comprising In-Patient services, a Day Clinic and Out-Patient and Domiciliary Visiting Services); by Liaison Services with other clinical Departments; and (in view of the mounting problems of the Public Mental Hospital) by Research and Training Facility in a Public Mental Hospital linked administratively to the Department. The Department should have its own ample laboratories for both experimental and clinical studies. These should, in part be staffed from within the department, but equally should provide space (either of the "Permanent" or "Guest" type) to members of the other Departments holding joint appointments with the Department of Psychiatry. This cross-representation could include all those Pre-clinical and Clinical Departments who would judge it mutually helpful to participle in the arrangements, it should, however, also include areas (such as Experimental Psychology, Sociology, Social Anthropology, Linguistics and Sciences of Communication) in other parts of the University.

Excessive mixing, for mixing's sake would, of course, have to be assiduously avoided. Nevertheless, it may be expected that carefully planned common Teaching and Research programs, the participation of psychiatrists in the work of other departments, common Seminar Schedules and a well – used Departmental Common Room could slowly lead to the growth of mutual understanding, and with it, of mutual respect between disparate areas of investigation. This process would take time, a period of five to ten years must be viewed as a mere beginning in such a process.

The creation of such a Department within a School of Medicine may have a number of simple consequences. It could, if successful, project a much clearer image of contribution of Neurobiology, Psychology and the Behavioral Sciences to an understanding of these Diseases than has been current hitherto. To the student, it could mediate (with other areas) a spirit of scientific humanism in an evolving medical curriculum. To the teacher, it could provide a challenge both in conceptualization and communication, keeping the teaching fresh, because of the constant controversy, which this growing edge of human knowledge engenders. To the research student it could present a field, still young and very open, and one reasonably assured of major reward.

PAPER 19

ON MEETING PSYCHIATRY:
A NOTE ON THE STUDENT'S FIRST YEAR[*]

Joel Elkes

Henry Phipps Professor of Psychiatry, Director, Department of Psychiatry and Behavioral Sciences, The Johns Hopkins University; Psychiatrist-in-Chief, The Johns Hopkins Hospital, Baltimore, Md

1. The Student Meets Him/Herself

It is trite to say that education is mutual education. Those who teach, know how much the student can be the teacher. The student mirrors the present, and senses the future. He/she has a habit of opening academic parcels and looking at what's inside. He/she may lose this habit as he/she grinds through the scholastic mill. But at the beginning, at any rate, enthusiasm and skepticism are his good companions. The green shoots of curiosity always press afresh. Curiosity demands a sense of order; order satisfied leads to a looking for more facts, connections, and discrepancies. Anyone who has engaged a group of first-year students in discussion will know the particular feeling, and the joy. Such *un*rest cures are highly recommended to teachers.

As he/she meets psychiatry, the student is prepared for yet another specialty. In this he/she is wrong. Psychiatry cannot compartmentalize: it deals in patterns and not pieces, in people and not organ systems. In making contact with the subject, the student brings to it his/her most important piece of portable equipment, namely him/herself. In his/her skull he/she carries a vast and fascinating laboratory of which he/she may be only dimly aware. He/she looks repeatedly to the bench sciences for analogies, and for the reassurance of fact and figure. He/she is apt to think in terms of logic, line, sequence, and compartmentalization of function. The concepts of "relationship", and "pattern" are more difficult to grasp. So is change in intricate patterns over time. Unless he/she has been prepared for the task in college, "behavior" remains to him/her a strange and unshapely beast, forever being fitted into the procrustean box of the bench sciences. Yet somehow he/she must be made aware, before he/she moves too far into his clinical training, that behavior and subjective experience are not only phenomena, but also instruments of high inferential value; that skill in observation of behavior, including his/her own behavior though more native to some than to others, can be both taught and

* This paper was delivered as part of a panel discussion on undergraduate education at the One Hundred and Twenty-First Annual Meeting of the American Psychiatric Association, May 8, 1965. It is published in the August 1965 issue of the American Journal of Psychiatry. In view of its topic it is included (also) in the March 1965 issue of Comprehensive Psychiatry by permission of Dr. Francis Braceland, Editor- in-Chief, American Journal of Psychiatry.
Reprinted with the kind permission of the American Psychiatric Association from The American Journal of Psychiatry 122: 121-128, 1965, and with the kind permission of W.B. Saunders from Comprehensive Psychiatry 8: 236-245, 1965

learned; that such learning requires conceptual tools of its own; that it can never be didactic and always has to be experiential; and that relative absence of hardware in clinical psychiatry and human psychology in no way reflect on its ability to measure, to conceptualize and predict. In short, the student must learn to respect the use of him/herself as much as his/her slide rule and statistical tables. In this self acceptance, and growing self. knowledge, there can be a source of much power. If acquired early, it will serve him/her well with his patients; and equally well should he/she choose a life in the laboratory rather than a life in the clinic. Adolf Meyer, in requiring autobiographies of his students, saw this quite clearly.

2. Four Strands of Theory: Human Development, Human Learning, Human Communication and Human Social Field Dependence

The past few years have seen major developments in neurobiology and the behavioral sciences: Neurobiology has witnessed the emergence of neurochemistry., behavioral pharmacology and neuroendocrinology as important branches of the neurological sciences. The animal behavioral sciences have developed powerful quantitative techniques for the control of stimulus situations, the analysis of the fine structure of behavior over time, the study of : the learning process, and the use of on-line computers in the control of. experimental situations. In the human behavioral sciences there have been; advances in developmental psycholinguistics, in the mathematical analysis of language, and other aspects of the sciences of communication, in the understanding of the learning process in children, and in the psychology of small (and particularly, family) groups. Contributions from these various areas to an understanding of the role of biological and psychosocial factors in the genesis of mental disorder and handicap can be reasonably expected. Yet, with a few notable exceptions, there has not been the kind of interaction between these various branches of science and psychiatry which would make for the evolution of common languages, common attitudes and common enterprises. Interdisciplinary approaches always stand in danger of becoming multidisciplinary institutions; and among these too few have focused on problems peculiar to the developing nervous system, and the evolution or patterns of individual and social behavior in animals, and in man.

The sources of these problems are not very difficult to trace. They rest primarily upon differences in the education of the biologist, and the behavioral scientist; and are poignantly reflected in the straddling position which the clinician, concerned with disorders of human behavior and symbolic function, occupies. Modern biology, has drawn for its greatest advances on biochemistry, biophysics, subcellular morphology and genetics: the languages it has developed are, by and large, based on these fields. To date, the languages of the behavioral sciences have developed relatively independently of advances in biology, the key departments often being situated some distance away from centers of biomedical training and research. Yet the need for interaction between the biomedical and behavioral sciences is urgent and real. It is apparent in psychiatry, in clinical and social psychology, psychophysiology, psychopharmacology, and psychosomatics, and, one would venture to suggest, in medicine at large; and nowhere is it more poignant than in the fields of normal and abnormal human development.

As is well known, a number of centers have developed important educational and experimental programs relating brain" to behavior'. By and large, these have attempted to bridge the gap through work in the adult animal, or grown man, drawing workers trained in one field (e.g., experimental neurology, neurochemistry or pharmacology) into collaborative efforts with workers in another (e.g., experimental psychology) . However desirable such attempts may be, they may not necessarily be the most efficient. Much that is complex in the adult nervous system can be studied more simply in the evolving nervous system. Much that is complex in some species can be studied more readily in less complex species. It is suggested that a program carefully planned to center on the biology of the developing nervous system, and its relation to the unfolding of patterns of behavior, could provide a most effective terrain for interaction between a variety of disciplines at an experimental, as well as a clinical level. It is furthermore suggested that such a direct, practical emphasis on developments in neurobiology, and developmental psychology is long overdue in psychiatry and could, in fact, provide a cornerstone of sound psychiatric theory. Psychiatry, having rightly stressed the importance of early life experience, and having accumulated a wealth of empirical data, has, by and large, viewed the phenomena of psychopathology through the inverted telescope of psychodynamic reconstruction. There are now heartening signs that this trend may be reversed, and that it may become less retrospective, and more prospective in its attitudes. Modern psychiatry may be ready, both conceptually and methodologically, to assimilate the findings of the developmental and comparative behavioral sciences into its own body of knowledge. The study of the genesis of patterns of behavior, and the effects of early environmental factors on their differentiation may provide a fertile ground for both education and investigation. Indeed, human development, human learning and human communication in a changing social field would seem to me to form the most solid starting points for the teaching of a science of man. What anatomy, psychology and biochemistry are to the clinical subjects, these subjects could be to psychiatry. They are the bedrock of good psychiatric theory; and whether we like it or not, much of our theoretical thinking (including psychoanalytic thinking) will have to find its place in this more general, and more satisfactory framework. There are signs that such a process may well have begun.

It is important to convey to the student quite early the principles of general evolution and the evolutionary history of man. With it should go an emphasis on the immaturity of his nervous system at birth, the continued development after birth, and the susceptibility of the developing nervous system to early environmental (sociofamilial) setting. Here pathology is often inclined to obscure the normal and healthy. Vulnerability is stressed a great deal. Potential, which is the obverse of vulnerability, is less emphasized. Students are sensitive to this defect in reasoning, and are quick to take one to task on this issue.

A consideration of Learning and Communication is inseparable from human development. Much is known about Learning. The experimental conditioning models (both classical and operant); the naturalistic data; the body of theory subserving modern pre-school education, including instrumental teaching, are all available; yet little is taught to medical students. The intelligent student has only got to look around him to realize that we all learn all the time; that our patients, in some manner, learn more slowly, and differently; and that we do not really understand why,. Learning, unlearning, and relearning (with regard to inner, rather than outer referents) are distinctly unfashionable words in the clinic. Yet in their profoundest sense they go to the root of change in a person. It is time, I think, that those terms were allowed to return from banishment.

Yet another term is communication. Here, for the sake of simplicity, the animal model is often invoked. The genetically coded signaling systems as described by ethologists form a good beginning. Yet the uniqueness, and subtlety of the human system of communication is that it makes possible a nongenetic transfer of information. Psychiatry and much of medicine deals with disorders of communication; psychotherapy is therapy by communication. Yet how many students are taught the elements of these communication processes? How many know something about the evolution and economy of message transmittal in gestures, and the complex type of motor activity known as spoken language? How many know of the mathematics of information transfer in artificial speech, of transmodal language prostheses? And, above all, how many know the realities and intricacies of the communication net in small groups; the pathogenic nature of double message communication in a family; or the inductive power of their own expectation in a casual conversation with their vis … vis, let alone in a therapeutic interview with their patients? How many are reinforced into a passive, frightened silence as a means of communication, leaning on an outdated model of nonparticipant neutrality? The problems and approaches to be taught in this area are legion: they go to the heart of psychiatry. They should permeate the course as a whole; only a mere beginning can be made at the introductory stage.

Linked to the concept of communication is the concept of social field dependence. Though we are all individual, none of us are alone. Man learns from, and communicates with others; and the family may well turn out to be man's most important school. Early awareness of this must be enhanced, as must be an awareness of the methods now available for describing and quantifying these intricate relationships. The psychology, sociology and pathology of small group interaction can be presented in a way which enhances self-awareness in the student and this awareness can be expanded into a broader sociological context of mental illness, for which available statistics provide eloquent marginal notes.

3. A Scaffolding of Neurobiology

Little has been said so far of the role of the biological sciences with which I began, and with which, through personal experience, I am familiar. This is intentional; for I believe that they belong at the end of an introductory course to psychiatry, and not at the beginning. It is the practice sometime to follow the logic of ascendancy from subcellular morphology to brain and behavior and hence the study of populations (by way of systems theory) . This oversimplification is unfortunate, for it does not allow for the qualitative inflections in evolution which have made man peculiarly what he is. Despite the usual cautionary caveat, a habit of mind is inclined to develop in the student which looks not for broad analogies, but for identities in processes which only share some features in common. Psychiatry, including experimental psychiatry, is clinical and human, or it is nothing. The animal experiment is supporting evidence, an evoker, provoker, and training ground in experimental technique. A science of man, however, to be true to itself, must remain peculiarly a science of man.

As elsewhere, to teach is to choose; and in considering the neural substrate of behavior, and of mental life, choices should clearly reflect a preoccupation with what is sometimes known as higher mental activity. The subject matter should touch on, and, in places go deeply into, the properties and processes which relate to the organization of man's affective and innately regulated behavior; his ability to perceive, to attend, to learn; his ability to speak, to read and to write, to reason; to register and to recall; to sleep, to dream and to invent.

The term "neuropsychology" is a useful guideline for considerations of this kind; and there is a wealth of data concerning Hypothalamic/Brain Stem/ Limbic/Temporal and Parietal Lobe relationships which bears upon the morphology (including subcellular morphology), the chemistry, electrophysiology, pharmacology, and experimental psychology of these areas, to make such a brief course inviting. Fuller study can come later, or during a period of summer work.

Psychopharmacology forms an especially useful binding agent. It ranges from behavior to the neural substrate of behavior; from the swift transactions of thought to the physics, chemistry and mathematics of the cerebral machinery. Another area, related to the above, is the genetics of mental defect and disorder; a third, (incidental perhaps, but useful and timely nevertheless) is the simulation of intelligence by the modern computer. There is thus no shortage of subject matter; it is the choices which give one a hard time; and in my own case, I confess, these choices are still largely unresolved.

4. An Exploratory First Year Course in the Sciences of Human Development and Behavior at Johns Hopkins

The Department of Psychiatry at Johns Hopkins is fortunate in having at its disposal some 100 hours of teaching time during the student's first year at the School of Medicine. It is also fortunate in another respect; namely, the inordinate strength of the developmental point of view in the institution as a whole. This is represented by the new and very modern Children's Medical and Surgical Center (Director, Dr. Robert E. Cooke); the Child Growth and Development Center; the important interdepartmental Kennedy Foundation Program for Research in Mental Retardation (which involves Senior Fellowships in the Departments of Pediatrics, Anatomy, Obstetrics and Gynecology and Microbiology); the new John F. Kennedy Institute for the Habilitation of the Mentally, and Physically handicapped child for which ground is to be broken very shortly; and the Disorders of Communication Program in the Department of Otolaryngology (Director, Dr. John E. Bordley). In the Department of Psychiatry, the Developmental point of view is represented by the Division of Child Psychiatry (Director, Dr. Leon Eisenberg), the Division of Adolescent Psychiatry (Director, Dr. Ghislaine Godenne), the Neurocommunications Laboratory (Director, Dr. Richard Chase), the Reading Disability Program (Director, Dr. John Money) as well as by access to related areas in the Pavlovian Laboratory (Director, Dr. W. Horsley Gantt), the Operant Conditioning Laboratory (Directors, Drs. B. Weiss and V. Laties), and the Ethological laboratories of the Department of Pathobiology of the School of Public Health (Director, Dr. William Sladen). The climate at Johns Hopkins is thus thoroughly propitious for teaching the principles of the sciences of human behavior from a developmental point of view.

During the period of September 1964 to the present, an exploratory modification of the existing course has been initiated, centering on the introduction of developmental, and specifically human material at an early stage of education and drawing upon resources in the Department of Obstetrics and Gynecology and Pediatrics for key contributions to the course. The planning of the course is entirely the work of a small committee consisting of Dr. Stanley Imber, Associate Professor of Medical Psychology; Dr. Leon Eisenberg, Professor of Child Psychiatry; Dr. Jerome Frank, Professor of Psychiatry; Dr. Richard A. Chase, Assistant Professor of Psychiatry; and myself. We are still feeling our way, and hope to submit a fuller account of our experience at a later date.

The course is conducted on Saturday, mornings, and, in as far as it is possible with a large (91) student class is designed to encourage student participation. This takes several forms. Selected papers are made available in the library as required reading for each lecture, and are taken as read. The lecture, in as much as possible, is conducted as a lecture conversation, with active encouragement of student questions during the presentation. The lecture, also, is either interspersed, or preceded, or followed, by either a demonstration (of films or patients), or an experiment in which the students are encouraged to participate (e.g. role playing, use of rating scales on patients or themselves, experiments in the fields of hypnagogic imagery, perception, registration, recall, experiments with speech and language, classical and operant conditioning in animals and man). In addition to these classes (which take place at the unpopular time of Saturday mornings), students are given the opportunity to meet with instructors in three groups on an elective basis after the class. Attendance at both classes and groups has been encouragingly and consistently high.

The course starts with a brief review of the history of psychiatry from its empirical beginning to its present-day status as an emerging clinical science. This is followed by a consideration of the constraints of language in description and communication. (J. Elkes) Then the concepts of incidence and prevalence in relation to mental illness are examined. Three issues are raised specifically in this discussion: Does prevalence vary with race? Has prevalence increased over the past century in relationship to increasing stress? What ecological factors are related to the prevalence of one important disorder, namely schizophrenia? (L. Eisenberg).

This is followed by an introduction to the concept of mental illness as a decompensation in the social functioning of an individual. The interaction of somatic and symbolic functions are reviewed with the help of suitable clinical examples. A consideration of suggestibility, and the part played by social conventions in defining illness form part of this presentation. (J. Frank) There follow then three presentations on the phenomenology of a mental illness (J. Frank). These review the conceptual and methodological bases underlying the classification of mental illness; the rationale, and the use of rating scales; and the use of a subjective rating scale by students on themselves during the subsequent week. The presentations also demonstrate successively, the principal features of organic brain disorders, the psychoneuroses, the schizophrenias, and the character disorders (with suitable case presentations). Also included are some elementary concepts concerning the bivalent nature of the neurotic process (in terms of self-perpetuation and self-defeat); the role of emotional arousal in relation to cognitive functioning; the concept of the "double bind" and its relation to the vicious circle of withdrawal into protective isolation; the concept of altered (or indiscriminate) arousal in the sociopathic personality; and possible physiological correlates thereof. This is followed by an exercise in role playing on the part of four students (where a "patient" and patient relative are interviewed by two "doctors" in front of four quartiles of the class. The realism and involvement in this exercise impresses one with the value of this method of experiential teaching.

It may be asked at this point why, at a time when the student is engaged in basic science studies (arid before he is introduced to the elements of psychopathology and human development), he should be given these vignettes of clinical phenomena, and of the areas to which they are related. It is the considered opinion of our committee that the students' grasp of the areas which follow is greatly enhanced by this early exposure. Many of the terms he is bound to hear later, come to life in these demonstrations. Also, at this stage he is unencumbered by theory and verbiage. He can observe, explore and describe at first hand; and most important, also, begin to look at himself as an active agent rather than a passive recipient. It is refreshing for teachers to observe the keenness of ear and eye of students, and to share the questioning "show me" attitudes which they maintain when discussion gets too abstruse. Their antennae are sensitive to quite subtle transactional cues. We regard these sessions not only as powerful reinforces of interest, but of capacity. Theory should follow phenomena and not precede them.

The tragedy of much of psychiatry is that the speculative `why has taken precedence over the "what", the "what, with" and the "how".

There follows, after this introduction to the broad phenomena of mental illness, a series of seven presentations on human development – four which view it in general terms (L. Eisenberg) and three which approach it from the specifically psychoanalytic point of view (A. McClary). The former series includes a general review of the theory of evolution and a consideration of the crucial steps in Hominid progression – bipedal locomotion, use of hands development of speech, and corresponding cranial development and the adaptive nature of positive social relationships. There is a discussion of response patterns of infancy, and their relationship to the development of distance receptors; of nursing habits, and the effects of interruption or change in these; of learning patterns in infants; of the genesis of intelligence as viewed particularly by Piaget; and the successive stages of personality development through adolescence as defined by Erikson. This is followed by a consideration of the psychoanalytic model along classical lines, and a discussion of mechanisms of defense (repression, reaction-formation, sublimation and somatization and cognate categories). At this point, too, there is a thorough discussion of the psychology of the female role (i.e., the biology of femaleness vis- -vis the imposed role of femininity) by the Director of the Department of Gynecology and Obstetrics (Dr. Allan C. Barnes). This is followed by a discussion of human sexuality and issues concerning sexual intercourse in man. The attentive seriousness and silence with which these matters are received by our students, and the thoughtful comments afterwards suggest that such teaching is entirely in place. This is followed by two discussions of various aspects of the process of aging (J. Birren).

There then follow two presentations on learning and memory (S. Imber) and two specifically on conditioning (J. Perez Cruet and V. Laties). These presentations build on material preceding them, and especially stress the difference between operant and respondent behavior. Part of the presentation deals with the clinical implications of learning theory; another part with experimental areas (such as differential reinforcement, extinction, chaining; multiple schedule reinforcement of fixed interval and fixed ratio type, etc.). The Pavlovian model deals with concepts of inhibition, excitation and induction, and the importance of the secondary signaling system in terms of semantic conditioning. Teaching films and live demonstrations on animal and human subjects serve to illustrate these points. This material also relates well to a presentation on the psychological theories of memory, with special reference to the selective nature of forgetting and the active, creative nature of the remembering process.

There then follow two sessions on the origin and nature of communication systems in lower species, as defined by ethological studies (with illustrative tape and film material), a discussion of the origins and building blocks of human speech, the implications of the term language, the sensorimotor control mechanisms subserving human communication, and the implication of modern techniques in the analysis of speech patterns and the synthesis of artificial speech (R. Chase). Here again practical demonstrations enhance the reality factor; and prepare students for some consideration of the processes of communication and miscommunication in small (and especially the family) group. This, in turn, is linked to role imposition, differentiation and role confusion in the family, and is also related to social learning, and mislearning in the family (R. Gordon).

By this time the students are well advanced in their courses in Anatomy, Physiology, and Physiological Chemistry and are ready for some material relating "Brain" to "Behavior." This is initiated by two presentations by the Director of the Department of Pediatrics (Dr. Robert E. Cooke) on the Biology of Mental Retardation and Handicap, and the lessons it holds for. the study of Human Development. It is followed by presentations on the general and regional metabolism of the brain in relation to a number of functional states; consideration of the regional chemical topology of the brain (including neuroendocrinology) in relation to instinctual and autonomic patterns of discharge; periodicity; sleep, wakefulness, arousal and focussed attention; some of the electrophysiological concomitants of these states and of processes of perception and conditioning; the role of inhibition as a structuring force in the nervous system; and some speculation on the molecular substrate of the storage of information by nervous tissue (S. S. Kety and J. Elkes). Since students are avid readers in these areas, it is well to keep the material reasonably up to date.

5. Needed: A "Praktikum" and Manual in Human Development and the Behavioral Sciences for Medical Students.

There are thus strong indications of the feasibility and usefulness of the developmental approach to the behavioral sciences in enhancing students" interests, specifically in human biology. However encouraging these indications may be, it is felt that our experiment so far falls far short of what could be attained and, indeed of what is desirable.

The principal weakness of the present course is its dependence on teaching to large groups. Although many of the lectures have developed into lecture-conversations, and although some of the demonstrations and exercises have required student participation, and problem-solving by students, there is need for a systematic organization of the material into a series of small group exercises (of the "personal research" or "problem-solving" kind) which would reinforce the presentation, demonstration, or assigned reading of a particular topic. It will have been noted from the material listed above that such exercises could take place in the laboratories and wards of several departments, though the Department of Psychiatry should be responsible for the major share of the facilities. The topics should be modified according to experience. The course should be self-renewing, and always up-to-date, and make fullest use of the resources within the University as a whole. A small instance may serve to illustrate this point. It is, for example, intended next year to introduce some practical exercises in game theory as applied to small group interaction; and, also, to arrange for exercises on artificial intelligence in conjunction with the Applied Physics Laboratory of Johns Hopkins. There are many other opportunities, as yet unexplored.

It is suggested that a course such as proposed above cannot evolve without the full-time commitment of at least one, and, if possible, two Senior persons. Such a commitment would involve the detailed planning of each item in the course, not only in terms of didactic content, but also in the invention of appropriate exercises (i.e., research problems in miniature) in a varied range of settings, and the coordination of these into a coherent, sequential, and meaningful whole. As has been mentioned, the exercises will involve several Departments. They may involve observations on the premature and new born well-baby wards and clinics, in nurseries and play rooms, in learning and language laboratories, in the schoolroom, in human perception, human psychophysiological (telemetering) laboratories, in sociological and small group laboratories, in an animal Pavlovian laboratory, in an operant conditioning laboratory, in a physiological, neuroendocrinological or neurochemical laboratory, or a computer facility. Clearly, a course such as this will make ever-changing demands. Yet, it is entirely feasible that within a few years it could lead to a *Manual in the Behavioral Sciences* for medical students which could embody cumulative experience of many students (and many students' notebooks) in a clearly repeatable "Praktikum", which could be made available as a text to others. All our experience suggest that such a practical guide, especially attuned to the changing demands of medical education, is urgently needed.

Thus, by way, of closing, we can only say again that we are encouraged by this small beginning. As expected, the student is proving an excellent teacher.

PAPER 20

MEDICINE AND THE BEHAVIORAL SCIENCES: THE JOHNS HOPKINS M.D.–PH.D. PROGRAM*

R.R. Rubin, J. Elkes, R.W. Maris, and P.E. Dietz

Department of Psychiatry and Behavioral Sciences
The Johns Hopkins University School of Medicine

There is a growing awareness of the potential contribution of the behavioral sciences to medical education research and practice (1–3). Few medical institutions however have demonstrated a long-term commitment to expended interdisciplinary activity through the provision of funds or the formation of durable administrative units. In American medicine as a whole, the current position of the behavioral sciences is that of a promising, but tentative liaison.

The future of the behavioral sciences in medicine will depend largely on the extent to which the methods and findings of these sciences can be integrated into clinical practice. Medicine's evolution has depended upon developments in appropriate "basic" sciences – anatomy, pathology, microbiology, biochemistry, pharmacology and genetics. These, in turn, increasingly depend upon more fundamental developments in molecular biology and in biophysics. A medical student is required to become familiar with both the established "basic medical" sciences and the natural sciences to which they relate. Yet the need for an equally firm foundation for the behavioral aspects of medical practice hasn't been met.

Behavioral factors are now known to contribute to all aspects of health and disease, not just to those illnesses traditionally within the domain of psychiatry, neurology and psychosomatic medicine. Just as all physicians need not be biochemists, all need not be behavioral scientists. Ideally, however practitioners would know something of the established findings in the behavioral sciences, just as they know something of established findings in biochemistry. Recent developments in neurobiology and behavioral pharmacology have indeed found a place in medical education and practice, but developments in other psychological sciences and in the social sciences in general are being assimilated so slowly as to suggest a malabsorption syndrome.

Growing attention to systems of health care delivery has increased the demand for interaction between medicine and the behavioral sciences in administrative and research settings. Such interaction occurring largely outside medical schools goes beyond joint efforts to deal with common and costly health problems such as alcoholism, drug abuse, violence, suicide and problems of the aged. Physicians and behavioral scientists are frequently partners in eval-

* Founded in 1971 by Dr. Elkes, Chairman of the Executive Committee, and Dr. Maris, Program Director, with the support of NIGMS grant 1 T01 GM02191, and of funds from the Grant Foundation, Inc., of New York City.
Reprinted with the kind permission of The Johns Hopkins University Press from The Johns Hopkins Medical Journal 136: 268-270, 1975

uating the effectiveness of health services as functioning organizations. They are also engaged in joint efforts to understand the role of cultural and class differences in patient cooperation and compliance and the implications of these differences for the efficacy of clinical practice.

While the biological sciences are strongly represented in medical institutions, the behavioral sciences still enjoy only "guest" or at best "consular" status. Their parent departments (Psychology, Sociology, Anthropology, Linguistics) are often remote from centers of medical education. Consequently, medical students' exposure to the basic behavioral sciences is often quite limited, though there is great diversity among schools (1, 2).

The growing appreciation of the relevance of the behavioral sciences to medicine hasn't yet resulted in the development of stable and open channels for cooperative work. Research workers who are not physicians are limited in their access to medical settings, whereas physicians are generally not prepared to carry out research requiring training in the behavioral sciences. These difficulties suggest the possibility that behavioral-medical research and teaching could be facilitated by providing selected individuals with doctoral training in the both fields.

THE HOPKINS M.D.–PH.D. PROGRAM IN THE BEHAVIORAL SCIENCES

In 1971, a small group of physicians and behavioral scientists of The John Hopkins University founded the M.D.–Ph.D. Program in the Behavioral Sciences, one of the first of its kind in the nation. The National Institute of General Medical Sciences provided funds for support of the program's fellows and for general administration. The Grant Foundation, Inc., provided funds for support of the program's core staff.

The school of Medicine's Department of Psychiatry and Behavioral Sciences and the Faculty of Arts and Sciences" Departments of Social Relations and of Psychology are the principal partners in the program. Faculty members of the School of Hygiene and Public Health's Departments of Behavioral Sciences, Medical Care and Hospitals and Pathobiology are also participants. From its inception, the Program's principal aim has been to provide concurrent, rigorous and integrated training in the medical and behavioral sciences, so as to promote truly interdisciplinary teaching and research within medical institutions.

Each year, two or three of the applicants who have been admitted to both the School of Medicine and the doctoral program in Psychology or Social Relations are selected by the M.D.–Ph.D. Program staff as M.D.–Ph.D. fellows. Fellows are provided with funds to cover tuition expenses and a stipend for up to four years of study toward the Ph. D. No funds are provided for training in the school of Medicine.

All fellows begin the program with the regular two pre-clinical years in the School of Medicine. The basic medical clerkships (surgery, medicine, pediatrics, obstetrics-gynecology and psychiatry) complete the M.D. Requirements in the joint degree program. The clerkships are undertaken either in the third year of study or after a year or two of study in the selected behavioral science department (Social Relations or Psychology).

One fellow has completed the program and twelve others are currently in residence, of these thirteen, seven have chosen to work toward the Ph.D. in Social Relations. Basic Ph.D. requirements are the same for joint degree candidates as for regular Ph.D. students, although M.D.–Ph.D. fellows have the additional opportunity of working with faculty in the School of Medicine to satisfy some of their degree requirements. Each fellow's dissertation research is supervised by a committee including faculty from both of School of Medicine and the Faculty of Arts and Sciences.

The core staff of the M.D.–Ph.D. Program consists of several behavioral scientists and a physician, who monitor the progress of fellows and provide supervision in the creation of *ad hoc* seminars, reading programs and research opportunities. The program's viability has always depended partly upon the full cooperation of Ph.D. – granting departments in the training of fellows of undeniable skills and ability but questionable commitment to the discipline *per se* as opposed to its medical applications. The full acceptance of core staff psychologists and sociologists in their parent disciplines is essential to insure that the program has a "friend in court" in the departmental councils, and to assure departmental faculty of adequate supervision for the program's unorthodox students. The acceptability of staff members in their parent disciplines has been assured by affording the participating departments a major role in hiring or designating core staff. All core staff have joint appointments in the School of Medicine and the Faculty of Arts and Sciences.

In June 1974 the first fellow to complete the joint degree program received his Ph.D. in Psychology.[*] This event confirmed the expectation that such training could be completed in six years, reducing by more than two years the combined average length of study toward the M.D. and Ph.D. degrees at Johns Hopkins. Six other fellows (three in the Department of Social Relations end three in the Department of Psychology) are now engaged in dissertation research and writing as a last step toward completion of the joint degree program. Research areas and residency training commitments of the seven advanced fellows are shown in table I. All seven fellows are utilising the opportunities provided by concurrent medical – behavioral training to conduct interdisciplinary research early in their careers.

The impact of the program upon the School of Medicine includes the development of courses in Behavioral Sociology, Behavioral Pharmacology and Response Process and the Analysis of Behaviour. Another course, Applications of Sociology to Clinical Medicine has been offered annually for three years as an elective track within the first-year Psychiatry course. In this seminar cases are presented by experienced clinicians and some possible contributions of sociological knowledge to case management are introduced by M.D.–Ph.D. fellows in Social Relations.

DISCUSSION

In 1973–1974 more than three-fourths of all American medical schools offered M.D.–Ph.D. programs (4). The vast majority involved Ph.D. training in one or more of the basic medical sciences – anatomy, biochemistry, microbiology, pathology or pharmacology. A smaller number involved Ph.D. work in such areas as biomedical engineering, biophysics, genetics and molecular biology. M.D.–Ph.D. programs are offered because individuals with joint degree training make special contributions to medical research, teaching and practice. In recent years, the potential contributions of the behavioral sciences to medicine have become more apparent and interdisciplinary research has increased. One indication of current thinking about the relevance of the behavioral sciences in medical education is the fact in 1973, for the first time, a Behavioral Sciences subscore was reported for Part 1 of the National Board Ex-

---

[*] The first fellows to enter the program had already completed two or three years of medical school.

aminations, along with those for Anatomy Board Examinations, and other basic medical sciences.

TABLE 1. Advanced M.D.–Ph.D. Fellows Ph.D. Department,
Research Area and Residency Training Commitments

Ph.D. Department	Research Area	Residency Training Commitments
Psychology	Biofeedback training to alter cardiovascular function	Internal Medicine
Psychology	Cognitive psychological and psycholinguistic aspects of aphasia	Neurology
Psychology	Long-term behavioral effects of drug tolerance and withdrawal	Psychiatry
Psychology	Testing procedures for cognitive functioning in human infants younger than six months	Psychiatry
Social relations	Social organization of psychiatric emergency care	Psychiatry
Social relations	Vocational experiences of physician's assistant	Surgery
Social relations	Relationship between psychiatrists' attributes and their choices among alternative therapeutic modalities	Psychiatry

There are now six schools of medicine that address the need for training in medicine and the behavioral sciences by offering M.D.–Ph.D. programs. These schools are Johns Hopkins, Harvard, Columbia, Indiana University, the University of Oklahoma, and the University of Missouri. The Hopkins program is unique in that it offers concurrent rather than consecutive training in the two disciplines. Insofar as concurrent training encourages interdisciplinary research in the formative stages of career development, it can be expected to increase the likelihood of continuing contributions at the interface between medicine and the behavioral sciences.

ACKNOWLEDGEMENTS
The authors wish to express their appreciation to the program's core staff, Drs. Karl L. Alexander, Daryl B. Matthews and David S. Olton for their helpful editorial assistance.

REFERENCES

1. Cope O.: Man, Mind and Medicine: The Doctor's Education. The Swampscott Study on Behavioral Science in Medicine, Philadelphia, Lippincott, 1968.
2. Webster TG: The behavioral sciences in medical education and practice. In Psychosocial Aspects of Medical Training. Edited by RH Coombs, CE Vincent. Springfield, Ill., Charles C. Thomas, 1971, pp. 285-348
3. Olmsted RW, Kennedy DA: Behavioral Science and Medical Education. A report on Four Conferences, National Institute of Child Health and Human Development. US Department of Health, Education and Welfare. DHEW Publication No. NIH 72-41
4. Association of American Medical Colleges. 1973. 1974. AAMC Curriculum Directory. Washington, D.C. Association of American Medical Colleges, 1973

PAPER 20

HEALTH AWARENESS AND THE MEDICAL STUDENT: A PRELIMINARY EXPERIMENT[*]

Leah J. Dickstein and J. Elkes

*Department of Psychiatry and Behavioral Sciences,
University of Louisville*

Summary

"Humanizing medical education" has remained a recurrent theme over the past fifty years in discussions concerning the training of physicians. The persistence of the theme attests to a stubborn paradox in medical education. As the biomedical sciences continue to evolve in a changing climate of new and powerful economic forces and a changing public awareness and concern, it seems appropriate to attend more closely to the physical and emotional health of the health-provider-to-be. Studies on the impaired physician and one important long-term longitudinal study of doctors suggest that the medical student is a person at risk; some of these risks are avoidable. Medical schools to date have not paid adequate pro-active (as against remedial) attention to student well-being. Humanism implies an awareness of self and others; other-care is best begun with self-care. Such skills, and relevant information, are best sampled early in one's career. Only steady practice can reinforce them.

A Health Awareness Workshop for incoming medical students, which grew out of the authors' respective experiences at Johns Hopkins and Louisville, is described. Its aim is to enhance self-awareness and to equip students with coping skills likely to maintain and improve their personal health and well-being while in medical school, and beyond. The workshop lasts four days. It is offered during the week *before* actual enrollment, on a purely *voluntary* basis. Participation over the last three years has been encouragingly high.

The workshop uses both a didactic and experiential mode, combining large presentations with small-group exercises. These events are led by previously trained sophomore students ("Health Tutors") and volunteer faculty. Topics covered include mode of life as a factor in illness and disability; the psychobiology of human adaptation, stress, and the stress response; the physiology of nutrition, exercise, and relaxation; the psychology of time management and study skills; listening, and the give-and-take of relationships; substance abuse and the impaired physician; and introductions to the ethics of medical practice and to the place of belief in healing. There is an attempt to maintain a balance between presentations of scientific evidence (including some very recent data) and a participatory, experiential "fun" approach to learning. A social network between student and student, and between student and faculty,

---

[*] Some material in this article is adapted with permission from Dickstein and Elkes, "A Health Awareness Workshop: Enhancing Coping Skills in Medical Students", which appeared in "Heal Thyself: The Health of Health Care Professionals". The book was edited by C.D. Scott and J. Hawk and published by Brunner/Mazel, Inc., 1986. Reprinted with the kind permission of the Fetzer Institute from Advances (Institute for Advancement of Health) 4: 12-23, 1987.

forms as a result of this interaction. This network has proven a useful support system in subsequent years.

It is suggested that such a workshop provides an unusual opportunity for long-term outcome research. The need for Laboratories (or Centers) of Student Health in medical schools is argued. Such laboratories, or centers, appropriately planned, equipped, and staffed could provide a growing data base on student health during medical training, and could monitor the effects of stressors at successive career transition points (for example, junior to senior, senior to internship, internship to residency, and residency to practice); and over time, could accumulate evidence as to whether the acquisition of a "pharmacopoeia of skills" affects attitudes and style of medical practice.

Students and physicians could provide a powerful source of long-term health data. As the design of curricula for the physician of the twenty-first century proceeds, student health should not be relegated to an asterisk of afterthought. Joy, enthusiasm, curiosity, and a sense of wonder are the most precious attributes of our students. In medical schools, they do not come free.

HUMANISM AND MEDICAL EDUCATION: A STUBBORN PARADOX

Some twenty years ago the Swampscott Conference examined "The Role of the Behavioral Sciences in Medicine" (1). Writing in his Chairman's summary, Oliver Cope, great surgeon and educator, put it this way:

> In medical schools understanding people should be a concerted project not left to chance. We should start with our own life rather than our patients' ... Personal experience is the laboratory of the Art of Medicine.... It must be a laboratory in which we can make observations, gather data, look for things which are comparable and ... for concepts of theory we can use in practice. An element of research will always be involved in the laboratory of the Art [of Medicine]... There is always more before us than we can see. (1)

The Swampscott meeting of leading educators, comprehensive in scope and temperate in expectations, addressed – need one say it? – the perennial problem of "humanizing" medical education. It argued for the recognition of the behavioral sciences, not only in psychiatry but in medicine as a whole, making them an integral part of human biology. It also stressed the value of subjective observation and self-awareness in the physician, alongside clinical skills and a dependence on laboratory data.

Rereading the proceedings of this meeting projects one's mind both backward and forward. The plea for "humanism" in medicine is as old as the Hippocratic Oath. It is reiterated wherever physicians are trained. In our century, Abraham Flexner, advocate of a scientific base for medical education and medical practice, and architect of the full-time system in medical schools, was quite outspoken on this point:

> For our purposes, science may safely be treated as a developing conception.... . At one point, practice lags behind theory, at another, theory has not yet overtaken practice. There is no pretense that science has as yet subdued either practice of education.
> There is a widespread impression that the scientific quality of medical education and medical practice is in some fashion dependent upon the part played by the laboratory. This is not the case ... Not only is the part played by the active senses the essential criterion of science;

one may go further – the vast and complicated paraphernalia of science are merely means of extending their scope. (2)

Creating a distance between "laboratory" and "human" approaches, between patient and physician, was not Flexner's intention. We need not here examine the forces that have led to a technologically advanced, test-dependent, and overspecialized medicine, and have interposed this technology between patient and physician. The gain has been worthwhile: a deepening understanding of pathology, and the emergence of rational therapeutics. The price has been – often, but not always – an impersonal mode of teaching, and of practice. All this has been said – and said very well – many times. We are, after all, "the youngest science." (3) It is merely reiterated to draw attention to a paradox that has simply not gone away.

We could point to other illustrations. In its 1932 report, the Association of American Medical Colleges' Commission on Medical Education recognized that in the educational process

the crucial element is the individual student, upon whose character, attitude, preparation, ability, and industry so largely depend the results of medical training. The aim [of medical education] is to develop minds capable of approaching evidence ... as well as methods of study which will prepare the student to continue his own education through his professional life. *The student and the teacher, not the curriculum, are crucial elements in the educational process.*

To achieve this the report advocates:

a distinct shift... toward placing greater responsibility on the student for his own training... The new methods are illustrated by the use of small teaching sections; personal contact between students and instructors; provision for reasonable free time for reading, individual work, and leisure... and opportunities of those who desire and are competent, to do independent work. (4)

A full fifty years later, the theme recurs. In its report, the Panel on The General Professional Education of The Physician and College Preparation for Medicine remarks that "Faculty pay little heed to personal growth and development or the emotional stresses students experience." The report recommends that medical faculties provide support and guidance to enhance the personal development of each medical student, and for counseling students in difficulties. This emphasis on the student's physical, mental, and social well-being seems to us a central feature of the report, which states:

The most compelling consequence of these deliberations will be restoration of *a sense of joy and enthusiasm of our medical student for the excitement, wonder, and future of the biomedical sciences and human medicine.* (5)

Sound ideas have a Darwinian persistence; they continue to surface until attended to. At times, they manifest themselves by way of a crisis born out of neglect. They also respond to the growth-enhancing forces inherent in changing times. The crises is by now well documented. The opportunity is equally apparent. The winds of change may well carry medicine into a rediscovery of the obvious and latent-familiar.

Increasingly, behavior is emerging as a major pathogen in our society (6). Health education, changes in attitudes, and day-to-day life habits (smoking, diet, exercise, self-regulation, and self-management of life stresses) are being taken seriously as factors in the maintenance of personal health. Family support programs and support in the workplace through Employee Assistance Programs are gaining their place as legitimate means of health maintenance.

Of these developments, however, the average medical student knows little. Once again, one cannot help being struck by a curious lag and paradox. For while corporate industry takes employee health seriously enough to make sizable capital investments to maintain health, well-being and morale (7, 8), the institutions training the health provider – schools of medicine – so far have left much of it to chance. Remedial counseling is available; of a preventive approach, health awareness, and personal health care we hear little. In medical schools, the behavioral sciences, despite their advances, still remain a poor relation to "proven" laboratory approaches.

A decade ago George Engel eloquently formulated a biopsychosocial model of disease (9), a model that has borne fruit in the transitional clerkship training at the University of Rochester and elsewhere. For two decades David Hamburg has lucidly argued for a major role for the behavioral sciences in the teaching and practice of medicine, and has drawn attention to the rich opportunities for long-term research in this area (10). The yield of such research is amply documented in the psychosomatic literature and has recently been comprehensively and critically reviewed by Weiner (11).

We would argue that psychobiology and the behavioral sciences are no longer "soft" areas of research; indeed they are "hardening" nicely. We would also argue that, while it may take time for the evidence to permeate the curriculum, such knowledge may be deeply relevant to the health and well-being of the individual student. Acceptance is enhanced by understanding and sound information. Such information is growing apace. The modern neurosciences are providing an increasingly precise understanding of mind/body relationships – the biochemical transcription of events outside the body to events within. Soma is being related to symbol in a measurable way – the society within the skin to the society without. A new body of knowledge concerned with states of well-being is slowly shaping, and may prove complementary to the traditions of medicine as we know it. This complementarity will grow, as the scientific base deepens. Neurochemistry, neuroendocrinology, neuropsychoimmunology; developmental, cognitive and social psychology; learning theory; the increasing understanding of the physiology of eating, exercise, sexuality, sleep and relaxation, and the psychology of work satisfaction, social play, and social support are steadily laying the foundation for what might be called a "psychobiology of positive states of being." Interestingly enough, the methods of investigation are the very methods that have given us a science of medicine. Applied to health, they may well enlarge the terrain of medicine itself.

Progress is usually signalled by institutional pain. We have drawn attention to some (perennial) sources of dis-ease and dissatisfaction in medical education and medical practice. We now add another – a focus of our attention in what follows – namely the problem of the impaired physician, and the factors that may contribute to it in schools of medicine. This serious problem, as we shall see, is another painful reminder of the difficulties besetting present-day medical education still at odds with humanism.

THE IMPAIRED PHYSICIAN:
POSSIBLE FACTORS OPERATING IN MEDICAL SCHOOL

A mounting literature attests to the reality of the impaired physician (12). The incidence and prevalence of depression, alcohol and substance abuse, marital difficulties, professional burnout, and attempted and completed suicide among physicians are by now well documented. In a pathbreaking prospective study, Caroline B. Thomas followed the careers of

1337 Johns Hopkins' medical students in the classes from 1946 to 1964 (13). This group became the core of the "Hopkins Precursors Study", which clearly demonstrated that medical students and physicians are at considerable risk; that hypertension, coronary artery occlusion, depression (including suicide), marital discord, substance abuse, and cancer represent what Thomas called "the dark side" of medicine (14). Thomas and her colleagues developed possible predictors of illness or of premature death. This work is now fully documented in over a hundred papers, and represents a courageous attempt – far ahead of its time – to understand the genesis of the so-called impaired physician.

Other authors have borne out these broad conclusions, repeatedly finding that the impairment began at least in medical school. Vaillant, Sobowale, and McArthur (15) studied physicians' earlier lives and found that vulnerability to impairment indeed antedates entry into medical school. Breiner (16) surveyed psychiatrists who had worked with impaired physicians and found that early warning signs commonly appear during medical schools. Gardner and Hall (17) reported that protracted stress syndromes, usually self-imposed, are seen in medical students. Linn and Zeppa (18), in a study examining stress in junior medical students, conclude that "since stress predictably will increase in residency and in the practice years, students should be exposed to stress management techniques to help prevent the known high consequences of stress such as substance abuse and suicide among practicing physicians." In 1978, the American Medical Association recommended two steps for long-term prevention of impaired physicians: to "humanize medical education" and to "teach coping skills" (19).

In a sensitive essay Bogdonoff comments on the nagging sense of dissatisfaction inherent in current medical education. Though "most of these very same students and faculty members believe that medical education in the United States ranks with the finest in the world," they "hold persistent doubt that perhaps all is not quite right with the process," that "it is a singular paradox that an educational realm which recruits its students from the scholastic top ten percent of college graduates and that promises a lifelong career of economic surety, societal prestige, and emotional gratification should be in any way significantly disquieted." Trying to define this sense of malaise Bogdonoff focuses on the *lack of collegiality* among students and faculty, and a lack of awareness of common purpose and mutual interest in each other's work. Students are too busy to be aware of each other, and competition creates distance. Bogdonoff does not recommend student faculty dialogues, "sensitivity seminars," or adding students to curriculum and administrative committees; but instead argues cogently for a continued sense of awareness of self and others; for continuity of contact with faculty and peers rather than the "staccato encounter of lectures, classes, shifting clerkships and the like." Yes, as he states, the opposite is still sadly true: the medical students is mired down in an overwhelming atmosphere of fierce competitiveness, unseemly haste, fragmentation, overscheduling, rote learning, overwork, examination pressure, insensitivity, awareness, and the inappropriate use of denial. In 1984 Murphy, Nadelson, and Notman, analyzing the perception of stress among first-year medical students, noted that medical school stresses as well as social stresses related to medical schools accounted for about two-thirds of the stresses mentioned by students.

Two examples of the types of programs suggested by Bogdonoff's comments are the educational formats developed at McMaster University in Canada and at Ben Gurion University in Beersheva, Israel, which remain eloquent examples of a successful blending of small group teaching and self-directed learning with exposure to clinical role models early in a student's career. A number of programs deal more directly with the experiences of stress by supporting students through their careers in medical school. Some have chosen high-risk students for attention. Others have experimented with random samples.

Flach, Smith, and Smith constructed a mentor program aimed to help students move from child–adult to peer–adult relationships; Hilberman et al., Cadden, Flach, and Blakeslee, and Rosenberg favor small discussion groups. Rosenberg reported "observable lessening of tension and growth of mutual respect between students and faculty." Goldstein suggested that medical schools should rate personal growth equally with knowledge of medicine, and Lief argues that developing attitudes is as important as acquiring information and skills. In 1952, Dingle, Bond, Bidder, Badgers, Ham, Hoerr, and Patterson at Western Reserve University began a significant evaluation of medical education at their institution. Their study focused on developing the student attitudes considered necessary for the physician.

At Eastern Virginia Medical School, Fletcher, Self, and Manning developed the Human Dimensions Program, based upon a prototype at the Center for Studies of the Person in LaJolla, California. Freshmen and faculty were invited to share weekend retreats as well as to meet in self-selected small groups for three months. The objective was to "help individuals develop their own sense of humanism… through learning to recognize, maintain, and develop personal characteristics which nurture compassionate and humanistic relationships with patients and colleagues."

We would draw particular attention to two recent programs which give us cause for much hope. On is the program developed at Mount Sinay by Gorlin and Zucker, the purpose of which, stated simply, is to help the medical student and resident understand how his or her feelings affect the treatment of patients. Once developed, "this understanding becomes a professional skill that encompasses all aspects of medicine." The program comprises four elements. The first is to expose students and residents to concepts of humanistic medicine in *every year of their training* with increasing emphasis during their clinical experience. The second is to design the program so that humanistic elements are intrinsic to the educational experience, and not separate exercises isolated from the main theme. The third is to provide sophisticated and sensitive role models for medical students and house staff. The fourth is to integrate the skilled faculty liaison psychiatrists who are comfortable with, and interested in, the complexities of biomedical care. These aims are achieved through a carefully guided program – partly didactic, but largely experiential – extending through undergraduate and graduate education. In this program allowance is made for the stresses operating in the young physician in training, and there is emphasis on accepting one's feelings in the face of "unacceptable pressures."

The second program includes studies reported in some detail in a recent outstanding volume <MI>Medicine as a Human Experience, by Reiser and Rosen. This book may be viewed as an eloquent, long letter to students anywhere, preparing to be physicians in the twenty-first century. It is both factual and personal, objective and existential. Using rich examples of actual and hypothetical cases, the authors draw upon their own teaching experience in pointing to the power of an integrated biopsychosocial model for teaching medicine, one that is both scientific and humane. As Norman cousins, who himself has eloquently pointed to the needs of the profession in this area, put it in the preface: "Integration is not a murky principle but expresses a need to affirm the importance of human spirit, dignity, fullness, and hope in the practice of our craft." Our own Student Hour program at the University of Louisville, which brings together faculty and students, has been a response in the same direction. In our experience, sharing concerns, "hassles," professional ambiguities, and worries, and getting to know other students and faculty can affect medical students' attitudes, improve performance, and reduce the sense of isolation and the risk of failing or dropping out.

All the above programs involve the student who is in medical school. In the program outlined below, the Health Awareness Workshop, our aim has been to impart to the student a sense of self awareness and some coping skills (based on solid information) *before* actual enrollment, and to make the offering *voluntary* rather than required. The program combines large presentations with small group discussions; it makes use of sophomore "health tutors" as group leaders and resource persons; it emphasizes positive student–student and student–faculty interaction at an early, sensitive stage in a student's career; it mixes didactic teaching with experiential exercises; it also shows students creative aspects of physicians" lives (art, music, literature) of which they may not be necessarily aware. However, the first and last aim of the Health Awareness Workshop is to be *useful* to students; and to emphasize effective functioning, coping, and competence, rather than pathology and disease.

As we already indicated, we feel that in this respect medical education may be still following rather than leading. Self-care and responsibility for personal health are clearly more than a fad. The existence of a huge self-care industry (of varying and questionable quality) reflects an increasing awareness on the part of the public that mode of life and behavior may be related to both disease and well-being. Medical schools cannot let the concept of well-being go by default: And there is no better place to begin than with the physician in training.

THE UNIVERSITY OF LOUISVILLE HEALTH AWARENESS WORKSHOP

Genesis of the Program

While one of us (J.E.) was at Johns Hopkins, he introduced in 1964, with several colleagues, a Behavioral Sciences course during the first year of medical school. The course involved the Departments of Psychiatry and Behavioral Sciences, Medicine, Pediatrics, and Obstetrics and Gynecology in joint presentations of the behavioral sciences as they related to medicine as a whole. A core message of the course was an opportunity for the student to meet him/herself. As J.E. put it at the time:

The Student Meets Him/Herself
As he meets psychiatry, the student is prepared for yet another specialty. In this he is wrong. Psychiatry cannot compartmentalize: it deals in patterns and not pieces, in people and not organ systems. In making contact with the subject the student brings to it his most important piece of portable equipment, namely himself. In his skull he carries vast and fascinating laboratory, of which he may be only dimly aware.

Yet somehow he must be made aware, before he moves too far into his clinical training, that behavior and subjective experience are not only phenomena but also instruments of high inferential value; that skill in observation of behavior, including his own behavior, though more native to some than to others, can be both taught and learned; that such learning requires conceptual tools of its own; that it can never be didactic and always has to be experiential; and that relative absence of hardware in clinical psychiatry and human psychology in no way reflect in its ability to measure, conceptualize, and predict.

In short, the student must learn to respect the use of himself as much as of his slide rule and statistical tables. In this self-acceptance and growing self-knowledge there can be a source of much power. If acquired early, it will serve him well with his patients and equally well should he choose a life in the laboratory rather than a life in the clinic.

This course, one of the first of its kind offered in a medical school, was built around four elements: human development, human learning, human communication, and the operation of the social field. It also comprised key concepts in psychobiology, and included didactic as well as experiential exercises. A workbook accompanied the course. It continues to this day, with a number of modifications and improvements.

Also while at Johns Hopkins, J.E. discussed with Dr. Caroline B. Thomas the desirability of taking her study one step further and moving out from a purely observational/epidemiological to an active, *interventive* approach. The opportunity arose when he came to Louisville, upon retirement from Johns Hopkins. At Louisville, he met Dr. Leah Dickstein who, in her capacity as Medical Director of the Mental Health Section of the Student Health Service (where she had treated some 300 impaired medical students) and, subsequently, as Associate Dean for Student Affairs, had introduced the "Student Hour" a support program for freshmen. The staff consisted of sophomores and faculty, the latter, chosen by the students for their above-average interest in the students" welfare. The sophomore staff was trained each spring in a series of meetings for the fall freshmen program.

Thus, the template for a Health Awareness Workshop already existed in Louisville. Not only was there a ready acceptance of the central idea, but there was a group of colleagues dedicated to conveying to freshmen a very practical message, namely, that both faculty and students *cared* about students' well-being. It remained to devise an approach that was nonintrusive to an already overloaded curriculum; non-threatening; and one that would mobilize student initiative, and make the effort itself – on both sides – its own reward. This is why we opted for a *voluntary* approach *before* students entered medical school. Out of the many preparatory discussions and training sessions there grew a program for a Health Awareness Workshop which was begun in 1981 and which has been offered yearly to incoming students since.

Structure of the Program

The program lasts four days and is offered to students in the week immediately preceding formal enrollment. It is open to the students, their spouses, and significant others (men or women living with but not married to an incoming student). Since the second workshop, a few students' mothers have attended every year. In 1984 a special program was initiated for students' children.

The offering is made by way of a letter of invitation from the Dean's office, sent during the spring semester to all students accepted to medical school during the year.

During the year preceding the workshop, sophomore students are instructed in skills pertaining to their future role as "health tutors," group leaders, and resource persons to 16-member freshmen groups designated as "unit labs." Faculty members, usually selected by the sophomore students, play a similar role. These small group "unit labs" provide an important counterpoint and "practicum" to the larger presentations that are given in the Freshman Lecture Hall of the School of Medicine.

One of the most heartening and surprising aspects of the workshops has been the degree of voluntary participation by freshmen. Despite the inconveniences of an early start (one week ahead of formal enrollment, the extra cost of lodgings, and so forth), the attendance has been notable: in 1981, 95 students out of a class of 138 (60 percent) and eight significant others; in 1982, 112 (90 percent) and 15 significant others; in 1983, 95 (68 percent) and 15 significant others; in 1984, 113 (93 percent) and 37 significant others; in 1985, 115 students (93 percent).

A special program was arranged for 10 children in 1984 and for 6 children in 1985. In 1986, 97 percent of the class and 16 significant others, including children, attended.

On the afternoon before the beginning of the workshop, a final planning session of student and faculty health tutors and workshop staff is held to coordinate the various activities. Registration takes place on the morning of the first day. At this time, students are given a variety of handouts, including a cookbook. (We describe this material more fully below.) The tutors wear a T-shirt stencilled with the emblem of the workshop. During the practicum, faculty wear these shirts as well. There are muffins and juice, and the group then adjourns to the auditorium for the introductory presentations.

These center on up-to-date evidence linking mode-of-life with illness and disability ("On Being Ill and Being Well: Awareness and Personal Responsibility," "The Psychobiology of Stress and the Stress Response"). There follow over the next few days, presentations on the physiology and role of exercise, the physiology of relaxation, on practical nutrition, effective coping in relationships, and on listening skills. Health checks are conducted during the each day of the workshop. The elements of efficient time management are presented, complemented by a presentation by sophomores on study skills. A Convention Bureau film introduces the out-of-town student to the city of Louisville, and an archivist presents the unique history of the medical school. Substance abuse is presented by way of the film, "Our Brothers' Keeper," followed by a panel discussion led by physicians from the State Medical Society's Committee on Impaired Physicians. There are presentations by senior colleagues on the importance of medical ethics and on the role of belief in healing. A special workshop is offered by a woman psychiatrist to significant others only, as an opportunity for them to voice concerns about living with and relating to theirs spouses as physicians. The children's program includes a tour of the medical center, a picnic at the center with their parents, and time to discuss a work-coloring book that helps the children envisage relating to their parents as medical students and future physicians.

The most significant aspect of the workshop is that throughout, it attempts to maintain a balance between scientific presentations of evidence, and a participatory, experiential "fun" approach to the exercise. The nutrition component, for example, includes the preparation of nutritious (and delicious) meals by sophomore students, under the guidance of an expert nutritionist, and the serving and eating of these meals in the form of a lecture -demonstration in the auditorium – a possible "first" in the annals of medical schools. Relaxation techniques are taught by faculty members in two separate sessions; the "Do's and Don'ts" of study skills are imparted by sophomores to their newcomer colleagues in life-like small satirical sketches and vignettes; a physicians' band plays for the students one evening after they have viewed a small physician-medical student art show, to make the point that here is room for leisure and recreation in the life a physician; there is a river cruise on the "Belle of Louisville," and on the last evening before formal enrollment, a picnic-sports festival in a public park (complete with student folk music) welcomes the students, their spouses, and their significant others to the medical school. In all these activities faculty and workshop participants engage freely. Strangers get acquainted, and some become friends. A sense of "welcome" and of "feeling at home" is nurtured. This "feeling at home" requires more than a quick tour of the Medical Sciences Center.

Handouts and Health Checks, Health Tutors and a Network of Support

The handout material given to each student on the first day of the workshop covers a wide range of practical information. It includes a statement of the basic philosophy of the Workshop; rankings of various medical school stresses; fifteen ways to substitute exercise for sedentary activities; a game to evaluate one's risk of heart attack; instructions for relaxation exercises; advice and a bibliography about accepting others" lifestyles and about communicating as women and men with others; a time management chart; study pointers from upperclassmen; advice and bibliography about married students" stresses; advice from senior medical students; charts listing fat, sodium, and calorie content of foods; recipes for protein-rich vegetarian foods; a menu-planning guide with sample menus; and grocery shopping tips with instructions for evaluating food labels. Along with the handbook students receive copies of Northwestern Mutual Life's "Longevity Game" (a life expectancy check list consisting of stress factors), information about Louisville from the Visitors Bureau, a list of University resources, a list of reasonably priced restaurants recommended by students and *A Survival Manual for Medical Students,* a publication by the Group for the Advancement of Psychiatry (38).

The health check, carried out in the outer office of the Associate Dean for Student Affairs, includes recordings of height, weight, blood pressure, and body fat measurement, carried out by senior students and sophomore health tutors. During the workshop registration and breakfast, all students complete four instruments to assess their response to stress: the Habits of Nervous Tension Scale, the Lorr Mood Scale, the Katz Social Adjustment Scale, and a questionnaire about drinking problems and leisure time art activities. More recently a Health Risk Appraisal instrument and stress scales have been added.

In all these activities the role of the sophomore health tutors is crucial. These students become very important resource persons during the exercise and thereafter. They do most of the legwork in the preparatory phase and during the workshop. Among their many activities, they prepare a practical version of the convention Bureau's introduction to Louisville, conduct surveys of facilities, and compile lists of medical students' favorite restaurants, banks with inexpensive checking accounts, and available apartments. They become attached to "their" freshmen, maintain contact, and check up on them during the year. They become a friend in need, and in deed.

The development of this human network of self-help support seems to us of crucial importance for the future. A medical school supporting mutual concern can hope to have this attitude reflected in the physicians it trains.

First Impressions: Need for Long-Term Follow-Up

The above experiment, essentially a pilot experiment based on voluntarism, was carried out on a minute budget. Fortunately, financial support for videotaping the actual workshop provided us with material by which we can judge the workshop retrospectively, to improve planning and content. The crucial question of long-term impact must, for the time being, remain unanswered. Some data are in the process of being gathered, and will be analyzed and reported when funds for such analysis are available. The next phase will include much more extensive use of health risk appraisal instruments and long-term (ten to fifteen years) follow-up, similar to the one carried out by Caroline B. Thomas (13); only such a program could give us a true measure of effectiveness. Nevertheless, such data as are in our possession from the students' feedback forms are highly encouraging. Students' comments were consistently positive. They found the relaxation exercises particularly helpful. They felt closer to classmates whose families they had met. They acknowledged attention to eating habits, and were grateful for sophomore study hints. Each year several letters from significant others express gratitude for being included and for the opportunity to discuss concerns.

In all workshops, participants found the information interesting and useful; none found it boring. Their comments on the scheduling of classes varied widely (too concentrated, not concentrated enough, too long, too short). We changed the format from four complete days to four half days, leaving time free for spontaneous group activity, and 84 of 95 evaluations reported that the length was optimal. We also took to heart students' advice about food, eating, exercise, and additional activities; for example, we turned over much of the introduction to the city to the sophomores, cutting down on the "public image" and presenting insiders' views instead. Only one student said that all the advice and warnings made him more nervous than before – a possible hazard of any approach that calls attention to anxiety. Everyone was pleased with the positive emphasis on active prevention and on coping with anxiety and stress.

The one feature of the workshop students mentioned most often, both spontaneously and in writing, was the chance to meet friends before school started. The immediate effect of the workshop is to form a social network. The freshmen were glad to have begun relationships with faculty and upperclassmen, as well as with each other, in the relative calm before the first term. We hope these relationships may further a sense of community in the years to come. There is always the hazard of students forming tight little groups of companions in misery, trying to "outwit" the faculty. We try to convey to students that faculty are their allies; that they are "there", that they care, and are available.

Some anecdotal evidence supports the positive written evaluations. In the freshmen photographs of previous years, students looked somber and severe. The class pictures taken at orientations since show many smiling faces. Students drop by the Student Affairs office more than ever, and watch out for each other as well as for themselves. For example, two students this year reported that two colleagues in their unit labs were in danger of dropping out of school, and that one was suicidal. They asked how to help, and persuaded their friends to seek help. Other students and a sophomore tutor, disturbed by seeing a classmate as a patient on a psychiatric ward, asked for guidance as to appropriate after-care support. These incidents highlight an *attitude*. It is probable that students help each other in many less dramatic ways that we do not even hear about.

A week is long enough to learn names and faces, to befriend one or two, to begin a social network, and to become aware of the importance of one's own well-being. We hope that the information we share with students and the experiences we go through with them may affect their skills in self care. It will take careful, rigorous design, and much long-term effort (and appropriate funding) to test the validity of our approach. So far, we and the students agree that the exercise taken at its simplest, is *useful.*

THE NEED FOR LABORATORIES (OR CENTERS OR INSTITUTES)
FOR STUDENT HEALTH

The Health Awareness Workshop differs from support groups and "orientation" sessions in several important respects. First, to repeat, it is a *voluntary* exercise, offered before the formal beginning of the academic year. Second, it mixes didactic and experiential programs. Third, the material offered goes beyond mere "survival"; it presents an introduction to some basic life skills (in terms of theory and practice) which we hope may "carry over" into the student's subsequent life and the way he or she views patients, and practice medicine. What is being offered is an opportunity to *learn*, with the full acknowledgement that changes in life-styles cannot really be taught. The best one can do is to present information in an engaging way, and offer the option of change through personal choice.

Students are impressed by the large body of data concerning epidemiology, cost, and consequences of the stressors operating in daily life. Furthermore, they are intrigued by modern insights into the physiology, biochemistry, and endocrinology of adaptation; and welcome these data – relative to theirs "laboratory within their own skin" – at an early stage of their education. They realize that prevention cannot be left to the accident of spare time. The Health Awareness Workshop is, of course, *pro* active. It avoids the pitfalls of depending on administrative supervision to identify impairment among students, an approach that can make an ostensibly helpful program just one more threat from "above." Further, the workshop treats all students equally; there is no focusing on "impairment." The social network starts from the first encounters and strengthens visibly during the four days of the exercise. The health tutors become resource persons, and in some instances, personal friends. There is throughout, a spirit of cooperation, sharing, and in the best sense, an "ethic of commitment."

There is, however, one other aspect of the program to which we wish to draw attention, namely, the research potential of such a workshop in terms of follow-up data. A medical student who appreciates the effort put out on his or her behalf by faculty and students may be willing to return the compliment by furnishing data, and respond to questionnaires as he or she goes through medical school and beyond. Physicians-in-training and in practice can be potent sources of health data. This was the core of Caroline B. Thomas's study. The difference in our experiment is that we intend to monitor the effectiveness of an *intervention*. However, we are the first to acknowledge (despite the encouragement and feedback we have received) our own dissatisfaction with our data to date.

What could emerge out of this workshop is the concept of a <MI>laboratory for student health (or a center or institute) engaged in long term studies of student health and in the development and appraisal of procedures designed to improve student health, morale and well being, in medical school and beyond. We realize that, at this stage, this may be a tall order for medical schools, requiring a re-definition of priorities and institutional emphases. Nevertheless we feel that the physician of the future should endeavor to be a role model to his or her patients; and that it behooves medical schools to take the lead in this regard.

Such endeavors should begin by recognizing and defining the need, and by viewing the need as an opportunity. Given a will for change, there could follow, in quick succession: (1)ÿ20the definition of a distinct organizational structure for such a center; (2) the allocation of space in appropriate locations within easy access of busy medical students; (3) the establishment of a distinct and adequate budget to meet initial outlay for equipment, staffing, and research personnel; and (4) the linkage of such a center to cognate facilities within the university. We would stress that a center such as we envision is no more "health clinic" or "counseling facility." Rather, it is intended to be a *legitimate and serious long-term laboratory for applied research into students' health and well-being.*

Studies seen at such a center, while drawing on established methodologies, could expand and codify new procedures, using modern data retrieval systems, and lead to the establishment of a long-term data base and a "scientific estate" capable of being carried on beyond the lifetime of principal investigators. More specifically, such studies could:

1. Appraise lifestyle and health risk in the incoming medical student.
2. Identify and codify the stresses operating throughout a student's career in medical school.
3. Equip students with coping skills in the face of identified stresses.
4. Develop a schema for successive learning and training opportunities offered at career transition points (which would include junior-to-senior, student-to-internship, internship-to-residency and residency-to-active practice). The experiments of Gorlin and Zucker, and Reiser and Rosen are fine examples of what can be done.
5. Create student/student and faculty/student social support groups to enhance coping skills.
6. Provide students with skills which could be carried over from their personal lives into the practice of their profession – a "pharmacopoeia of skills."
7. Initiate experiential educational experiments in other health care personnel in the institution.
8. On the basis of data, and by osmosis and example, influence teaching methods and curriculum design and introduce the principles of "health behavior" and "behavioral medicine" in the parent medical institution.

In sum we feel that an informed concern for the health of the healer is timely and that "humanism," "personhood," "self-awareness," and "well-being" are closely related. We suggest that as the design (and re-design) of curricula for the twenty-first century proceeds apace, student health not be relegated to an asterisk or afterthought. Joy and enthusiasm, curiosity and wonder are indeed the most precious attributes of our students. In medical schools they do not come free.

REFERENCES

1. Cope O, ed. Man, mind, and medicine: The doctor's education, a chairman's view of the Swampscott Study in Behavioral Science in Medicine, 23 Oct – 4 Nov, 1966. Philadelphia: J.B. Lippincott, 1968.
2. Flexners A. Medical education: A comparative study. New York: Macmillan, 1925. Pp. 4-5.
3. Thomas L. The youngest science: Notes of a medicine-watcher. New York: The Viking Press, 1983.
4. Rappleye WC. Medical education: Final report of the commission on medical education. Association of American Medical Colleges Commission on Medical Education, 1932. (Quoted in: Physicians for the Twenty-First Century – The GPEP Report). Washington, DC: Association of American Medical Colleges, 1984, pp. XIV, 34.
5. Emerging perspectives in the general professional education of the physician. The AAMC Project on General Professional Education of the Physician and College Preparation for Medicine (Special Report). Washington, DC: Association of American Medical Colleges, 1983, p. 8.
6. Elkes J. Toward a science of health: Thoughts on brain, behavior, and wellbeing. Paper read at Symposium "Optimum Utilization of Knowledge in Service of Health" at AAAS Annual Meeting titled, "Science and Engineering: Toward a National Renaissance," Detroit, Michigan, May 26-31, 1983.
7. Pelletier KR. Healthy people in unhealthy places: Stress and fitness at work. New York: Delacorte Press, 1984.
8. Fielding JE. Corporate Health Management. New York: Addison-Wesley, 1984.
9. Engel GL. The need for a new medical model: A challenge for biomedicine. Science 1977; 196:129-36.
10. Hamburg DA, ed. Psychiatry as a behavioral science. Englewood Cliffs, NJ: Prentice-Hall, 1970.
11. Weiner H. Psychobiology and Human Disease. New York: Elsevier-North Holland, 1977.

12. Scheiber SC, Doyle BB. Emotional problems of physicians: Nature and extent of problems. In: Scheiber SC, Doyle BB, eds., The impaired physician. New York: Plenum, 1976, pp. 3-10.

13. Thomas CB. The precursors study: A prospective study of a cohort of medical students. (5 vols.) Baltimore: Johns Hopkins University School of Medicine, 1959-83.

14. Thomas CB. What becomes of medical students: The dark side. Johns Hopkins Med J 1976; 138:185-95.

15. Vaillant GE, Sobowale NC, McArthur C. Some psychologic vulnerabilities of physicians. NEJM 1972; 287: 372-5.

16. Breiner S. The impaired physician. J Med Ed 1979; 54:673.

17. Gardner ER, Hall RCW. Protracted stress syndrome in health care providers. Texas Med 1980; 73: 63-65.

18. Linn BS, Zeppa R. Stress in junior medical students: relationship to personality and performance. J Med Ed 1984; 59:7-12.

19. Robertson JJ, ed. Proceedings of the Third AMA Conference on the Impaired Physician, September 29–October 1, 1978 (No. 55). Chicago; Department of Mental Health: American Medical Association, 1980.

The author apologizes sincerely for the absence of references beyond reference 19. Unfortunately they have been irretrievably lost.

Part Eight

FIVE LECTURES

PAPERS

22. J. Elkes: The Salmon Lectures. *Chemistry, Awareness and the Imagination. Lecture I: Altered states of consciousness: Some experimental approaches. (Abstract)*
    Thirty-first series of the Thomas William Salmon Lectures. Delivered on Thursday, December 5th, 1963 in the afternoon at the New York Academy of Medicine.
23. J. Elkes: The Salmon Lectures. *Chemistry, Awareness and the Imagination. Lecture II: Chemistry and the imagination. (Abstract)*
    Thirty-first series of the Thomas William Salmon Lectures. Delivered on Thursday, December 5th, 1963 in the evening at the New York Academy of Medicine.
24. J. Elkes: Harvey Lecture. *Subjective and objective observation in psychiatry.*
    Reprinted with the kind permission of Academic Press from The Harvey Lectures, Series 57 (pp. 63–92). New York, Academic Press, 1963
25. J. Elkes: Jacob Bronowski Memorial Lecture. *On the neurosciences, awareness, choice and the good day.*
    Delivered on January 19, 1978 at the Salk Institute, La Jolla, California
26. J. Elkes: Distinguished Psychiatrist Lecture, American Psychiatric Association. *On psychobiology and communication: psychiatry and the future of medicine.*
    Reprinted with the agreement of Elsevier Science from B.T. Taylor and I.J. Taylor (eds.) Psychiatry: Past Reflections – Future Visions (pp. 75–107). New York: Elsevier, 1990

These invited lectures present some overviews and perspectives. They stray into areas, which are not directly of the substance of psychopharmacology; yet, in Elkes' view, are implicit in a broader view of the field.

In his Salmon Lectures, of which only the abstracts are available, Elkes had just moved to Johns Hopkins and was preoccupied with administrative matters. Elkes refers to his long standing interest in the biological correlates of altered states of consciousness, and implicitly, in the spontaneous play of the creative imagination. He refers to the role of families of naturally present regulatory compounds ("neurotransmitters") derived from old evolutionary lineage, which are unevenly and regionally distributed throughout the brain. He considers the possible role of local chemical shifts in nodal areas of the brain in the regulation of states of consciousness; he suggests that these same molecules may also play a role in the encoding and evocation of the affectively laden memory trace.

The theme of subjective phenomena experienced in fluctuating states of consciousness and in drug induced states is also taken up in the Harvey Lectures (Paper 24) delivered in 1962. This paper addresses some core issues about the adequacy of language in describing subjective and objective phenomena in psychiatry as manifesting in self-observation, the dyadic interaction, and in groups. It points to the critical role of the evolution of appropriate mathematical languages in the development of modern physics, and the lack of such languages in psychiatry.

The author draws on Whorf's and Susan Langer's theories of language, distinguishing between its "sequential" and "presentational" attributes. He argues that we have "tried to force discursive languages on phenomena in which they have no business." He refers to the emergence of concepts of "complementarity" in physics and suggests, some years before the advent of classical research on interhemisphericfunction, that the nervous system is endowed with power for both "serial" and "parallel" processing of information, and that "counting" and "pattern" proceed simultaneously in self-organizing systems. He argues for the need for new languages for describing the flux of subjective phenomena; and suggests a long-term investment in small, carefully conceived "Inner Space Laboratories" and the long-term training of "Intronauts" capable of self-observation to whom "unfamiliar phenomena have become as familiar as foreign territories are to seasoned travelers." He hopes that such Laboratories will involve cooperation between psychiatrists, pharmacologists, psychologists, linguists, mathematicians and communication engineers; and that persons trained in one discipline could be trained in another – a recurrent theme in the author's hopes for psychopharmacology.

The Bronowski Lecture (Paper 25) delivered in 1978 in honor of Jacob Bronowski – creator of the award-winning Documentary series "Ascent of Man," mathematician, poet, philosopher of science, and student of Blake – was given as a Memorial Lecture at the Salk Institute where Bronowski had been a Fellow-in-Residence. The lecture draws on some of the author's earlier papers; examines regional specificity and the overriding role of discriminate chemically mediated inhibition in both perception and performance. It suggests some ways of looking at chemically mediated signal detection, and maintenance of homeostasis. It speaks to the possibility of evolution of symbolic forms, by a kind of Darwinian process of natural selection, using communicating cell populations as ensembles. The possibility is suggested that the small molecules we know as neurotransmitters may have something to do with the labeling of functional decision points at the neuron surface, building specific organelles which respond to specific interrogation – a kind of molecular transponder. These may be transferred from cell to cell by "a sort of transneuronal infectious process."

Phenomena of such staggering magnitude and subtlety also suggest the possible operation of some underlying thermodynamic field effects related to quantum phenomena. Modern molecular biology is perhaps a prelude to the study of information processing at this level.

The lecture ends with a distinct applied aspect. Jacob Bronowski was a fierce advocate of the democratization of science. The author argues that modern neuroscience provides a sound basis for an understanding of the powers of self-regulation, and the working of the body's own Inner Pharmacy. He sees Awareness (both of self and others) as central to living one good day at a time. Given present-day knowledge and decent education, a person's body/mind could indeed become a "laboratory for the self," and "every day an experiment."

The Distinguished Psychiatrist Lecture (Paper 26) delivered before the American Psychiatric Association in 1991 draws on previous material, but emphasizes communication as a central issue in psychobiology, and psychiatry. Molecular communication is key to managing energy and information within the body; Symbolic communication – preverbal, verbal, and the metalanguages of the body/mind are the business of psychiatry. Modern psychiatry is the only branch of medicine which can take a comprehensive view of Communication as it applies to man – from molecular signaling to the languages and metalanguage used in human intercourse. It has the power to offer a comprehensive Science of Man. Adolf Meyer's hope was just that.

PAPER 22 and 23

THE SALMON LECTURES
CHEMISTRY, AWARENESS AND THE IMAGINATION

Joel Elkes

Henry Phipps Professor of Psychiatry,
The Johns Hopkins University School of Medicine,
Psychiatrist-in-Chief, The Johns Hopkins Hospital

Lecture I: Altered States of Consciousness: Some Experimental Approaches (Abstract)

Recent years have seen an enhanced interest in the investigation of a number of altered states of consciousness. Their study, as a part of continuum of human experience, is far from new; present day experimental methods, however, allow a more discrete analysis. The demands made by subjects compel the evolution of new and appropriate languages.

Though possible neurophysiological correlates of some altered states of consciousness have been suggested, principally in terms of changes in the reciprocal, inhibitory play between brain-stem, diencephalic and limbic cells assemblies, and alteration in patterns of single cell discharge, their chemical correlates, both within and without the brain, remain obscure. The existence in the Central Nervous System of small families of compounds selected by evolution, and capable, by mutual interaction, of governing the regional gating mechanisms subserving basic states of consciousness has been previously suggested by the author. These small molecules (as exemplified by the catechol amines, indole amines and the membrane active amino acids) have been variously regarded as neuro-humoral transmitters, modulators, or inhibitory substances. While this may be true, they may also be endowed with more pervasive attributes. The possibility is suggested that these molecules, or allied members, may, by interacting with proteins, play a key part in the encoding and evocation of the memory trace.

Lecture II: Chemistry and the Imagination (Abstract)

The use of substances, principally of plant origin, in the induction of altered states of consciousness is as old as recorded culture and probably older. It may well have played a part in the origin of religions. Various compounds, including some synthetic analogues will be briefly considered and theories as to their mode of action discussed. The evidence suggests regional effects on the binding, release and disposition of some physiologically occurring small molecules, with which these compounds also share with structural affinities.

Some aspects of the phenomena induced by the dysleptic drugs compel comparison with hypnagogic states, the dream state and the play of the creative imagination. An attempt will be made to view these as a continuum in the elaboration and condensation of transforms by the brain in various functional states. If learning and the imagination be aspects of the evolution of symbolic forms, some chemical traces of this evolution should, in time, be discernible. The drugs now available provide instruments for such inquiries, which, inexorably, post an ethical dilemma to science at its most poignant.

PAPER 24

HARVEY LECTURE
SUBJECTIVE AND OBJECTIVE OBSERVATION
IN PSYCHIATRY[*]

Joel Elkes

*Clinical Neuropharmacology Research Center, National Institute of Mental Health,
Bethesda, Maryland and St. Elizabeths Hospital, Washington, D.C.*

I have given much thought to the choice of subject for this lecture and was sorely tempted, at one stage, to examine some aspects of the physiology and pharmacology of the brain, inasmuch as they relate to behavior. I would have been much more comfortable in such a course; for at least, it would have given me the benefit of familiarity, arising out of personal experience over some years. Yet, central to any statement concerning a pharmacology of behavior, there is a description of behavior. Behavior is not an epiphenomenon, but the major phenomenon; not only a phenomenon but an instrument. In the strange no-man's land now extending between somatic chemical process and symbolic transaction, familiar rules and assumptions are strained, an new rule still in the making. For not only does neurobiology demand precision from a description of behavior, but the elaborateness of behavior makes demands on neurobiology, which, so fat, it cannot even remotely meet. This interaction, and this deficiency are rendered peculiarly poignant in the clinical field, where intracerebral chemical process can be guessed only inferentially, and where the varieties and subtleties of behavior challenge established techniques. If, therefore, I have chosen to dwell on the assessment of clinical phenomena in psychiatry, and have selected such phenomena from among the drug-induced states, this is done for a double reason. I happen to think that in the foreseeable future patients will still be seen by physicians; whatever the reliance on test procedures, and electronic data reduction techniques, the interpersonal clinical transaction will still be cornerstone of treatment. I also happen to believe that psychopharmacology (as the subject has been sanguinely called) is forcing many issues which have lain dormant in psychiatry since its inception, and which are relevant to its aspirations as a clinical science. I have therefore intentionally omitted reference to the wealth of material that is pertinent in psychometrics. Nor do I wish to refer, except in passing, to some so called psychophysiological equivalents. These have been amply reviewed (Lacey 1956). My twin themes are thus an examination of the value of subjective and objective observation as sources of information in clinical psychiatry; and the ways and means by which we communicate this information to one another.

---

[*] Reprinted with the kind permission of Academic Press from The Harvey Lectures, Series 57 (pp. 63\'c492). New York, Academic Press, 1963

SUBJECTIVE AND OBJECTIVE OBSERVATION: SOME TRENDS
IN NINETEENTH CENTURY PSYCHIATRY

On the day after Christmas, in 1799, young Humphry Davy, twenty years old, made the following note following a self-experiment with nitrous oxide which he had carried out in his laboratory in the company of one, Dr. Kinglake (Davy 1800): "I felt a sense of tangible extension, highly pleasurable in every limb; my visible impressions were dazzling, and apparently magnified. I heard distinctly every sound in the room, and was perfectly aware of my situation. I lost all connection with external things; trains of vivid images rapidly passed through my mind, and even connected with words in such a manner, as to produce perceptions perfectly novel. I existed in a world of newly connected and newly modified ideas. I theorized; I imagined that I made discoveries. When I was awakened from the semidelirious trance by Dr. Kinglake who took the (gas) bag from my mouth, indignation and pride was the first feeling produced by the sight of persons about me. My emotions were enthusiastic and sublime: and for a minute I walked about the room perfectly regardless of what was said to me. As I recovered my former state of mind I felt an inclination to communicate the discoveries I had made during the experiment. I endeavored to recall the ideas, they were feeble and indistinct; one collection of terms, however, presented itself: and, with the most intense belief and prophetic manner, I explained to Dr. Kinglake – 'Nothing exists but thoughts!' – the universe is composed of impressions, ideas, pleasures and pains."

In one bold empirical step, thus, young Davy revealed the power of an anesthetic not only to obtund, but to enhance sensations, and to manifest aspects of mental life only sparingly used in normal waking existence: The features he described are common enough in such states. The intensity of personal feeling, the heightened perception, the connectedness among things normally disconnected, the synesthesia (i.e., the evocation of one sensory modality by another), the fusion, the feeling of devotion, of identity, and attempt to communicate the experience except in metaphor and allusion. A number of drugs have shared this power to evoke and to transcend: it is no accident that, throughout their long history mescalin (Klüver 1928) and the mushroom poisons (Wasson and Wasson 1957) were used in complex religious rites in remote and inaccessible regions. In Europe, for reasons which have been examined elsewhere (Elkes 1961), things happened more slowly. DeQuincey's confessions on the effects of opium were published in 1822. In 1845, Moreau wrote in this monograph on marihuana (hashish): "By its mode of action on the mental faculties, hashish gives him who submits himself to its strange influence the power of studying on himself the moral disorders which characterize mental illness, or, at least, the principal intellectual modifications which are the points of origin of all kinds of mental disturbances." (Moreau 1845)

Some thirty years later, in 1874, Benjamin Blood, stimulated possibly by his predecessors, described "anaesthetic revelations" brought about in himself and his friends by the inhalation of ether. Lewin rediscovered mescaline (Klüver 1928) in the Mexican hills; Kraepelin (1883) was experimenting with drugs in his newly founded laboratory, a trend continued by Weir Mitchell in England (1896), and by the Heidelberg School of Beringer (1932) and Mayer-Gross (Mayer-Gross and Stein 1926) in Germany. The chemical divining rod was thus found useful; it brought forth riches wherever it touched. In 1943, there occurred in the laboratory of Hofmann, in Basel, the accidental discovery of lysergic acid diethylamide (Stoll 1947), a drug which in the infinitesimal amount of 50 μg. by mouth will produce marked mental changes in man. There followed the rediscovery of psychoactive mushroom poisons, the identification of psilocybin (Hofmann et al. 1958) and a host of synthetic derivatives, including other trypt-amine derivatives (Szara 1956), the N-substituted piperidyl benzilates (Abood et al. 1959) and l-(l-phenylcyclohexyl)piperidine (Luby et al. 1959), to mention, but a few. We who have learned to live with psychopharmacology know that we are still witnessing a mere beginning.

I mention this chemical path, trodden by many, to draw attention to a quieter way which, at any rate in medicine, was sought by relatively few until the turn of the century. For coincident in time with the above observations, there were others centering on subjective phenomena experienced without chemical aids, and sharing with drug-induced states their intensely personal, private, averbal, and incommunicable nature. Mentioned here may be the early observations of Johannes Müller (1848) on the so-called hypnagogic phenomena – experiences any of us know in the brief twilight states between wakefulness and sleep; or the analysis, at the hands of Frederick Galton, the father of medical genetics, of what he called "Visions of Sane Persons" (1881) and the "Statistics Mental Imagery" (Galton 1880). In 1896 Weir Mitchell published his account of mescaline intoxication, observed in himself; and it is of interest to compare this account with Ladd's account on so-called "Visual Dreams" published four years earlier (Ladd 1892). Hovering over the field, but still very much at the periphery of medicine, there was the concept of unconscious or preconscious mental activity. Thus, there is Carus, writing, in 1846, on the "Developmental History of the Soul"; von Hartmann, 1869, on the "Philosophy of the Unconscious" (von Hartmann 1869); Fechner (1860), Helmholtz (1863), and Wundt (1862) speculating and experimenting on perception and threshold states of consciousness: and Carpenter laying down his "Principles of Mental Physiology" in 1874. Towering over others are the figures of Titchener (1909) and William James, who regarded Benjamin Blood's "Ether Dreams" (1874) as a stepping stone in this own thinking (James 1912). Indeed, much that went before culminates in James and the titles of his essays: "The Varieties of Religious Experience" (1901), "A Pluristic Mystic" (1912), and "The Stream of Thought" (1890), tell their own tale. In his preoccupations with subjective phenomena (while incidentally building the first Experimental Psychology Laboratory at Harvard), he significantly deviated from the principal paths of nineteenth century science. As he says in this well known quotation: "What must be admitted is that the definite images of traditional psychology form but the smallest part of our minds as they actually live. The traditional psychology talks like on who should say a river consists of nothing but pailsful, spoonfuls, quartpotsful, barrelsful and other moulded forms of water. Even were the pails and pots all actually standing in the stream, still between then the free water would continue to flow. It is just this free water of consciousness that psychologists resolutely overlook. Every definite image in the mind is steeped and dyed in the free water that flows round it. With it goes the sense of its relations, near and remote, the dying echo whence it come to us, and the dawning sense whither it is to lead (James 1890).

These "echoes", and this "dawning sense" of knowing is, as we saw in Davy's description, not unfamiliar in the drug-induced experience; and it is these private, subjective, personal, and incommunicable elements which rendered chemical devices so useful for purposes of religious rites. Somehow, then, it appeared, even in the nineteenth century, as though certain functional modalities which are part and parcel of the repertoire of human experience, but normally used only transitorily and sparingly in the waking state, could be chemically locked by drugs into more persistent manifestations. One would hesitate to claim identity among these various processes; there is, however, a family resemblance. The changes observed more recently in hypnosis, in sensory isolation (Solomon et al. 1961), in the dream process (Kleitman 1961), attest to this affinity to this day.

In parallel which these developments, and complementary to them, there took place in psychiatry another development of great consequence. We know Philippe Pinel as the spirited Director of the SalpétriŠre who, under the impetus of the French Revolution unshackled patients in his native France and thus presaged the era of humane care of the mentally ill. Yet, it was he, also, who said right at the beginning of his "Treatise on insanity published in English translation on 1806: "Nothing has more contributed to the rapid improvement of modern natural history than the spirit of minute and accurate observation... (With this in view) ... I therefore resolved to adopt a method of investigation which has invariably succeeded in all departments of natural history, viz. to notice successively every fact without any other object than that of collecting material for further use, and to endeavor as far as possible, to divest myself of the influence, both of my own prepossessions and the authority of others" (Pinel 1806).

Pinel's work forms the first major descriptive treatise of the forms of insanity. Across the Atlantic, Benjamin Rush, Professor of Chemistry at the Medical School in Philadelphia, guiding spirit of the Revolution, Treasurer of the Mint, published his "Observations on Disease of the Mind" (Rush 1812) a volume which for decades remained the major available textbook of psychiatry in the United States. Pinel's pupil Esquirol (1772–1840) coupled the reform of mental hospitals with a major descriptive work of mental illness (Esquirol 1838). The English school flourished under Tuke, Haslam, Prichard, Conolly, and. later, Maudsley; but is was not until Kraepelin (1856–1926) that a definitive nosology of psychiatric disorder was developed (Kraepelin 1906). The exploration of subjective experience, and the classification and taxonomy of mental disorder thus proceeded in parallel within roughly the same century. There was overlap between the two approaches and a searching out of subjective elements in objective presentation and vice versa; There were shifts in emphasis; yet, with certain exceptions, the two lines exemplified attitudes -attitudes which are with us to this day.

There is, however, a third trend running through our field, the outlines of which can, in retrospect, be clearly distinguished. The implicit recognition of unconscious process at the hands of Carus (1846), von Hartmann (1869), and Carpenter (1874) has already been mentioned. Yet it was not until Charcot's studies on hypnosis and hysteria (1892) that the clinical implication of this process were given their full due. Charcot's "lessons" were attended by many: Babinsky, Binet, Janet, Marie, and of course, Freud. In 1893, Breuer and Freud published their preliminary communication on hysteria stating, quite simply, that "hysterics suffer mainly from reminiscences." The repressed, affectively laden memory trace thus emerged not only as a subjective phenomenon welling up randomly in dreams or in drug-induced states, but as a clinical entity, capable of affecting sensorimotor or visceromotor function. The exteriorization of the subjective memory into overt behavior (coupled, at a later date, with the concept of "acting-out" in a transference situation), assumed therapeutic as well as theoretical implications. Psychoanalysis and psychosomatics were thus cast in the same mold, psychoanalytic theory attempting to provide a conceptual link between subjective experience and overt behavior. We are not here concerned with the validation or otherwise of the theory. What we would rather note are the many modifications at the hands of its originator which is underwent, emphasizing its tentative and empirical nature; and the minute serial observations of subjective states of mind over time, on which it was based.

PHYSICS, AND THE FUNCTION OF LANGUAGE IN SCIENCE

Discoveries such as these, however, fitted ill the brash innocence of a young emergent materialist science. An age set firmly in the framework of classical physics, wedded to the meter rule, the clock, and the kilogram, secure in its concept of space, time, matter, and causality, and propelled by the idea of evolution: such an age did not readily accept introspection as a source of evidence, or behavior as a phenomenon in its own right. Matter was the primary reality; and the studies of its properties – living or dead, silent or articulate – were judged the proper objectives of science. Physiology, though recognizing homeostasis and the self-regulatory properties of living systems, was wedded to chemistry and physics; and the inventiveness of the Russian schools of neurophysiology, leading to the evolution of the Pavlovian method, while providing penetrating techniques for the analysis of behavior, did not have the backing of present day neurobiology and mathematics to enable it to realize its full yield. Yet, as is well known in retrospect, forces of quite another kind were at work in that same age. The concept of the electromagnetic field... so new to a period preoccupied with the mechanical motion of matter... was consequent upon Michael Faraday's experiments. In 1856 Clerk Maxwell published his equations on Faraday's lines of force. It was the same Maxwell who, in his paper on "Atoms" for the Encyclopedia Britannica (Maxwell 1874) wrote: "There are thus two models of thinking about the constitution of bodies which have had their adherents both in ancient and modern times. They correspond to two methods of regarding quantity... the arithmetical and the geometrical. To the Atomist is the true method of estimating the quantity of matter in a body is to count the atoms in it. To those who identify matter with extension, the volume of space occupied by a body is the only measure of quantity in it."

Clerk Maxwell's ideas were followed by Ernst Mach's "Die Mechanik" (1897), in which Mach questioned Newton's definition of space and the concept of absolute rest. (It is incidentally, the same Ernst Mach who in 1886 published his "Analysis of Sensations, and the Relation of the Physical to the Psychical," and who, by implication, influenced the development of gestalt psychology.) What followed is well told by the men who partook of the change (Einstein 1934, Bohr 1958, Heisenberg 1958). Within three decades, the theory of relativity way established and quantum mechanics was in being. Probability and chance had entered into the definition of the state of physical systems; and the concepts of "complementarity" of mutually exclusive states (such as particle vis ... vis wave, position of particle vis ... vis velocity and momentum) (Heisenberg 1958, p. 49) was found to be productive and substantially workable model in the descriptions of the fine structure of matter. As Heisenberg dryly observes, "the possibility of playing with different complementary pictures has its analogy in the different transformation of the mathematical scheme; it does not lead to any difficulties" (Heisenberg 1958, p. 50). There is a profound truth in this fit of phenomenon, and statement about the phenomenon.

I have dwelt briefly on these developments in turn of the century physics because, in a way which, at least to me, is far from clear, they may well bear upon the evolutionary forces now at work in neurobiology, and the biology of behavior. I do not mean here the mere cracking of a crust of certainty by the expanding root of doubt. The dialectics of the process go deeper, What appears significant is that while denying subjective observation of fluid, multiple, phenomena as a source of valid data, and forcing overt behavior into a materialistic frame which fitted it ill, that same frame – rigid, formidable, buttressed by the enormity or its industrial product – underwent a loosening and expansion which, within a few brief decades, presaged a new age. Concepts, strangely familiar, yet never rigorously applied to behavior were being quietly incorporated into mathematical statements concerning the structure of matter. What had been regarded as universal statements (such as Newtonian mechanics and Euclidean geometry) were reduced to special instances of statement of even greater validity. States regarded as mutually exclusive, were assumed, in Weizs"cker's timely phrase, to coexist (Heisenberg 1958, p. 185). The mathematical scheme of quantum theory expanded the tenets of classical logic, the concepts of "either or" giving way to the "also" and the "and", making classical logic a providence of quantum logic. The deliberately open, probabilistic, mathematical statements were found, in the light of experiment, to provide a more precise description of reality than older and more circumscribed rules. Above all – and from the point of view which we are considering most important – a mathematical language for mechanics which had to serve the varied needs of the theoretician, the experimental physicist, the technician, and the engineer was treated more discretely, new symbolic inventions serving the needs of fine structure of matter and older devices remaining in use to run trains and to heat buildings. As with Berzelius' (1779–1848) invention of a formal shorthand for chemistry, it is the evolution of a new, appropriate language which made modern physics what it is.

I suppose that whether we like it or not, we have now arrived at a crucial point in our discussion. For if behavior is to be described in a way accurate enough to predict its attributes, either in the individual or the group; if subjective experience is to be conveyed even to oneself, in terms which clearly and strongly apprehend its significance and meaning, languages are required to model and symbolize the processes with which they are concerned. I hope, as we proceed, to give some instances of such devices in current usage, if only to point to the pain which goes into their making and the limitations from which they suffer at present. A thorough exploration of the limits of language is presented in Susanne K. Langer's writing (1942, 1957); and the problem of communication and validation of subjective clinical data has been examined by Henry K. Beecher in his recent monograph (1959a). I have learned a great deal from reading these sources and gladly acknowledge my debt to them.

There can be little dispute of the attributes of language. Language is "our most faithful, and indispensable picture of human experience" (Langer 1942, p. 76), a heuristic symbolic instrument shaping mode of observation and interpretation, and interpenetrating deeply with experience. Phonemes and morphemes condense meaning into words, and the relation between word-symbols is regulated by rules of syntax and grammar. Such rules – rules of astonishing logic and economy – go, as Whorf showed (1956) into the fabric of even the most primitive language. They make for the smooth use of language as an instrument of social adaptation and communication. They order the relation of the fact-symbols to each other, and to the world which they represent. To serve such adaptive functions, the rules imposed by syntax must be strictly followed, and the symbols presented in a certain order. It is evident that "Tom followed Harry" does not mean the same as "Tom follow Harry" or "Harry followed Tom." Conventional logic imposes a liner, sequential quality, which has come to be known as "discursiveness" (Langer 1942, p. 77), and it is in this sense that the laws of reasoning and logic are sometimes known as "the laws of discursive thought" (Langer, 1942, p. 77).

There is, however, another quality in words implicit in the one just discussed. For, while carrying certain meanings in one context, words carry a totally different meaning in another; and even standing alone they may – as anyone who has traced the origin of a word in a dictionary – carry on accretion of different meanings in a sort of strange algebra and calculus of their own. This economy, this logic, this dependence on context is characteristic even of the most primitive language (Whorf 1956). Words are thus not mere labels, cards, stacked for reference in one of Broca's areas; they are states, sets, depending on relation, and context: they carry multiple meaning. Carnap, in "The Logical Syntax of Language" (1937), has examined the capacity for expression of any given linguistic system. What is remarkable in that analysis is how little our ordinary means of communication measures up to the standard of meaning which a serious philosophy of language, and hence a logic of discursive thought, demands.

It would thus seem that there are large areas in communication and in self-communication (i.e. the symbol making not exteriorized in overt behavior) which are not represented by ordinary language. For whereas grammar and speech are essentially sequential, linear, and discursive, the characteristic of these other subjective states is the multiple simultaneous presentation of internalized objects and relations. The form of the "unspeakable" is as different from the "speakable" as the structure of a dream, or even a day dream, is from the structure of deliberate action. In such symbolic forms totality is apprehended simultaneously at different levels; mutually occlusive elements coexist; time is of no consequence; and serial ordering in time, that backbone of causal reasoning, gives way to simultaneously perceived relationships. The philosophy of language tends to dismiss this type of presentational activity as falling into the sphere of subjective experience, emotion, and feeling. As Russel (1927) put it: "Our confidence in language is due to the fact that is shares ... the structure of the physical world. Perhaps that is why we know so much of physics and so little of anything else."

I would submit that we know so little of that large "anything else" because, all to often, we have tried to force discursive language and method on phenomena in which they have no business. Nor is a relegation of such matters to the mystique of intuition at all helpful. There is nothing mystical, for example about recent developments in sensory physiology. Here the data suggest a unique capacity of the brain to build up a central representational system through the juxtaposition of simultaneously coded transforms of multiple sensory inputs, modulated and gated by an interplay between central and peripheral, specific and nonspecific systems (Livingston 1958). Sense experience is thus a fundamental way of creating form; and a mind working with meaning must have organs that supply it with forms (Langer 1942, p. 84).

Having said as much, I now want to consider some empirical approaches to the problem of measurement in clinical psychiatry with special reference to the effects of drugs on human behavior. Time allows only a few examples, a mere listing, in fact. The various approaches have been ably reviewed (Uhr and Miller 1960).

SUBJECTIVE AND OBJECTIVE OBSERVATION IN THE SINGLE SUBJECT

Take, for example, the sensation of pain and its relief by analgesics. Like other subjective experience, pain can manifest in motor behavior; however, it need not. It is a sensation difficult to define operationally; one "known to us by experience, and described by illustration" (Lewis 1942). There are other puzzling features about pain. In the single individual it can be estimated by a variety of experimental procedures, registering the so-called pain threshold (Beecher 1959a, p. 92). Yet a careful review of the fields leads Beecher to the surprising conclusion that "Some 15 groups of investigators have utterly failed to demonstrate any effectiveness of morphine on experimental pain threshold" (1959b). This sounds odd, in view of the patent usefulness of the drug in the clinical situation, a usefulness which is confirmed when the drug is tried in a carefully controlled clinical setting. Here there is remarkable agreement between data from Lasagna and Beecher's laboratory (Beecher 1959b, pp. 104–105; Lasagna and Beecher 1954) and from the group of Houde and Wallenstein (1953) concerning the effectiveness of 10 mg. morphine in pain of different origin (postoperative vis-…-vis metastatic cancer), and agreement concerning the reproducibility of data in successive experiments extending over three years by different groups of investigators in the same laboratory (Beecher 1959b, pp. 104–105). In reviewing the effect of morphia on wound pain (Beecher 1959a, p. 164), Beecher quotes evidence how attitudes to a wound determine the need for the drug. Thus, soldiers, to whom a wound can be the symbol of survival (rather than evidence of injury), require less morphine than civilian postoperative patients, to whom (despite far less tissue damage) the operation may signify severe disability. The subjective reaction to the injury, the "psychic processing" (Beecher 1959a, p. 158) in a total behavior situation modifies not only the original sensation, but evidently its reaction to pharmacological intervention. Mood and attitude are thus all pervasive; and the measurement of change of mood is an all pervasive problem in psychiatry.

There are a number of scales to quantify mood; anxiety and depression, being common symptoms, have been particularly studied in this respect. Taylor (1953) and Cattel have developed instruments for the measurement of anxiety: Cattel isolated a "universal index" and a number of more discrete factors. A number of scales have been elaborated for estimating depression (Grinker et al. 1961, Hamilton 1960). Such scales although still in the process of trial appear to be reliable (Hamburg ct al. 1958), there being good agreement among raters, and also between subjective self-assessment and objective observation.

Another method, founded on the work of Nowlis and Nowlis (1956) has recently been developed by Clyde (1960). It makes use of a list of adjectives describing various mood states in simple, nontechnical terms, found empirically to be least ambiguous. Each term is printed on an IBM punch card; the subjects is asked to sort these cards into four piles to describe the degree to which they describe his feelings, ranging from "not at all" to "extremely." Patients like this card sorting task, and prefer it to a check list. After sorting, the cards are fed directly into an electronic computer, for scoring, and analysis. Specific categories of mood and behavior (such as "friendly", "aggressive", etc.) can be arrived at according to the grouping of words which describe them. Above all, subjective self-ratings can be compared with observer's ratings. By having a central clearing house for the cross validation of this and other scales (such as is available at the Psychopharmacology Service Center of the National Institute of Mental Health under Dr. Jonathan Cole's very able leadership), confidence levels for various instruments can be determined and clinical reaction forms (as manifested by clustering of items) agreed upon. These scales have a further advantage. Being self-administered, they make possible the careful study of fluctuation over time in a single case; and particularly of diurnal variation and variation on successive days. These variations can be quite marked, and, can vitiate baseline readings (Knight 1963). It is also possible to use these scales to gauge interaction between personality structure and the effect of a particular medication. Time does not permit a consideration of this most important area. That has been recently reviewed (Lindemann and von Felsinger 1961). In any event, pain, anxiety, anger, and depression, all common enough clinical symptoms, can at present be approached in quantitative terms.

It is much more difficult to quantify other symptoms, such as the disorders of perception or of cognitive function manifested, for example, in the states induced by dysleptic ("psychosomimetic") drugs. For here, as we saw, the flux, the speed, the intensity, the variety, the strangeness defies ordinary language. Silence can be more eloquent than words, and the small guttural noise can carry the quintessence of meaning. The experience can be projected in a drawing, or in a poetical condensation. It can also be item analyzed, in a self-rating question-naire. Some 47 items have been listed by Abramson, Jarvik et al. (1953); some 300 in a card sort test used by Ditman (1960). Yet here a difficulty arises. Answering a questionnaire re-quires attention; attention breaks continuity; the very act of attending, or of speaking, may al-ter the phenomena; the answers, even if they are informative are only partial answers; ant the more trained the subject and observer, the more familiar with the inner space which he is ex-ploring, the more informative the answers. Such item analysis, however, has great merit. It gives rank order and pattern to individual responses and maps the distribution of symptoms over time. A shorthand can be devised to describe various categories and their fluctuation over time, and such categorization can be reinforced by retrospective self-description and the play-ing back of tape-recorded responses. The symptoms can also be related to striking alteration in the sense of time, noted in these states (Boardman et al. 1957). One other advantage of this longitudinal approach is that symptom intensity can be correlated which metabolic findings. Thus, in our laboratory Dr. Szara has attempted to correlate symptom intensity produced by diethyltryptamine, a powerful dysleptic, with the pattern of excretion of its metabolite, 6-hydroxydiethyltryptamine. There are some, admittedly slender, indications of a possible correlation between symptom intensity and the excretion of 6-OH-diethyltryptamine in man (Szara and Rockland 1962).

What is the objective counterpart to this kind of subjective observation in the single sub-ject? The sensory or social isolation experiments demand such observation (Solomon et al. 1961). There, the throat microphone, the closed-circuit television camera are useful technical devices. However we may briefly note one situation in which the behavioral output of an iso-lated individual is continuously monitored in a controlled situation. This approach, known as the operant conditioning approach, is based upon Skinner's (1938) classical studies. It allows a piece of behavior to "operate" upon the environment in the light of past occurrence, so as to "obtain" a "reward" or "avoid" "punishment": the behavior thus determines the consequences of behavior. The "reward" and "punishment" can be presented at regular ("fixed") or irregular ("variable") intervals, altering the levels of expectancy. Moreover the reward can be actual (Lindsley and Skinner 1954) (candy, visual displays) or symbolic (points, won or lost, as in a game). Dr. Weiner, in our laboratory, favors the latter course; he is also exploring the rela-tively unknown area of the influence of "cost" in human operant behavior (Weiner 1962). By suitable automatic programming, the "cost" of each response intended to procure a reward can be altered (i.e. the apparatus set so as to ensure that points are *lost* every time the subjects seeks his reward); the economy with which a subjects uses resources at his disposal can thus be assessed. The task is essentially a vigilance task – the detection of a light on a frosted glass panel, for which the subject is allowed to look by pressing a lever. Gain of points is signified by a bell. The responses are recorded on a cumulative recorder. The behavior under "cost" and "no cost" conditions is strikingly different; and already individual differences between sub-jects in terms of handling "cost" and "no cost" contingencies are apparent. This approach may, in time, give one an insight into the way individuals of different personality structure, (or, for that matter, psychopathology), handle the very rapid transitional states (i.e. changes in anticipatory set) which some of the procedures demand. They also may teach one something of the individual variation in the experience of time; of the individual meaning of "gain," "loss," "reward," and "punishment." It has been of great interest and encouragement to Dr. Weiner. Dr. Waldrop, and their colleagues that patients respond to "symbolic" incentives more readily than to actual minor material rewards; and that performance remains remarkably stable in certain contingencies. With the equipment now available at the Behavioral and Clinical Studies Center of Saint Elizabeth's Hospital a number of patients can be tested simultaneously on different schedules. Printed circuit computer components make for an economy and flexibility of gear which would have been difficult to achieve with older devices. Moreover, a careful clinical study of the same patient and an inquiry into subjective states of mind during actual performance can proceed in parallel with the operant experiment. The data both warrant and are amenable to mathematical analysis.

NONVERBAL AND VERBAL BEHAVIOR IN THE DYADIC TRANSACTION; CUE AND EXPECTATION IN RELATION RESPONSE

There are thus some clinical responses in the single subject which, though unsatisfactorily, can be expressed in quantitative terms. It is significantly more difficult to measure a piece of behavior in an interpersonal field. The psychiatric interview or the analytical session are the prototypes of this situation. Much has been written on the nature and analysis of this transaction (Hilgard et al. 1952, Masserman 1958); and it has, correctly in my view, been described as a system of expectations as well as of communication (Lennard and Bernstein 1960). The interaction is here created by a continuum of individual signals – gestures, nonverbal sounds, words, sentences – each of which carry symbolic meaning. These are subjectively perceived and put out behaviorally, there being a constant interplay between subjective and manifest elements. The moment-to-moment input into this system is thus enormous; and the devices developed to reduce randomness and sources of variance can, to date, but mark a well-intentioned beginning. The traditionally "neutral" attitude of the psychoanalyst is such a device. The study of nonverbal cues in a transaction is another.

Gestures have been viewed by some as the most economical way of communication (Critchler 1939), and have been examined with a view to disturbances in communication (Ruesch and Kees 1956, Ruesch 1957). A notation system for analysis of body motion and gestures known as "kinesics" has been developed (Birdwhistell 1952). Separate silent and sound film analysis of a transaction presents another approach. A method has recently been introduced for the analysis of motion picture records by accurate geometrical fixation in successive planes. (Dierssen et al. 1961). These techniques – because of the specialization and also the expense they involve – have so far been used only sparingly in psychiatry. Nevertheless, they may quantify cues which are of the oldest in the body of clinical medicine.

There are similar and more varied attempts to quantify aspects of verbal behavior; analysis of the nominative, connotative quality of words is but one of such analyses. There is suggestive evidence (through the use of appropriate filters) that the frequency spectrum alone – robbed of any connotative quality – can convey the affective quality of a speech sample (Hargreaves and Starkweather 1962). Respiratory function during speech is another index (Goldman-Eisler 1955) giving evidence of striking regularities in relation of patterns to speech production, and particularly in regard to verbal output (syllables) per expiration. An extension of this time analysis of speech production is provided by the interaction chronograph (Chapple 1940, 1949). Used in a standard nondirective interview situation, this has already yielded valuable results. In essence, this instrument is an automatically controlled electronic stopwatch, measuring total speech time (irrespective of words) designated as action, pauses, silences, tempo, and other variables in both subject and observer. The coupling of the apparatus to data reduction devices increases the yield and makes possible the derivation of further measures, such as initiative and dominance. These measures have proved reasonably reliable (Matarazzo et al. 1956, Tuason et al. 1961), and there are indications that they may be sensitive to change, including drug-induced change (Tuason et Guze 1961). *Time* of action thus emerges as an important element in communication, providing, with pitch, the matrix in which the detail of connotative meaning is embedded. Another feature may be noted at this point; as in operant conditioning behavior, time analysis forms and important element is verbal behavior. Verbal behavior is, in fact, operant behavior, a probabilistic symbolic game in which a piece of behavior operates on one's environment and determines outcome of behavior: verbal conditioning (Luria 1961) makes it possible to examine these contingencies experimentally. In this reciprocal feedback system of an interpersonal transaction it is not easy to separate patient behavior from therapist behavior; both therapist and patient are, in a sense, participant observers of each other, and the total transaction is the behavior of a two-group, or dyad (Lennard and Bernstein 1960). It is in these contextual terms that the detail of verbal symbolic behavior must be viewed.

Some analysis of the naturalistic therapeutic transaction has been proceeding for some time and is beginning to bear fruit (Leary and Gill 1959). The microscopic analysis of samples of speech with regard to word type, grammatical and syntactic structure, the themes referred to, and the context of such themes, suggests that the technique is sensitive to drug effects (Gottschalk et al. 1956). Moreover, it is possible to assess, in a preliminary way the relationship between the specificity of a therapist's remarks and the expansion of constriction of the patient's statement which follows (Lennard and Bernstein 1960). Patients talk more directive and constrictive the quality of activity, the more likely the negative reaction.

Buried in this obvious statement, there is another aspect of the same phenomenon. If linguistic transaction is in fact a system of mutual expectations, the expectation should influence subjective experience, as manifested in language. These expectations can be experimentally altered. There is, for example, some evidence (in need of much more detailed study) that the mere presence of an observer in an experimental analytical situation significantly influences the imagery in psychoanalytic free association (Colby 1960). In a more direct way expectation, manipulated either by direct instruction or by implied association, can markedly influence the subjective effect of a drug. This is most obvious in the old, old remedy of the placebo (Beecher 1959a, p. 65). Moreover, when a drug (e.g., pentobarbitone) effect is compared with *both* placebo and untreated control, diametrically opposite results have been reported leading to the conclusion that "because of the several varieties of placebo reaction, as well as their potential for interaction with pharmacodynamic effects of drug, this dynamic quality, which is inseparable from the act of drug administration in man, must be taken into account, and controls must be used which identify the direction as well as magnitude of the placebo effect. For this it may be necessary to use the *unblinded no drug-at-all control* to complement the usual identical dummies in the double blind setting" (Modell and Garrett 1960). A cognate approach is to examine the interaction between paradoxical instructive set and effect of a drug (for example, the administration of amphetamine with instructions appropriate to a barbiturate or vice versa). Such experiments are in progress (Fischer 1962).

GROUP INTERACTION, WARD SETTING, AND THE CLINICAL TRIAL

It is obvious from the foregoing that forces which powerfully influence a dyadic social field are bound to be manifest in an amplified degree in larger groups. The subject of small group interaction has been thoroughly reviewed (Hare et al. 1955, Nowlis 1960), and classified for such factors as group size, the communication network, the personal and social characteristics of members, role differentiation, initial expectancy of members with respect to each other, and setting, as important input variables. Various methods have been used to approach the subject. For example, the communication network can be controlled by varying the sequence of communication between subjects (Christie et al. 1952). A topographical system of notation (chain, wheel, star, circle) (Christie et al. 1952) have been introduced and quantification is possible by means of devices such as the transmittance matrix (Roby and Lanzetta 1958), linear graph analysis (Cartright and Harary 1956) or measure of centrality (Leavit 1951) or independence. The mathematical problems in the analysis of small group behavior have also been recently considered (Solomon 1960). A psychical task (e.g., getting a ball up spiral plane) can be arranged to depend upon the collective skills and cohesion within a small group. In one such instance, such a task was found to be sensitive to sleep deprivation and medication (Laties 1961). Even in the absence of a definitive task there are striking changes in the interpersonal field following medication. Thus one study (Rinkel et al. 1955) on the effects of LSD-25 reported a significant increase in avoidance, withdrawal, hostile, punitive, competitive behavior, while friendly reciprocal, equalitarian behavior was clearly reduced. The effect of a drug on behavior must thus be considered in a social field. The same drug, in the same dose, in the same subject will produce different effects according to the interpersonal and motivational situation in which it is given. This, particularly, applies to moderate doses of drugs.

It is much more difficult to study interaction is a large group, such as a ward population. Here both overt observation, and observation by a participant observer assuming a patient role (Caudill) has been practiced. In our own laboratory, and arising out of the need of the clinical trial, a method known as the Social Interaction Matrix was developed by Kellam (1961). This device makes use of a suitably marked grid to record the amount and kind of social contact between patients on the basis of regular and frequent observations on the ward during the day. It is a scale deliberately designed to measure the amount of social mobility among patients, and one of the several instruments available to quantitate behavior on a psychiatric ward.

There are many such devices, and around them center some of the liveliest controversies in psychiatry. Should rating scales be used or should one rely on clinical observation only? If rating scales are to be used, who is to use them, how often, and why? Is the physician's rating based on a half-hour interview once a week more reliable than that of the Nursing Assistant, potentially having access to the patient for 8 hours? How should raters be selected, and how trained? Upon whose vocabulary is the rating scale to be built? What are minimal criteria for scale validity in terms of content and construct? When do criteria become predictive? These and many other questions continue to be asked, and have been authoritatively reviewed (Lorr 1960). One can draw comfort from such opinions. It is possible, for example, to record serially, and adequately, behavior in a metabolic unit (Beauregard et al. 1961). The reliability of some scales is high, so much so that by careful selection of items of high information content, a reliability of 0,9 can be archived with as few a 12 items (Lorr 1960). Moreover, when such scales are used in a formal controlled clinical trial of several phenothiazines (Kurland et al.

1961), the conclusions regarding rank order of the various compounds compare not at all badly with an open, non-blind, clinical assessment (Freyhan 1959).

The native clinical experience evidently is still a match for artificial intelligence, and the computer we carry in our skull is at least equal to its metal counterpart. Somehow the experienced, sensitive, and skeptical clinician collates data for internal consistency and error simultaneously at many levels, arriving at a formulation which represents a creative act of very high order. It is humbling that, despite its limitations, ordinary language should be able to convey its message so clearly in such a formulation. Rating scales thus have their place, but should be used only where there is clinical judgment. It is, in fact, when rigid assessment precludes continuous observation of clinical process over time; when observation of the outer shell of behavior presumes either to ignore or to infer subjective states of mind, that it is well to send one's young colleague back to the ward to write a long anecdotal history. Refined statistical manipulation will not mask poor case selection, or coarse rating scales, or poor inter-rater agreement. Sooner or later truth will out. In this age of restless manipulation it is well to learn to stare at phenomena in the ward; to take up the fragment, and the detail, only after having had a sense of the subtlety of the whole.

ON THE NEED FOR NEW SYMBOLIC SYSTEMS
IN PSYCHOBIOLOGY AND PSYCHIATRY

In 1854, George Boole, a man who self-taught had risen to a Royal Society Medal and a Chair in Mathematics at Queens College, Cork, published his "Investigation of the Laws of Thought". In this work, as in an earlier one – "The Mathematical Analysis of Logic" (1847) – he examined the ability of symbols to express logical propositions, "the laws of whose combination should be founded upon the laws of mental processes which they represent". In searching for such outward representation, he invented the theory of classes and sets and the nonassociative relation between them, divising a symbolic algebraic shorthand for the expression of these relations in which concepts such as product, complement, inclusion, and a number of others are clearly represented.

Boole's path-breaking contributions led by way of Frege (1879), Jevons (1964), Peirce (1880) to Whitehead and Russels's "Principia" (1910–1913) in our day. One may note, in passing, the titles of some of these earlier works. Jevons named his work "Pure Logic, or the Logic of Quality apart from Quantity." Frege called his study a *Begriffschrift* – a "formula language, (Formelsprache)" of pure thought. Somehow the inexpressible, the suggestive qualities which in other circumstances we would call intuitive grew into communicable notations and symbols of great propulsive power; and opened a world of relations hitherto considered closed. It is outside my competence to examine the influence, of Boolean algebra on modern experimental physics. However, the relation of a theory of sets and classes to communication and information transfer is nearer at hand. For the very word "communication" (from "communicare") implies sharing – i.e., the sharing of properties; and any encoding process depends upon the apprehension of such shared properties among sets and classes. It is by this sharing, too, that redundancy, far from being wasteful, serves in the transfer of information; redundancy provides context and thus minimizes error; it is a safety device – a reserve – in the flow of information (MacKay 1961); a reserve, incidentally, amply encountered in biological systems.

Yet how independent are the demands of a subject, and the demands of a language for a subject. When chemistry, or electrical engineering needed appropriate symbolic forms of notation, such systems were duly invented: and when turn of the century physics felt constrained by Newtonian mechanics, it was modified according to need. However, so young is the biology of mental phenomena (which we will call psychobiology) that its great discoveries were made, using a linguistic apparatus leased from chemistry and physics, and from the language of every day use. This hybrid arrangement has served for a time: no one will deny the many advances made so far. Nevertheless, it is clear that demands of quite a different order are pressing on the biology of our day. Interaction in macromolecular systems, and the control mechanisms inherent in such systems are evidently of a different order from reactions between simple inorganic compounds; any accounting for the flow of information in such systems (as, for example, in the obvious instances of the gene or the immunological specificity of proteins) demands a language in which mere chemical or descriptive language is no longer sufficient. Woodger (1952) has indeed attempted to define the elements of a concise formal language for some aspects of genetics and evolutionary theory: a difficult but enormously worthwhile task.

It is the fortunate, if embarrassing, feature of the phenomena of behavior and of mental life that by their very nature they brook less compromise in such matters than any other branch of biology. The purely physical and chemical analogies do not hold: and the psychochemical correlates demand, as we have seen, a much more detailed specification and description of behavior, and of concomitant chemical change, than is currently available. For behavior implies multiple simultaneous change of a system in time, and *form* in behavior is really a topology in time. Discursive, linear, metric language does not apprehend such patterns. Presentational, experiential language suggests intricate simultaneous relationships, but does not define them. Yet it is the characteristic of every culture that is has invented symbols for such subjectively experienced relationships; it is significant, too, that in its own evolution physics (and the branch of mathematics known as topology) has developed a shorthand for the apprehension of cognate simultaneous relations in the so-called outside psychical world.

Could it, thus, be that in behavior and subjective experience we could see – if we wished to look see most clearly and cogently the "laws of thought" of which Boole spoke and which govern our understanding of the physical world? And could it be that the two uses of language which we distinguished represent two mutually complementary ways – one multiple, simultaneous, and another serial, successive by which the brain constructs its models of reality? I have elsewhere (Elkes 1961b) tentatively examined the possible relation of schizophrenic thought disorder to information processing, or misprocessing, by the brain. In this scheme I suggested that transformations proceeded simultaneously at different yet closely interrelated neural levels, and distinguished between an ability to organize information serially in time – to structure in time – (in terms of the immediate adaptive demands of the "Here" and "Now") and a much more pervasive function of nervous tissue which depended upon its ability to organize simultaneously changing multiple inputs into a temporal topology of high information content. In this context the distinction between "serial" and "parallel" programming of computers concerned with pattern recognition is of special, if topical, interest (Selfridge and Neisser 1960). Essentially, the distinction is one between asking questions serially one at a time, i.e., letting each answer determine the next question by successive elimination; or asking, as Neisser put it (1962), all the questions at once. It is found for example, that in the recognition of patterns of letters of different calligraphic quality the multiple, parallel method is more economical and effective. The silicon intelligence thus turns up with a familiar linguistic problem; and there is at least inferential evidence that, at one level of its organization, the nervous system has the capacity of asking many questions all at once. The multiply connected reticular mixing pool may provide a substrate for precisely such transactions. The illogical thought process of intense subjective experience, of the dream, and so-called "primary" process (Freud 1900) may thus have its parallel in presentational language, in the "geometric" thinking of Clerk Maxwell, the principles of complementarity and coexistence of physics, and the multiple (or "parallel") approach of the modern computer; the logical, structured, sequential pattern of conscious deliberate action (sometimes called "secondary process") may be mirrored more closely in discursive language, the arithmetical approach, the scale, the serial analysis. Counting and pattern, rating and correlation, are thus at opposite ends. One feeds into the other, and science draws on them both. This process is well illustrated in Harvey's famous passage in Chapter VIII of "De motu cordis" (1628) where, following the minute sequential observation described in the preceding parts, the "movement, as it were, in a circle" is first conceived. "Movement in a circle" implies an intuitive seeing of a relation in time. Indeed, time would appear to be the main axis around which we build our models of reality; and nowhere is this more apparent than in the models we construct to represent behavior, including human behavior.

It would seem advisable, in view of the foregoing, to give early thought to the development of adequate new symbolic system in the study of interpersonal processes, and to relate such attempts, whenever possible, to existing instruments in the natural sciences. The creation of such new systems would require long-term planning within small groups. It would require highly trained observers and highly trained subjects, capable of self observation to whom unfamiliar phenomena have become familiar through practice, as foreign territories are to seasoned travelers, and who are capable of developing operational definitions of states experienced and observed. Such an endeavor would require close cooperation between psychiatrist, psychologist, mathematician, and communication engineer; it may require training of one discipline in the skills of the other, to ensure a most direct personal contact with the phenomena. It will require much debate, and much crude trial and error. Yet, the history of sciences suggests that once such a beginning is made, progress can be quite rapid. It may be not too much to hope that concepts only partly or inadequately covered by present day language may, before very long, find a more adequate expression in new symbolic systems of greater precision and power. The usefulness of such systems may – and I would venture to say, will – not be confined to the study of behavior. For the phenomena of behavior pose, in a most poignant way, some fundamental issues in biology, particularly in regard to the storage and transfer of information in living systems. Indeed, the chief merit of behavior may perhaps lie in its intolerance to facile analogies borrowed from other branches of science, and its compelling need for rules in its own right. The Behavioral Sciences, and that vast body of experience known as Clinical Psychiatry, thus need not look apprehensively over their shoulder; having been nourished by the natural sciences, they may well be in a position to repay a longstanding debt. It is one's hope – and, if pressed, would be one's contention – that a science of Clinical Psychiatry is in the making in our day; and that in its growth it will enlarge the realm of the very sciences on which, quite properly, it still depends.

REFERENCES

Abood, I.G., Biel, JH. and Ostfeld, A.M. (1959). In: Neuropsychopharmacology, Proceedings of First International Congress (P.B. Bradley, P. Deniker, and C. Radouco-Thomas, eds.) pp. 433-437. Elsevier, Amsterdam.

Abramson, H. A., Jarvik, M.E., Kaufman, M.R., Kornetsky, C., Levine, A., and Wagner. M. (1955). J. Psychol. 39, 3-60.

Beauregard, R.M., Wadeson, R.W., and Walsh, L. (1961) J. Chronic Diseases 14. 609-628.

Beecher, H.K. (1959a). Measurement of Subjectives Responses. Oxford Univ. Press. London and New York

Beecher, H.K. (1959b). In: Quantitative Methods in Human Pharmacology and Therapeutics (D.R. Laurence, ed.) p. 102. Pergamon, New York

Beringer, K. (1932) Nervenarzt 5, 346-357.

Birdwhistell, R.L.(1952) Introduction to Kinesics. Univ. of Louisville Press. Louisville, Kentucky

Blood, B.P. (1874) The Anaesthetic Revelation and the Gist of Philosophy. Amsterdam, New York.

Boardman, W. K., Goldstone, S., and Lhamon, W.T. (1957). A.M.A. Arch. Neurol. Psychiat. 78. 321-327.

Bohr, N. (1958) Atomic Physics and Human Knowledge. Wiley, New York

Boole, G. (1847) The Mathematical Analysis of Logic. Cambridge.

Boole, G. (1854) An Investigation of the Laws of Thought. Walton and Maberly, London.

Breuer, J., and Freud, S. (1893) Neurologisches Zentr. 12, 4-10

Carnap, R. (1959) The logical Syntax of Language. (Reprinting of 1st English edition, 1937, Routledge, Kegan and Paul, London) Littlefield, Adams, Paterson, New Yersey.

Carpenter, W. B. (1874) Principles of Mental Physiology. H.S. King and Co., London.

Cartright, D., and Harrary F. (1956) Psychol. Rev. 63, 277-293.

Carus, J. F., Lasky J. J., Klett, C. J., and Hollister, L. E. (1960) Am J. Orthopsychiat. 22. 314-334.

Chapple E.D. (1940). Genet. Psychol. Monogr. No. 22. 1-247.

Chapple, E.D. (1949) Personnell 25, 293-307.

Charcot, J.M. (1892) Leons du Mardi a la Salpetrire. L.Bartaille, Paris

Christie, L. S., Luce, D. R., and Mary, J., Jr. (1952) Communication and Learning in Task Oriented Groups. Technical Rept. No. 321 Cambridge, Massachusetts. Research Laboratory of Electronics, MIT

Clyde, D. J. (1960) In: Drugs and Behavior. (L. Uhr and J.G. Miller, eds,) pp. 583-586. Wiley, New York.

Colby, K. M. (1960) Behavioral Sci. 216-232.

Critchley, M. (1939). The Language of Gesture. Edward Arnold, London.

Davy, H. (1800) Researches, Chemical and Philosophical, Chiefly concerning Nitrous Oxide of Dephlogisticated Nitrous Air and its Respiration. Biggs and Cottle, Bristol.

DeQuincey, T. (1822) Confessions of an English Opium Eater. Oxford Univ. Press. London.

Dierssen, G., Lorenc, M., and Spitaleri, R. M. (1961) Neurology 11, 610-616.

Ditman, K. S. (1960). In: The Use of LSD-in Psychotherapy. (H. A. Abramson, ed.) p. 118. Josiah Macy, Jr Found. New York.

Einstein. A. (1934) Essays in Science. Philosophical Library, New York.

Elkes, J. (1961a) Psychotropic drugs Observations on current views and future problems In: Lectures on Experimental Psychiatry (H. Brosin.ed.). pp.65-113. Univ. of Pittsburgh Press. Pittsburgh, Pennsylvania.

Elkes, J. (1961b). In: Chemical Pathology of the Nervous System (J.Folch Pi. Ed.), pp. 648-665. Pergamon, Oxford.

Esquirol, E. (1838). Des Maladie Mentales, Considerées sous les Rapports Médical Hygiénique et Médico-Légal. Balliere, Paris

Fechner, G. T. (1860). Elemente der Psychophysik. Breitkopf und Hartel, Leipzig.

Fischer, S. (1962) Personal communication

Frege, G. (1879). Begriffschrift eine der Arithmetischen Nachgebildete Formelsprache des reinen Denkens. Halle

Freud, S. (1900). The Interpretation of Dreams. Reprinted (1938). In: The Basic Writings of Sigmund Freud. p. 525. The Modern Library, New York

Freyhan, F. (1959) Am. J. Psychiat. 115. 577-585.

Galton, F. (1880) Mind 5, 301-318.

Galton, F. (1881) The visions of sane persons. Popular Sci. Monthly (New York) 19, 519-531.

Goldman-Eisler, F. (1955). Brit. J. Psychol. 48, 53-63.

Gottschalk, L. A., Kapp F.T., Ross, D. W., Kaplan S. M., Silver, H., MacLeod, J. A., Kaaahn, J. B., Van Maanen. E. F., and Achesib G. H. (1956) J. Am. Med. Assoc. 161, 1054-1058.

Grinker, R. R., Miler, J., Saabshin, M., Nunn, R., and Nunnally J.C. (1961) The Phenomena of Depressions. Hoeber, Harper, New York.

Hamburg, D. A., Sabshin, M. A., Board, F. A., Grinker, R.R., Korchin, S. J., Basowitz, H., Jeath, H., and Persky, H. (1958) A.M.A. Arch. Neurol. Pychiat. 79. 415-425.

Hamilton, M. (1960) J. Neurol. Neurosurg. Psychiat. 23, 56-62.

Hare, P., Borgana, E.F., and Bales, R. F. (eds.). (1955) Small Groups Studies in Social Interaction. Knopf, New York.

Hargreaves, W.A., and Starkweather, J. A. (1963) in press.

Harvey, W. (1628). Exercitatio anatomica de moru cordis et sanguinis in animalibus. G. Fitzer, Frankfurt.

Heisenberg, W. (1958). Physics and Philosophy. Harper, New York.

Heimholtz, H. von (1863). On the Sensation of Tone as a Physiological Basis of the Theory of Music. English translation by A. J. Ellis (1954). Dover, New York

Hilgard, E. R., Kubie, L. S., Pumpian-Mindlin, E. (eds.) (1952). Psychoanalysis as Science. Stanford Univ. Press, Ca.

Hofmann, A., Heim, R., Brack, A., and Kobel, H. (1958) Experientia 14, 107-109.

Houde, R.W., and Wallenstein, S.L. (1953). Drug Addiction and Narcotics Bulletin. Appendix F. p. 660. National Research Council, Washington, D.C.

James, W. (1890) Principles of Psychology. Vol. I. Henry Holt, New York, Reprinted (1950) by Dover Publ, p. 255.

James, W. (1901) The Varieties of Religious Experience, A Study in Human Nature. (Gifford Lectures on Natutal Religion, 1901-1902). Reprinted (1928) by Longmans, New York.

James, W. (1912). A Pluristic Mystic. In: Memories and Studies, pp. 371-411, Longmans, Green, New York.

Jevons, W. S. (1864). Pure Logic, or the Logic of Quality Apart from Quantity. London.

Kellam, S. G. (1961). J. Nervous Mental Disease 132, 277-288.

Kleitman, N. (1961). In: The Nature of Sleep. (G.E. Wostenholme and M. O'Connor, eds.). pp. 349-364. Ciba Foundations Synposium. Little Brown, Boston.

Klüver, H. (1928). Mescal. The Divine Plant and its Psychological Effects. K. Paul, Trench, Trubner, London.

Knight, R. A. (1963). In: Specific and Non-specific Factors in Psychopharmacology. (M. Rinkel, ed.) in press.

Kraepelin, E. (1883) Philosoph. Studies, I, 573-605.

Kraepelin, E. (1906). Lectures on Clinical Psychiatry. Balliere, Tindall and Cox, London.

Kurland, S. A., Hanlon, T. E., Tatom, M. H., Os, K.Y., and Sinopoulos, A. M. (1961). J. Nerv Ment Dis 133, 1-18.

Lacey, J. I. (1956). Ann. N.Y. Acad. Sci. 67, 123-163.

Ladd, G. T. (1892). Mind (N.S.) 1, 299-304.

Langer, S. K. (1942). Philosophy in a New Key. 9th printing (revised, 1958). New American Library, New York.

Langer, S.K. (1957). Problems of Art. Scribner, New York.

Laties, V. G. (1961). J. Psychiat. Research 1. 12-25.

Lasagna, L., and Beecher, H. K. (1954). J. Pharmacol. 112, 306-311.

Leary, T., and Gill, M. (1959). In: Research in Psychotherapy. (E. A. Rubinstein and M. B. Parloff, eds.), pp. 62-93. American Psychological Association, Washington, D.C.

Leavit, H. J. (1951). J. Abnormal Soc. Psychol. 16, 38-50.

Lennard, H. L., and Bernstein, A. (1960). The Anatomy of Psychotherapy. Columbia Univ. Press, New York.

Lewis, T. (1942). Pain. Macmilian, New York

Lindemann, E., and von Feisinger, J. J. (1961). Psychopharmacologia 2, 69-92.

Lindsley, O. R. and Skinner, B. F. (1954). Am. Psychologist 9, 419-420.

Livingston, R. B. (1958). In: Handbook of Physiology. Section I: Neurophysiology (J. Field, H. W. Magoun, and V. E. Hall, eds). Pp. 741-760 American Psychological Society, Washington D.C.

Lorr, M. (1960). In: Drugs and Behavior. (L. Uhr and J. G. Miller, eds). Pp. 519-539. Wiley, New York.

Luby, E. B., Cohen, B. D., Rosenbaum, G., Gottlieb, J. S., and Kelley, R. (1959). A.M.A. Arch. Neurol. Psychiat. 81, 363-369.

Luria, A.(1961). The Role of Speech in the Regulation of Normal and Abnormal Behavior. Liveright, New York.

Mach, E. (1886). The Analysis of Sensations and the Relation of the Physical to the Psychical. Translated from the 1st German ed. by C. M. Williams: Open Court Publishers, Chicago, 1914.

MacKay, D. M. (1961). The Science of Communication. Inaugural Lecture at University College of North, Keele, England.

Masserman, J. H. (ed.) (1958). Science and psychoanalysis. Grune & Stratton, New York.

Matarazzo, J. D., Sasslow, G., and Guze, S.B. (1956). J. Consult. Psychol, 20. 267-274.

Maxvell, J. C. (1874). Article on "Atoms" for Encyclopedia Britannica. In: Scientific Papers of J.C. Maxvell. (W. D. Nive, ed. 1890, Cambridge). Vol. I. pp. 155-229.

Mayer-Gross, W., and Stein, H. (1926). Z. Neurol. 101. 354-361.

Mitchell, S. W. (1896). Brit. Med. J. II. 1623-1629.

Modell, W., and Garrett, M. (1960). Nature 185, 539.

Moreau, J. (1845). Du Hachisch et de l''aliénation mental. tudes psychological. Librairie de Fortin. Masson. Paris.

Müller, J. (1848). The Psychology of the Senses, Voice, and Muscular Motion with Mental Facilities. (translation from German, Müller's Elements of Psychology). pp. 849-1419. Taylor. Walton & Maberly, London.

Neisser, U. (1963). Psychol. Rev. in press.

Nowlis, V. (1960). In: Drugs and Behavior. (L. Uhr and J. G. Miller, eds.). pp. 563-581. Wiley, New York

Nowlis, C., and Nowlis, H. H. (1956). Ann. N. Y. Acad. Sci. 65, 345-344.

Peirce, C.S. (1880). A. J. Math. 3, 15.

Pinel, P. (1806). A Treatise on Insanity. Cadell & Davis, London.

Rinkel, M., Hyde, R. W., Solomon, H. C., and Hogland, H. (1953). Am. J. Psychiat. III. 881-895.

Roby, T. B., and Lanzetta, J. T. (1958). Psychol. Bull. 55, 88-101.

Ruesch, J. (1957). Disturbed Communication. Norton, New York.

Ruesch, J., and Kees, W. (1956). Nonverbal Communication. University of California Press, Berkeley, California.

Rush, B. (1812). Medical Inquiries and Observations upon the Diseases of the Mind. Kimber and Richardson, Philadelphia, Pennsylvania.

Russell, B. (1927). Philosophy. p. 265. Norton, New York.

Selfridge. O.. G., and Neisser, U. (1960). Sci. American 203, 60-68.

Skinner, B. F. (1938). The Behavior of Organisms. Appleton-Century, New York.

Solomon, H. (ed.) (1960). Mathematical Thinking in the Measurement of Behavior. Free Press of Glencoe, Illinois.

Solomon, P., Kubzansky, P. E., Leiderman, P. H., Mendelson, J. H., Trumbull, R., and Wexler, D. (eds.) (1961). Sensory Deprivations. Harvard. Univ. Press. Cambridge, Massachusetts.

Stoll, W.A. (1947). Schweiz. Arch. Neurol. Psychiat. 60, 279-323.

Szara, S. (1956) Experientia 12, 441.

Szara, S., and Rockland, L. H. (1962). Proc. 3rd. World Congr. Psychiat. I, 670-673. Univ. of Toronto Press, Toronto.

Taylor, J. A. (1953). J. Abnormal Social Psychol. 48, 283-290.

Titchener, E. B. (1909). Lectures on the Experimental Psychology of the Throught Process. Macmillan, New York.

Tuason, V., and Guze, S. B. (1961). Clin. Pharmacol. Exptl. Therap. 2, 152-156.

Tuason, V., Guze, S.. B., McClure, J., and Beguelin, J. (1962). Am. J. Psychiat. 118, 438-446.

Uhr, I., and Miller, H. G. (eds.) (1960) Drugs and Behavior. John Wiley, New York.

Von Hartmann, E. (1931). Philosophy of the Unconscious. (Reprint of 1st edition, 1869.) Harcourt Brace, New York.

Wasson, V.P., and Wasson, R. G. (1957). Mushrooms, Russia and History. Pantheon, New York.

Weiner, H. (1962). J. Exptl. Anal. Behavior 5, 201-208.

Whitehead, A. N., and Russell, B. A. W. (1910-1913). Principia Mathematica. 3 vols. Cambridge Univ. Press, London

Whorf, B.J. (1956). Language, Thought and Reality. Selected Writings. (1927-1941). Wiley, New York, and The Technology Press, Massachusetts Institute of Technology. Cambridge. Massachusetts.

Woodger, J. H. (1952). Biology and Language. Cambridge Univ. Press. London and New York

Wundt, W. (1862). Beitrge zur Theorie der Sinneswahrnehmung. C. F. Winter, Leipzig.

PAPER 25

JACOB BRONOWSKI MEMORIAL LECTURE ON THE NEUROSCIENCES, AWARENESS AND THE GOOD DAY*

Joel Elkes

*Department of Psychiatry and Behavioral Sciences,
The Johns Hopkins University*

I. INTRODUCTION

Jacob Bronowski was a vast continent of a man, cognisant of his own map and deeply aware of his own geology. Through three cultures in his youth, and four settings for his work – one would hesitate to speak of career in the case of Jacob Bronowski, but simply refer to "ein Leben" – a *life* – he traveled the length and breadth of the territory that was him, searching for what Goethe called Gleichnis – a simile, a unity in the hidden likenesses of nature. Reading his life, his plays, his essays, his poetry, and above all, his study of Blake, I have the feeling that – no matter how far-ranging his gaze, how deep his excursions into the corners of the universe, – he walked his own land firmly every day. In this daily walk he had the companion of truth, with whom he made a lifelong contract. He saw through the trappings of mind which disguise truth. He was never taken in by the shape of categories and classes, by their logical beauty or their contradictions; but would merely point to their constraint and their potential tyranny; and his vision of likenesses was never diffuse, but had the sharpness and elegance of a line drawn by a master. It is commonplace to say that to Bruno Art and Science were of a piece. To him, they represented deep rules by which things living went about their business. Nor was insight into these connections to be the privilege of the few. In the developing tissue that is mankind, it was, he felt, given to the few to enact their awareness; but only so as to evoke the dormant universals of knowing in the many. Art and Science was there to be touched and used, and enjoyed, and it was that touching, and that joy of knowing, which was to make mans day a good day. It was this deep respect for every man, and for the fundamental truth in people, that made him the passionate messenger he became. He saw the sinews of truth showing through all the illusions and follies of mankind, and saw the follies and illusions as detours and mutations, markings on the road which inevitably led back to truth, to the way things were in nature. It is this deep conviction which nourished the wellsprings of his hope, and his humor. And his dreams were good dreams, because they were possible.

He was a deeply aware and deeply observant man. He saw awareness as a gateway to choice. He used his language not as a screen, not a foil, nor a shield, nor a weapon; but quite

---

* Delivered on January 19, 1978 at the Salk Institute, La Jolla, California simply, as an extension of himself – a hand – a strong hand, stretched out in warmth and in friendship. We feel its firm grasp still.

To the end of his day, he was preoccupied with the nature of illusion, and the nature of truth, and the place of the imagination in the genesis of both; and with the organ which related knowledge, to the image of the world to the image of the self. The brain drew him like a magnet. Had he lived, I have no doubt that is where his next quest would have taken him.

He knew that illusions were important to man; for, strangely, his rites and dreams are the germ plasm of his efforts at understanding. To paraphrase Thomas Huxley, science does not only start in knowledge, harden into dogma and end up in superstition; it has often begun in superstition, become science, and ended in dogma. Superstition and dogma differ from science in that the latter is backed by shared evidence, rather than mere shared feeling. In the old days, the evidence of the senses was enough. Experiment, however, relied increasingly on instrumental extensions of the senses, and developed a complex scientific technology to observe, understand, and enact the phenomena of nature. Yet, to this day, feeling states are the forces which bind and part men. Feeling states are shared at first hand. No telescopes or microscopes are needed for men to know or to deny one another. Man's unaided senses are his sensors, and the detectors are carried within his skin and skull. Not so with the natural sciences. Here a vast array of exosomatic extensions of ourselves have created the bulk of our culture. Within a mere hundred years or so – the briefest moment in man's total existence – these inventions have totally and radically transformed our physical environment and firmly established the dominance of our resourceful and dangerous species on this planet. In our own life, they have made change the only constant, and excess a state of body and a state of mind. Excess, that is, of material product, coupled with gross unevenness in its distribution. Excess of people, newly born, and newly preserved, coupled with excess power to kill, leading to the absurdity of nuclear overkill; an undreamt technological inventiveness, coupled with a deep loss of the person. We are choked by our own abundance, yet puzzled by the strange hollow ring within. We are at once more active, and more passive, more connected and more separated, more interdependent and more lonely. The product of science bind us; but science in the service of man has blurred the image of man. The concept of the self is becoming increasingly outer-dependent and diffuse. For the symbols of science are alien to immediate experience, and often encased in special languages known to the few rather than the many. Our perception of ourselves and of each other: on the other hand, – even of a world changed so radically by science – are still fairly direct. Experience still determines expectation, and expectation induces both action and outcome. Fear still engenders fear, and friendliness still engenders friendliness. We still, fundamentally, like others in the measure that we like ourselves; and yet tend to depend on our self esteem and on the judgment of others. Our self-image propels or bars us; our self image, that is, reflecting the image of ourselves in others. Life, thus, in large measure would seem to be *other people*. Whether we like it or not, we are as Jacob Bronowski put it, both social and solitary. Man's evolution is non-genetic social evolution. Somehow this capacity to evolve – to represent, to connect, to enact, – is related to a unique power to model the world in sight and sound to communicate, (from the Latin "communicare," i.e. to share) attributes among things diverse, and test them for adaptive value. This sharing, we agree, is due to the peculiar organ which we carry in our skull. Man's species-specific uniqueness is his brain: symbols, signifying things and events and the relation between them. This brain then, during its very short evolution, could learn and adapt to a changing environment long after birth; it developed a capacity to model the outside world in sight and sound; to transfer these models to other members of the species, and ultimately from generation to generation. When tools appeared in evolution, they appeared suddenly in great abundance. Models assumed independence of their bodily substrate, and became more related to each other. Culture became possible, and man's adaptation became not a passive adaptation to environment, but a sort of active conversation between the brain and its products; a process which has continued exponentially and explosively to this day. If we were to count the emergence of our species as one day, the events related in Jacob Bronowski's "Ascent of Man" would occupy a fraction of a second. In stressing this new tack in evolution – exosomatic, as we call it – do not let us neglect and bury something simply because of its obviousness. However, intricate, awesome and alien man's inventions, however huge the products – whether they be Blake's Satanic Mills, or the Viking or Apollo Spacecraft – the models thereof are originating as maps inside our skull. Thus, this strange tissue is the shaper of man's destiny.

II. EMERGENCE OF THE NEUROSCIENCES

ll too slowly for the pace of modern technology we are learning what this organ is all about;and we are learning by observation from without and by observation from within. Observation from without uses the technological tools of science, and observation from within notes events by way inward vigilance and awareness. We call this the objective and subjective approaches. They are, to be sure, tools of rather different kinds, used by different people for different purposes. Again, and again, as I read and reread Jacob Bronowski, I am conscious of his passionate preoccupation with the relationship of the without to the within, and of the within to the without; of the objective to the subjective, and the place their mysterious, incandescent points of fusion in the evolution of man. He knew the place of both observation and the place of awareness, and lived his poetic day fully, by maintaining both inward and outward vigil, feeling that truth – his truth, any truth – demanded uncompromising, free commerce between these two modes of knowing. To the end of his life – as I said – he was preoccupied with the brain, and its tool of tools, language. If I may I would like to examine briefly some aspects of brain function, dwelling mainly on aspects of chemical communication within the brain; to look at subjective observation in relation to both brain and language; and to examine some practical consequences flowing out of these two approaches. If I do so in a personal idiom, I hope you will forgive me. It is, quite simply easier for me to think of it that way.

In this year of 1978 with large national and international bodies representing the neurosciences and psychobiology, with societies and colleges flourishing in many countries, with major journals devoted to new findings, and huge industries invested in their application, it is hard to realize that the field, as we know it, is barely a quarter of a century old. To be sure, it rests on the arms of giants. Claude Bernard, who far ahead of his time, foresaw self-regulation, the negative feedback, and the systems approach to homeostasis. Hughlings Jackson, who put the evolution of ascending functional hierarchies in the central nervous system in their place, and clearly recognized the overwhelming role of inhibition emanating from the cerebral cortex. Charles Sherrington who wove the principle of reciprocal inhibition into the very fabric of integrative action, showing that the contraction of one muscle group depended on an exquisitely organized precise, concomitant and *active* relaxation of its opposite member; and I. Pavlov who demonstrated that symbols and memories are *structures*, capable of affecting profoundly bodily functions. It was Charles Sherrington who wrote in 1951:

The body of a worm and the face of a man alike have to be, taken as chemical responses. The alchemist dreamed of old that it might be so. The dream, however, supposed a magic chemistry. There they were wrong. The chemistry is plain everyday chemistry. But it is complex. Further the chemical brew in preparation for it, time has been stirring unceasingly throughout some millions of years in the service of a final cause. The brew is a selected brew.

This dream was uttered in a different way by the founding father of neuro-chemistry, Wilhelm Thudicum, who spoke of the effects upon the brain substances fermented within the body. These attitudes are still with us to this day, but with better reason.

For the chemistry of which Sherrington and Thudichum spoke developed, not in the brain, but in peripheral nets, the simpler neural nets of the heart and gut, and giant fibres of invertebrates – giving us an idea of the action of chemical messengers such as acetylcholine and norepinephrine, and ionic fluxes at the neuron membrane. Here we are still in the company of giants; Otto Loewi, Henry Dale, Allan Hodgkin, John Eccles: things were dormant and things were ready, until the boot of empiricism sent some of us reeling with new facts of great clinical significance. The discovery of LSD-25, which in the remarkable low dose of 25–50 micrograms by mouth (that is in the dose of the order a hormone) could induce striking temporary mental changes in man; and of Chlorpromazine and the anti-depressants in the early fifties, demonstrating striking effects in the mentally ills. I still remember vividly our first trial – as it turned out to be, the first blind, controlled trial of Chlorpromazine – in the City Mental Hospital in Birmingham, England, which proved to be an encouraging exercise in all kinds of ways. The dialectic, however really began when the new facts began to hunt for an explanation; and it is here that the evolution of new *methods* brought us to the position we are in today.

III. METHODS IN THE NEUROSCIENCES

These methods were in part anatomical and physiological, in part chemical, in part behavioral, and in part clinical. They combined subjective with objective observation. In this respect, psychobiology or psychopharmacology brook no compromise, and like no other fields compel a continuous conversation between various disciplines and approaches: in essence, it is a conversation between the somatic and the symbolic, a conversation extending from the deepest recesses of subjective awareness to behavior, and the neurobiology of behavior. This conversation may be silent, implied or articulate. It can take place in one head, one team, one group or preoccupy a whole institute. We know that from the time he began serious writing, this passionate dialogue proceeded in the mind of Jacob Bronowski.

I said earlier that the methods which brought us to the position which we are in today are in part anatomical, physiological, in part chemical, in part behavioral, and in part clinical. It was a combination of anatomy, physiology and a study of behavior which slowly bared the mosaic of sub-systems governing the control centers of respiration and circulation, and energy exchange, located in the very old part of the medulla, brain stem and hypothalamus, which Paul McLean terms the neural chassis. It was the same approach which defined the physiological anatomy of the subsystems subserving sleep and wakefulness, arousal and focussed attention, and of sexuality, prey killing, and territorial, repetitive, stereotype behavior located in the so-called reptilian brain.

And it was the same combination, coupled with microphysiological approaches which led to an understanding of the role of convergence; filtering and funneling of signals in peripheral sense organs (such as the retina), integration at high central level, and the assignment of significance and value in relation to memory, in what we call affective terms, in the pathways, and structures of the Limbic System. It is here, too, by way of self stimulation experiments, that the organizing power of the Reward and Punishment Systems emerged; through thee works of Jim Olds, with still other areas of the organization of discriminate sensory fields and the sequential ordered motor performance which we know as speech being related to respectively the parietal cortex and temporoparietal cortices of the two hemispheres.

If all this sounds like the language of the cerebral localizers of the nineteenth century – a sort of phrenology of the brain – it both is – and isn't. The brain, to be sure, is an assembly of suborgans, a system of systems, a mosaic of biassed homeostats: the Medulla; the stereotype Reptilian brain; the Limbic Systems, and the huge cortical mantle are such homeostats. The brain has its nodal areas, its cables and connections; and presumably, in certain respects, is wired for a purpose. But the wiring, and the concept of control centers, should not mislead. For equally clear and emerging from recent evidence, are diffuse and generalized effects. Coursing through large areas of the brain, or the brain as a whole. Phenomena of modulation, gating, and slow potential drifts. It is these which may be related to the now established fact of differential cell populations in even small areas of the brain; and the influences, by way of widespread projections of nodal midline areas (such as the locus coeruleus) over such large areas.

IV. CHEMICAL MAPPING AND REGIONAL NEUROCHEMICAL SPECIFICITIES

While these developments were proceeding, a chemical map was being quietly superimposed upon functional anatomical findings. It started with painstaking dissection of gross areas of the brain and bioassay. It proceeded to the sampling of ever smaller areas, and the analysis of single cells. The use of radio isotopes added to this dimension, and further elucidated the regional chemical organization within Central Nervous System. But it did more. For by taking down the regional process to the organization of sub-cellular components, by showing up the astonishing precision and economy of the processes governing release, reuptake, and storage of specific small molecules, it related spatial subcellular organization to turnover *in time*. It added the concept of quantal discharge of transmitters by differential synaptosomal populations, thus, introducing a much needed *statistical, probabilistic* element into our thinking. It also made much real the concept of heterogeneous cell populations. Between 1953 and 1957, I suggested that: "Perhaps rather than thinking in unitary terms, it might be advisable to think in terms of the possible selection by chemical evolution of small families of closely related compounds, which by mutual interplay would govern the phenomena of excitation and inhibition in the central nervous system." I spoke of the operation of chemical fields in nodal regions of the brain which would depend on the rate of liberation, diffusion and destruction of locally-produced neurohumoral agents; and proposed that the agents in question may be either identical with or, more likely, derived from neuro-effector substance familiar to us at the periphery – substances such as Acetylcholine, Norepinephrine and Serotonin. I felt, as I put it, "The number of those substances was probably small, but their influence upon integrative action of higher nervous activity could be profound, and that the basic states of consciousness might well be determined by variations in the local concentration of these agents."

These speculations were based on the time-consuming bioassay of brain extracts and inferential evidence on the electrical activity of the brain in the conscious cat, as studied by my colleague P.B. Bradley. Isotopes had not yet been used, and synaptosomal fractionisation was not yet in being. But as methods grew, so grew precision in data. Like the Cloud Chamber in Physics we have now a number of inferential approaches which allow us to monitor chemical events at subcellular, cellular and inter-cellular levels. These are the subcellular fractionation, and radioactive update techniques, giving us a fairly precise picture of intra- and pericellular kinetics; the radio immune approaches allowing cyto-chemical localisation of components in different parts of the cell; the literally illuminating Swedish fluorescent and immuno-fluorescent techniques showing up special neuron populations and pathways according to putative neurotransmitters associated this them; and the path-breaking combination of radio isotope techniques with multi barreled micropipette and electron microscopy in single cells, pioneered by Dr Floyed Bloom and his colleagues, making possible a mapping of chemical susceptibility in different cell populations. We now have the most elegant extraction, fractionation and purification techniques for brain prohormones and peptides developed by Guillemin and his group. Added to this there are pharmacological tools to interfere selectively with the natural process; there are agents which can specifically inhibit syntheses, and destruction; selectively deplete intra cellular pools; block specific reuptake; or act as false transmitters. Already these agents have found their way into behavioral pharmacology, and into general medicine as anti-hypertensive agents; and into psychiatry as antidepressants.

These methods have yielded rich harvest. They have clearly confirmed that principles of *regional economy* in the central nervous system can be carried to the chemical specificities of the individual cell itself. They have linked certain enzyme systems with certain structural components; they have also made possible the detailed step-by-step analysis of the informational flow, the feedback, as we say, between product and enzymatic machinery governing production; between release and uptake, between release and disposition. We now even talk of auto-receptors within the individual neuron. When such findings are applied to neurons exerting a scanning, filtering, condensing and integrating function, our analysis of that rather vague term "modulation" becomes possible, not only in a neurophysiological, but also in chemical terms. What is even more exciting is, that by placing single cell monitoring devices judiciously along particular pathways in the learning animal, a monitoring of electrical and electro chemical events *preceding* behavior becomes possible. There is evidently a chemistry of intention and attention; as there is a chemistry of learning.

The picture, which is emerging in terms of chemical control systems, thus, already exceeds our early naive assumptions. To be sure, there are families of compounds. There are the adrenergic pathways related to norepinephrine and the dopamergic pathways related to dopamine coursing, through the brain stem and the Limbic System. They have been related, a little prematurely, perhaps, to the genesis of depression, and the functional pathology of schizophrenia. Behind these, however, stand the cholinesters and indolamines; and relatively simple amino acids, such as GABA in the cortex, and Glycine in the spinal cord, which exert very powerful and selective inhibitory influences. There are the effects of second generation compounds like the prostaglandins, possibly acting as secondary transmitters; and now, the breathless detective story of the endorphins, – "Novel peptides of brain and hypophyseal origin with opiate like activity" to use Guillemin and Bloom's phrase. We have all witnessed the pathbreaking developments now coming from the laboratories of Robert Guillemin and Floyd Bloom and their colleagues of this Institute, on the chemistry of these new chemical messengers produced by the brain. Thanks to this work, the brain now emerges as a huge organ of internal secretion, trafficking in small molecules eliciting very specific effects. The role of β-lipotropins as a prohormone, and the chemical and physiological characterisation of the five principal members of the endorphin group has now proceeded apace. The effects of β-endorphin on prolactin and growth hormone secretion, its predominantly inhibitory effects on many neurons, yet its significant, excitatory effects on the hippocampus and the behavioral effects in producing an apparently highly vigilant state of immobility, resembling catatonia in the experimental rat, suggest that new and very important guests have arrived at the party, and that the neurotransmitter conversation is likely to get, to say the least, animated. Conversation may be a useful term in this context. For if there be one overriding principle emerging from this stimulating confusion, it is the *interactive, and therefore, conditional nature of the chemical grammar of the brain.* Like words, these chemical states depend on context. What a particular substance will do to a cell, or a cell group, depends very much on what other substance is there, or has been there at about the same time. This applies to the interaction of the catecholamines with steroids, and neuroactive ions including lithium (an ion found very useful in the treatment of mania), or between acetylcholine and serotonin. Moreover, as has been shown in critical studies by Bloom and his colleagues, there is an exchange between signals at the cell membrane and a switch-on mechanism in the cell interior; the catecholamines, by way of adenylcyclase, influencing cyclic AMP, and, thus, affecting protein and glyco-lipoprotein synthesis. Add to this the suggestion that muco-polysaccharides at the cell surface may be related to specific encoding, and one has an idea how complex a term neuronal specificity has become. It cries out for a systems approach. There must be clearly both genetic and acquired labelling of the neuronal surface or interface, and the incorporation of specific recognizers or transponders (that is structures answering to interrogation) into the cell surface.

V. CHEMICALLY MEDIATED HOMEOSTASIS; THE EVOLUTION OF SYMBOLIC FORMS WITHIN THE BRAIN

What then is emerging is a picture of the brain as an exquisitely organized system of electrochemically mediated detectors and homeostats arranged in ascending fashion, roughly concentrically and rostrally around the mid line. Some areas are integrating, nodal, and widely connected, exerting profound effects on wide cell population all over the brain. The discriminate analysers, on the other hand, (in the cortex and cerebellum, for example) comprise a layered, laminar arrangement of cell sheets, which process and condense information from layer to layer by way of vertical cell columns. Programs are both fixed (so to speak, prewired), and continuously evolving. The fixed programs have proven organismic and species survival value, and are also used as referents in sensory analysis. The evolving programs encode and transmit ongoing, experience by non-genetic means.

There are clear indications of chemical specificity in some of the inborn fixed programs. There is, for example, chemical specificity for the sexual response depending on the incorporation, the fit so to speak, of specific steroids on to specific command cells in the hypothalamus. There are indicators for a chemistry of territoriality and aggression. Above all, thanks to our late Jim Olds and men like Larry Stein, and much collateral evidence, we are now getting to know something about the chemistry of those grand selectors in the learning process, reward and punishment, and by implication, the organizing power of positive and negative moods. Pleasure may be governed by the catecholamine and possibly, as was lately suggested by Stein, the endorphins. Again there is suggestive evidence for a regional chemistry involving the Raphe nuclei and the Nucleus Coeruleus in the stages of sleep, dreaming and wakefulness, with serotonin, the catecholamines and GABA playing important parts. There is evidence for sharp hormone fluctuations in blood and brain throughout the 24 hour cycle, a sort of chemical setting of the Circadian Clock. In any event the neurohumoral coding of these old inborn regulatory functions is remarkable for its rugged stability and high specificity in terms of molecular configuration. The same applies to genetically coded patterns in non-vertebrates.

The chemistry of learning, on the other hand, presents problems infinitely more complex. We do not yet rightly understand the chemical processes which make naive neurons informed neurons. The work of Kandel on the simple marine organism Aplysia, and of Agranoff on fish, is beginning to give us some clues as to the cellular basis of learning. Clearly some chemical labeling must take place. I have steadily held the view that the small molecules we have, so far considered may have something to do with the labelling of the junctional decision points at the neuron surface. Learning involves discrimination and specific recognition, therefore one must assume the presence of organelles on the cell surface which respond specifically to interrogation – we would say the presence of specific transponders. The mystery is how these Transponders are built up, and how membranes of widely separated cell groups can be discriminately labelled. It would seem likely that some active transfer of materials must take place from cell to cell, possibly by way of the neurotubules – a sort of trans-neural infectious process. Growth in the nervous system, therefore, carries with it specificity. The resemblance to tissue immune responses will not have escaped you. It is also possible that in recognition and the apprehension of redundancy some new thermo-dynamic principles may be involved of which so far we have only the dimmest notion. A holographic model has been suggested by Pribram. Let us remember that electricity was discovered by Galvani watching the twitch of a frog's leg.

To put it in another way, the simpler the brain, the more stereotype the response and the clearer the chemical coding. The larger the brain, the higher the redundancy, the more discriminate the selection, and the more massive the selective banking of the inappropriate and the irrelevant. It is this massive capacity to selectively delay, inhibit and ignore which makes decision and discriminate performance possible. In the mammalian brain, and particularly in the brain of man, learning implies the ability to construct and code at tremendous speed a series of successive transforms condensing more and more information into less and less. I have suggested elsewhere that these transforms employ shifting and highly discriminate inhibitory mechanisms in laminar cellular hierarchies in the elimination of redundant information; that they are matched for fit against stored programs, and, tested in a sort of internal rehearsal for aptive value to the organism, until a decision and commitment is either imagined, or enacted. The final product, thus, – be it a percept, or a motor act, or an "idea" – represents a condensed symbolic model of a succession of operations which always, always comprise informational traces – shared properties – of the antecedent phases in a temporally coded pattern. There is, in the brain, continuous communication, i.e., sharing of properties – matching, weighing, voting – and the operational use of electrochemical languages in these processes. To put it another way, there proceeds, in the brain, a continuous evolution, by natural selection, of symbolic forms, using communicating cell populations as ensembles. This evolution of informed cell assemblies, is, of course, non-genetic; and in man can be transferred from generation to generation in symbols in sight and sound. Languages, thus, appear to be used as the tools within and without the head. The number of bits of information which can be potentially processed by the brain is truly prodigious; it has been estimated as two to the power of ten trillion. The sensory or recollective funnel is very wide: the enactment is selective and narrow. It requires, as we say, focussing, inhibitory control and selective attention. We know from the work of Evarts and of Mountcastle of the extraordinary organizing power of this process of selective attention. It can be mobilised by a percept: but importantly it can be also organized – held in place, – by a firmly held disciplined, recollected memory or image. I will return to this aspect a little later; for I believe it to have important implications for both psychosomatic disorders, and the maintenance of personal well being.

Be it as it may, we know, as yet, little of the chemistry of learning in the adult. There are however, significant clues from learning in the immature and developing animal. There is now mounting evidence to suggest that early social experience, (e.g., play, separation, loneliness, and loss) is chemically transcribed. Social experience leads to enzyme induction, both in the acetylcholine system (Rosenzweig) and the catecholamine system (Bruce Welch) early separation and loss has chemical consequences. The relation to adult depression is still far from clear; but, in Homo sapiens, the long post-natal immaturity and the chemical plasticity of the nervous system, make him particularly vulnerable. Slowly we are beginning to see the outline, albeit, in a broad silhouette, not only of the chemistry of separation and loss, but potentially the chemistry of coping and of competence. The ability to cope is learnt early, and the chemical correlates of these early rehearsals for adult life are probably reflected in both brain and blood. I say brain and blood because, as we noted earlier, the brain is emerging as a formidable organ of internal secretion, trafficking both within itself into the cerebro spinal fluid, and by way of special portal arrangements, into the blood stream. The small molecules we mentioned, and particularly the oligopeptides are here to stay; they clearly influence the response to stress, are concerned with pain and pleasure, reward and punishment; but also, as shown by De Wied, play a part in learning. The economy of this functional arrangement, with giant prohormone molecules yielding specific fragments, code words, so to speak, is awesome in its economy and beauty. Hans Selye speaks of stress, distress and eu-stress; within a decade or less, it should be possible to put chemical name and number alongside such concepts.

VI. SOME PRACTICAL CONSEQUENCES

The practical consequences of these discoveries flow deeply into biological psychiatry. In the past, we used to intervene, then speculate and infer; the fit now is much closer; and the blunderbuss chemical hammer is slowly giving way to discriminating specific probes. In a few lucky instances we have even inferential indicators of the processes predominantly affected. The catecholamine deficiency hypothesis of depression, and the dopamine hypothesis of schizophrenia are beginnings in this respect. They are sure to be revised, but have yielded valuable guidelines in the design of clinically useful drugs. Gradually psychopharmacology is edging closer to its mother source – physiology – and in so doing is baring a working principle which may, seem a little strange to the classically trained pharmacologist. For whereas in peripheral organ pharmacology we see compounds with a single overriding and highly specific property, the psychoactive drugs appear more likely to be *sharers of* several properties; and skill in drug design rests often around changing the proportions of these various effects – for example, anticholinergic vis-...-vis dopaminergic properties in the phenothiazines. In view of what we said of interplay and *inter*action of small molecules in the central nervous system, this is hardly surprising.

However, administering a drug is one thing; drawing inferences from the assay of hormones and metabolites in blood and urine is a more hazardous procedure. Such fluctuations, may only palely reflect central events, which involve highly localized, formidably shielded cell groups in the brain. Fortunately, however, the field looks less forbidding than even a decade ago. There are metabolites like MHPG, which reflect central, rather than peripheral turnover. There is the possibility of using stable-isotope labeled materials in man. Quite possibly, also, we may come upon peripheral enzyme systems (such as monoamine oxidase and catechol-O-methyl transferase in blood elements) which may serve as genetic markers in the patients' families. If alongside, one were to put the wide range of specific metabolic loading procedures (precursors, specific inhibitors and the like) one obtains an idea of how useful these methods could eventually be in defining specific psychophysiological patterns of reactivity. Already in the study of the affective disorders, or the schizophrenias (and, even, potentially in disorders of the senium), there are indications of metabolic imbalances which may distinguish subgroups within a given syndrome in terms of individual reaction patterns to a given chemical load. If one were to begin to combine such metabolic studies with systematic studies of stress responsiveness, and graded performance, one could, while monitoring physiological responses, also establish quantitative threshold responses to particular drugs. The interaction between the phenothiazines and prolactin secretion is a case in point. Slowly, thus, one is beginning to approach what one might call *Psycho-Chemical Diagnostic Procedures.* A Space Age Technology awaits to be used; and in our lifetime such psychochemical screening procedures may well become a routine admission procedure for patients, and provide a rational basis for diagnosis, therapy and even new drug design. Let me venture another aside in this context These response patterns may cut clearly through cozy conventional diagnostic nosologics, and define much more accurately and operationally levels of functional integration of the states of consciousness which we know as mental order or disorder. Thus, I believe that we may be standing on the threshold of a new taxonomy of mental disorders, drawing upon a deeper biological understanding of both function, and dysfunction. We should also be able to identify at-risk populations more readily.

VII. ASPECTS OF SUBJECTIVE OBSERVATION

You will have noted in all we have so far said that it rests on objective observation. Such observation looks from without, and infers the within. The data, as we say are consensually validated; the knowledge is public knowledge.

There are however, aspects of knowledge only inadequately covered by the instrumental approach. Perhaps, an extreme example will serve to make the point:

> On the day after Christmas, in 1799, young Humphry Davy, twenty years old, made the following note following a self-experiment with nitrous oxide which he had carried out in his laboratory in the company of one, Dr. Kinglake (Davy 1800): "I felt a sense of tangible extension, highly pleasurable in every limb; my visible impressions were dazzling, and apparently magnified. I heard distinctly every sound in the room, and was perfectly aware of my situation. I lost all connection with external things; trains of vivid images rapidly passed through my mind, and even connected with words in such a manner, as to produce perceptions perfectly novel. I existed in a world of newly connected and newly modified

ideas. I theorized; I imagined that I made discoveries. I was awakened from the semi-delirious trance by Dr. Kinglake who took the (gas) bag from my mouth, indignation and pride was the first feelings produced by the sight of persons about me. My emotions were enthusiastic and sublime; and for a minute I walked about the room perfectly regardless of what was said to me. As I recovered my former state of mind, I felt an inclination to communicate the discoveries I had made during the experiment. I endeavored to recall the ideas, they were feeble and indistinct; one collection of terms, however, presented itself: and with the most intense belief and prophetic manner, I explained to Dr. Kinglake – 'Nothing exists but thoughts' – the universe is composed of impressions, ideas, pleasures and pains."

In one bold empirical step, thus, young Davy had revealed the power of an anesthetic not only to obtund, but to enhance sensation, and to manifest aspects of mental life only sparingly used in normal waking existence: the features he described are common enough in such states: the intensity of personal feeling, the heightened perception, the connectedness among things disconnected, the synesthesia (i.e., the evocation of one sensory modality by another), the fusion, the poetical feeling of devotion, of identity, the sense of insight and truth; and, above all, the incommunicability of the experience except in metaphor and allusion. A number of drugs have shared this power to evoke and to transcend. Intense religious experiences have been linked to the ritual use of mescaline and cohoba. De Quincey and Coleridge chewed opium. In France there were the "Hashishiens", and in England, the "ether revelations" of Benjamin Blood. The chemical divining rod was thus found useful; and its the modern sequelae, from LSD-to DMT are well known.

I mention this chemical path, trodden by many, to draw attention to a quieter way which, at any rate in medicine was sought by relatively few until the turn of the century. For coincident in time with the above observation, there were others centering on subjective phenomena experienced without chemical aids and sharing with drug-induced states their intensely personal, private, averbal and incommunicable nature. Mentioned here may be the early observations of Johannes Müller (1848) on the so-called hypnagogic phenomena – experiences any of us know in the brief twilight states between wakefulness and sleep; or the analysis at the hands of Frederick Galton, the father of medical genetics, of what he called "Visions of Sane Persons" (1881) and the "Statistics Mental Imagery" (1880). In 1896 Weir Mitchell published his account of mescaline intoxication, observed in himself; and it is of interest to compare this account with Ladd's account on so-called "Visual Dreams" published four years earlier (Ladd 1892). Hovering over the field, but still very much at the periphery of medicine, there was the concept of unconscious or preconscious mental activity. Thus, there is Carus, writing, in 1846, on the "Developmental History of the Soul"; von Hartmann, in 1869, on the "Philosophy of the Unconscious"; Fechner (1860), Helmholtz (1863), and Wundt (1862) speculating and experimenting on perception and threshold states of consciousness; and Carpenter laying down his "Principles of Mental Physiology" in 1874. Towering over others are the figures of Titchener (1909) and William James, who regarded Benjamin Blood's "Ether Dreams" (1874) as a stepping stone in his own thinking (James 1912). Indeed, much that went before culminates in James; and the titles of his essays; "The Varieties of Religious Experience" (1901), "A Pluristic Mystic" (1912) and "The Stream of Thought" (1890), tell their own tale. In his preoccupations with subjective phenomena (while incidentally building the first Experimental Psychology Laboratory at Harvard), he significantly deviated from the principal paths of nineteenth century science. As he says in his well-known quotation:

"What must be admitted is that the definite images of traditional psychology form but the smallest part of, our minds as they actually live. The traditional psychology talks like one who should say a river consists of nothing but pailsful, spoonfuls, quartpotsful, barrelsful and other moulded forms of water. Even were the pails and pots all actually standing in the stream, still between them the free water would continue to flow. It is just this free water of consciousness that psychologists resolutely overlook. Every definite image in the mind is steeped and dyed in the free water that flows round it. With it goes the sense of its relations, near and remote, the dying echo whence it came to us, and the dawning sense whither it is to lead." (1890)

These "echoes", and this "dawning sense" of knowing, is, as we saw in Davy's description, not unfamiliar in the drug-induced experience; and it is these private, subjective, personal and incommunicable elements which rendered chemical devices so useful for purposes of religious rites. Somehow, then, it appeared, even in the nineteenth century, as though certain functional modalities which are part and parcel of the repertoire of human experience, but normally used only transitorily and sparingly in the waking state, could be chemically locked by drugs into more persistent manifestations. One would hesitate to claim identity among these various processes, there is, however, a family resemblance. The changes observed more recently, in sensory isolation and in hypnosis attest to this affinity to this day. Hypnosis was used by Charcot in his studies on hysteria. Charcot's "lessons" were attended by many; Babinsky, Binet, Janet, Marie; and of course, Freud. In 1893, Breuer and Freud published their preliminary communication on hysteria stating quite simply, that "hysterics suffer mainly from reminiscences." The repressed, affectively laden memory trace thus emerged not only as a subjective phenomenon welling up randomly in dreams or in drug-induced states, but as a clinical entity, capable of affecting sensorimotor or visceromotor function. The exteriorization of the subjective memory into overt behavior (coupled, at a later date, with the concept of "acting-out" in a transference situation), assumed therapeutic as well as theoretical implications. Psychoanalysis and psychosomatics were thus cast in the same mold, psychoanalytic theory attempting to provide a conceptual link between subjective experience and overt behavior. We are not here concerned with the validation or otherwise of the theory. What we would rather note are the many modifications at the hands of its originator which it underwent, emphasizing its tentative and empirical nature; and the minute serial observations of subjective states of mind over time, on which it was based.

VIII. PHYSICS, AND THE FUNCTION OF LANGUAGE IN SCIENCE

Discoveries such as these, however, fitted ill with the brash innocence of a young emergent materialist science. An age set firmly in the framework of classical physics, wedded to the meter rule, the clock, and the kilogram, secure in its concept of space, time, matter and causality, and propelled by the idea of evolution: such an age did not readily accept introspection as a source of evidence, or behaviour as a phenomenon in its own right. Matter was the primary reality; and the studies of its properties – living or dead, silent or articulate – were judged the proper objectives of science. Physiology, though recognizing homeostasis and the self-regulatory properties of living systems, was wedded to chemistry and physics; and the inventiveness of the Russian schools of neurophysiology, leading to the evolution of the Pavlovian method, while providing penetrating techniques for the analysis of behaviour, did not have the backing of present day neurobiology and mathematics to enable it to realize its full yield. Yet, as it is well known in retrospect, forces of quite another kind were at work in that same age. The concept of the electromagnetic field – so new to a period preoccupied with the mechanical motion of matter – was consequent upon Michael Faraday's experiments. In 1856, the year of Freud's birth, Clerk Maxwell published his equations on Faraday's lines of force. It was the same Maxwell who, in his paper on "Atoms" for the Encyclopedia Britannica (Maxwell 1874) wrote:

> "There are thus two modes of thinking about the constitution of bodies which have had their adherents both in ancient and modern times. They correspond to two methods of regarding quantity – the arithmetical and the geometrical. To the Atomist the true method of estimating the quantity of matter in a body is to count the atoms in it. To those who identify matter with extension, the volume of space occupied by a body is the only measure of quantity in it."

Clerk Maxwell's ideas were followed by Ernst Mach's "Die Mechanik" (1897), in which Mach questioned Newton's definition of space and the concept of absolute rest. (It is, incidentally, the same Ernst Mach who in 1886 published his "Analysis of Sensations, and the Relation of the Physical to the Psychical", and who by implication, influenced the development of Gestalt Psychology.) What followed is well told by the men who partook of the change (Einstein 1934, Bohr 1958, Heisenberg 1958). Within three decades, the theory of relativity was established and quantum mechanics was in being. Probability and chance had entered into the definition of the state of physical systems; and the concepts of "complementarity" of mutually exclusive states was found to be a productive and substantially workable model in the description of the fine structure of matter. As Heisenberg dryly observes, "the possibility of playing with different complementary pictures has its analogy in the different transformation of the mathematical scheme; it does not lead to any difficulties." There is a profound truth in this fit of phenomenon, and statement about the phenomenon.

I have dwelt briefly on these developments in turn of the century physics because, in a way which, at least to me, is far from clear, they may well bear upon the evolutionary forces now at work in neurobiology, and the biology of behaviour. I do not mean here the mere cracking of a crust of certainty by the expanding root of doubt. The dialectics of the processes go deeper. What appears significant is that while denying subjective observation of fluid, multiple phenomena as a source of valid data, and forcing overt behaviour into a materialistic frame which fitted it ill, that same frame – rigid, formidable, buttressed by the enormity of its industrial product – underwent a loosening and expansion which, within a few brief decades, presaged a new age. Concepts, strangely familiar, yet never rigorously applied to behaviour were being quietly incorporated into mathematical statements concerning the structure of matter. What had been regarded as universal statements (such as Newtonian mechanics and Euclidean geometry) were reduced to special instances of statements of even greater validity. States regarded as mutually exclusive, were assumed, in Weizscker's timely phrase, to coexist. The mathematical scheme of quantum theory expanded the tenets of classical logic, the concepts of "either/or" giving way to the "also" and the "and", making classical logic a province of quantum logic. The deliberately open, probabilistic, mathematical statements were found, in the light of experiment, to provide a more precise description of reality than older and more circumscribed rules. Above all – and from the point of view which we are considering most important – a mathematical language for mechanics which had to serve the varied needs of the theoretician, the experimental physicist, the technician, and the engineer was treated more discretely, new symbolic inventions serving the needs of fine structure of matter and older devices remaining in use to run trains and to heat buildings. As with Berzelius' (1779–1848) invention of a formal shorthand for chemistry, it is the evolution of a new, and appropriate language which made modern physics what it is.

I suppose that whether we like it or not, we have now arrived at a crucial point in our discussion. For if behaviour is to be described in a way accurate enough to predict its attributes; if subjective experience is to be conveyed even to oneself, in terms which clearly and strongly apprehend its significance and meaning, languages are required to model and symbolize the processes with which they are concerned. The capacity and limitations of language have been examined in a most searching way by Roman Jacobson, and in a different idiom by Susanne Lange and Noam Chomsky; to them I am deeply indebted.

There can be little dispute of the attributes of language. Language is "our most faithful and indispensable picture of human experience" (Langer), a heuristic symbolic instrument shaping modes of observation and interpretation, and interpenetrating deeply with experience. Phonemes and morphemes condense meaning into words, and the relation between word symbols is regulated by rules of syntax and grammar. Such rules – rules of astonishing logic and economy – go, as Whorf showed (1956) into the fabric of even the most primitive language. They make for the smooth use of language as an instrument of social adaptation and communication, and make it the discursive, narrative instrument it has become.

There is, however, another quality in words implicit in the one just discussed. For, while carrying certain meanings in one context, words carry a totally different meaning in another; and even standing alone they may – as anyone who has traced the origin of a word in a dictionary – carry an accretion of different meanings in a sort of strange calculus of their own. This economy, this logic, this dependence on context is characteristic even of the most primitive language; it is also at the very heart of the poetic allusion. The german word for poet is "Dichter" from Dicht (dense) – a condenser of meaning. Words are, thus, not mere labels, cards, stacked for reference in one of Broca's four areas; they are states, sets, depending on relation, and context; they carry multiple meaning. Carnap, in "The Logical Syntax of Language" (1937), has examined the capacity for expression of any given linguistic system. What is remarkable in that analysis is how little our ordinary means of communication measures up to the standard of meaning which a serious philosophy of language, and hence a logic of discursive thought, demands.

It would thus seem that there are large areas in communication and in self-communication (i.e., the symbol making not exteriorized in overt behavior) which are not represented by ordinary language. For whereas grammar and speech are essentially sequential, linear and discursive, the characteristic of these other subjective states is the multiple simultaneous presentation of internalized object and relations. The form of the "unspeakable" is as different from the "speakable" as the structure of a dream, or even a day dream, is from the structure of deliberate action. In such symbolic forms, totality is apprehended simultaneously at different levels; mutually occlusive elements coexist; time is of no consequence; and serial *ordering* in time, that backbone of causal reasoning, gives way to simultaneously perceived relationships. The philosophy of language tends to dismiss this type of presentational activity as falling into the sphere of subjective experience, emotion, and feeling. As Russell (1927) put it: "Our confidence in language is due to the fact that it shares … the structure of the physical world. Perhaps that is why we know so much physics and so little of anything else."

I would submit that we know so little of that large "anything else" because, all too often, we have tried to force inappropriate languages and methods on phenomena in which they have no business. Nor is a relegation of such matters to the mystique of intuition at all helpful. There is nothing mystical, for example, about the work of George Boole, the inventor of Boolian algebra, who in his "Investigation of Laws of Thought", "The Mathematical Analysis of Logic" (1847) examined, as he put it, the ability of symbols to express propositions, "the laws of whose combination should be founded upon the laws of mental processes which they represent." In searching for such outward representation, he invented the theory of classes and sets and the nonassociative relations between them, devising a symbolic algebraic shorthand for the expression of these relations in which concepts such as product, complement, inclusion and a number of others are clearly represented.

Boole's path-breaking contributions led by way of Frege (1879), Jevons (1864), Peirce (1880) to Whitehead and Russell's "Principia" (1910–1913) in our day, and in a sort of branch line on to the theorems of Godel and Tarski. One may note, in passing, the titles of some of these earlier works. Jevons named his work "Pure Logic, or the Logic of Quality Apart from Quantity." Frege called his study a Begriffschrift – a "Formula Language (Formelsprache)" or pure thought. Somehow the inexpressible, the suggestive qualities which, in other circumstances, we would call intuitive, grew into communicable notations and symbols of great propulsive power; and opened a world of relations hitherto considered closed. It is outside my competence to examine the influence of Boolian algebra on modern experimental physics. However, the relation of a theory of sets and classes to communication and information transfer in the brain is nearer at hand. For the very word "communication" (from "communicare") implies, as we saw, sharing – i.e. the sharing of properties; and any encoding process depends upon the apprehension of such shared properties among sets and classes. It is by this sharing, too, that redundancy, far from being wasteful, serves in the transfer of information; redundancy provides context and thus minimizes error; it is a safety device – reserve – in the flow of information (Mackay 1961); a reserve, incidentally, amply encountered in all biological systems.

Yet how interdependent are demands of a subject, and the demands of a language for a subject. When chemistry, or electrical engineering needed appropriate symbolic forms of notation, such systems were duly invented; and when turn of the century physics felt constrained by Newtonian mechanics, it was modified according to need. However, so young is biology as a science, and so much younger still is the biology of mental phenomena (which we will call psychobiology) that its great discoveries were made, using a linguistic apparatus leased from chemistry and physics, and from the language of every day use. This hybrid arrangement has served for a time; no one will deny the many advances made so far. Nevertheless, it is clear that demands of quite a different order are pressing on the biology of our day. Interaction in macromolecular systems, and the control mechanisms inherent in such systems, are evidently of a different order from reactions between simple inorganic compounds; any accounting for the flow of information in such systems (as, for example, in the obvious instances of the gene or the immunological specificity of proteins) demands a language in which mere chemical or descriptive language is no longer sufficient. Woodger (1952) had indeed attempted to define the elements of a concise formal language for some aspects of genetics and evolutionary theory; and Roman Jacobson has done so quite recently. – A difficult but enormously worthwhile task.

It is the fortunate, if embarrassing, feature of the phenomena of behavior and of mental life that by their very nature, they brook less compromise in such matters than any other branch of biology. The purely physical and chemical analogies do not hold; and the psychochemical correlates demand, as we have seen, a much more detailed specification and description of behaviour, and of concomitant chemical change, than is currently available. For behaviour implies multiple simultaneous change of a system in time, and *form* in behaviour is really a topology in time. Discursive, linear, metric language does not apprehend such patterns, Presentational, experiential language suggests intricate simultaneous nonlinear relationships, but does not define them. Yet it is the characteristic of every culture that it has invented symbols for such subjectively experienced relationships; it is significant, too, that in its own evolution, physics (and the branch of mathematics known as topology) has developed a shorthand for the apprehension of cognate simultaneous relations in the so-called outside physical world.

IX. LANGUAGE, AND INTERHEMISPHERIC RELATIONS

Could it, thus, be that in behavior and the analysis of subjective experience we could see if we wish to look most clearly and cogently the laws of thought of which Boole spoke and which govern our understanding of the physical world? And could it be that the two uses of language which we distinguish represent – as in Clark Maxwell's double definition of quantity – two complementary ways: one multiple and simultaneous and another serial, and successive, by which the brain constructs its models of reality? All we know of the respective functions of the right and left hemisphere from the seminal studies of Sperry and Bogen to the recent developmental studies, including those of Sandra Witelson, suggest that we do indeed carry two complementary organs of information in our head. The right hemisphere appears to apprehend shapes, relationships and simultaneous configurations. It can handle many data all at once; its access to memory stores is rich. It functions best when the doors of perception are ajar or closed – as in the day dream, the dream, the untrammeled flow of fantasy. It is, if you will, the lobe which is inwardly aware.

The left hemisphere is concerned much more with analytic and linear operations: it abstracts, eliminates, sequences, groups, maps action into temporal order, and enacts its plans. Far more than the right lobe, it depends on selective attention. It is outwardly vigilant, locked to perception, – as we would say, attentive and appropriate.

That our brain should have created two huge special organs to handle these two aspects of knowing, suggest that there is something pretty basic about this relatively simple complementary arrangement. We will also note that whereas awareness is private, action is public; and that whereas awareness can be self sufficient, action is usually linked to control, and to power. Awareness uses feelings as a powerful source of knowledge. The narrative blueprint of instrumental technology, on the other hand, views feeling as a source of error. Yet – as we said at the beginning – in human life, unaided feeling states are powerful sources of knowledge, signifying congruence, fit and appropriateness, or lack of such fit. They are signals of whether total communication in the organism, is *in* order, or *out* of order. Pain – physical or mental – signifies incongruity, separateness, distancing – the part being a-part, out of phase with the whole. Anxiety carries the message of a problem awaiting solution, of continuing rehearsal, until a solution is found. And pleasure signifies wholeness, harmony and well-being. The quality which we know as the quality of life would appear to be closer to awareness and organismic self sufficiency, than to the objective products of life instrumental. It is closer to awareness and self control than "other" control, to self regulation rather than "other" regulation, to autonomy rather than outer directedness. To being rather than having.

X. TOWARDS COMPETENCE AND WELL-BEING

Now it is curious that at this time, both in the neurosciences and in inquiries into awareness, there is a convergence into a shared interest in some areas of personal coping and functioning. In the remainder of the time I would like to touch upon this aspect; it is what one might call an understanding of the roots of competence and the biology of well-being.

We have already noted how neuropharmacology is edging us to source – to physiology – and how all we know, and are about to know of the brain as an organ of internal secretion emphasizes its extraordinary powers of compensating restitution and self regulation in the *absence* of outside chemical prostheses. The brain informs and is informed to the farthest corners of the organism; and by way of its distance receptors, and instrumental extension of its biological organs, can scan deep, deep into the universe. Within the skin it guides internal organs securely along their way; it regulates generalized responses to assault and invasion; it regulates immune responses; it regulates healing. It is, we will admit, a brilliantly comprehensive health care system, encasing its messages in relatively simple chemical code.

We have earlier examined the implications of the neurosciences, for the understanding of some forms of mental disorder; but beyond the mental disorder lies the whole field of mental *order,* and the dormant knowledge of a chemistry of coping and of competence. Here I confess the line between what is pleasurable and what is desirable becomes thin and precarious; for whereas one would wholly subscribe to a true physiology of well-being, one would hesitate to further its pharmacology unless it was physiologically rooted. The body has a way of reacting to untoward chemical intrusion, as the effects of cortisone on ATCH secretion well illustrates. There is justifiable reaction against the chronic use of analgesics and hypnotics and mild antidepressants, through self medication. Dependence travels in many guises; and I for one, positively abhor the idea of a happiness pill. Yet I cannot but hope that research in to successful coping and well-being, from its genesis in the rehearsals of infancy and childhood, to its sustenance in maturity and old age, will be taken as seriously at research into the psychobiology of depressive disorders and schizophrenia. What, we could ask, are the hormonal and neurohormonal consequences of adequate work and fulfillment? Of physical exercise, which notoriously affects mood? Of rest and recreation? Of play, and above all of simply and quietly being oneself? What are the hormonal differences between compulsively taken vacation, and truly and deeply taking time out to reassess priorities and values, and perhaps to rearrange one's life? How do the parents of children, of healthy families differ biochemically from families notoriously under stress? The family, after all, is still the principal school of Homo sapiens. Why do some families share both joy and pain and even in uncertainty, while others rage, or hurt, or cut-off? Why, among the older, do some stay young and others wither early? We will note in passing that studies such as these require an alliance between laboratory methods and work carried deeply into daily life. Only by making the consumer the sharer and potential beneficiary can one hope to develop the kind of open and cooperative partnership between the research and the consumer. This would give such work the social significance it potentially holds. In this Institute, the similarity of this approach and preventive vaccination will not have escaped you. For such applied research gently merges with health education, aiming at an informed consumer-client. It is out of such studies that physiologically based restitutive procedures and compounds may emerge. After all, vitamins and mega-vitamins, have been on the average breakfast table for some time. Who knows what FDA approved food additives junior, will take a decade hence?

Whether such physiological additives will lead to a chemical extension of known physiologically boundaries in man, we do not really know. Recent symposia have examined the portents of the psychochemical revolution, probable or otherwise. Clearly drugs are already at hand which affect fertility; others are close which may influence sexual desire and sexual performance. There are the drugs which influence hunger and pain; there are drugs which physiologically affect the sleep cycle. The circadian clock could be conceivably manipulated to a 48 hour day, and there is a possibility to chemically induced long hibernation. The counterpart of prolonged feats of physical endurance can also be envisaged. Equally, the potential chemical enhancement of attention and of learning ability and overall intelligence, is certainly conceivable. There is, as we saw, suggestive evidence of the relation of protein synthesis to the consolidation of the memory trace and to neuronal sprouting and growth. The implications for our mounting geriatric population in this respect are quite obvious. In sum, the neurosciences have made their point; their achievements over so short a time have been stupendous, and their future looks bright indeed.

XI. INNER AWARENESS AND COMPETENCE. SELF REGULATION AND BEHAVIORAL MEDICINE

Yet it is a sobering fact that despite these dazzling insights, and technological advances, our culture should abound in all manner of strange and profoundly significant experiments and movements, emphasizing awareness and direct *personal* experience rather than objective knowing by way of the tools of conventional science. In centers, practically all of them significantly outside of academia, elaborate methods are being developed to guide people to be themselves, alone, or in small groups. The methods may vary; so may setting and the relative emphasis on negative and positive affects, and the means of their expression. But again, and again common ingredients emerge, all aimed at enhancing awareness, genuineness; truthful and direct contact with feelings as sources of knowledge, and contact with one's body as a sort of memory bank of feelings. These techniques make use of altered states of inner attention. They use guided imagery in waking, or twilight states to evoke feeling states and the somatic correlates of such states. At their best, they are experienced as profoundly healing. Clearly these phenomena have a deep biology of their own, the regularities of which we are just beginning to emerge.

Equally, there is another area emerging in parallel. Body language techniques are returning after being banished to the closets of faddism. Stance, posture, gait, the appropriate use of one's own weight, the systematic training of sensory acuity, and of hand/eye coordination are being developed to enhance the enteroceptive and proceptive vocabulary of the individual, using their own body as a source of awareness. Much inventiveness is going into these approaches, and many unusual and strange phenomena will no doubt be discovered as they continue to be used. All this is not new – the East has always regarded the body as a planet worthy of exploration. There is in these exercises great slowness and deliberation, great discipline, great beauty; there is also a clear engagement, and a disciplined use of selective attention. In these deeper states, there are levels of concentration in which communication by "ordinary" language is clearly inappropriate, and where visceral function is profoundly altered. These states of meditation and deep concentration show striking shifts in physiological measures. In terms of information processing, it would seem that they are characterized by a gradual change in selective attention, and that the perceptual process is, so to speak, pushed back in reverse. Information, in these states is, as Tart observes, "state specific."

But to the neuroscientist there is, even at this early stage, one thing distinctly familiar about these states; for it is quite clear that the brain, unaided by any chemical prostheses, can induce huge autonomic shifts in the organism through well defined inner learning procedures. The neurobiologist will note that respiration – the only autonomic function under control, and one strikingly sensitive to the endorphins is evolved in these training procedures – and that energy demands and sensitivity to oxygen lack is reduced. He will also observe that the training instructions, if carefully followed, involve a deliberate training of selective attention, with an increasing shutting-out of sensory impressions, of memory traces, a desidentification from obsessionally recurrent ideas, a cultivation of non-intrusive emptiness, and the deliberate training of muscle groups and of blood vessels, of heart into states which spell calm, rest, and a deep sense of acceptance and *allowing*. Muscle groups and viscera appear to have, of their own learning, curves in these states. The results, so far, suggest that these training procedures are beneficial in a wide variety of stress induced disorders, from hypertension to disorders of peripheral circulation, such as Raynaud's disease. What is also impressive is the evidence on the coupling of this internal learning to monitoring devices displaying autonomic activity to the subject while the subject engaged in such is learning. I am, of course, referring to biofeedback, about which a great deal has been written of late. Here the instrumentation is an important training tool, and one often abandoned when training reaches criterion. It is simply, a special case of a general principle. Self regulation is clearly possible: self regulation depends on awareness of visceral signals, either displayed or perceived. Images and cognitive structures held firmly in the mind, attitudes, and will can powerfully influence the body's internal economy. To be more aware makes it possible to choose, and to act on a choice. To be more aware makes it possible to choose, and to act on a choice. To be more aware means to be less afraid, more competent, more non-dependent. There is clearly healing power in the imagination, provided one befriends it.

Now, it is a curious thing that, in every religion, irrespective of origin or culture, phenomena such as we are describing have been at the center of devotional practices, and that the healing powers of these states has been fused with the traditional healing powers of the physician-priest. Placebo, you will say. But then, in Heaven's name, what is the placebo, and why does it work?

I have, over the past few months, with the aid of able guides like Dan Goleman and Charles Tart and William Brown been trying to read myself into descriptions of the various stages of Eastern concentration exercise. It is like poring over medieval maps of the Ottoman Empire. The continents are in place, their shape and outline look very familiar, though the projections by our coordinates seem off. As one reads one marvels at the detail of self observation and the patience of the training. For thousands of years men have clearly traveled in these strange lands.

In view of what we saw these lands beckon to be visited by modern man, and the modern neuro- and psychological sciences are ready to do just that. Skills of inner observation, skills of notation, skills of communication and of recording are needed, and can be best developed in closely knitted small groups. Some fifteen years ago I suggested the creation, of what I then called "Inner Space Laboratories", to study and develop operational definition of altered states of awareness and attention, which are clearly of enormous value to the organism. Such laboratories could nurture a species of Inner Space Observers – I called them "Intronauts" – to whom the strange territories of inner life are as familiar as the Australian Reef is to the divers of Jean Cousteau. Such an endeavor would require close cooperation between psychiatrists, psychologists, linguists, mathematicians, and communication engineers. It may require training of one discipline in the skills of the other. It will require much debate, and much true trial and error. Yet, the history of science suggests that once such a beginning is made progress can be quite rapid. It may not be too much to hope that concepts only partly or inadequately covered by present day languages, may before very long find a more adequate expression in new symbolic systems of greater precision and power. The usefulness of such systems may, and I would venture to say, will, not be confined to the study of behavior, or subjective experience. For the phenomena presented by these states pose in a most poignant way some fundamental issues in the organization of information-sharing among symbolic systems which we know as innovation, and creativity. My physicist friends tell me, that their mathematical insights require, as they put it, "a sort of peculiar state" to manifest; they appear to be readied deeply in the unconscious. It would be nice to known a little more: though I still think that a walk on the bluff is a pretty good laboratory exercise.

Let me add a practical element – the term "Inner Space Laboratories" is not quite apt; for it conveys a sort of isoteric isolation; yet, to me the promise of such enterprises is precisely the opposite. For essentially we are still talking about levels and degrees of awareness and their value in applying such knowledge to daily life. In this respect we are caught in a dilemma. For our fragmented health care system is essentially a passive sickness centered system and has done little to shift the incentive for personal well-being from the system to the person. Yet, health incentives, health enhancement, and preventive health care, are clearly what the future portends, and they must, to my mind, be best based in experimental learning by all of us at first hand. By and large we are still only dimly aware of the control we can have over our own well-being, provided we hearken the signals of body and mind, and develop personal listening for the incentives and for the enhancement of our own well-being. The day need not be a day blindly followed or passively enjoyed. Awareness is a quality which can make a day truly shine: and the skills for the training of awareness, for pacing one's activities, for self management, and self regulation, for following naturally the deep rhythms which our chemistry dictates are beginning to be defined. They can be taught and can be learnt. Some of us call this self regulation and health enhancement, some self-care; some behavioral medicine. A huge technology, from self-report and self monitoring to the videodisc stands ready to draw upon ancient knowledge, rooted deep in our biology, to help people to become more competent and caring for their own personal house. As we move into Jonas Salk's Epoch B this informed responsible self care is bound to grow very rapidly. In immunological terms, we are talking of the active enhancement of individual psychobiological competency, rather than transient *passive* immunisation – a challenging but immensely worth while task.

XII. CLOSING

We have, in a sense, come full circle. We began by considering the structure and geometry of the brain in relation to a regional chemical organization of its interconnected parts; and ended by examining, in admittedly broadest terms, the possible relation of symbolic functions to chemical coding devices used by the brain. We mentioned that connectivity in the central nervous system is chemically specific, and that learning, particularly in the early developmental period depended in such specific connectivity. We considered that hormones of known chemical composition apparently code innate forms of behavior; that simple chemical substances may, by their interplay influence the acquisition, storage, and flow of information within the central nervous system. We mentioned that the rhythms of our biological clocks and waking and sleeping may be chemically mediated, and that the mood disorders, such as depression, or thought disorders, such as schizophrenia may have their chemical counterpart. We felt that such knowledge already provided the footings for a future rational therapy of these disorders; and we considered the implications this knowledge of the brain's chemical economy in the enhancement of competencies, and personal well-being. Throughout we examined the fundamental role of language – be it a chemical transcript or an ensemble of symbols invented by man – as a propulsive force in evolution, and the place of communication, that is the process of recognizing and sharing hidden likenesses, and using them in new combinations as a basic rule of biological growth.

In all these phenomena we have, I hope, come to regard the brain and its environment as one. The brain detects, codes, reflects, and fashions its environment all at once. In a way, I suppose we have looked at possible ways in which symbolic forms could evolve in the teeming cell population in the central nervous system – former very tiny, yet immensely powerful, capable not only of representing, but, in the case of man, decisively fashioning his environment. The variety and stability of these forms is stupendous and it is man's unique capacity to pass them from generation to generation which has made human heredity radically and qualitatively different from other species, and human culture the outstanding biological reality of this planet. We do not at all know what chemical selectional pressures were at work to bring about the development of the human nervous system; but as we have seen, are getting at least the beginnings of a working knowledge as to the ways in which it can influence somatic and symbolic function in man. In such studies, the phenomena become their own witness, and their own instrument; the richness and subtlety of subjective phenomena defy objective instrumentation, which is developing apace. New languages, and, I would repeat, particularly new mathematical languages *are* needed. In this respect, science merely shows the earmarks of its own evolution. To understand symbols, new symbols have to be invented: the evolution of science is merely the evolution of languages of science. Thus, physicists and mathematicians in our field would be most welcome – and the sooner the better.

That such knowledge may pose an ethical dilemma is evident; yet it is far from evident that this ethical dilemma is more special, more poignant, more urgent than in the growth of any area of new knowledge.

For the concepts of Good and Evil, and of Choice are inherent in any evolving biological system; and go to the marrow of science itself. Evolution always compels choices; evolution in gene populations chooses genes of high adaptive value, making these choices laboriously and, as we say, blindly over many generations, resulting in the "good" of identical or near identical populations. In man things are different. His ability to map and model his environment with reasonable accuracy has made it possible to bypass genetic mutation and transfer new knowledge in prodigious amounts. We are apt to forget how young these qualities are. Roughly a million years or less for toolmaking, 50.000 years for social organization, and agriculture; 7.000 years or so for written languages; 300 odd years for modern science. Cultural and social evolution is, a direct product of science; and we have only to look around us to see the staggering acceleration of cultural evolution, compared with biological evolution.

This evolution has always involved choices, necessitated by adaptation. For our science is human science: its core is subjective – in the last analysis, all our experience is profoundly subjective, and its power rests in its ability to achieve consensus by way of validation – a sharing, as we say, of evidence. What is shared is seen as true; what is not shared, or not validated is seen as freak or false. Integrity, truthfulness is the cement of science. So far, this truthfulness is shared in the physical and bench sciences through shared special instruments and special languages. But in the field of psychobiological and social reality – human social biology, if you will, – it is a little different. As we said our perceptions are apt to be at once more direct more distorted. For as truth is perceived about our relation to each other, and the origin of these relations, the principles of social adaptation are beginning to look more and more like the ancient truths which every culture has enshrined in its religions to ensure its own survival. These rules we know as moral principles – rules rooted deep in the biology of systems. Life, it would seem, is being oneself with others; community is sharing; and science – even if it starts as a game of solitaire in the single inventive mind – is a social game, played by social rules. Human knowledge, single or complex, individual or social, is linked to choice. Choice is the watershed which separates knowing from action. And our ethics are as much an adaptive product of our nervous system, as our ability to know; indeed, it is upon ethical choice that the very survival of our knowledge depends. Earlier we spoke of the biological correlates of mental life, and of communication. That a chemical text should carry the imprint of experience and partake in its growth in no way diminishes the place of the infinitely more important rules which keep us aware, sharing, communicating, loving and human. In this respect we are at a juncture. We talk of hard sciences and soft sciences, of technologies and human engineering. We talk of the morality of science, when, perhaps, we should be talking of a science of morality. Here we do not have to go far. For Morality grows out of awareness, and its truth is inherent in the very marrow and structure of Science itself.

In this age of change and future shock, morality is no longer an ideal, but a necessity. A Moral Society, small or large – team, tribe or nation – is the only rational alternative to the death of a society – inexorably – albeit by way of huge historical byways, excursions, and mutations, and extravagances. Social evolution is nudging, or bumping, or bludgeoning us that way. Natural selection is a rugged rule.

It is this sense of deep connectedness between Awareness, Knowledge, Truth, and Moral Choice which informs the passionate journey that was the life of Jacob Bronowski. It is a story of loving and of knowing, of an informed and loving giving of what he knew to his fellow men. Like Goethe he sensed that there was a Gleichnis, a likeness of the universe in us all; and like Plotinus he deeply understood the concept of "Adequacy": "Knowing," said Plotinus, "demands the organ of knowing fitted to the object"; "knowing demands that the understanding of the knower must be adequate to the thing known." Bruno sensed that we carried within us all that is potentially to be known about our universe. And that while our adequacies, with respect to knowledge varied, it was important to advance them by the best means available to make the use of knowledge, not arbitrary, but just. That he should have made the Salk Institute his home and should have guided its Council on Biology in Human Affairs, simply expressed an alignment of Jacob Bronowski with himself. He was a deeply practical man; he apprehended from the beginning the clear, deep vision of the Institute's Founder, and the joint Purpose of its fellows, and Trustees. Here, again, there was Timeliness, "Adequacy", Congruence between purpose and act. He sensed the streams that were flowing from the natural sciences into social biology: and knew that they were flowing potentially to bring man a Better Day. As he says, at the end of his essay on William Blake, speaking of Freedom to Learn:

> "Men who are denied the right to dissent are no longer full men, and do not make a Society worthy of men. The right to ask and to be answered, truth; the right to judge and to choose, dignity; these and justice, and pity, and love, and reason are of the shape of man's mind."

Here you have it all; and here he walks amongst us – clear, strong, warm and smiling.

PAPER 26

DISTINGUISHED PSYCHIATRIST LECTURE AMERICAN PSYCHIATRIC ASSOCIATION ON PSYCHOBIOLOGY AND COMMUNICATION: PSYCHIATRY AND THE FUTURE OF MEDICINE[*]

Joel Elkes

Department of Psychiatry and Behavioral Sciences
University of Louisville

I. INTRODUCTION: ADOLF MEYER AND PSYCHOBIOLOGY

In an age of revolutions, one gets used to revolutions. As in the headlong rush, continents disappear, and new continents emerge and merge, one looks at old maps to get one's bearings. At such times language obliges – and as in political life – new acronyms appear to denote new relationships, connections and emphases.

In recall, for example, how novel – how mysteriously novel – the term "Biochemistry" – a chemistry of life, no less – seemed to me as a medical student some sixty years ago. I recall, too, how, in the mid-fifties, some of us – in the proverbial smoke-filled room – debated the merits of the term "Psychopharmacology vs. Neuropsychopharmacology" to describe our new, exciting, yet poorly defined, and still empirical, field. Today molecular genetics and molecular biology have profoundly remade modern biology; and, happily, modern genetics and modern molecular biology are deeply woven into the fabric of modern psychiatry. We rightly pride ourselves, not only on our firm foundation in the neurosciences, but our decisive contribution to the evolution of these very sciences. Look around you, in the program of this very meeting, put together so thoughtfully by Dr. Tasman and his colleagues. And, please, also recall that some of the most significant discoveries in the neurosciences in the last two decades were made in laboratories and Institutes founded and funded by a prescient NIMH and ADAMHA.

But something else happened which I find disturbing. I refer to an undue shift of emphasis from the Art of Psychiatry to the Science of Psychiatry, even if there be a science of the Art; a lack of proportion; a veering away from our central and unique position in medicine to that of a mere specialty within medicine. I remember feeling this unease when I first came to Hopkins in 1963. I had been asked to establish a Neuroscience Program in Psychiatry, but – against the

---

[*] Delivered at the Annual Meeting of the American Psychiatric Association on May 14, 1991, in New Orleans, Louisiana.

The ideas expressed in this paper were also presented at the Taylor Manor Hospital Psychiatric Symposium, held March 31\c4April 2, 1989, in Baltimore, Maryland.

Reprinted with the agreement of Elsevier Science from B.T. Taylor and I.J. Taylor (eds.) Psychiatry: Past Reflections \c4 Future Visions (pp. 75\c4107). New York: Elsevier, 1990

considerable protest of my biological colleagues – proceeded to name our department "The Department of Psychiatry and *Behavioral Science*." Here, again, one looked back to older maps. For, through the door of my office at the Phipps Clinic, there was the Phipps Clinic library., established by Adolf Meyer in 1913 and named for him by us on the anniversary of his birth. There were also visitors with whom it was good to share one's concerns. I remember, particularly, a wonderful three hour discussion with Dr. Karl Menninger, who visited me soon after he had published his "Vital Balance". *Balance* – Balance in Psychiatry – The Balancing Wheel of Psychiatry in Medicine – that was what our discussion was about. And in that library, there was another volume, which gave me solace in those anxious and important days. It was the American Journal of Insanity, Vol. 69. which describes the dedication of the Henry Phipps Psychiatric clinic of April 13, 1913.

It was a ceremony in the grand manner attended by Osler, McDougall, Eugen Bleuler, Cushing and Ernest Jones, among others. Speaking briefly on the purposes of a psychiatric clinic, Adolf Meyer said:

"For the first time in English speaking countries, a university and large general hospital serving a medical school received, as not merely affiliated, but as an intrinsic part of its facilities, a well equipped clinic to take care of its patients with mental disorders… At last science begins to take up with new and forceful methods the great problems of mental life… This work does not stop in the sanctum of the investigator. Just as bacteriology studies the water supply, air, and food of communities, schools, and homes so we psychopathologists have to study more the community, and the atmosphere… from which patients come and to which they must return." (1)

There was a comprehending comprehensiveness about Adolf Meyer's vision of Psychiatry. Brain, body, thought and behavior were to him a biological continuum; and symbolic life, an aspect of general biology. He connected, like few before him – and long before the life sciences were ready for such a connection – Psychiatry to the Life Sciences, and the Life Sciences to Psychiatry, probing the relation of Claude Bernard's Inner Environment, and later, Cannon's homeostasis, to the forces and influences playing upon an ordinary person's life, from birth to maturity, into old age. He emphasized early bonding in human development and learning, and saw the family as the most important school of man. He recognized the web of social support as a healer of great power. Long before the present emphasis on life events, he focussed, by way of the autobiographical essay, on life events. Long before cybernetics, autoregulation, social field theory and the analog computer, he sensed, and thought, and wrote about the importance of systems in human affairs. He traveled light and he traveled far, crossing boundaries – from his neuroanatomical laboratories (which literally comprised brains from lizards to elephants) to the clinic and to mental hygiene in school and community, and back again; and did so with great élan and vitality. In a word, he saw *connections* between the disparate fields which, in his day, related medicine to psychiatry and psychiatry to medicine. Soma and Symbol, the society within the skin and the society without, were to him aspects of a vast realm of communication which he termed "Psychobiology". All his life he struggled valiantly with the awesome comprehensiveness of the term. His Salmon Lectures on the subject were delivered in 1932 but not published until several years after his death in 1957 (2). Yet, long before modern neurochemistry, molecular biology, and concepts that we take totally for granted today, Adolf Meyer had a view of Psychiatry which remains astonishingly modern. Communication was to him at the heart of Psychobiology; communication reaching beyond psychiatry into the body of medicine at large. It is this theme of communication in relation to psychiatry and medicine which I would like to address. For Psychiatry is about communication. Intercellular communication by way of special signal molecules in brain and body; communication and coding in neural and immunological nets; communication between brain and organ systems, and brain and the world, including the duplicate world we encode in our symbols. I would like to examine some of the attributes of the languages – molecular and symbolic Å which make up the matrix of modern psychiatry; point to certain features which these languages may have in common; examine the implications of this new knowledge for our day-to-day practice and training in psychiatry, and in related areas of medicine, and point to a steadily lessening contradiction between brain chemistry, its exquisite susceptibility to environment, and the so called psychosocial approaches. The observations I wish to put before you are by now well known and well established; I will merely try to relate them to each other. Also, since they have affected my own life, I hope I may be forgiven some personal recollections and repetitions (3–8).

II. MOLECULAR COMMUNICATION, SYMBOLIC COMMUNICATION, AND THE PRESERVATION OF THE SYMBOLIC SELF

A Society Within the Skin

The society of cells residing within the human skin forms an entity which throughout evolution has continued to function with remarkable smoothness, efficiency, and resilience. This entity, making up a man's body, is built up of parts of varying size and complexity – from cell constituents like mitochondria, microsomes, and membranes to cell ensembles, tissues, organs and organ systems. These units interact and communicate; the whole is informed of the part and the part is informed of the needs of the whole. In a word, the biological machine is a self organizing system. In the exchange of matter and energy, precise information is the key. Information, in turn, is linked to time and timing. It is information arriving at the right place at the right time which appears to be the cardinal rule of biological order. Somehow, cell ensembles have developed plans and schemata for cooperation – a sort of inner altruism. Homeostasis and constancy are achieved in the face of the opposite, namely, continuous change and exchange. The primary goal of this remarkable arrangement is the maintenance of the intactness of that society. Normally we take this arrangement totally for granted. Only when we are ill, are we shaken out of our insensibility, to become aware of the ever renewing miracle within us.

Communication within the skin is effected by the exchange of electrochemical signals between cells coded for function through specific genetic instructions. These are very precise. The advances in our understanding of intercellular communication has been very rapid. Cells govern themselves by signals from membrane to interior (the first and second messenger system) or from membrane to membrane. The agents are relatively small molecules, some of them remarkably simple in structure, which interact with receptors of specific configuration. The interaction conveys precise instructions which initiate and terminate a specific process, be they ion fluxes across a membrane or the transport or induction of an enzyme in a specific plan of protein synthesis. The action is usually optimal for the conditions which pertain at the time.

While cell to cell communication pertains in plants and marine organisms, and operates in ourselves in regulating and limiting growth, we are endowed with three broad systems which decisively influence intercellular and intracellular message transmittal. One is a fixed system which, like a giant plant emanating from a central trunk and core, pervades the farthest reaches of the body through its finest tendrils and arborization. I speak, of course, of the nervous system and its broad division of voluntary and autonomic control. The second system is composed of clusters of specialized fixed cells contained in glandular tissue like the Pituitary, Thymus, Pineal, Thyroid, Adrenal, which release signaling molecules into the blood stream; reaching their target receptors by that route. This system is the endocrine system. The third is made up of colonies of cells which are partly fixed and partly mobile, which carry out a surveillance function for the body and scan for molecular information which is "foreign" to the body. This system – the immune system – comprises the thymus, spleen, lymph nodes, bone marrow and lymphoid tissue scattered in mucosa and elsewhere – a vast array of especially endowed cells, and Macrophages, Lymphocytes, T cells, Killer cells and the like. Both, the nervous system and the immune system have memories operating at the molecular level. The weight of the brain is about three pounds, the weight of the immune system, about two, and the weight of the endocrine system, less than a pound. Yet, it is these systems which guard our identity and preserve our biological and symbolic self – the immune guarding our biological identity and the nervous system our symbolic identity. There is not a cell in the society within the skin which is not irrigated by blood, bathed by lymph, and exposed to continuous fluxes of the autonomic nervous system. The final common path of these convergent communication systems is the exquisite micro apparatus of the cell membrane. The numbers operating in these processes are stupendous. Twelve to fourteen billion neurons, each capable of making some two hundred connections, 10^{12} lymphocytes. Some hundred million billion antibodies produced per second. All this tremendous variation is derived from a relatively small genetic pool. The three communication systems are, in turn, internally connected. The nervous system, by way of the hypothalamic pituitary axis, guides the endocrine system; and the endocrine system, in turn, transduces information from the nervous to the immune system. More direct pathways between the nervous and the immune systems both ways have been recently identified (13). The sympathetic nervous system, for example, innervates spleen, bone marrow, and lymph glands; and chemical messengers of the nervous system turn upon the surface of cells of the immune system. Integrity, coordination and decision making Å the right information at the right time – are all of a piece. The linking of the society within the skin to the society without involves a miraculous piece of chemical engineering.

III. THE BRAIN: MOLECULAR COMMUNICATION, SYMBOLIC FORMS AND THE SENSE OF SELF

The human brain emerges as the most remarkable biological machine to appear in the evolution of this planet. In the briefest moment of human history it has radically transformed our ecology and established the dominance of our able and dangerous species on earth. The exosomatic extensions which have become the instruments and agents of our technology and culture are products of the brain; it is to these that our body/mind must now adapt.

The organ in question is relatively young and carries within it the regional chemical footprints of its own evolution. It is a system of systems, an ensemble of homeostats, which has grown exponentially in cellular mass and cytoarchitectural elaboration in the last few minutes (a mere two million years or so) of the evolutionary calendar of life on this planet. Despite its complexity, its, and the teeming interneuronal molecular traffic, certain functional, regionally organized groupings can be clearly distinguished.

The so-called amphibian brain, located in the brain stem, connected to the hypothalamus pituitary apparatus subserves decisions concerning individual survival – hunger, thirst, sexuality, territoriality and the like. It is here that we find the centers which subserve the rhythms and tides of life – the ebb and flow of respiration, the beat of the heart, sleep wakefulness, arousal, attention. The plans here are genetically "wired", the sensory cues extraordinarily elaborate and precise; the responses released by very specific cues are swift, stereotyped and effective. Like any neural net it can learn. There is more latitude in the programs of the Limbic System (14), concerned with *species* survival. The behavior patterns related to sexuality, pair bonding, tropism of attraction and repulsion – pleasure and displeasure, love and hate – in short the cardinal functions of emotional arousal attack, anger, withdrawal, flight, affection and joy – appear to be coded by cell ensembles which, as has been shown by Nauta (15), have deep and pervasive connections into the lower brain stem, the spinal cord, and upward into the thalamus and the neocortical mantle. However, the explosive growth of the neocortex remains man's most characteristic acquisition; a process re-enacted ontogenetically in remarkably sped up fashion in intrauterine and early postnatal life. This, as has been said many times, makes for plasticity and vulnerability of immature man.

With cortical development came an ability to code, store, and model perception and forms of behavior in symbols; and through myriads of inner schemata and maps, create a duplicate inner representation which made it possible to be aware, to make tools to learn, to plan, and to think. Body Image, or to use a better term – Henry Head's *Body Schema* (17) is the primary representative map of the world within the skin. We suspect that visceral representation is laid down and stored relatively early, only to intrude when disturbed in illness, or brought into awareness through biofeedback and visceral training. The world without is scanned through distance receptors, and modeled through sound, images, pictures (ideograms) and the emergence of language. And it is in these early stages of the evolution o modern man, the Pleistocene Period (roughly from 70.000 to 8.000 B.C.) that we must look to the origins of both language and art.

This continuous modeling engages distinct, hierarchically organized cell groups in successive convergence, transformations and condensations of information (19). Such concepts owe a great deal to the study of the process of perception and learning in primitive organisms. The simpler the brain, the more stereotyped the responses, the clearer the chemical coding. The larger the brain, the higher the redundancy, the more discriminate the selection, the more massive the selective inhibition and "banking" of the inappropriate and the irrelevant. It is this massive capacity to selectively delay, inhibit and ignore which makes decisive and discriminate performance possible. The human brain, indeed any brain, in a series of successive transforms, condenses more and more information into less and less. I have suggested elsewhere (20) that these transforms employ shifting and highly discriminate inhibitory mechanisms in laminar, cellular hierarchies in the elimination of redundant information; that they are matched for fit against stored programs, and tested in a sort of internal rehearsal for adaptive value to the organism until a decision and commitment is either imagined or enacted. The final product, the emerging whole – be it a percept or a motor act, or an idea – represents a condensed symbolic model of a succession of operations which always, always comprise informational traces – shared properties – of the antecedent phases in a temporally coded pattern.

There is thus in the brain, continuous communication; a sharing of properties; a matching, weighing and feature extraction using electrochemical languages in these processes. To put it another way, there proceeds in the brain a continuous evolution, by natural selection, of symbolic forms which employ communicating cell populations, or groups, or ensembles in sort of Neural Darwinism (21). This evolution of informed cell assemblies is, of course, non-genetic; and in man can be transferred from generation to generation in sight and sound. Languages – silent or articulate – are the tools of evolution. We are what we are because of the continuous evolution proceeding in our head. If you will, the brain may be regarded as a fashioner of wholes.

We will note too, some aspects in these successive transformations. The process operates both in series and parallel modes, asking and answering the questions., one at a time, and asking the questions all at once. It operates – in albeit very rapid – almost automatic stages: A search; a scanning for fit against coded or genetically or cognate acquired schemata; a recognition and affective labeling in terms of adaptive value of the schema to the organism; inhibition of other inappropriate response repertoires; re-entry to test for validity; commitment to move a particular cell ensemble to a particular course action; and action through speech, or another motor act. We will note two features of this sequence: first, the key role of informed inhibition in structuring a response. What is not happening – banked, as it were – is as important as what emerges. Second, the inexorable nature of commitment – a stage which, once reached, is difficult to reverse.

The process of inner communication and evolution and non-genetic transmittal of information has populated our world with the exosomatic products of our culture. From brain, to libraries, to computers, communication remains our principal attribute. In this respect the brain underwent an interesting evolutionary twist. For quite early, it distinguished and parcelled out two modes of operation in information transfer – putting the sequential (digital-linear) and the parallel-analogous mode into two separate hemispheres, interacting by way of the corpus callosum. Something else probably happened as well. Just as species specific behaviors appear to have been stored and encoded for reference in the amphibian and limbic system, so culturally valuable schemata – rituals, ceremonies, myths, racial memories if you will – may have found their repository in the right hemisphere, leaving the left hemisphere to plan and enact – by way of sequential speech – the ever present *NOW*. While we know a good deal of the dominant hemisphere and its role in the genesis and maintenance of consciousness, we know far too little of the non-dominant hemisphere. Far from silent, it speaks to us distinctly in our trade. Dreaming and day-dreaming may be related to its activity. Symbolic form-constants emerge impressively, from James Frazer (22) to Jung (23) to Campbell (24), and lately, Stanislav Grof (25). These symbolic forms, in their incessant transformations, are accessed, not through words but through means of communication which are both pre-verbal and – forgive the term – post-verbal metalanguages of the inner self. Dreaming, day-dreaming, music and dance, painting and poetry, deep meditation and religious experience, practiced individually or in a group, are our avenues to them; and, strangely significant, experiencing them gives us a feeling of a loss restored, a sense of completeness, wholeness, connectedness, communication and knowing. We must ask why this should be so. What is it about art that restores? Restores to what? What is it about the best of religious practice that communicates and makes whole like nothing else? What is the "a-part-ness" that is healed? We must suspect that ancient psychobiological processes, pervading the whole structure of the Body/Mind, from Soma to Symbol, are at play in the experience and expression of these states; and conclude, then, that their study is very much the business of modern Psychobiology.

IV. IMMUNITY: MOLECULAR COMMUNICATION AND
THE PRESERVATION OF THE BIOLOGICAL SELF

The explosive growth of modern immunology, stimulated by advances of molecular genetics and the pressing exigencies of AIDS, coincides with a mounting recognition of the connection between the nervous system, the endocrine system and the immune system, and the influence of psychological and behavioral factors on immune function. The pioneering work establishing these connections has now been documented (26–29). It records a story with profound implications for the behavioral scientist. As findings accumulate, the vast array of specialized cells comprising the immune system (we will recall the numbers mentioned earlier) emerges as an exquisitely balanced, self monitoring information network, communicating by chemical signals. It monitors the invading "without" against the "familiar" within. This network employs strategies reminding one of the processing of information by the nervous system; and, even more than the nervous system impresses by its stupendous biological reserve, manifesting as "degeneracy" and redundancy (21). Somewhat like the construction of the body image and visceral schemata, self recognition and other recognitions proceed continuously; the molecular intactness of the biological self is preserved through a miraculous, continuous process of inner communication. I may perhaps be forgiven if, in an informal discussion some years ago, I referred to the immune system as a "Liquid Brain," an all-pervasive embodiment of mind.

It is beyond my scope here to detail the different functions assigned to different kinds of cells. There are some excellent reviews for the general reader (28, 29). Nossal uses six key words to capture the task confronting the system. They are *Encounter, Recognition, Activation, Deployment, Discrimination* and *Regulation.* "The invading antigen must *encounter* cells capable of responding ... molecular mechanisms of *recognition* must exist... the system must possess the capability of responding to any conceivable antigen, including "new" substances synthesized by man... Having recognized the antigen, lymphocytes must be *activated* to respond either by producing antibodies or by. acting in the inflammatory response... They have furthermore to *cooperate* in an elaborate *deployment* strategy, amplifying and distributing defense functions... The evolutionary process has ensured that the system can *discriminate* between self and non self, thereby avoiding autoimmune damage... The mechanisms establishing such tolerance are part of a wider series of control loops that constitute immune *regulation* in which the intensity of the immune response is corrected for a particular antigenic load." (30)

More and more it looks like a coordinated *network* (12, 26). The network has an afferent pathway comprising a specific recognizing and a non-specific parallel set – indeed, the immune system has been called a sensory organ, scanning for molecular fit (31). One can also envision an efferent "imaging" component and an effector loop which is held in check by a process of internal inhibition. This is selectively modulated to lead to clonal selection and proliferation of the appropriate lymphocytes. Scanning, recognition, selection, modulation and selective inhibition, leading by way of a sort of internal rehearsal to *commitment*, are steps which remind one of communication in the nervous system. Induction of antibody production is an irreversible commitment once it has occurred, and is remembered for the future.

Moreover, a two way connection between the nervous, endocrine and immune systems is now established (32). Selective damage or stimulation of brain areas, particularly hypothalamus, affects immune function (33). The sub-organs of the immune apparatus (thymus, spleen, lymph nodes, bone marrow, mucosal parenchyma) receive rich autonomic innervation from both the parasympathetic and sympathetic systems (34, 35); communication goes both ways. There is also *afferent* communication *back* from the immune system to the nervous system, particularly the thymus (32). Most significantly, too, as shown in the now classical studies, the immune system responds to environment and can be conditioned (36). Alteration in immune function is seen in stress (e.g. examination stress, 37), and related to style of coping (38). There is evidence suggesting impaired immune function in depression (39, 40). The complex field of the relation of personality type, coping style and emotion to the onset or remission of cancer is full of promising leads and inconsistencies (41–44) which should be resolved in the next decade. The same applies to the old/new field of possible immune dysfunction in the genesis of schizophrenia (45, 46). On a slightly different note, one cannot leave this field without referring to the enormous benefit experimental neuroscience has derived from the advent of the fluorescent antibody techniques, making, literally, regional neurochemistry shine in the dark.

V. FAMILIES OF NEUROREGULATORY COMPOUNDS AND "INFORMATIONAL SUBSTANCES"

"The body of a worm and the face of a man alike have to be taken as chemical responses. The alchemist dreamed of old that it might be so. The dream however supposed a magic chemistry. There they were wrong. The chemistry is plain everyday chemistry. But it is complex. Further, the chemical brew in preparation for it time has been stirring unceasingly throughout some millions of years in the service of a final cause. The brew is a selected brew (47).

The chemistry of which Sherrington spoke began, not in the brain but in the gut and in the heart. It began with Acetylcholine, Histamine, and later Norepinephrine and Serotonin. It is hard, in an age which takes ligand techniques and the *in vivo* PET scanning of metabolic pathways in the brain totally for granted to grasp how improbable forty years ago, a coherent chemistry of the brain seemed. I, for one, was warned by my elders; they told me that the brain was a "sticky mess" which would prove one's professional undoing. Yet, I still recall vividly the excitement with which I read the classical paper of Feldberg and Vogt (48) questioning the universal transmitter role of acetylcholine in the brain, and listening to Marthe Vogt as she presented her evidence for the distribution of norepinephrine in the very areas of the brain where (on electrophysiological evidence) Bradley and I suspected the existence of a biogenic amine. Those were heady days, labor notwithstanding. It took two Ph.D. students two years to map the distribution of an enzyme system in the brain.

Between 1953 and 1957 (50, 51) on the basis of electrophysiological and neurochemical evidence I suggested that "perhaps rather than thinking in unitary terms, it might be advisable to think in terms of the possible selection by chemical evolution, of small *families* of closely related compounds which by mutual interplay would govern the phenomena of excitation and inhibition in the central nervous system." I spoke of the operation of chemical fields in nodal regions of the brain which would depend on the rate of liberation, diffusion, and destruction of locally produced neurohumoral agents; I stressed the uneven distribution of cells with different chemical endowment in various areas of the brain – some cells condensed in nodes, others colonizing particular layers, some scattered randomly; I proposed that the agents in question may be either identical with, or more likely, derived from neuro-effector substances familiar to us in peripheral neural nets. I stressed the importance of *inter*action, and *inter*dependence between molecules governing and modulating the gating, storage and flow in self-exciting neural loops. As I put it, "The number of those substances was probable quite small but the influence upon the integrative action of higher nervous activity could be profound; the basic states of consciousness might well be determined by variation of local concentration of these agents." (52)

The substances we knew at the time were acetylcholine, norepinephrine, serotonin and GABA. We all know what has happened since. We are no longer talking of small families, but hierarchies perfected by evolution; generations of families of compounds, from GABA, Glycine, and cyclic AMP to prohormones, peptides and opiate like substances. The brain is emerging as a huge organ of internal secretion, and to synaptic transmission there is now being added the very important concept of *para*synaptic communication… local hormone-like effects of messenger substances, reaching brain cells through the extracellular fluid bathing the cell surface.

In a seminal paper, F.O. Schmitt, a towering figure in modern neuroscience, has proposed as a working hypothesis the concept of Informational Substances as molecular regulators of brain function (53). His list of classical neurotransmitters number about 10, comprising members of the small families to which I earlier referred. The lists of neuropeptides and neuro-hormones, as we know, comprise some forty members; it has grown considerably since. The import of this paper is twofold. First, it traces the evolutionary origin of the neurotransmitters, suggesting that they may have evolved from being intracellular messengers, to a role in rapid intercellular communication through synaptic discharges. Secondly, it argues for a twofold mode of communication: a precise, familiar mode of neuron-to-neuron synaptic transmission (we will recall that each neuron carries about 200 junctional sites); and a more direct information transmission "in parallel" or alongside (not instead of, or in competition with) neuronal circuitry. This may take place through the release and diffusion of informational substances through extracellular fluid, and their attachment to ligands on the cell surface, coding for a particular behavioral repertoire (as in sex hormone releasing behavior) or for components of a mosaic which makes up the repertoire. It is this combination of serial, synaptic, and parallel parasynaptic communication which makes for extraordinary flexibility in the repertories of a particular neural net. Scanning, analysis, recognition and discharge would seem to depend on recognizers for a particular configuration being in place. There appears to be "crosstalk" between recognizing sites as well. Once again, one is reminded of the immune system.

The awed sense of wonder grows as some of the very same informational substances familiar to us in the nervous system turn up on the surfaces of lymphocytes. Lymphocytes have receptors for acetylcholine, epinephrine, norepinephrine, histamine, dopamine, testosterone, insulin and a number of other hormones. The list is growing steadily (54).

In these electrochemical conversations between different sites, another very important principle emerges. Somehow the informational substances act in concert; their effect depends on the presence of each other. Like in spoken language, not only do molecules signal, they communicate and interact; the net meaning depends on *context*. What a particular substance will do at a particular time, at a particular site, will depend who and what else is, or has been, there at that time. This brings to mind early observation on the interaction between acetylcholine and norepinephrine at peripheral receptor sites (55). One grapples for an analogy which could comprise both space and time. The image of a molecular combination code – a sort of evanescent combination lock – spread throughout the body provides a rough approximation of an idea.

VI. MOLECULAR LANGUAGES IN THE TRANSCRIPTION OF MIND/BODY EVENTS

The pervasive presence of neuroregulatory and informational substances throughout the body makes it possible to think of the transcription of symbolic events in molecular terms. The classical studies of Kandel in a simple organism, aplysia (56), have furnished us with one molecular model of a memory trace. This model emphasizes the role of calcium as a critical regulator of transmitter release. However, the molecular transcription of psychosocial cues is evident in other areas (57, 58). Social factors, especially in early life, influence drug responsiveness and affect enzyme induction, with deep influence on an organism's social reactivity. Handling, stroking, and touch may affect growth hormones, liver enzymes and development (59). More significantly, hormones abound in the autonomic nerve endings of viscera; even the heart has its hormones (64).

In an important series of papers, Rossi (66, 67) has argued that learning, any learning, is conditioned by the chemical state of the organism – particularly the brain – in which it occurs. The model which is derived from the study of addiction is that of *State Dependent Learning.* Behavior learned under the influence of drugs are exquisitely susceptible to these same drugs, or related social cues (68). Similarly, it is argued that behaviors and/or memories, or visceromotor responses acquired during a particular state of neurohormonal arousal (a particular hormonal "mix") are susceptible to cognate cues. Such memories, in Rossi's experience, are evoked in low arousal states by the use of an Eriksonian approach of gentle hypnosis and guided imagery. The somatic specificity of such responses is certainly impressive; and suggests widespread cell communication, and extensive representation and discrimination in the memory trace. Whether this is due to a widespread dissemination of molecular recognizers (62), or a peculiar and specific chemical wiring, or some form of molecularly conditioned, transcellular "resonance", or (to my mind, quite likely) electromagnetic and/or electrochemical fields (69), is unknown. One is, however, certainly reminded of tissue hypersensitivity.

VII. DISEASE AS A DISORDER OF MOLECULAR AND SYMBOLIC COMMUNICATION

The evidence briefly reviewed above brings us to the point with which we began. The society within the skin emerges as a miraculously coordinated communication system in which the whole is informed of the part, and the part is informed of the whole. Constancy of body function is maintained throughout adult life through an extraordinary array of signal exchange. Evolution in man manifests daily in symbolic life. The core and content of our life is symbolic; and – be it in soma or symbol – we consciously sample only the tiniest fraction of the ancient symbolic structures with which we are endowed and which inform our day-to-day being.

The messaging system of the body/mind is truly stupendous. The chemical languages, honed by many millions of years of biological evolution – far transcending our species – are extraordinarily precise. Compared with the precision of these messages, our language, developed as a tool of social evolution, is paltry, clumsy, and imprecise in the extreme. The parable of the Tower of Babel still holds. Just listen to the verbal clutter invading our living room every night.

Within our skin and skull then, there exists a vast laboratory of symbolic forms in ongoing transformations which we only dimly perceive unless things go very wrong or very right. When things go wrong we "know it in our body." When things go right we are inwardly aware how good things can be. In the first we say we are uneasy, concerned, anxious, angry, furious or depressed; in the other we experience the joy of simply being. We are signaled when communication is out of phase. Anxiety is a warning, and signifies that a problem is unsolved and demands solution. Depression is an act of adaptive coping by not coping; pain (including mental pain) signals severing of organisms integrity; an invasion or an incipient (or actual) parting of the part from the whole. As Bakan put it, "disease is estrangement" (70); and healing, as the word implies, is a restoration of communication – a coming together, a return to wholeness. When communication is good, we amble along. When it falters, we are warned to attend to it; when it is impaired or lost, we get sick". Curious that in our profession we know so much about anxiety, pain and depression, and much, much less about joy. We know more about the biology of despondency than the biology of expectation and hope. A Science of Sorrows is still waiting for a Science of Joys.

In a significant paper, still in press, Herbert Weiner (9) has argued that disease may in fact be a manifestation of disturbed intercellular and organ communication. He regards an altered relationship between messenger, mediator and receptor as crucial; and postulates several levels of organization at which this might occur. A cognate model has been very ably argued by Cunningham (71). Rubenstein too has examined the suggestive evidence, speaking of diseases related to defects in intercellular communication (10).

The examples of this model in somatic diseases, though still sparse, are suggestive. There is Graves disease caused by a circulating autoantibody binding preferentially to the receptor for thyrotropin and interrupting the normal feedback loop to TRH; myasthenia gravis, where the ACh receptor is blocked by an autoantibody, impairing neuromuscular transmission and ultimately destroying the receptor; a deficiency for low density lipoprotein LAL receptor which leads to dangerous elevation of cholesterol in familial hypercholesteremia, and reduction of the number of insulin receptors in diabetes in relation to stressful life events (10).

But surely the richest field in support of this thesis is our own field of biological psychiatry. For here, through the evolution of modern psychopharmacology and the refined methodologies of receptor identification and purification *in vitro*, the elegant ligand techniques (72, 73), metabolic loading techniques and brain imagery have given us a plethora of new findings and generation upon generation of working hypotheses.

For evidence, I refer you to the section on Biological Psychiatry of *Psychopharmacology: The Third Generation of Progress*, edited by Herbert Meltzer and published in association with our own American College of Neuropsychopharmacology on its 25th Anniversary (74). The volume numbers 1,840 double columned pages – a one volume encyclopedia. The section on Biological Psychiatry covers 541 pages by distinguished invited authors and comprises forty-one articles with up-to-date statements on the biology of the affective disorders, schizophrenia, psychiatric disorders of childhood, dementia, and anxiety, among others. Norepinephrine, dopamine, serotonin, acetylcholine, opioid peptides, corticotrophin, somatostatin and thyroid hormone appear involved in affective disorders; Dopamine, GABA, the prostaglandins and peptides, and prolactin and growth hormone in schizophrenia; Norepinephrine in attention disorders in children, cholinergic, serotonergic, and neuropeptides in Alzheimer Disease. The locus coeruleus, with the implied deregulation of the norepinephrine system and the GABA, benzodiazapine receptor complex appears to be involved in anxiety and panic. Again and again the same players turn up.

Some years ago, at the 3rd International Neurochemical Symposium in Strasbourg in 1960, I considered possible chemical factors which, in schizophrenia, might interfere with the information processing in the brain. I spoke of "a fundamental organizing process which during wakefulness in the normal,. and at tremendous speed, registers, codes, matches, and correlates new against stored information, and in a succession of such transactions computes the probabilities which are of optimum service to the adaptive needs of the organism." I furthermore suggested that "these transformations proceed simultaneously at different, yet closely interrelated neural levels; that they employ shifting reciprocal and highly discriminate inhibitory mechanisms in a successive elimination of redundant information." In the same paper I speculated on the chemical topology (involving the norepinephrine/dopamine/serotonin system) possibly underlying a *mis*processing of information, emphasizing interplay and interaction, possibly involving the Globus Pallidus and Caudate Nucleus.

We did not really have the help of the computer modeling of information processing at the time; and the chemicals in question were a mere handful. Today one is deeply encouraged by what has happened. For the various disorders we know as mental diseases may indeed turn out to be manifestations of de-regulation of molecular communication in the regionally organized, chemically mediated organ of information which we carry in our skull.

VIII. RESTORING COMMUNICATION: MOLECULAR LANGUAGES, VERBAL LANGUAGES AND THE METALANGUAGES OF THE INNER SELF

It would seem then, that the core element of our work is to restore communication, to re-pair, to re-connect the parted parts into a smoothly functioning whole. At the level of intercellular and inter-organ commerce the organism evidently employs precise molecular languages. These have been selected by evolution to exercise these functions. The symbolic "releasers" of innate and specific behaviors are probably chemically coded. The verbal languages used in day-to-day human commerce are much, much younger, and much less precise. They are also the backbone of modern psychotherapy. Younger still is the astonishing array of the languages of science which, over the shortest span of evolution, have given us the products of our technology; and beyond these, as a sort of common ground of our humanity, there are the ancient symbolic metalanguages treasured by our species from culture to culture. These have special reflective attributes; for used in appropriate settings – be it individual, be it in a group – they have the power to evoke certain unmistakable experiences of wholeness, identity, selfhood, and meaning. In some strange nonverbal way, these metalanguages appear to restore and reconnect. Art, religion and spirituality are the terms reserved for this realm. One is tempted to inquire into their mode of operation. Here one moves away from the realm of traditional science: Asking "how" is more appropriate than posing an immodest "why".

I submit that at a molecular level of communication we are way ahead. The astonishing explosion of knowledge, evident at this meeting, has carried the *in vivo* regional chemical topology of the brain from anatomical and histochemical to the molecular level. It has given us insights into regional metabolic shifts in relation to thought and intention. Now receptor configurations amenable to precise analysis; a taxonomy, a sort of periodic table (75) of informational substances is afoot. Add to it modern genetic engineering, the isolation of genes fashioning receptors, and the crafting, literally harvesting of transmitters and receptors *in vitro* and you have the advent of a rational chemotherapy of mental disorders which none of us thirty years ago would have dreamt of in our philosophy.

However, as we enter the area of verbal communication and the languages of psychotherapy, things become at once, more human and more complex. For languages, while depicting and reflecting experience, also shape experience. The rules governing their structure are ancient rules; quite probable, the brain is coded for them at birth (76). These rules – rules of astonishing logic and economy – go, as argued by Whorf (77), into the structure of even quite primitive languages; they order the fact.-symbols to each other and to the world they represent, and make for the smooth use of language as an instrument of social adaptation and communication. Again, as in molecular languages, we come up against the key concept of *context*. Conventional logic imposes a linear, sequential, discursive quality upon them which seriously limits their informational power. For while carrying certain meanings in one context, words may carry a totally different meaning in another; and even standing alone they may... as anyone who has traced the origin of a word in a dictionary can see... carry an accretion of different meanings in a strange calculus of their own. Words are, thus, not just labels; cards stacked for reference in one of Broca's areas. They are states, sets, depending on relation and context. They carry multiple meaning. The "unspeakable" metalanguages of the inner self are as different from the "speakable" as the structure of a dream is from deliberate, planned action. In such symbolic forms totality is apprehended simultaneously at different levels; mutually occlusive elements co-exist; time is of no consequence; and serial ordering in time... that backbone of causal reasoning... gives way to simultaneously perceived relationships. I have elsewhere examined these issues in relation to the languages of physics (5). In this context, listen to William James (78):

> "What must be admitted is that the definite images of traditional psychology form but the smallest part of our minds as they actually live. The traditional psychology talks like one who should say a river consists of nothing but pailsful, spoonsful, quartpotsful, barrelsful and other moulded forms of water. Even where the pairs and posts all actually standing in the stream, still between them the free water would continue to flow. It is just this free water of consciousness that psychologists resolutely overlook. Every definite image in the mind is steeped and dyed in the free water that flows round it. With it goes the sense of its relations, near and remote, the dying echo whence it came to us, and the dawning sense whether it is to lead."

IX. TRADITIONAL AND NON-TRADITIONAL PSYCHOTHERAPIES

Jerome Frank, in his classic <MI>Persuasion and Healing (79) and a thoughtful series of papers (80, 81) and McHugh and Slavney, in their monograph on *Perspectives on Psychiatry* (82), have examined the qualities and limitations of language in psychotherapy. Dr. Frank has argued for a comparison of psychotherapy to both rhetoric and hermeneutics. Rhetoric may be defined as the use, of words to form attitudes and induce actions: clearly this is an active mode. Hermeneutics is interpretive – the original word pertains to the interpretation of a religious text to discover intended meaning. In rhetoric, there is a common ground of emotional arousal followed by a cognitive process of argument. In hermeneutics, the patient is read like a text. Patient and therapist jointly engage in a quest to improve communication within. Contradictory aspects of functioning, forgotten memories and subpersonalities are engaged in conversation. A web of *meaning* is arrived, which represents the best schema to account for past and present difficulties, and offers an alternative interpretation of the future. This meaning is not absolute: on the contrary, it is relative and individual. Yet, with meaning comes a sense of connectedness, and with this connectedness and communication, a reduction of despair and a raising of morale, competence, and a return of hope. The biology of these positive states is relatively unknown. I suggest that they present a central theme for a psychobiology of the future.

Now it is deeply significant that in this quest for a sense of wholeness, for meaning, modern psychotherapy does no longer wholly depend on the verbal transaction. To the analytical interpretive, and the deeply significant developments in cognitive therapy (83), there have now been added the group approaches (84), where, as in a lens, interpersonal forces of great power are focused on individuals in a group (especially when led by a professional who is also a peer; 85) and interpreted – as in psychosynthesis – with special reference to establishing communication between subpersonalities. The Gestalt "Body" and Movement techniques mobilize somatic memories "frozen" into a "body armor" (86); the powerful techniques of guided imagery in low states of arousal mobilize the imagination and illuminate true needs and choices (87); approaches which deliberately call on the devotional and sacred elements in a person's life are experienced as healing (88). We will readily admit that some of these approaches are a long, long way from the sciences which inform traditional medicine; yet, since they are reported to work, they should be included in our future agenda of research. Significantly, too, they provide. bridges to the other ancient modes of self communication invented to allay the travails of the spirit. The arts and religion have been old partners in the practice of healing: like few branches of modern medicine, they have provided avenues into meaning which emerge as cornerstones of modern psychotherapy. We must ask why they have persisted; what has been their biological function for so long (88, 90). I have never understood the so called contradiction between the practice of science and an acceptance of religion. I suspect it is contrived by persons who do not understand either science or religion. If the need for belief has so long an evolutionary history, religion – not doctrine, but faith – the need to believe is surely the business of psychobiology.

X. ARTS, AND THE SPIRITUAL ELEMENT

It would require a separate paper to review the place of the Arts in therapy. Their time-honored role in psychiatry is well established; professional associations and journals attest to their effectiveness. What is regrettable is that they have remained at the periphery of medicine. Music, for example, is establishing for itself a firm place in therapeutics. Analgesic, anxiolytics and hormonal effects of music have been noted (92, 93), as have effects of music and imagery on adrenal corticosteroid and circadian rhythms. Moreover, certain temporal musical patterns have grammatical patterns akin to other languages (91), and appear to be related to certain common emotional states, the so called sentic cycle (94).

Similarly, the languages of the visual and plastic arts are related to therapy and have been used for at least a century, and offer a fascinating field of inquiry lying in the borderlands of sickness and creativity (95).

A spiritual element can be central to a patient's life. As healers, we should inquire after this dimension in our patients. A recently introduced Spiritual Inventory for the Medically Ill Patient takes stock of this important dimension in the medically ill (96). It inquires how one's patients see and interpret the meaning of their illness: Do they see it as a challenge? An Enemy? A Punishment? Weakness? Relief? It asks how they see their Values, their Belief and Faith; the function of love in their lives; the place of forgiveness, and the place of prayer; the capacity for private meditation, worship in a group. As we said earlier: if restoration of meaning be central for successful psychotherapy, these aspects of inner life would appear central to meaning. I suggest that we seriously look beyond the traditional therapies into the restorative and healing powers of these old/new approaches, and that we do so in a systematic way, by established tools of biomedical research. Private institutions have an extraordinary opportunity in this regard. Nor can we do it alone. New professions, new mixes of professions are needed: Of necessity, they will emerge in time.

XI. TOWARDS A SCIENTIFIC HUMANISM: THE CATALYTIC FUNCTION OF PSYCHIATRY IN A MEDICINE OF THE FUTURE

Psychiatry as a Statement of Human Biology

I hope that by now we have noted some attributes of our field, which at once are a source of difficulties and of high promise. ours is a peculiarly personal science. There may be impersonal medicine, but there cannot be impersonal psychiatry. However "biologically oriented," we may be the *person* is central to our trade. Meaning is not an asterisk, an after-thought, but at the very heart of what we do. Medicine may have got into its present difficulties by failing to distinguish between disease and illness (97). Psychiatry brooks no such distinction. It is a specialty as well as a "generality," a vast continent of a discipline, extending from the deeply molecular to the deeply human. Bridging such realms of knowledge is quite a task. Psychiatry has always forged alliances with other disciplines: and no discipline which has worked with psychiatry has failed to be enriched by contact with us. Whether it be genetics and neurobiology or developmental, experimental and social psychology, anthropology, the social sciences, or linguistics, the gain has always gone both ways. Psychiatry poses obstinate questions at the very core of medical practice. Some twenty-five years ago, when I was invited to take up my post at Johns Hopkins, I wrote a memorandum to the Search Committee outlining my hopes for our field (98). Looking around at this meeting in 1991, one is comforted by progress. I submit that what Psychiatry is today will be very relevant to a medicine of tomorrow.

In dealing with disorders of communication, psychiatry has, provided the outlines of an understanding of the role of information transfer in psychosomatic exchange. It has done so at the molecular, the interorgan and the symbolic level. It has addressed the individual, the dyad and the group. It has inquired into the evolution of values and belief systems, and contributed to our understanding of their beneficent function in coping and healing. It has even begun to address the biological origins, correlates, and role of spiritual elements in life, and the arts as potential agents of healing. The ancient functions of physician as a teacher and a facilitator of hope are beginning to make a great deal of biological sense. Indeed, we may be witnessing a profound revolution, of which modern psychiatry may be the forerunner. It has been called the information revolution or Info-medicine (99). The concept of single-cause disease is giving place to causes seen in *context*. Analytical thinking is being exposed to a non linear cybernetic model in which the study of the whole and the part are inexorably linked. More and more the society within the skin appears to have its congruencies and correlates without.

I suggest, in the light of the foregoing, that modern psychiatry already provides us with a more complete and comprehensive description of the mind/body connection than any branch of medicine, and that it can help us to insights concerning the inner mechanisms of recovery and healing which may only be on the peripheral field of vision of conventional medicine. It already excels at fashioning molecular models of mental disorder. Its models of illness are broader. Person, meaning, coherence (100), coping and competence are at the very core of its work. To the biophysical model, it now adds an attitudinal ("spiritual") element, and is ready to inquire into these aspects of healing by accepted methods of biomedical research. Its models of illness inexorably lead it to models of health; the techniques which have given it an understanding of the negative emotions stand ready to be applied to the study of positive states of being. Psychiatry, in trying to comprehend, outlines a truly comprehensive kind of medicine. I submit that, even as it is today, its peculiar amalgam of disciplines provides the best introduction to human biology that we have.

I suggest that it is time to consider how we can best put this new knowledge to the service of medicine and society. We must begin with ourselves, our own profession, and the professionals who are our colleagues. We must also recall that a powerful democratization of knowledge is afoot, especially through the media. The American public seems to be going to medical school. In our field, it behooves us to exercise quality control and ensure that the information is sound, up-to-date, and above all, useful.. Within the scope of this paper I can only indicate some possible trends, and illustrate them with a few examples out of my own experience.

XII. THE NEW BIOBEHAVIORAL SCIENCES: THEIR ROLE IN HUMANIZING MEDICAL EDUCATION

"Humanizing medical education" has been a recurrent "cri de coeur" echoing through reports on medical education reform for the past fifty years (101–104). Those of us who have participated in the paste and scissors operation of curricular reform, know how hard it is to merge the clinical and human element into an overcrowded, overworked curriculum. Far reaching experiments in self directed learning are attempting to weave preclinical sciences into experiential, clinical practice (105–108). I suggest that the new knowledge concerning Mind/Body communication provides an excellent teaching "spine" for an introduction to medicine. It also enhances a student's awareness of him/herself as a fascinating portable biological laboratory; and helps to put this knowledge to use in the great laboratory of everyday life. It is important that such exposure occur early in the curriculum. I refer you particularly to the pioneering experiments initiated in Rochester by George Engel and his colleagues (107, 108); and will tell you a little about two experiments which my colleagues and I began: one at Hopkins some twenty years ago, and one more recently, still in progress in Louisville, Kentucky.

In 1964, Dr. Richard Chase, a group of colleagues and I initiated an introductory Behavioral Science course at Hopkins, taught in the second year (109). Four themes recurred through the course: Human Development, Human Learning, Human Communication and The Social Field. Biology – psychobiology – was related to each; we tried to make it both theoretical and clinically applied; and both didactic and experiential. A major feature of the course was that three departmental chairmen – of the Department of Pediatrics, Obstetrics, and Gynecology and myself, and several senior teachers from the departments of medicine and surgery participated in the course. As Dr. Engel, R. Reiser and Dr. Rosen had done (108), we tried to make it interdisciplinary, clinically relevant and symbiotic, demonstrating, we hope, the pervasive influence of psychiatry in modern medical practice.* The course was well received, and, I was delighted to learn, that it has provided a template for a more contemporary and advanced version under the inspired leadership of Dr. Paul McHugh.

At Hopkins I had the good fortune to meet Dr. Caroline Thomas who, in following a cohort of 1,337 medical students over 16 years, had developed her famous Precursors Study (110) on the basis of psychological profiles, and had identified certain predictive risk factors in medical students for stress related disorders, including hypertension, coronary heart disease, depression and cancer. It occurred to me at the time that an intervention *preceding* those stressful years might be worth trying. The opportunity arose in Louisville when I had the good fortune to meet Dr. Leah Dickstein, associate Dean of Students in the School of Medicine, and our newly elected Vice President of the APA. Again, the Department of Psychiatry, with Dr. John Schwab's unwavering help and support, became the sponsor of what has now become known as "The Louisville Experiment (111)."

The idea is really very simple: it is a week long event, known as the "Health Awareness Workshop", offered to medical students during the week *preceding* their official enrollment in August. Last year, out of a class of 124, 122 students, including spouses and some eight children, attended this offering. The exercise is staffed by voluntary faculty and student volunteers. These act as "health tutors" and student mentor-colleagues in subsequent years.

The idea is to communicate to students the practical reality of the Mind/Body connection, and to provide them with coping skills to master the competitive obstacle race which awaits them in their training. The exercise is partly didactic and partly small-group experiential. It includes overviews of the psychobiology of stress and coping, attention to nutrition, exercise, relaxation, time management, study skills, listening skills, spouse and sexual problems, substance abuse, medical ethics and the place of faith, hope and humor in healing. We judge the experiential element to be very important. The health check and health risk appraisal is carried out by the students themselves. (We have, incidentally, discovered several early hypertensives in each of our classes). Nutrition is taught through the preparation and serving of nutritious meals in the medical school auditorium, and a student-authored cookbook; Relaxation is taught through two elementary one-hour exercises, carried out by the whole class; Time management and exam tips are presented by senior students through humorous sketches. The sense of learning and sharing in joy and in *fun*, permeates the whole exercise. Staff and students wear identical T-shirts embossed with an attractive "Ways to Health" logo. As behooves our field, the arts are very much in evidence. There is an exhibit of staff and student work; an award for an original contribution; a concert; and at the end, the Doctor's Jazz band, made up of prominent physicians, ushers the student towards formal enrollment into their career. By

---

* See also papers 18, 19 and 21, on pages rspectively, in this volume.

the time the Dean greets them in welcome (on the last day of the exercise), social support groups have gathered spontaneously and networks have formed. No student is a stranger to colleagues or to staff. We believe that carried in follow-up, we have in this exercise the makings of an important epidemiological health laboratory for physicians-in-training, and in subsequent practice. We try to convey the idea to the student that within his or her own skin there is a magnificent mind/body laboratory: that every day can be an experiment, and that a training of awareness is a key element to living a good day, one at a time.

More recently we have added another component, namely a program in the Arts and Medicine safely housed in the Division of Attitudinal and Behavioral Medicine in the Department of Psychiatry. The principal objectives of the program are:

1. To introduce the practice and appreciation of the Arts as an accepted therapeutic modality into treatment settings.
2. To study and assess the effectiveness of such interventions by accepted methods of biomedical research.
3. To enhance the practice of art forms in health care personnel as an effective means of self-exploration.
4. To identify and attend to the special treatment needs of practicing artists which would enhance their personal well-being and creativity.
5. To develop educational programs to bring to the attention of the health community the place of the arts as an effective non-invasive therapeutic intervention.

We have in our group representation in Painting, Sculpture, Music, Drama, Poetry, Storytelling and Humor. Work is proceeding in the effectiveness of Expressive Therapies in the Posttraumatic Stress Syndrome; the usefulness of psychodrama and role playing in adolescent disorders; the use of music in Alzheimer's Disease; the usefulness of relaxation and imagery in dealing with performance anxiety; and the therapeutic use of humor.

I have furnished these examples to which others could be added from the literature, to make a central point, namely, the catalytic role which psychiatry can, and should, play in shaping attitudes and patterns of care in a medicine of the future. It is not accidental that an offering such as we put together in our Behavioral Science course and in the Health Awareness program should emanate from a department of psychiatry. To repeat, so far, only psychiatry, among medical disciplines, spans a coherent body of knowledge extending from mind to body, from the molecular to the symbolic, from disease to recovery, to coping, to wellbeing. I suggest that we have not even begun to exercise our full influence in the training of physicians, in the planning of a humane health care system, or in bringing our knowledge into the vast, pervasive laboratory of everyday life. For far too long we have spoken only when spoken to.

I hope you have noted that the arguments and models I have put before you, while conjectural, have a distinct practical side. Explained to the average person – to *any* patient – such communication about mind/body can carry a powerful rationale for enhancing personal initiative and coping. our place is then, not only in participating with our clinical colleagues in joint practice and research, but in explaining, and training people who could explain what we know; in planning treatment facilities which would "do it better," and differently; and in fashioning, with the best that present day medical science has to offer, approaches which take us beyond disease into prevention, and thus lay the groundwork for a science, not only of illness, but of well-being.

We must become more visible in care and education, and go beyond well meant consultation-liaison work. Mode of life is emerging as the major pathogen in our society. Behavioral factors are emerging as *the* risk factors in the plagues of our time, from alcoholism and AIDS to hypertension, cardiovascular disease and, possibly, cancer. We must take our place firmly alongside, and even ahead of, other specialties in treatment, research and prevention. We must enter into joint major enterprises with our colleagues; join in Grand Rounds, with major research and educational programs, particularly in relation to the stress related disorders, substance abuse, AIDS, adolescent disorders, and chronic diseases. We need good studies to test the cost effectiveness of the interventions we offer, particularly on mobilizing self efficacy and speeding recovery. I submit that industry is ready to provide the dollars: but we – not others, but *we* – must take the initiative. Third party carriers are still mean in recognizing the value of our services. We must make money talk. Our hard-won body of knowledge can be put to practical use; and if we are too busy to serve as educator-doctors, we should give thought to the training of professionals who could function as "explainers" to mobilize a patient's physical and psychological resources to optimize and speed recovery. There are many nurses, counselors and social workers who innately and intuitively possess these qualities and exercise them when given a chance. But I do not know of any training anywhere which offers the peculiar mix of a strong and modern theoretical foundation and applied practical experience which one would call adequate, In my mind, I have named such professionals, provisionally, "explainers" or "attitudinal counselors", and the branch of medicine which they would represent, "Attitudinal Medicine". Don't misunderstand me. I do not see them as robust, rosy-cheeked Mrs. Cheerfuls, sweeping into the sickroom to spread light and laughter. Warmth, to be sure, is a requisite; but with it should come maturity, high intelligence and ability to master the varied body of new knowledge now forming; toughness and resilience in the face of suffering; ability to share, to communicate with others (from physicians and colleagues to patient's families, work settings and friends); and, above all, an ability to sustain a realistic optimism in the face of disappointment. Some years ago my former wife, Charmian Elkes, began at Hopkins a program for training mental health counselors. The program, drawing upon the native abilities of mature women coming from different backgrounds, trained them into highly successful professionals (89) who subsequently won high acceptance in the Maryland Mental Health community. A Masters degree in Mental Health Counseling was offered. Attitudinal counselors who explain as they encourage, and encourage as they explain, could be powerful factors in raising patient morale, not through exhortation, but through participation, understanding and insight. It may be worth trying.

I believe that through applying the principles of communication which are at the heart of our field, we can provide leadership in the transformation of the medical environment, fashioning a true partnership between provider and consumer, reducing apprehension and fear, and enhancing hope. Could waiting areas be Learning Centers? Could the media in patients' rooms be arranged to provide choice of channels to include relevant technical information, well set out in lay languages, or mixes enhancing positive attitudes through information, through art, through humor? Could all that we know about groups be put to use in medical wards to speed recovery? Could all that we know about families become the therapeutic rule, rather than the exception in an emergency? And moving to the outpatient setting, could a referral to a psychiatrist be robbed of its stigma, and accepted, again, as part of a well explained, comprehensive therapeutic plan?

When, long before HMO's or group health were "in", we started on a prepaid system of medical care in Columbia, Maryland (112), psychiatry was seen as a *primary* care giver, together with Pediatrics, Medicine and Obstetrics and Gynecology. The offices were adjoining; a modest sliding fee scale limited to 10 sessions ensured acceptance. These thoughts are offered in the hope of a diffusion of what we know into the body of general medicine. Psychiatry should have the courage to use its knowledge, and use it comprehensively.

Psychological Medicine, Behavioral Medicine, Attitudinal Medicine – all imply the application of what we already know in modern psychiatry – to the ills, almost any ills – endemic in modern society. We should not be shunted aside: we bring with us a comprehensive and human approach. There is a need for "hospices" for the living as well as for the dying. Modern psychiatry knows enough to help in their design.

XIII. TOWARDS A SCIENCE OF WELL-BEING – THE PERSON IN THE LABORATORY OF EVERYDAY LIFE

As we move to the role of Psychological medicine in the arena of everyday life, we detect a costly paradox. For, whereas leading health planners are calling for a recognition of attitudinal behavioral interventions as factors in reducing health. cost (113) and diminishing the incidence of disease; whereas industry is making major capital investments in attempting to influence changing life habits in the workplace, and already reaping clear financial return on its investment (114, 115), we in medicine still stand at the periphery – preoccupied, hesitating, and "awaiting", as we say, "the evidence". Neither our curriculum nor practice reflects these urgent societal needs. Yet, modern psychiatry is already broad enough and strong enough to be in the lead. For the very methods and sciences which have given us medicine's most brilliant advances and have led us to precise diagnoses and rational therapeutics, now stand ready to be applied to the much less well mapped terrain of personal competence and well-being. To the ward and clinic and long term care facility we now add the laboratory of everyday life. It is beginning to prove an immensely rewarding area of investigation.

I suggest that modern psychiatry must go public with its knowledge, and that the public is ready and eager to learn what we already know. The success of media events like the PBS series on the Brain and Mind, where leading psychiatrists participated; the enormous sales of books on the Mind/Body/Brain connection; the emergence of powerful advocacy groups like the Schizophrenia foundation, the Alliance of the Medically Ill, N.A.R.S.A.; the pressures put on our state health services by the recent enactment of the 1987 Law; these all serve to build both negative and positive pressures to move the needs of our field into the public awareness. We have an opportunity to create an *informed constituency*. I am amazed by the timeliness, sense of newness and power, and appeal of our work; work whi.ch, in our parochial way, we have been taking totally for granted. Investment in particular diseases may be a powerful propellant; yet, in our case it could benefit from a broader base. I recall meeting recently with a prominent person to discuss needs for public support. "The Bloom is off the medical rose. We have heard, and heard, and heard about diseases", he said. "But the Mind/Brain/Body connection – that is new, fascinating stuff. It applies to disease as it does to health. You fellows must tell the public what you know already; communicate about communication – molecular, verbal, symbolic, social; about inside the skin and out. Their eyes will light up!"

We would do well to take note of my friend's sound advice.

REFERENCES

1. Meyer A: The purpose of the psychiatric clinic. AM. J. Insanity, 1913, 69, 835-860.
2. Meyer A: Psychobiology, A Science of Man. Springfield, IL: Charles C. Thomas, 1957.
3. Elkes J.: Psychopharmacology: On beginning in a new science. In: Ayd F.J. and Blackwell B. (eds.)
4. Elkes J: Behavioral pharmacology in relation to psychiatry. In: Gruhle HW, Jung R, Mayer-Gross W., and Mueller M. (eds.) Psychiatrie der Gegenwart. Berlin: Springer Verlag, 1962, pp. 929-1036
5. Elkes J: Subjective and objective observation in psychiatry. The Harvey Lectures, Series 57. New York: Academic Press, 1963, pp. 63-92
6. Elkes J: Epilogue and foreglimpse: Letter to a young colleague considering a career in psychopharmacology. In: Clark WG and de Guidice J (Eds.). Principles of Psychopharmacology. New York: Academic Press, 1978, pp. 741-53
7. Elkes J: Towards a science of health: Thoughts on brain, behavior, and wellbeing. Paper read at Symposium Optimum Utilization of Knowledge in Service of Health, at AAAS Annual Meeting titled, "Science and Engineering Toward a National Renaissance." Detroit, Michigan, May 27, 1983
8. Elkes J: On awareness and the good day. In: Ng LKY and Davis DL (Eds.) Strategies for Public Health: Promoting Health and Preventing Disease. New York: Van Reinhold, 1981, pp. 71-85
9. Weiner H: The organism in health and disease: An attempt at an integrative medical model. Paper presented at the Conference on New Models of Health, Illness and Disease: Implications of Psychoneuroimmunology, Lake Arrowhead, CA, 1987
10. Rubenstein E: Disease caused by impaired communication among cells. Sci Amer, 1988, 242, 102-121
11. Edelman GM: Topobiology: An Introduction to Molecular Embryology. New York: Basic Books, 1988
12. Jerne NK: The generative grammar of the immune system. Nobel Lecture. Hioscience Reports 1985, 5, 439-51
13. Spector NH: Interactions among the nervous, endocrine and immune systems. In: Frederickson RCR, Hendrie HC; Hingtgen JN and Aprison MH (Eds.) Neuroregulation of Autonomic, Endocrine and Immune Systems. Boston: Martinus Nijhoff Publishing, Inc., 1986, pp. 329-41
14. Mac Lean PD: The limbic system ("visceral brain") in relation to the central and reticulum of the brain stem. Psychosomatic Med 1955, 17, 355
15. Nauta WJH: Hippocampal projections and related neural pathways to the midbrain in the cat. Brain 1958. 81. 319
16. Craik KJW: The Nature of Explanation. London: Cambridge University Press, 1952
17. Head H: Aphasia and Kindred Disorders of Speech. London: Cambridge University Press, 1926
18. Miller NE: Learning visceral and glandular responses. Science. 1969, 163, 434-45
19. Edelman GM, Mountcastle V: The Mindful Brain: Cortical Organization and the Group-selective Theory of Higher Brain Function. Cambridge: ICT Press, 1978
20. Elkes J: Schizophrenic disorder in relation to levels of neural organization. In: Folch-Pi J. (Ed.) The Chemical Pathology of the Nervous System. London: Pergamen Press, 1961, pp. 648-65
21. Edelman GM: Neural Darwinism: The Theory of Neuronal Group Selection. New York: Basic Boocs, 1987
22. Frazer JG: The New Golden Bough. New York: Criterion Books, 1959
23. Jung CG: Man and His Symbols. Garden City NY: Doubleday, 1964
24. Campbell J: Historical Atlas of World Mythology. New York: Harper and Row, 1987
25. Grof S: Beyond the Brain. New York: State University of New York Press, 1985
26. Amkraut A, Solomon GS: From symbolic stimulus to pathophysiologic response. Internat J. Psychiat In Med. 1975 5, 134-56
27. Ader R: Psychoneuroimmunology. New York: Academic Press, 1981
28. Nossal GJV: Current concepts: Immunology. New Eng J. Med. 1987, 316, 1320-25
29. Locke SE, Colligan D: The Healer Within. New York: E.P. Dutton, 1987
30. Nossal GJV: Loc. Cit., p. 1320
31. Blalock JE: The immune system as a sensory organ. J Immunol. 1983, 132, 1067-70
32. Hall NR. McGillis JP, Spangelo BL, Goldstein AL: Evidence that thymosins and other biological response modifiers can function as neuroactive immunotransmitters. J. Immunol. 198, 136, 806-11
33. Keller SE, Stein M. Camerino MS, Schleifer SJ, Sherman J: Suppression of lymphocyte stimulation by anterior hypothalamic lesions in the guinea pig. Cell Immunol, 1980, 52, 334-40
34. Felten DL, Felten SY, Carlson SL, Olschowka JA, Livnat S: Noradrenergic and peptidergic innervation of lymphoid tissue. J Immunol. 1985, 35, 755-65
35. Bullock K, More RY: Innervation of the thymus gland by brainstem and spinal cord in mouse and rat. Am J Anat. 1982, 162, 157-66
36. Ader R, Cohen N: Behaviorally conditioned immunosuppression. Psychosom Med. 1975, 37, 333-340
37. Kiecolt-Glaser JK, Garner W, Speicher C, Penn GM, Holliday J, Glaser R: Psychosocial modifiers of immunocompetence in medical students. Psychosom Med. 1984, 46, 7-14
38. Locke SE, Kraus L, Leserman J, Hurst MW, Heisel S, Williams RM: Lifestress changes, psychiatric symptoms and natural killer cell activity. Psychosom Med., 1984, 46, 441-453
39. Linn BS, Linn MW, Jensen J: Degree of depresssion and immune responsiveness. Psychosom Med. 1982: 44, 128

40. Stein M, Schleifer SJ, Keller SS: Stress, depression and immunity. In: Fredrickson CA, Hendrie HC, Hingtgen JN and Aprison MH (Eds.) Neuroregulation of Autonomic, Endocrine and Immune Systems. Boston. Martinus Nijhoff Publishing, Inc.; 1986, pp. 329-41

41. Riley V, Fitzmaurice MA. Spackman DM: Psychoneuroimmunologic factors in neoplasia studies in animals. In: Ader R (Ed.). Psychoneuroimmunology, New York: Academic Press, 1981

42. Levy S: Host differences in neoplastic risk behavioral and social contributors to disease. Health Psychol, 1983, 2, 21-44

43. Lloyd R: Possible mechanisms of psychoneuroimmunological integrations. Advances, 1984, 1, 43-49

44. Levy SM (Ed.): Biological Mediators of Behavior and Disease: Neoplasia. New York: Elsevier Sciences Publishing, 1982

45. Heath RG, Krupp IM: Schizophrenia as an immunologic disorder. Arch Gen Psychiat 1967, 16, 1-9

46. Solomon GF: Immunologic abnormalities in mental illness. In: Ader R. Psychoneuroimmunology, New York. Academic Press. 1981

47. Sherrington CS: Man on His Nature. Cambridge (Engl.): Cambridge University Press, 1951, p. 104

48. Feldberg W, Vogt M: Acetycholine synthesis in different regions of the central nervous system. J Psysiol (London), 1948, 107, 372

49. Bradley PB. Elkes J: The effect of atropine, hyoscyamine, physostigmine and neostigmine on the electrical activity of the brain of the conscious cat. J Physiol (London), 1953, 120. p. 14

50. Bradley PB. Elkes J: The effects of some drugs on the electrical activity of the brain. Brain, 1967, 80, 77-117

51. Elkes J: Drug effects in relation to receptor specificity within the brain: Some evidence and provisional formulations. In: Wolstenholme GEW and O'Connor CM (Eds.) Neurological Basis of Behavior. CIBA Found- ation Symposium, London, 1957. London: J & A Churchill, 1958, p. 303

52. Bradley PB, Elkes J: The effects of some drugs on the. electrical activity of the brain. Op. cit., pp. 113-14

53. Schmitt FO: Molecular regulation of brain function: A new view. Neuroscience, 1984, 13, 991-1001

54. Keiss W, Hall DR: Psychoneuroimmunology and endocrine mediated evolution of the immune system. In: Hesch D (Ed.) Handbook of Endocrinology, Munich, West Germany: Urban and Schwarzenberg, 1989

55. Bulbring E: The action of adrenaline on transmission in the superior cervical ganglion. J. Physiol. 1944. 103. 55-67

56. Kandel ER: Cellular meahanisms of learning. In: Kandel ER. and Swartz JM (Eds.) Principles of Neuroscience. New York: Elsevier Sciences Publishing, 1985

57. Reite M, Field T: Psychobiology of Attachment and Separation. Orlando: Academic Press; 1985

58. Hanin I, Usdin E: Animal Models in Psychiatry and Neurology, New York: Pergamon Press, 1977,

59. Evonink GE. Kuhn CM, Schanberg SM: The effect of tactile stimulation on serum growth hormone and tissue or-nithine decarboxylase activity during maternal deprivation in rat pups. Communic Psychopharmacol. 1979, 3, 363-70

60. McGaugh J: Preserving the presence of the past: Hormonal influences on memory storage. Am Psychologist, 1983, 38, 161-73

61. Black IK, Ader JE, Dreyfus CF, Friedman WJ, LaGama EF, Roach AH: Experience, neurotransmitters plasticity and behavior. In: Meltzer H (Ed.) Psychopharmacology: The Third Generation of Progress. New York: Raven Press, 1987, pp. 63-70

62. Pert CB: Neuropeptides, the emotions and bodymind. Noetic Sci Rev, 1987, 2, 8-13

63. Nienwenhuys R: Chemoarchitecture of the Brain. New York: Springer Verlag, 1985

64. Cantin M, Genest J: The heart as an endocrine gland, Sci Amer, 1986, 25 (2), 76-81

65. Selye H: History and present status of the stress concept. In: Goldberger L and Breznitz S (Eds.), Handbook of Stress, New York:, McMillan, 1982, p. 7-20

66. Rossi E: From mind to molecule: A theory of mind body healing. Advances, 1987. 4, 46-60

67. Rossi E: The psychobiology of Mind-body Healing. New York: W.W. Norton, 1986

68. Overton D: Major theories of state-dependent learning. In: Ho B, Richards D and Chute D (Eds.) Drug Discrimination and State Dependent Learning. New York: Academic Press, 1978, pp. 283-318

69. Becker RO, Selden G: The Body Electric: Electromagnetism and the Foundation of Life. New York: William Morrow, 1985

70. Bakan D: Disease, Pain and Sacrifice. Chicago: University of Chicago Press, 1968

71. Cunningham AJ: Information and health in many levels of man. Advances, 1986, 3, 32-45

72. Snyder SH: A marriage of molecules, mind and medicine. In: Ray OS, Wilkes-Ray D (Eds.) American College of Neuropsychopharmacology, Anniversary Anthology, Nashville, TN: ACNP Publication, 1986, pp. 153-57

73. Bloom FE: Are pharmaceutical futures necessaril a prophetless commodity. In: Ray OS, Wilkes-Ray D (Eds.) American College of Neuropsychopharmacology, Anniversary Anthology: Nashville, TN: ACNP Publication, 1986, pp. 141-45

74. Meltzer HY (Ed.): Psychopharmacology: The Third Generation of Progress. New York : Raven Press, 1987

75. Barchas JD: Considerations for a future psychopharmacology. In: Ray OS, Wilkes-Ray D (Eds.) American College Neuropsychopharmacology, Anniversary Anthology. Nashville, TN: ACNP Publication, 1986, pp. 135-39

76. Chomsky N: Language and Mind. New York: Harcourt, Brace and World, 1968

77. Whorf BJ: Language, Thought and Reality. New York: Wiley, 1956
78. James W: Principles of Psychology. New York: Henry Holt, 1890. Reprinted by Dove Publications, New York, 1950, Vol. I. p. 255
79. Frank J: Persuasion and Healing (2nd edition), Baltimore, Johns Hopkins University Press, 1974
80. Frank JD: Psychotherapy, the transformations of meanings. J. Royal Soc Med, 1986, 79, 341-46
81. Frank JD: Psychotherapy, rhetoric and hermeneutics: Implications for practice and research. Psychotherapy, 1987, 24, 293-301
82. McHugh PR, Slavney PR: The Perspectives of Psychiatry, Baltimore: Johns Hopkins Press, 1983, pp. 1-26 and 125-34
83. Beck A: Cognitive Therapy and the Emotional Disorders. New York: International Universities Press, 1976
84. Yalom ID: The Theory and Practice of Group Psychotherapy. Second Edition, New York: Basic Books Inc., 1975
85. Rhodes J, Foard T, Dickstein L: Professional peer group counseling in the management of rheumatoid arthritis: A clinical trial. In: Hall RCW (Ed.) Recent Advances in Psychiatric Medicine, Orlando, FL: Ryandic Publishing, 1989
86. Reich W: Character Analysis. New York: Orgone Institute, 1949
87. Singer JL, Pope KS: The Power of the Human Imagination: New Methods in Psychotherapy. New York: Plenum Press, 1978
88. Hiatt JF: Spirituality, medicine and healing. Southern Med J. 1986, 79, 736-43
89. Elkes C, Godenne G.D. and Stone R.: The making of Mental Health Counselors. 1971. MSMHA Reports 86, pp. 307-313
90. Spingte R and Droh R.: Music in Medicine. Basel, Editiones Roche, 1985
91. Jackendoff R, Lerdahl F: Grammatical parallel between music and language. In: Clynes M (Ed.) Music, Mind and Brain. New York: Plenum Press, 1982, pp. 83-118
92. Shehhati-Chafai G, Kau G: Comparative study of the anxiolytic effects of diazepam and music in patients during operations in regional anesthesia. In: Spingte R and Droh R. Loc Cit, pp. 231-236
93. Tanioka F, Takazawa T, Kamata S. Kudo M, Matsuki A, Oyama T: Hormonal effect of anxiolytic music in patients during surgical operations under epidural anesthesia. In: Spingte R and Droh R. Loc Cit, pp. 285-291
94. Clynes M: Sentics: The Touch of Emotions. New York: Doubleday (Anchor) 1977
95. Adason E: Art as Healing. York Beach (Maine): Nicholas-Hays, 1984
96. Kuhn CC: A spiritual inventory of the medically ill patient. Psychiatric Medicine, 1988. 6, 89-100
97. Kleinman A: Patients and Healers in the Context of Culture, Berkeley, Los Angeles, Univ. of Calif. Press, 1980
98. Elkes J: Self regulation and behavioral medicine: Early beginnings. Psychiatric Annals, 1981, 11, 2, p. 54/27
99. Foss, L, Rothenberg K: The Second Medical Revolution – from Biomedicine to Infomedicine. Boston, Shambala Publications, 1988
100. Antonowsky A: Health, Stress and Coping. San Francisco, Jossey Bass, 1980
101. Rappleye WC: Medical education: Final report of the commission on medical education. AAME Commission on Medical Education,. Washington, DC: Association of American Medical Colleges, 1932
102. Cope D (Ed): Man, mind and medicine – The doctor's education, a chairman's view of the Swampscott study in behavioral science in medicine, 23 Oct – 4 Nov, 1986. Philadelphia J.B. Lippincott, 1968
103. Physicians for the twenty-first century. The GPEP report, Washington DC: Association of American Medical Colleges, 1984
104. Cousins N: Physician as a humanist. In: Reiser, DE and Rose, DH. Medicine as a Human Experience. Baltimore, University Park Press, 1984, p. ix
105. Neufeld VR. Barrows HS: The McMaster philosophy and approach to medical education. J. Med: Ed., 1974, 49, 1040-1050
106. Prywes M: The beer sheva experience: Integration of medical care and medical education. Isr J Med Sci, 1983, 19, 775-79
107. Engel GL: The need for a new medical model: A challenge for biomedicine. Science, 1977, 196, 129-36
108. Reiser DE, Rosen DH: Medicine as a Human Experience. Baltimore, University Park Press, 1984
109. Elkes J: On meeting psychiatry: A note on the students first year. Am J. Psychiat., 1965, August, 121-8
110. Thomas CB: What becomes of medical students: The dark side. Johns Hopkins Med. J., 1976, 138, 185-95
111. Dickstein LJ, Elkes J: Health awareness and the medical student: A preliminary experiment. Advances, 1987, 4, 11-23
112. Stone EM, Greenblatt M: The Columbia Plan: An interview with Joel and Charmian Elkes. Semin in Psychiatry, 1971, 3, 199-206
113. Knowles JH (Ed): Doing Better and Feeling Worse: Health in the United States. New York: W.W. Norton and Co., 1977
114. Fielding JH: Corporate Health Management. New York, Addison-Wesley, 1984
115. Pelletier KR: Health People in Unhealthy Places: Stress and Fitness at work. New York, Delacorte Press, 1984

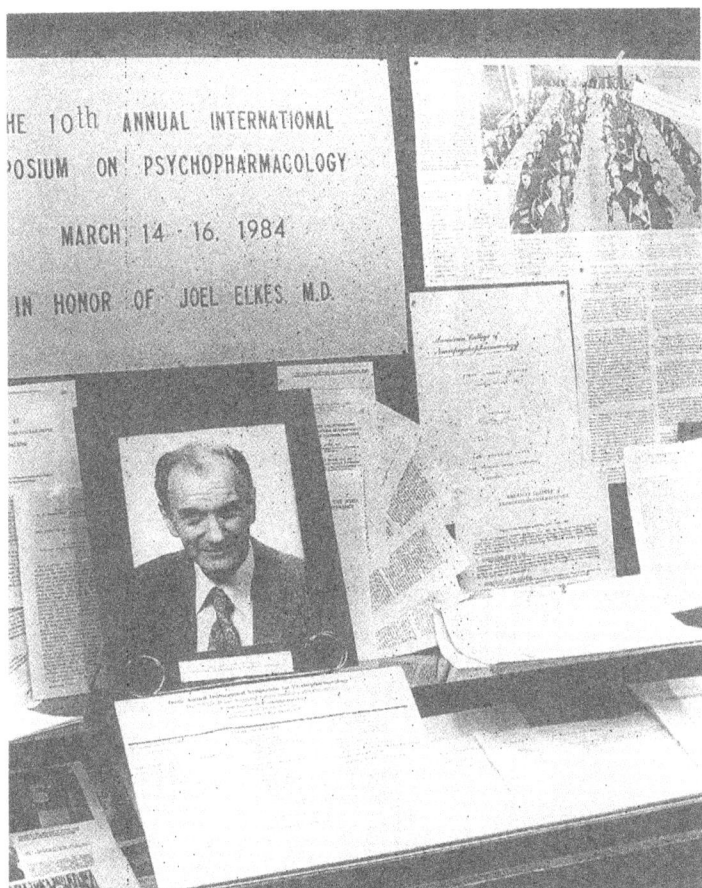

Tenth Annual International Symposium on
Psychopharmacology
Louisville, 1984, Library Display

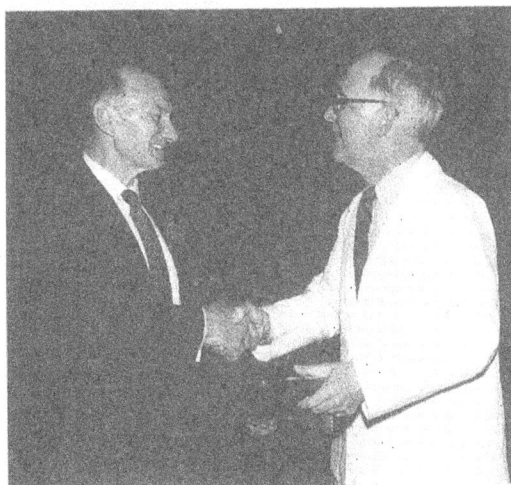

Receiving the Dedication Plaque from Paul McHugh,
May 18, 1988

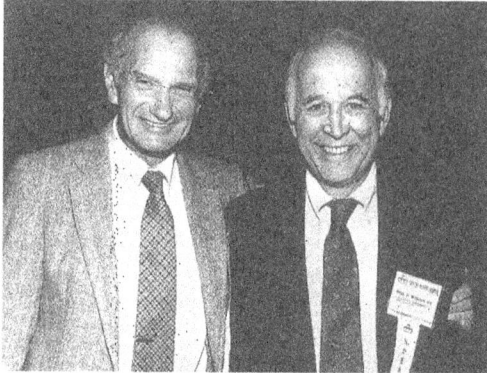

At Taylor Manor Symposium
with Paul McHugh

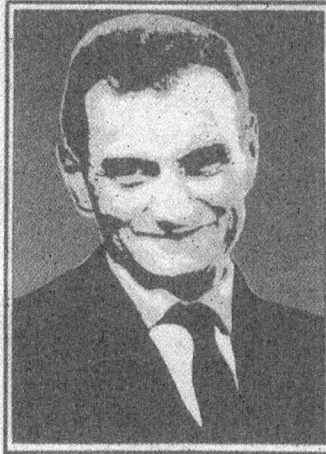

Dedication of the Joel Elkes Research Laboratories
and 75th Anniversary of the Founding of the
Department of Psychiatry and Behavioral Sciences
Johns Hopkins University and Hospital

Joel Elkes, M.D.
*Henry Phipps Professor and Director, Department of Psychiatry
and Behavioral Sciences*
1963-1975

Moderator	Speakers
Paul R. McHugh, M.D.	Joseph V. Brady, Ph.D.
	Solomon H. Snyder, M.D.
	Robert G. Robinson, M.D.
	Marshall F. Folstein, M.D.
	Joseph T. Coyle, Jr., M.D.
	Paul R. McHugh, M.D.

May 18, 1988   2:00 - 5:00 P.M.
Scientific Meeting, Turner Auditorium

5:00 - 6:00 P.M.
Tours of the Meyer Building

Announcement of Dedication of Joel Elkes Research Laboratories, May 18, 1988

Part Nine

THE COMMUNITY
AS AN AGENT OF PROACTIVE
HEALTH CARE
AND HEALTH ENHANCEMENT

PAPERS

Ever since his medical student days, Joel Elkes has been interested in the role of community-based health centers in pro-active health care, health education and health enhancement. When an opportunity presented itself in 1937 to study, at first hand, a novel experiment in prospecive health care in a working class London Borough, he seized it eagerly. The experiment was known as the *Peckham Experiment:* his comments on the subject, to a 1985 reissue of the book, describing this pioneer experiment are given in Paper 27.

The theme of social responsibility of psychiatry and the crucial role of the family in health maintenance and health enhancement did not leave him when he moved to Johns Hopkins in 1963. He spoke of this to the Baltimore Mental Health Association at the time.

In 1964/1965 Elkes learned of the plans by the Rouse Company for creating, *de novo*, a planned city between Washington and Baltimore. This city, Columbia, in Howard County, Maryland, was to be designed as a series of five to nine confluent villages, each with its own Family Life Center, schools within easy walking (or bicycling) distance and an array of educational, recreational and religious facilities. Columbia was to present the face of the "New America." It offered unprecedented opportunities for providing cost-effective medical services (including mental health services) emphasizing prevention and prompt mental health intervention without stigma; and also the prospect of a wide range of psychosocial research. Joel Elkes participated in the early conversations in 1964-65 between Johns Hopkins and the Rouse Company.

In July 28, 1966, he wrote to James W. Rouse, visionary developer, and Chairman of the Rouse Company. The letter (Paper 28), printed here, proposes the creation of a Center for the Study of Human Development as a joint venture between the Department of Psychiatry and Behavioral Sciences at Johns Hopkins and the Columbia Association.

Dr. Charmian Elkes, the wife of Joel Elkes was appointed the first chief of psychiatry at the Columbia Clinic. Her pioneering work there made Psychiatry (with Pediatrics, Internal Medicine and Gynecology and Obstetrics) a *primary,* rather than secondary specialty – an unusual arrangement at the time. Emergency and limited-term therapy were offered for a modest co-payment; and Mental Health Counselors, trained by Charmian Elkes and colleagues at Hopkins, offered effective intervention at an affordable price.

An interview with Joel and Charmian Elkes about the Columbia Plan and the Columbia Clinic is included (Paper 29).

PAPER 27

PAST/FUTURE CONJOINED:
NOTE FROM USA ON THE PRESENT EDITION
OF THE PECKHAM EXPERIMENT[*]

Joel Elkes

Distinguished Service Professor, Emeritus, The Johns Hopkins University and Professor of Psychiatry, Emeritus, Universities of Louisville, and McMaster University

It was a warm summer day in 1937. We had heard of The Peckham Experiment while on student rotation under Aleck Bourne, Chief of Obstetrics and Gynecology at St. Mary's Hospital, London. A man of deep human sympathy, and far ahead of his time, he had a clear vision of where medicine was going. A novel experiment in prospective health care was apparently proceeding in a working class London Borough. There was not much interest in our little group, except for one other student and myself. So on that warm summer day the two of us set out to see for ourselves.

We arrived in the late afternoon. Nearly fifty years later, I still recall the first impression of the building – a feeling of access and transparency: glass walls, glass doors, story-high open spaces. The classrooms and playrooms abutted the gym, and the swimming pool. The kitchen, the cafeteria, the reading room, even the pathology labs were visible from the passage way. Only the interview rooms we shielded from view. Children of all ages were everywhere, playing in crŠches, nurseries, and playrooms. Some were with their parents, some with "sister" (nurse) – some solo, some in clusters doing their thing on ropes, or roller skates, or engaged in quiet study or games. On the terrace-cafeteria, overlooking the pool, there were parents – mainly mothers, some of whom might be seen again in the evening joined by their husbands or friends. There was also a sprinkling of grandparents here and there. We noticed one other aspect: as the hours passed, more and more teenagers joined in. I remember thinking at the time how remarkable it was to have parents, children, teenagers, and even grandparents, all under one roof, and all clearly enjoying themselves. If there was "staff," it was hard to tell who was who.

Dr. Scott Williamson set aside the evening to explain his basic hypothesis, and let us sit in on a family health examination. We also looked at the record system – from laboratory tests, spirometer readings, and tonoscillograms, to the number of times a particular family had purloined roller-skates or hockeysticks. In these days of computerized health risk appraisal, this indeed appears a prescient vision enacted. I kept coming back to that unique human laboratory, participating, watching, and learning.

---

[*] Reprinted with the kind permission of the Scottish Academic Press from I.H. Pearce and L.H. Crocker's The Peckham Experiment: A Study of the Living Structure of Society (pp. 25–27). Scottish Academic Press, Edinburgh, 1985

The Peckham Experiment is contemporary and relevant. I was reminded of this when I came to Johns Hopkins, where a distinguished predecessor of mine, Adolph Meyer, had opened, in 1913, the building in which we all were to work later. As he said at the time:

> "At last science begins to take up with new and forceful methods the great problem of mental life… This work does not stop in the sanctum of the investigator. Just as bacteriology studies the water supply of communities, schools, and homes, so we psychopathologists have to study more effectively the atmosphere of the community; and must devise safeguards in the locality from which patients come, and to which they are to return." (1)

I have a feeling that, although they may not have agreed in detail, Adolf Meyer and Scott Williamson would have liked each other. Both were what the Germans call "Naturforscher," searchers of Nature, keen observers of things natural, students of the human condition-in-context. Both recognized the limitations of the purely analytical approach. Both sought languages to express novel relationships, and found existing languages wanting. Long before the birth of formal Systems Science, both were "Systems" men to their marrow.

A slight shift in focus can open a universe of new contours and connections. The depth of the obvious calls for a special kind of vision. Scott Williamson was endowed with that special vision. He looked deeply into the obvious and, like good painters, made the familiar glow anew. Instead of studying Health in the context of Disease, he and Innes Pearse resolved to study Disease in the context of Health and Ease: "Ethology rather than Pathology."

They put the terms of "living" and "dying" into context. "A whole lifetime may be spent in the process of dying." they argued. "Survival" isn't living; nor is health the mere absence of disease, but a dynamic, continuing, lifelong state of growth. Health, so contemporary (and so abused) a term is a subject worthy of scientific study. They studied the family as the appropriate biosocial unit, in its home, not as a material fabric, but a live zone for the interchange of social nutrients.

The Pioneer Health Centre was a strange hybrid of a Center, in part a Leisure Centre, in part a Health Surveillance Clinic (serving to identify, but not to treat, incipient disorders); in part a Family Club; a Baby and Children's Care Center; a Nutrition Learning Center; and, in part, a school: but first and foremost it was their laboratory for the study of health.

The incisive simplicity of the approach may be noted in another respect. The baby care center was emphatically *not* a "day-care center." It functioned on afternoons, when mothers could bring their children and enjoy each other's and their children's company on the premises. The staff was sparse and very competent.

If all this has a familiar ring, it is simply because what has been hidden in medical care has become obvious. Behavior and mode of life-lifestyle, as we say – have emerged as major pathogens in our society. Galloping health costs have forced planners to shift emphasis from high technology care to cost containment at primary sources nearer home. Industry, usually ahead of the general public, is taking very seriously Employee Assistance Programmes, Health Awareness, and Preventive Education in the workplace. A lively stress management industry – of highly variable quality – is offering all manner of comprehensive approaches to the willing buyer. A "Wellness" wave – complete with workshops on jogging, nutrition, yoga, and all – is sweeping through homes and institutions; the general public is going to medical school by way of evening classes, books and cassettes. Yet, in all this "Wellness" frenzy a central theme is both subsumed, and lost by default. That theme is, The Family as a School. In changing times, to be sure, families will change; but even in post-industrial times, one would venture to predict, families, schools, neighbourhoods will become more, rather than less important. More work will be done in the home, and telecommuting to work (rather than body-commuting) will be commonplace. Leisure will be a main byproduct of a shorter work-week. Longevity will call for more, rather than less, intergenerational contact. The neighbourhood of the future could indeed be very different: it could be infinitely more human and humane than the present suburban sprawl. All that is needed is Vision and Data.

It is this need which makes the challenge of Peckham so thoroughly contemporary. For if the megaproviders, megamanagers, and megaconsumers of the future took a cognate approach, a data base for sound, enlightened, participatory, practical planning could quickly emerge. The megaproviders are the Government, the Corporate giants in Health Care Delivery, and the Insurance Industry. The megaconsumers are Corporations, to whom good employee health simply means good business. Developers of urban renewal projects, or of new urban and suburban neighbourhoods, and of factory towns, have a special opportunity.

It would be simple and relatively cheap to build neighbourhood Family Life and Health Centers into such developments; similar centers could also be set up in existing neighbourhood renewal programs in conjunction with local authorities, physicians, community agencies, churches, and the like. In these days of computerized family records, families could generate data deeply significant to their *own* health and wellbeing. For health data have a social function: they should not be consigned to Ph.D. theses, but be returned to the consumer to be tested in the laboratory of everyday life. In the field of health, Search and Re-Search, Discovery and Proof, while distinct phases, go hand in hand as a single enterprise.

Moreover, the scientific biomedical base is broadening. Modern psychosomatics is becoming a fascinating experimental science. Bodymind is no longer two words, but one. The laboratory within one's skin is becoming accessible to Everyman.

To all of which I would add another term, which I heard in quiet hours at Peckham. There they talked of the Healing Community, and of Comm-Union; and as I listened, I agreed that it does not come free.

REFERENCE

1. Meyer, A. The Purpose of the Psychiatric Clinic. (American Journal of Insanity: special number in celebration of the opening of the Henry Phipps Psychiatric Clinic: Vol. LXIX, No. 5:858: Baltimore, Johns Hopkins Press, 1913.)

PAPER 28

LETTER TO JAMES W. ROUSE

July 28, 1966

Mr. James W. Rouse
President
The Rouse Company
The Village of Cross Keys
Baltimore, Maryland 21210

Dear Mr. Rouse:

I have given a good deal of thought to our several conversations and am writing to explore with you further the possibility of creating, at an early date, Center for Human Development in Columbia under the joint aegis of this Department and the Columbia Association. Such a Center could conveniently be known as the Columbia Hopkins Center for Human Development, though other names maybe judged more appropriate.

Over the past decade I have become increasingly concerned over the failure of academic psychiatry to "deliver" in the area of prevention of mental disability, and (with certain notable exceptions) to interest itself in problems of health rather than sickness. The traditional approaches of psychiatry have been remedial and retrospective, rather than preventive and prospective. Studies of mal-development and breakdown still outweigh, by far, studies of successful coping and of social adequacy. This emphasis on pathology rather than Well-Being has powerfully affected general medical education, the education of psychiatrists, and a host of paramedical professions, and has hardened into attitudes and institutions which, to my mind, have left a sad imprint on the American way of life.

Yet there is need in our society to define and test operationally those factors and forces which, used appropriately, and in concert, could make for the growth of human initiative and ability, the enhancement of social responsiveness and the evocation of capacities inherent in us all. It would seem to me that a community such as Columbia could offer the Behavioral Sciences an opportunity to engage in research which could become very meaningful to that community. It would also offer an opportunity to train leaders in evolving techniques, and in new professions. The manpower problem is sure to loom large in the years to come: anything that can be done to anticipate the needs of communities-to-come would certainly be timely.

The Center which I am proposing should not be too large. Size is inversely proportional to communication. It should be strong in theory *and* in practice. Its staff should comprise some six (or at most eight) behavioral scientists chosen not only for their academic distinction, but their proven ability to render their discipline socially useful. Among the disciplines so represented could be Sociology (and/or Social Psychology), Cultural Anthropology, Education (and/or Educational Psychology), the Study of Family life, the Study of Small Group Process, Computer Technology, Epidemiology and Biostatistics. Naturally, such representation would depend on the availability of suitable people. Such people are scarce. Yet, I am hopeful that, given sufficient funds and adequate facilities, we could compete reasonably well.

It would seem advisable, during the initial formative period (of, say, five to seven years) to link the Center administratively to our Department and the Johns Hopkins University, while at the same time establishing an active working relationship between the Center and the Columbia Association. The academic and the applied sides of the Center would thus be nicely balanced. The link with our Department (where it would occupy major "Divisional" or "Center" status, for which there is precedent) would make it possible for the principal figures to hold appropriate academic rank in the University, and to train students (both predoctoral and post-doctoral). It would also make available the abundant facilities of the Johns Hopkins School of Medicine, the Johns Hopkins Hospital, with its major investment in Columbia, the School of Hygiene and Public Health and the facilities on the Homewood Campus, where there is considerable interest in Columbia. Moreover, our own planned study of underprivileged negro population in Baltimore could provide valuable reference populations for comparison with re-settled negro families in Columbia.

The interface with the Columbia Association, on the other hand, could amount to a working partnership between an academic institution and an evolving community. The Center could interact with the experimental school programs, the Family Life Center, the Neighbourhood Center, the Churches' Social Action Program and the abundant continued education activities. Through judicious use of the data it gathers, the Center would share in the shaping of the community of which it would be an organic part. It is to be hoped that a good many scientists would live in Columbia and thus would function as scientist-citizens. Studies and Experiments could be initiated in a number of variants; and the lessons learnt in one phase of development applied to the next.

You may well inquire after the reasons for my own deep interest in your program. In part, I have stated these, in somewhat negative terms, at the beginning of this letter. On the more positive side, I believe that a major involvement of the Behavioral Sciences in medical education and medical practice is inevitable, and that an interaction between clinical psychiatry and the behavioral sciences, and between psychiatry and education is long overdue. The name of this Department expresses this trend. Moreover, it seems likely that studies of Human Development, of Human Learning (including social learning), Human Communication and of the Social field will make up much of the matrix of future psychiatry. In our Department we have stressed Child and Adolescent Psychiatry, Educational Therapy, and laboratory studies of the genesis of language, of communication, and the processes of cognitive functioning, attention and learning in children. We will take up Small Group Process studies and Family Studies as soon as we obtain suitable personnel. The family would still seem man's most important school. The Behavioral Sciences have much to contribute to our understanding of the mal-functioning of human institutions; but they must be given a chance to engage, evolve, and learn at the same time.

It is, I suppose, an affinity between these general trends, and the ideas expressed at the meetings to which you so kindly invited me, which prompt one to suggest to you the creation of an Academic Center at Columbia. Please regard this proposal as the most preliminary of statements; and feel free to call on me for any further details which you may require.

Sincerely yours,
Joel Elkes, M.D.
Henry Phipps Professor of Psychiatry
Director, Department of Psychiatry and Behavioral Sciences
The Johns Hopkins University
Psychiatrist-in-Chief
The Johns Hopkins Hospital

PAPER 29

THE COLUMBIA PLAN: AN INTERVIEW WITH JOEL AND CHARMIAN ELKES*

Evelyn M. Stone and Milton Greenblatt, M.D.

Massachusetts Mental Health Center

Columbia, a planned new city, situated half-way between Washington, D.C., and Baltimore, was first conceived by Mr. James Rouse and his wife Libby, of Baltimore, and came into being in 1966. It is designed as a series of nine confluent villages (each with its own village center), surrounding a downtown central core, and fringed by well-planned industrial areas, housing more than thirty different kinds of industries, including distributing, light manufacturing, and research and development enterprises. There is abundant parkland enclosing artificial lakes, bridle paths, and golf courses, and a large array of recreational facilities, ranging from an open-air Symphony Pavilion (seating 5000) to community halls and small theatres, workshops, and artists' studios. At present there are about 10,000 people living and working in Columbia. The anticipated yearly growth rate is about 10,000, with a goal of about 110,000 inhabitants by 1980.

On October 1, 1969, the Connecticut Life Insurance Company and the Johns Hopkins Medical Institutions joined in forming the Columbia Hospital and Clinics Foundation which undertook to provide a prepaid comprehensive insurance health plan open to all citizens of Columbia. The present psychiatric coverage (under a total monthly medical premium of $51.00 per family) provides for 15 visits at a co-payment of $2.00 per visit, and any number of visits under a co-payment of $10.00 per visit until the end of a given calendar year (when a co-payment of $2.00 per visit for 15 visits resumes).

Q.: We are curious to know how Johns Hopkins, and you, specifically, became involved in the Columbia Plan.

J.E.: The idea of a medical service in Columbia arose originally in a conversation between Dr. Russell Nelson, the President of Johns Hopkins Hospital, and Mr. James Rouse, the developer of Columbia. In November, 1964, a meeting took place at which Mr. Rouse, Dr. Nelson, Dr. Paul Lemkau (Professor of Mental Hygiene, the John Hopkins School of Hygiene and Public Health) and I discussed the idea further.

Q.: Are physicians usually called in the planning of a new city?

J.E.: No, not usually; but then, Mr. Rouse is a most unusual man. It was he and Mrs. Rouse who conceived the idea of completely planning a new city (rather than a mere development). Nor did they stop at the mere physical phase of planning, important and attractive though this

---

* Joel Elkes is Henry Phipps Professor and Director of the Department of Psychiatry and Behavioral Sciences, The Johns Hopkins University School of Medicine, and Psychiatrist-in-Chief, The Johns Hopkins Hospital, Baltimore, Maryland.

Charmian Elkes is Associate Professor of Psychiatry, The Johns Hopkins University School of Medicine, and Psychiatrist, Columbia Hospital and Clinics, Columbia, Maryland.

Reprinted with the kind permission of W.B. Saunders from Seminars in Psychiatry 3: 199-206, 1971.

may be. They were equally concerned with the way in which social institutions in Columbia could be designed to enhance the quality of life. Mr. Rouse and his associates created a number of study groups to examine various aspects of health, education, communication, etc. The central idea was to plan the City around a group of confluent villages, each with its own idiomatic community life. Mr. Rouse was also taken with the idea of the old "Pechham Experiment" in London (in which, it so happens, I participated as a medical student before World War II).

When Mr. Rouse invited me to join his various planning groups from 1964 forward, I was delighted at the opportunity.

Q.: What we find provocative is that psychiatrists (you and Dr. Lemkau) should be consulted in the initial planning stage.

J.E.: Mr. Rouse believed that psychiatry could take a somewhat more comprehensive view of problems of health maintenance, and prevention, than a conventional clinical" model was likely to provide. Since modern psychiatry is family and community centered, I certainly agree.

Those early planning discussions in the Rouse Company's offices between 1964 and 1967 were extraordinarily rich and varied. Many outside experts and consultants participated. At the same time, Dr. Nelson and our former Dean, Dr. Thomas Turner, and their colleagues were slowly, moving the Johns Hopkins Medical Institutions toward the idea of operating a new kind of enterprise (a prepaid medical plan) in Columbia. Our present Dean, Dr. David Rogers, and his colleague, Dr. Robert Heyssel, Director of the Johns Hopkins Office of the Health Care Programs, have given a vivid account (2, 4) of what transpired before the Johns Hopkins Medical Institutions finally accepted the Columbia plan. All manner of arguments were mounted against it; yet the soundest of all was that the institution should not accept responsibility for a plan in Columbia without developing a comparable plan for the community in our immediate neighbourhood in East Baltimore. I felt strongly, that it should be "double or nothing", and said so. In the end, good sense prevailed: We now have two plans; one (just about to be implemented), for East Baltimore, the other in Columbia. Between them, they provide an unrivaled experimental terrain for the operation of health care delivery systems, and opportunities for developing new professional skills, mixes, and indeed, new professions. I am sure that Charmian will want to refer later to her part in the training of new types of psychiatric personnel.

Q.: What constitutes the Johns Hopkins Medical Institutions in this context?

J.E.: The Johns Hopkins University School of Medicine, the Johns Hopkins Hospital, and the Johns Hopkins School of Hygiene and Public Health.

To go back, while all this was happening, Columbia was acquiring its first citizenry who were asking for medical help. Also, at the same time, some critical negotiations were proceeding with the Connecticut Life Insurance Company. What came forth was a remarkable agreement. The Connecticut Life Insurance Company undertook to underwrite the developmental costs of the program over the first 5 years; this gave our Institutions the monies to move forward.

Q.: Would that include building the clinic now at Columbia?

J.E.: The clinic now functioning in Columbia is housed in a temporary building. The clinic of the future is envisioned, ultimately, as a 180-bed hospital, the first phase of which – a 60-bed general hospital unit and outpatient facilities – should be completed within about 18 months. The present clinics function under the aegis of the Office of Health Care Programs, of which Dr. Robert Heyssel is Director. My wife, Dr. Charmian Elkes, who is at the clinic, is employed by the Columbia Medical Group.

But to go back a little to 1967 and 1968. I have already mentioned my work on Mr. Rouse's advisory committees. At the beginning of 1968, requests for more advice in the area of community development came in. In response to these demands, Dr. William Hausman (now Chairman of the Department of Psychiatry, University of Minnesota, who, at that time, was Director of our Student Mental Health Service at Hopkins) established a field office at Columbia. This served three purposes. First, he was available for the occasional clinical consultation. Second, he could engage in planning activities with local community resource personnel. And, third, the planning of the modest psychiatric component of the Columbia plan could also proceed.

To make planners understand the assigned place of psychiatry was not easy. For one thing, there are very few prepaid plans which include psychiatry, and there was thus little in the way of guidance available. For another, I think, one probably also dealt with a state of mind which traditionally viewed the role of psychiatry as looking after the "sick" psychiatric patient. The catalytic and preventive role of modern family centered psychiatry in a comprehensive family centered health service was more difficult to accept, because of its unfamiliarity.

Dr. Hausman and I also set up the Columbia Council, a community council on which major institutions of Columbia are represented. This was the first time that major county officers, education officers, police, and the clergy began to formulate plans in which their interests overlapped.

Q.: How did you finally convince people of the need for a psychiatric service?

J.E.: By just quietly talking, and, hopefully, showing the economic of it; and by the spareness and reasonableness of our demands. Please remember, there is not a penny of grant money in either our Service or our Mental Health Counselor Training Program. Dr. Hausman, in his discussions with the Council, referred to the integrating function of psychiatry in achieving a family centered service. Psychiatry provides the common ground between specialties, which properly used, can reduce medical costs.

Q.: Were you also trying to sell the concept of preventive psychiatry at that time?

J.E.: Yes. However, the Columbia Plan is a Sickness and Health maintenance plan – witness the annual physical check-up, and well baby care. Prevention in the area of mental illness has to reach deeply into the school, into the family (which is the most important school of all), into social institutions, and into recreation. I am, as you know, firmly committed to the concept of the self-helping society. Such activities as I mentioned, therefore, must be coordinated in a manner to be complementary to the services provided by the Columbia plan. I am formally Director of Mental Health Services for the City of Columbia, and am now engaged in a major planning effort to develop such complementary community-centered services. Charmian is the head of the psychiatric component of the Columbia Hospital and Clinics. It is quite clear that the two will overlap.

The Johns Hopkins Medical Institutions regard the Columbia and East Baltimore programs as their main laboratories for experimentation in health care delivery systems. The role of the applied behavioral sciences in health education and health care delivery is becoming steadily more apparent – to some, at any rate.

Q.: What do you consider the major obstacles in setting up the Columbia program?

J.E.: Well, there were institutional obstacles, and there were some attitudinal obstacles. In other words, one had to really convey the role of psychiatry in the context of day-to-day primary care practice, rather than its role as a secondary care specialty for referral patients. This is a different image from the way in which psychiatry is often regarded. Psychiatry is, in my view, a primary care resource. Also, one must fit psychiatry into an economic budget; and there, the kind of service which Charmian has developed, using mental health counselors, is very significant, and, in my view, far-reaching.

Q.: Before discussing the services, we would like to hear from Dr. Charmian Elkes something about the people who live in Columbia. Is it essentially a middle-class community?

C.E.: Yes, I would say so. They would be sociologically speaking about Class III, with many college-educated people. There is a racial mixture, about 15% blacks, also largely middle-class. However, there are plans for industrial growth in Columbia, including a major factory of General Electric, which will employ about 10,000 people. Many will then come from lower socioeconomic classes which will change the present composition of Columbia.

Q.: When did you first become involved with Columbia? Was it from the very beginning?

C.E.: No, I became involved in July 1969, and the clinic actually started operation in October. We started out with a small group of physicians: two internists, two pediatricians, one obstetrician-gynecologist, one radiologist, and a psychiatrist. Joel is right in what he said about the role of psychiatry in the clinic to begin with. The rest of the staff were not accustomed to having a psychiatrist around, and as I had not worked in a general medical setting for many years, it was strange for me, too. From almost the first day, the clinic was busy and it has grown more so during the first year. Of the members, 80% have made use of the clinic, and we now have about 6000 members. Now the population of Columbia is something over 10,000.

Q.: Membership meaning those in the prepaid plan?

C.E.: That's right. They may join the plan if they are residents of Columbia; and, in addition, the population of most of Howard County and adjacent areas are eligible if their employers offer the plan through group coverage.

Q.: How long were you in operation before you had your first psychiatric patient?

C.E.: I had my first Columbia patient that first month, and then the services increased rapidly. Initially, most of the patients were self-referred; but recently more and more of them have been referred by physicians. We have a very easy and informal way of meeting and discussing problems back and forth. You know, I would like to talk a little about how the psychiatric department became a part of the clinic. Psychiatry was really neglected at first; however, over the months, just by being there and sort of quietly mingling and being available, the other physicians have become more accepting.

Q.: The resistances were from the medical staff then and not from the community?

C.E.: Initially, yes; but, I would say, they have largely disappeared. I think the resistance was due to lack of experience on the part of the medical and administrative staff with this kind of participating psychiatric service. From the community there seems little resistance except from the teenagers. I think the reasons for our acceptance on the clinical level are first, that the clinic is still a small unit, and second because of our geographical position in the clinic. The clinic is built like a horseshoe; the internists and gynecologists on one side, pediatricians on the other, and psychiatry in the middle, so that we can't avoid each other. I think this has been a very great benefit to the patients. The physicians ask me for consultations, and refer and discuss patients whom they would not refer if they did not have someone so easily available.

Q.: You see both children and adults?

C.E.: Yes. It was only myself to start with; and then in December one of the mental health counselors (1) joined me for 1 day a week. In January we had a child psychiatrist 1 day a week and one of the Phipps (Johns Hopkins) residents 3 hours a week. He was donated for the whole year; we did not pay him. The child psychiatrist was also partly donated for a time so that our outlay for psychiatric care was pretty small.

Almost immediately we had a great problem of dealing with children. The pediatricians were anxious for a child psychiatrist. When he came, he evaluated children and also visited one of the nursery schools as a consultant. We had an arrangement with the Howard County School system whereby he could consult with them, but that fell through. Because of the Howard County experience we haven't become too much involved with the schools, but fortunately we have a Phipps resident who acts as a consultant to the schools. He also has contact with the probation officers, public health nurses, and others who are peripheral to school consultation.

I would like to say a word about the mental health counselors. One of the aims of the clinic is to provide comprehensive health care within an economical, budget. The use of paramedical personnel is one way to do it. In the psychiatric service we have been able to implement this plan by the use of mental health counselors, women who have received an intensive 3-year training in psychotherapy at the Phipps Clinic. This program has been in operation since 1966 and has recently been approved for a master's degree in mental health. It is modeled on a pilot training project which was carried out at the NIMH 10 years ago (3).

Q.: Does a community, where everyone is putting down roots, so to speak, pose any unique psychiatric problems?

C.E.: I believe so from my experience in Columbia. One fact of this community is that many people know that they need psychiatric help. It is not uncommon for people to say they have wanted it for a long time but have not been able to afford it. Our utilization rate in the first year has been nearly 4%, which I believe is rather high in relation to other comparable plans. I read a paper from HIP of New York reporting 1.1% utilization for their psychiatric services.

Q.: Are there any emotional hazards in living in such a closed community?

C.E.: One of the emotional hazards might be that everyone has just moved and moving is a disruption; it is really a traumatic experience. It's my impression that these people are very often the pioneering sort of people who have the energy and the initiative to get up and go to a new place. But they also have very much the "grass is greener" attitude, and then they suffer a letdown. I think we're dealing with that quite a bit. The structure of the population means that we have a lot of referrals because they are very sophisticated, well-educated, psychiatrically-oriented people, and many of them come to us saying they need help with their marriage, for example.

Q.: What happens when you see a patient who is frankly psychotic? You have no facility to take care of such a patient at Columbia. Where do you send him?

C.E.: We try to admit to Phipps. If he can't be admitted there because of the bed situation, he would be taken care of in another hospital.

Q.: Do you see that patient at Phipps or do you just hand him over?

C.E.: The situation is such that I know most of the staff there and am part of the staff, so that yes, I could always see him. The limiting factor is time, so mostly I might just visit and then accept the patient back when he is discharged. We've had eight or ten people admitted to Phipps in the last year.

Q.: Is yours a 24-hour emergency service?

C.E.: No, I see patients from 9 to 5, and after that I'm on call.

Q.: What would be Columbia's priority for mental health services? Is it to stamp out drug abuse? Or improve race relations? Or what?

C.E.: We have been asked mostly for direct clinical service, and sometimes for participation or leadership in discussions on community projects. The community itself takes care of some of their mental health problems. There are a number of on-going sensitivity-type group discussions, often led or organized by various religious groups in the community. I have heard of black-white confrontation groups in this context, but it doesn't seem to me that racial tension is high in Columbia. People have told me that they come to Columbia so that their children may grow up in a mixed community, and intermarriage is not uncommon. It may be that there is a tendency to deny the existence of a black-white problem, but I really don't now about that.

There is a difficult problem with drug abuse among teenagers, but we don't see many of them at the clinic. Our patients are mostly young to middle-age adults and children. However, a group of students from the Columbia branch of Antioch College received a state grant to set up a drug abuse program for teenagers. They deal with a variety of kids, many of whom come from outside. Columbia is a new place and has become a congregating area from all over the place for teenagers, including Washington and Baltimore. This program is called "Grass Roots".

Q.: Pretty appropriate name wouldn't you say?

C.E.: Yes. They actually deal most of the time over the telephone with disturbed teenagers, who by no means all want help with drug problems. They are also runaways and kids with family problems. The students who run "Grass Roots" are rather loosely associated with us. Some of us sit on their Advisory Committee, but they are not too keen on formal supervision. Actually, I've been rather favorably impressed with their work so far.

Q.: Do you have a waiting list for your clinic?

C.E: I'm afraid so. Apart from urgent cases, people sometimes wait 4 or even 6 weeks for an appointment. I don't like waiting lists, but with our small staff it's unavoidable at present. I'm at the clinic 3 days a week; Dr. Lazaroff, the child psychiatrist, 1 day; and three mental health counselors, a total of 4 days. Our services range from single-visit consultations, crisis intervention, continuing short and long-term therapy, to follow-up of people with medication. The number of visits per patient has averaged 5.7 in the first year. One of the things I regret is that we've not been able to do more group work. We only have one group at present, a married couples group; we do a lot of work with couples and also family therapy. We will have to wait for more staff before expanding the group work.

Q.: Would you at any point consider the idea of using somebody who lives in Columbia as one of your mental health counselors or would you just eschew that as a matter of confidentiality?

C.E.: No, no. One of our mental health counselors does live there, actually. There are, however, problems with that. We have to be careful about whom she sees, that it is not someone with whom she is socially familiar; but this has worked out all right.

Q.: How do the patients feel about your counselors? Do they resent being seen by a counselor and not by you? Has there been any objection?

C.E.: I have not heard of any. Some people ask for me by name; they might do that because they don't want to see a counselor. But on the other hand, some people ask for them by name, too. I haven't heard any complaints about them. Acceptance by patients and physicians is very high.

Q.: What would be the optimum staff for you right now?

C. E.: I was just thinking about that, because of estimating for staff for next year and I was also again looking at the HIP reports. They had a staff of 12 full-time people for a membership of 65,000 and an utilization rate of 1.1%. Somebody did the arithmetic for me and that would have meant for us the equivalent of 3 $^1/_2$ full-time people, and we have the equivalent of 1.7. I think 3 1/2 will be overstaffing and I estimate the optimum at present would be 2 $^1/_2$ full-time staff.

Q.: What rate of growth per year do you envisage for the Columbia Plan?

C.E.: This is extremely hard to estimate, but we are planning with the expectation of 15,000 members by the end of 1972.

Q.: In the permanent hospital that's being built, will you have any beds allocated to you?

C.E.: Yes. There will be four available, but that won't mean that they're just kept for psychiatric patients. But they will be available if we need to keep anyone for observation. I don't want a psychiatric unit in the hospital. I think it would be too costly and I hope we can continue to admit to Phipps.

J.E.: We intend to build a small unit in Columbia, as soon as this becomes feasible.

Q.: What do you call small?

J.E.: 25 to 50 beds. Thus, a long-term facility at Columbia would be complementary to our facility at Phipps. We also intend to develop the closest possible links with representative persons and institutions of the community, i.e., the consumer, and have a feedback system from the consumer to us to ensure quality control. The areas of prevention and health education work with schools, families, and the interfaith center will be developed as our department becomes more active in Columbia and the surrounding county. The beauty about Columbia is that it's a very modern city growing, in its own idiom, in a county which is thoroughly rural; a sociological and human point and counterpoint, a challenge which continues to intrigue.

REFERENCES

1. Elkes, C.: The training of mental health counselors: An account of three program. World Mental Health Assembly, Washington, D.C., November, 1969.
2. Heyssel, R. M.: The Johns Hopkins Columbia Medical Plan. Med. Opinion 6:30, 1970.
3. Riocb, M., et al.: NIMH pilot project in training mental health counselors. Public Health Service Publication 1254, 1964.
4. Rogers, D. E., and Heyssel, A M.: One medical school's involvement in the development of new health care delivery models: Its problems and its pleasures. Unpublished.

Part Ten

HOLOCAUST AND ISRAEL

PAPERS

30. J. Elkes (1985) *Remarks made at the holocaust commemorative ceremony.*
    Kentucky Center of the Arts. April 17, 1985
31. J. Elkes (1996) *Charles E. Smith and the possible dream.* Introductory remarks at the 25th
    Anniversary Symposium of the National Institute for Psychobiology in Israel in Memory
    of Charles E. Smith[*], April 18, 1996
    Reprinted with the kind permission of the National Institute for Psychobiology in Israel
    from the booklet prepared by the Institute

Joel Elkes received his high school education (from 1922 to 1930) in Kovno, Lithuania. The
school was unusual in that all subjects (from trigonometry to Voltaire) were taught in modern
Hebrew. Academic standards were very high. The teachers were masters of their subject, and
devoted to their task. When textbooks in Hebrew were lacking, the teachers wrote them during
the summer vacation and distributed the material on stenciled sheets. The school's aim was to
prepare students for a constructive life in the then Palestine... a future homeland, and ultimately State, of the Jewish people.

Joel Elkes' father, Dr. Elchanan Elkes, was a prominent physician in Lithuania. He sent
Joel Elkes and his sister, Sara, to England in 1931 and 1937, respectively. He and his wife,
Miriam, stayed behind. The German occupation of 1941 brought the Holocaust to Lithuania.
Ghetto Kovno was established in August 1941. Dr. Elchanan Elkes as elected head of that
Ghetto by the Jewish community – one of the very few Jewish leaders to be so elected, rather
than appointed by the Germans. By the end of 1941, some 137,000 Jews had been killed in
Lithuania, including nine members of Joel Elkes' family.

Against impossible odds, a portion of the small community of Ghetto Kovno survived almost to the end of the war. This was due to the leadership of the Ghetto Council, headed by Dr.
Elchanan Elkes. Civic structure, work, and cultural life were maintained to an extraordinary
degree: Dr. Elchanan Elkes' dignity and bearing in dealing with the Germans is now a legend
in the Annals of the Holocaust.

In October 1997 there opened a major exhibit at the National Holocaust Museum in Washington, D.C. to honor the extraordinary community of Ghetto Kovno, and its leadership. The
Exhibit was up for two years, and was seen by approximately two million people. A two-hour
film, narrated by Sir Martin Gilbert, distinguished historian, and biographer of Churchill, was
commissioned by the History Channel, and shown at the same time. Joel Elkes wrote a Memoir on his father to coincide with this exhibit. (See face sheet, p. . .). Dr. Elchanan Elkes died
in Dachau in October 1943. He had gone on a hunger strike on a matter of principle. Dr. Elkes'
mother survived Stutthof concentration camp and died in Israel in 1965.

The above gives the context of the Memorial address (Paper 30). It was delivered in Louisville in remembrance, not of Kovno, but of the concentration camp Theresienstadt. It also provides the context of Joel Elkes' work in Israel over the past forty years.

Joel Elkes serves on the Board of Governors of the Hebrew University and Haifa University. In 1970, with the sustained and generous support of Charles E. Smith and his family, of

---

[*] The National Institute for Psychobiology in Israel was founded by the Charles E. Smith Family.

Washington, D.C., he founded the Israel Center for Psychobiology, which has grown since into the National Institute for Psychobiology in Israel. The story of the creation of this Institute, its unusual cooperative structure, involving four universities and two major research institutes, is recalled in Paper 31. The Institute has played a highly significant role in the development of laboratory and clinical research, and the cultivation of talent in the neurosciences and in psychobiology in Israel. Some leading neuroscientists in Israel received support from this Institue in their youth.

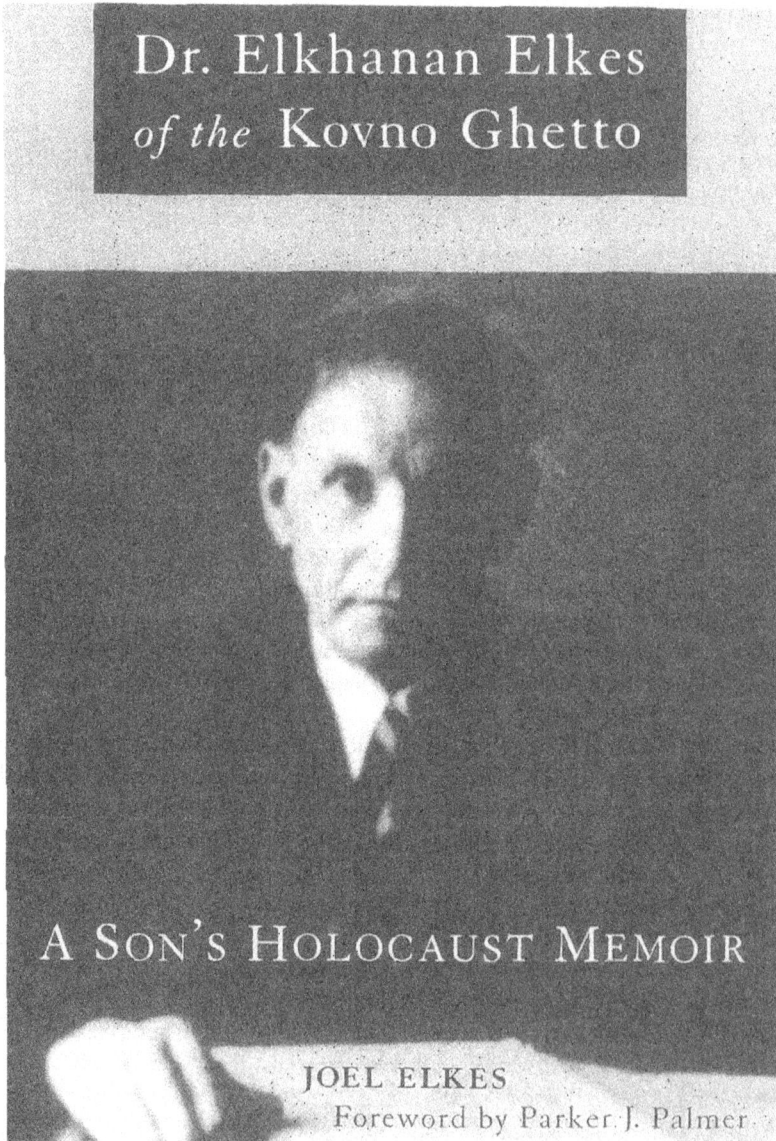

Book cover of "Dr. Elkhanan Elkes and the Kovno Ghetto"

PAPER 30

REMARKS MADE AT THE HOLOCAUST COMMEMORATIVE CEREMONY
Kentucky Center of the Arts, April 17, 1985

Joel Elkes

Distinguished Service Professor, The Johns Hopkins University
Professor of Psychiatry and Behavioral Sciences,
University of Louisville

It is a word of three syllables and two meanings conjoined into un-nameable darkness. The roots are Greek, – "Holo-Caust" – signifying "Whole Burning", absolute destruction to the last remnant and residue. "Burnt Offering" – that too comes to mind.

Images and words are not made for such stuff. One can smell and hear. One refuses to see and to utter. A decade passes – two, three, four. Voices, letters, diaries, scripts, messages, messengers – for it takes time for messengers to speak and to be heard. There are the gatherings of survivors – registries, archives, special places – where memories are, and will be, sanctified. Yet, as our murderous century thunders on, we manage to pretend that it is business as usual, sustained by a mix of hope and denial. Hope has its own mysterious waters which save it from final burning; and the anodyne of denial helps us to move through our days, one at a time. Sanity is maintained at huge cost – the six o'clock news notwithstanding. Society, it appears, has no choice but to wait it out; and in the waiting there appear – like wondrous plants, as they always have through man's history – kindness, generosity, decency, duty, responsibility, joy, compassion, and passion. These qualities have proved miraculously resilient. In this alone there is a powerful message about our nature. But we all agree that time is running short.

There are names and numbers for the un-nameable. From the chasm of deepest despair come reasons for deepest hope. Ravensbruck, Sachsenhausen, Flossetburg, Bergen-Belsen, Theresienstadt, Buchenwald, Stutthof, Dachau, and Auschwitz: these we know as places marked for industrialized murder. But we could add hundreds upon hundreds of towns where Poles and Czechs and Russians died in their millions. We could add the killing fields of Cambodia, the Dustbowls of Ethiopia, and the Bamboo Archipelago of Malaysia. We could add, and go on adding, and still there would be no end to killing through human intent, or human indifference. Yet, planned, industrialized genocide stands as something on its own, strictly an invention of our century. The Wannsee conference, attended by a mere sixteen officials on January 20, 1942, estimated the "product" of the planned operation as 11 million dead Jews, including, incidentally, 330,000 Jews from England and 34,000 Jews from my own country of origin, Lithuania – an estimate which, in the case of Lithuania, fell 200,000 short of those actually killed.

You can also stare at maps. Martin Gilbert's *Atlas of the Holocaust* (written by Churchill's biographer) carries 316 such maps, densely dotted with names and numbers, its routes and arrows of human transports flowing like roads and rivers across the length and breadth of Europe. They give one, again, visual statistic of the unimaginable. In introducing his atlas, Gilbert presents one map in some personal detail. He writes:

> "The map below shows the places of work, deportation, and execution of 17 jews who were murdered during the war years. If similar short references were made to each jew murdered between 1939 and 1941, 353,000 such maps would be needed. To draw these maps at the author's and cartographer's fastest rate, would take 967 years."

Names, numbers, maps. – As the mind grapples desperately with the unthinkable, it comes to know the tools of industrialized killing. But the enemy's most powerful tool proved our most uniquely human attribute. For to carry out the unspeakable, one must think, speak, and write in a certain way. Even executioners must sleep, greet their wives and children at breakfast, and be ready for the next day's work. So language is put into SS uniform. The instructions for the death transports read like shipping orders. The statistical columns are clear, meticulously ruled, and the reports duly dated, signed, and countersigned. Death trains run on time, and even have priority. At the time of the collapse of the Reich, while the Wehrmacht was desperately crying out for rolling stock to move troops, Eichmann's trains got through by special order.

And then there is the language of official silence – allied silence – loud and clear. Two conferences to consider allied intervention led to nothing. Weizmann's plea to the British foreign office for a bombing of Auschwitz was declined for "technical reasons." Numbers, maps, statistics. They give us a dimension. But only individuals can take one where we fear to go. As McAfee Brown puts it in his splendid book on Elie Wiesel:

> "To speak out becomes an impossible
> necessity. To speak jointly, a duty,
> despite the terrible paradox.
>
> For the event took place, but defies
> description: one cannot speak
>
> The event supports an alternative. one can,
> choose silence
>
> The event precludes silence; one must
> become a messenger.
>
> The event supports a certain kind of messenger – a teller of tales."

The telling can never be complete. Yet, in this telling and retelling, one bears witness, one *testifies*. Being a witness to the past makes one a witness to the present. History may be a series of accidents on a gigantic scale, but at least we are not blindly destined to repeat them.

We fear the pain of the telling. Pain, indeed, may presage death. But as physicians know, pain may also herald a deep constructive rearrangement which we know as healing; the repair of life's fabric and the maintenance of life's continuity. Remembering can warn: Remembering can heal.

In his darkest allegory, our deepest teller of tales Elie Wiesel, utters a warning surely felt by most of us. The destruction of "Kol Village" is Kol Village – Every village Everywhere – like medieval Everyman. We are getting too used, he tells us, too numbed, too cconditioned to man-made death We scream and kick, and shun and avoid, to remain human. World War I and II, all that happened before between and since, *could* be a rehearsal. Again, listen to the language. "Theater of War" implies actors and spectators. Realists know better. The script of the last play, with its thousands suns, is participatory theater. The inscription carved on the cenotaph of Hiroshima reads: "Rest in peace, for the mistake will not be repeated." But can we be sure?

To say it again: Figures, statistics overwhelm. They do not tell the central tale. They do not make for hope. Hope, first and last, is people – people remaining human despite the monstrously inhuman. Through journals, diaries, books, recollections, drawings, photographs, the images and voices speak to us this day. They tell unbelievable tales. We learn of communities functioning as communities, to the very point of extinction; of safe houses and escape routes for children. We learn of the heroism of non-jews helping jews at the risk of their own lives – Raoul Wallenberg, priests, nuns, managers, office workers, people in the street, ennobled by acting on their human duty. We have consecrated a special place for them in Israel. We learn of day to day accounts being smuggled out, to be used at future trials of war criminals. We learn of resistance – feeble at first, but stronger towards the end: Mordechai Anilevicz, and the Warsaw uprisings; the Resistance in Vilno: the Partisans in the forests of my native Lithuania. These we recall today, in deepest respect and gratitude. The Ghetto Kovno, led by my father, Dr. Elchanan Elkes, was mentioned in the introduction. There will be another occasion to recall the life and fate of this remarkable community. It survived, in its remnants, long after many communities had ceased to exist, maintaining its faith, maintaining its structure and inner dignity despite, yes, always <MI>despite its inevitable fate, well known to its members.

But we are here to celebrate yet other voices. "When man in his grief falls silent", Goethe said somewhere, "God gives him the strength to sing of his sorrows". We are here to celebrate those who sang in their sorrows, in conditions without precedent, and beyond human belief.

The tiny township of Theresienstadt nestles in beautiful countryside quite close to Prague. A few buildings; a post office, stores, and a tavern and soldiers' barracks commemorate the empress Maria Theresa. But in World War II it became the waystation to the crematoria of Auschwitz. It also became a grotesque instrument of Nazi deception. For it is in Theresienstadt that the SS stage-managed particularly cruel charades, duly filmed for the benefit of the Red Cross, to document the humane ways of the Third Reich. Of the one million – yes, *one million* children killed in the holocaust, many passed through Theresienstadt. Their story is impossible to tell. If you are strong enough, you can read it. Education was forbidden; but they attended makeshift schools, where punishment was to miss a lesson. They wrote and acted imaginative plays, produced a children's opera, drew pictures, wrote poetry, and above all, *observed.* They saw beauty with he innocence of youth. They saw reality with the harsh clarity which escaped many of their elders.

Yes, and there was music at Theresienstadt. One cannot name all the musicians. Their deeds are recorded in appropriate places. But we will recall Gideon Klein, and Truda Solanova, Arnost Weiss, Karel Ancerl, Rudolf Franck, Karl Berman and Carlo Taube, among the many. Their own records, and records about them, tell – need one say it again – an unparalleled tale of courage, and of hope. There was, of course, no piano. But Gideon Klein discovered an ancient rump of a piano in an attic. It had no legs – it stood on trestles – string and keys were missing. He secretly managed to rebuild it into a usable instrument. The "Appasionata" and "Waldstein" were performed on that piano. Score papers had to be ruled meticulously by hand, to copy parts. Rehearsals were carried on in attics, in low voice. Mozart's A major violin concerto was performed to the accompaniment of an accordion. There was Carlo Taube's Terezin Symphony; there was "Brundibar", an opera performed in large part by children. And there, in Theresienstadt, yes *Theresienstadt*, there was sung Verdi's "Requiem". Let me read you an extract from Karl Berman's recollections.

"On the platform stood the 150-member mixed chorus, before them the soloists Marion Podolier, Heda Aronson-Lindt, David Grunfeld and myself, below the platform the two pianos. Behind one of them, Gideon Klein; behind the other, Editha Kraus, and in front of us all, on a little box, stood Rafael Schachter, who knew the difficult score perfectly by heart. It was a revolutionary and militant feat that had no equal."

He adds:

"The Requiem had to be rehearsed three times in all because after every first performance a large part of the chorus left in one of the transports."

The transports, one assumes, were for Auschwitz. He ends by saying:

"If the historians one day succeed in writing the cultural history of the ghetto of Terezin, mankind will be amazed. Grown-ups and children, in constant expectation of death, lived a full, noble life between outcries of pain and anxiety, among hunger and misery, among the hundreds of corpses of those that died daily, among hearses taking the corpses out of town and bringing back bread. Under constant great physical exertion, they lived a life that was a miracle under the given conditions.

Indeed, few of those who survived the Nazi hell realize today what strength was necessary for man not to lose his human dignity, not to lose faith in man; to write, to calculate, to sing and recite, even though he had lost his name; to philosophize and think realistically, though he had become a mere number."

There are members in this room who know whereof we speak. Our distinguished guest, Ms. Freed, was born in Israel. Her mother lives in Israel: Ms. Freed's mother was in Auschwitz.

So we recall; and without denying what occurred, continue to affirm. We take heart that such men, women, and children lived. Images come as I speak; a chain of hands reaching from them to us, across forty years – telling us through their grip, and warmth: "Hold on, It is Possible." Then, into the images meld voices, children's voices, and voices of their elders. "We must believe in man", they say, "despite man, for he is us, and we are still a very young and immature species". And beyond the voices, the voice of silence.

Each year, this memorial day (and eight hours ago this day) the whole land of Israel falls silent for a few minutes. In Tel Aviv, and Haifa, and Jerusalem the traffic stops, as if frozen in memories; in the Kibbutzim, in the villages, in fields and factories, in the farthest army outposts in Galilee and the Desert: in schools and places of learning people cease whatever they are doing, so as to better listen to the silence. Believers and non-believers affirm together: The way to God – anyone's God – is through Man. No one is alone in such an hour. We connect what was to what is; and remember in awed gratitude those whose courage continues to light our Hopes.

I would ask you now to join me in observing this silence.

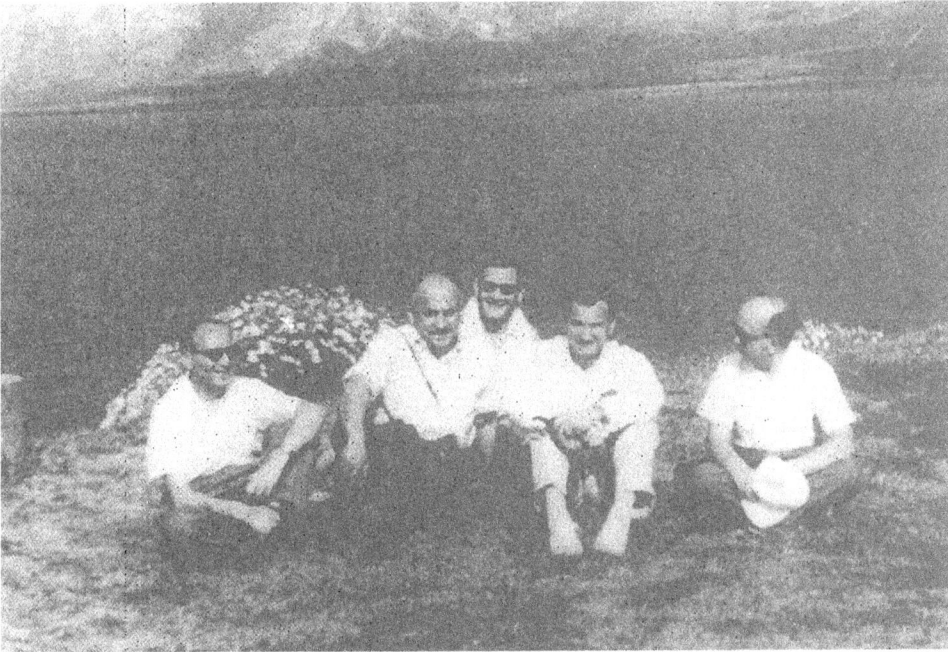

Before the Founding of Israel Center of Psychobiology.
Joel Elkes with Israeli Colleagues. Shore of Sea of Galilee, 1968

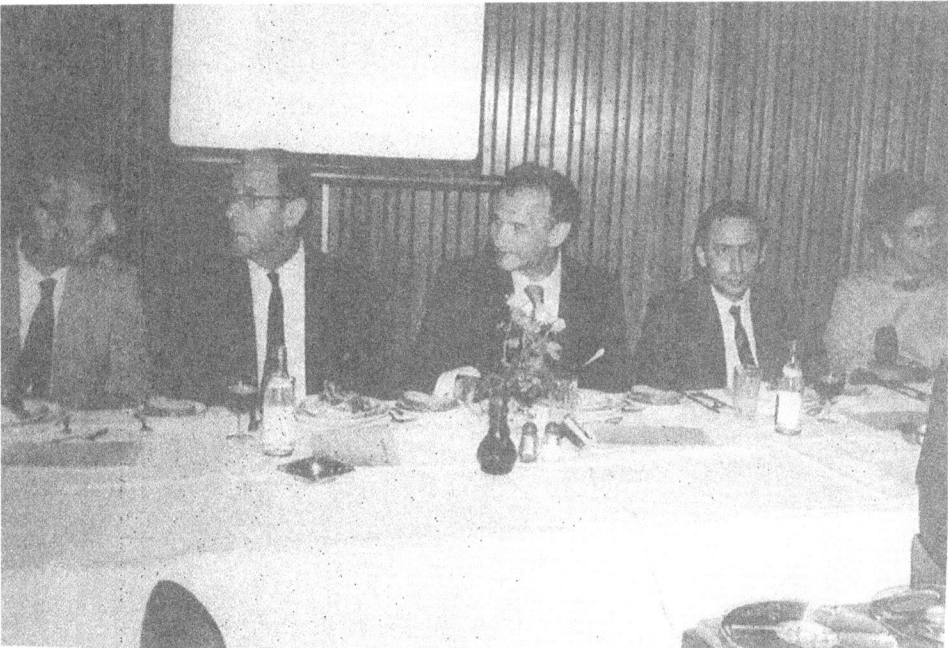

At Foundng Dinner Israel Center for Psychobiology, April 1970.
From left to right: M. Prywes, J. Magnes, J. Elkes, A. Charmon, H. Sharon

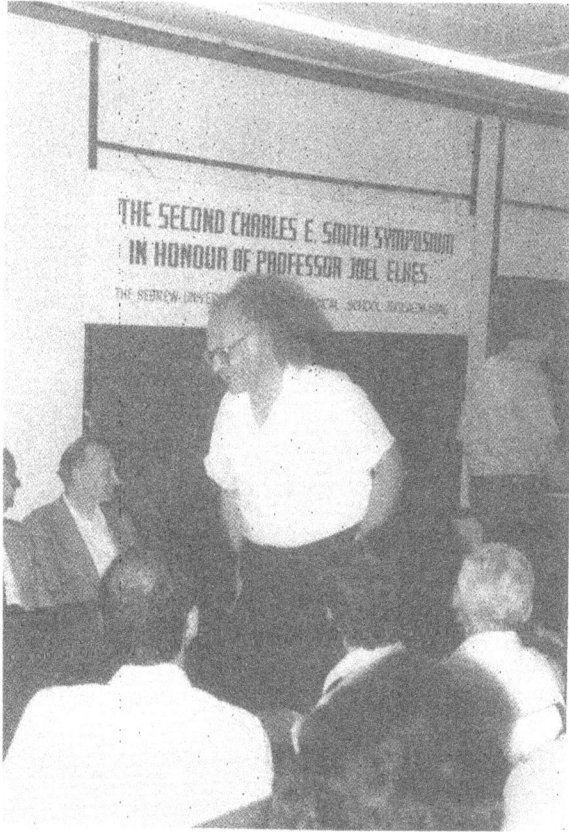

The Second Charles E. Smith Symposium, Jerosalem, Israel, 1985.
Professor Rami Rahamimoff greeting guests

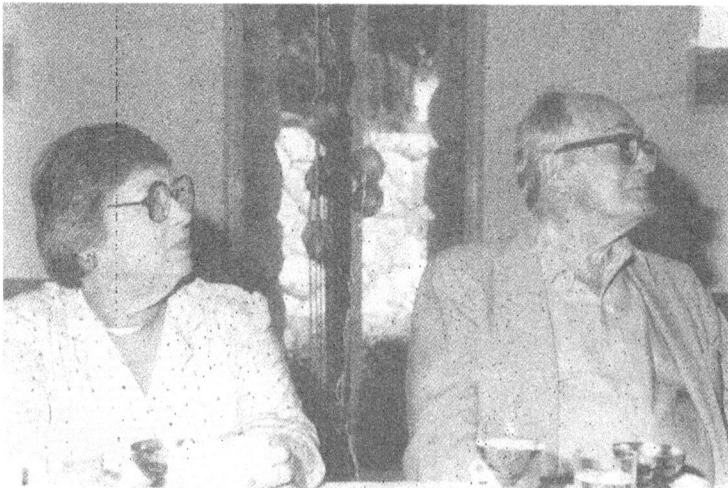

Josephine and Seymour Kety, Jerosalem, 1985

PAPER 31

CHARLES E. SMITH AND THE POSSIBLE DREAM
Introductory remarks at he 25th Anniversary Symposium
of the National Institute for Psychobiology in Israel
in Memory of Charles E. Smith[*], April 18, 1996

Joel Elkes

Chairman, Board of Trustees and Founding Director,
The National Institute for Psychobiology in Israel

Reprinted with the kind permission of the National Institute for Psychobiology in Israel
from the booklet prepared by the Institute

It is with a poignant mix of joy, gratitude and remembrance that I join Hanoch Gutfreund, President of the Hebrew University, in opening this meeting to mark the 25th Anniversary of the Israel Center for Psychobiology (since 1980 the National Institute for Psychobiology in Israel) dedicated to the memory of our beloved and unforgettable, Charles E. Smith.

The real giants in this world walk unseen; and meeting Mr. Smith casually – slight in frame, soft in voice, gentle, warm courteous in manner, a welcoming smile partnering a twinkle in his eye – one would not readily know the measure of the man. Yet, in Washington you have only to look around you to perceive his presence. Anyone flying into the city will see, immediately adjacent to the National Airport, the gleaming skyline of Crystal City, conceived, built, owned and operated by the Charles E. Smith Companies. As you move around the town, you will see his name on buildings and institutions. As the Washington Post observed in its tribute to him on January 1, 1996, "There are few, if any individuals who have had more influence on where and in what surroundings Washingtonians live and work than Charles E. Smith." Yet, these vast enterprises would only be an outer attribute of the man we knew. Charles E. Smith was a Master Builder in the deepest sense of the world. He built buildings and built lives; he built true and built strong. And no matter what or whom he touched, the plumbline – the vertical – always ran through Charles Smith, the person.

In his autobiography, *Building My Life,* edited by his grandson, David B. Smith, Charles Smith tells the story of his life, in a spare, simple, direct, and utterly compelling way. Born in 1901, in the tiny hamlet of Lipnick, Russia and raised in a hut with a dirt floor, he spent his first 11 years in his native Russia. His father, Reuven was a carpenter and farmer. He also owned a windmill. Reading his memoir, one feels that God was a house guest in the Smith's cottage. At all times – good and bad – the family addressed him as a Person. When one night the windmill caught fire and burnt down, the Rabbi told Charles' father that this was a sign – a "seeman" – for him to up and go, and leave Lipnick. He came to New York in 1908 and Charles and the family followed him in 1911. Charles was self taught and learned fast. At his Bar Mitzvah, he delivered speeches – in English (which he had just learned) and Hebrew. His

---

* The National Institute for Psychobiology in Israel founded by the Charles E. Smith Family.

father became a builder and Charles, braving the Depression and several starts in other professions, rose to become a builder too. Starting small, he moved from New York to Washington and, during World War II, began his extraordinary career as a builder and contractor in the nation's capital. Before long he was to become deeply involved with the community in which he lived. He built concentrically; from Self to Family; from Family to Community – Jewish and non-Jewish; and from Community to Israel. These do not necessarily represent an order of priority, but rather a deep organic web of connections, centered on Charles E. Smith, Builder of Buildings, and Builder of Lives.

"He who occupies himself with the needs of the community is as though he occupies himself with the Torah," so says the Talmud Yerushalmi. In a sense, Charles Smith was engaged in daily study and worship. He served his community and Israel with devotion, a deep joy and a totally natural humility. A passionate interest in education and learning informed his life. Schools, universities and community centers have all felt his beneficent influence. The Charles E. Smith Day School in Rockville, Maryland, which combines Jewish education with general education of an extraordinarily high standard, remains to this day the prime school of its kind in the United States. There were others: major contributions to George Washington University, where an Athletic Building is named after him; the Jewish Theological Seminary; the Crippled Children's Fund; the National Conference of Christians and Jews; all bear the marks of his wisdom and generosity. His honors were many, but I never learned of a single one from him directly. He did his work imbued by a deep sense of the history of his people and the central place of the Jewish Ethic in a rapidly changing society.

Without formal prayer, Charles Smith lived with his God day by day. For example, he recalls in the chapter on his childhood how two of his siblings died of diphtheria which he survived. He did not take his survival for granted, but simply asked "Why?", believing that he was put on earth for a purpose. He had a deep sense of mission and spoke to me of this mystic premise candidly and openly; without the slightest embarrassment, as a simple fact of his life. His measure of success was not wealth or institutions but bringing out the best in people. Education – from Educere to bring out – giving people a sense of worth, dignity, and self-respect became a lifelong quest to him. As pointed out by Rabbi Rabinowitz and Rabbi Hartman at the service held in his memory on January 2nd in Washington, his name, too, bears a sign. For Charles stands for his Hebrew name, Tsuriel. It is an unusual name; and it appears in the Bible only once, in the book of Numbers. Its meaning is "God is my Rock". The duty assigned to this original Tsuriel was to take responsibility for the construction and maintenance of the ancient Tabernacle of Moses; again – building in God's good company. We talked about this a good deal – this relation of building communities to the building of lives. When I stayed with him, he would spend hours in the study of the writings of our sages. He always carefully selected the material the night before. He believed in going to bed with a good sentence.

I will always remember the plane trip from London to Tel Aviv one April day in 1969, during which Charles Smith and I began talking about Brain, Biology and Behavior. "What is Psychobiology?", he asked, "It's a long word, isn't it, too long a word for me." "Psychobiology is the study of the relation between the sciences of life and the science of mental life", said I. "The relationship between Body and Brain and Brain and Behavior, between Behavior and Thought and Thought and Feelings, Disturbed Thought and Disturbed Feelings, Disturbed Behavior and Disturbed Body Function." "Something of necessity, pretty broad," said Mr. Smith. "Are there any more precise leads?" he continued in his precise, businesslike way. I could – even then, in 1969 – reply with an honest affirmative. "Yes," I said, "a good deal is becoming known about the chemical steering mechanisms of the brain, and chemical and hormonal imbalances which govern life in health and in disease. About the chemistry of waking and sleeping and even possibly dreaming; about neurochemical correlates of mood, aggression, mania and rage; of feeling low, feeling high, or feeling simply happy. There were emerging ideas about the operation of regional chemical fields in the brain. (No CAT Scan, no PET Scan in those days!) Genetics was emerging as a rewarding field both in relation to schizophrenia and manic depressive illness; genetic markers in patients could possibly lead to the detection of high risk members in disease-prone families. There was, I said, even at that time, progress in understanding the way in which proteins in the brain could transcribe and encode an impression or an idea into a memory trace, both transient and long term; of the way stresses in early development, playing on a highly plastic nervous system; could critically influence an organism's capacity to cope in later life. "Yes, I said on that plane ride, there were bridges being built, between Mind and Body, not on the basis of conjecture, but on the basis of evidence. Mind and Body and Body and Mind were becoming not two words, but one; the term Psychobiology really expressed this deepening relationship between the Life Sciences and the Sciences of Mental Life."

"Very interesting", commented Mr. Smith. And then came the key question, "Were there any scientists in Israel who were active in the field?" Here, again, I could reassure Mr. Smith. I had started coming to Israel on a regular basis in 1953, having been first invited, by Professor Moshe Prywes, at that time Associate Dean or the Medical Faculty in Jerusalem. Some of us, Professor Moshe Prywes, Profesor Seymour Kety, and the late Heinrich Waelsch – Professor of Neurochemistry at Columbia –, the late Professor Jonathan Magnes, and the late Professor Ernst Bergman, the brother of Professor Felix Bergman, Professor Halpern, and Professor Alex Keynan and I had met some colleagues working on the brain. Professor Shaul Feldman, Professor David Samuel, Professor Rami Rahamimoff, Professor Raphael Mechoulam, Professor Felix Sulman, Professor Peter Hillman, Professor Barry Berger were also members of our initial group. There was a wonderful symposium at Ohalo (I believe in 1956 or 1957 – I do not recall which) that brought us all together. At those meetings, we were impressed by the talent existing in the country, as well as the lack of opportunities for developing this talent; by the assets as well as gaps, by duplication as well as genuine deficiency. Traveling up and down the country I had met some colleagues "on location"; the quality of the work was most impressive, the potential for a pharmaceutical industry in Israel very evident, even then.

On the plane trip, I shared these impressions with Mr. Smith. "Could anything be done to advance these possibilities in Israel?" he asked in his direct way. Again, I replied in the affirmative, outlining very briefly the idea of a nationwide cooperative enterprise based at the Hebrew University. "Let me think about it," said Mr. Smith, "and let me discuss it with my family." I was deeply encouraged by the immediacy and readiness of Mr. Smith's response.

As I reflected upon this conversation with Mr. Smith, the idea of a National Center, functioning under the aegis of our oldest university, began to take shape. Psychobiology is a transdisciplinary discipline. It extends from fundamental molecular neurobiology by way or animal behavior techniques and reaches deeply into the clinical field and an understanding of the nature of health and wellbeing; in short, it is a field which demands cooperation.

In a memorandum written to Mr. Smith on November 1, 1970, I set out the broad objectives of the Center.

"The Israel Center for Psychobiology is not a conventional scientific society, nor is it a conventional institution. It represents an attempt to create a nationwide network of Israeli scientists engaged in research on various aspects of Psychobiology and to support such work in a manner which encourages optimal use of available resources. Israel is a small country; resources are scarce and precious; there are often complementary approaches and techniques. It is with a view of identifying and furthering cooperative programs within and between existing institutions and training scientific manpower in the area of psychobiology that the Center is created. The aims of the Center are:

1. To identify workers engaged in research and psychobiology in Israel.
2. To create mechanisms to ensure regular and steady communication between them.
3. To support cooperative and individual projects in selected areas of the subject.
4. To provide a mechanism for bringing to Israel a few selected leading workers for extended periods and ensure a wide exposure of the membership to these visiting scientists.
5. To provide a complementary mechanism for sending Israeli workers to leading laboratories to require approaches and techniques in which Israel is deficient at the present time.
6. To establish a base at a major American University (e.g. Johns Hopkins) so as to ensure a continuing working relationship with agencies in the United States.
7. To participate increasingly on the international scene in the area of Psychobiology.

I remember the occasion when Mr. Charles Smith and I presented the idea to President Abraham Harman of the Hebrew University. He felt, at first, that the Center should firmly function within the confines of the Hebrew University; I, on the other hand – at first gently – and then more firmly – introduced the idea of creating a cooperative network in which the Universities of Haifa, Tel Aviv, Beer Sheva, Bar Ilan, the Weizmann Institute, and the Israel Biological Research Institute, Ness Ziona and various hospitals were also to be represented. Abe Harman was doubtful at first; it took quite an argument to convince him of the validity of the idea. "Will they really cooperate?" he kept on asking. "If you, as President of our oldest University, are there to lead, they will," I said. And so Abe became our ally, our champion and our deep friend. No matter where and when, I could always call on his help, his wisdom, experience and judgement at any time. In fact, I remember once meeting him at his hotel in Philadelphia at six o'clock in the morning before, I believe, he was to see Mr. Annenberg. The matching funds from the University – so much at the core of our budget – were due to Abe Harman; and the exemplary key role played by the Hebrew University was his work.

The first grant to the newly created Center for Psychobiology was made by Mr. Smith and his family in 1971. In that year, we had the great good fortune to have Professor Amiram Carmon join us as Associate Director – and later as Director and our dear Hadassah Sharon, central pillar and mainstay of the Institute since its founding – joined us in the same year as Executive Secretary.

After the first grant had been made, another piece of luck came our way. The Office of Research and Development of the Prime Minister's Office, where I had visited before (in the hope of encouraging interest in a Pharmaceutical Industry), commissioned us to prepare a survey of existing facilities and resources in Psychobiology in Israel – a map much needed if we were to pursue an intelligent policy of support and cooperative funding. How I relish the memory of those days when Amiram Carmon and I, separately and together, traveled up and down the country. In the wonderful Summer and Fall of 1972 and 1973, we visited every laboratory, every clinical unit, every animal house, and saw every major piece of equipment used in the Neurosciences in Israel. In time, we came to know every worker in the field. Some had already established national or international regulations; some were on their way of building the reputation which they enjoy it the present time. The survey on the state of Psychobiology in Israel prepared by Amiran Carmon, Danny Dagan and myself was presented to the National Council for Research and Development, the Prime Minister's Office, in November of 1974 (Drugs, Brain and Behavior, NCRD 7-76, Jerusalem). It considered Psychobiology in terms of its future as an interdisciplinary science; catalogued its present status in Israel in terms of Clinical, Research and Teaching programs; and emphasized particularly the need for student and post-graduate training in Psychobiology. There were separate considerations of selected areas, namely Neurochemistry, Neurophysiology, Human Neuropsychology, Psychophysiology and Physiological Psychology. There followed operational recommendations for the future development of Psychobiology in Israel in terms of manpower, research facilities and research programs. The tables and statistics of the report make interesting reading, particularly in retrospect. Rereading it 20 years later, I find an aside on page 72:

"The usual argument advanced is for more people. The Survey suggests a somewhat different mandate with regard to manpower, namely that rather than spending money on additional positions, it may be appropriate to invest in a small number of gifted individuals, insure their adequate training, and, through the creation of appropriate career ladders, provide them with settings in which their work, and especially their collective work, is recognized and duly rewarded, thus encouraging them to apply skills for the solution of mental health problems which are sure to face our country in the years to come. We would, therefore, argue for expenditure of limited funds to make the use of large existing funds more efficient. This could be done through taking a nationwide, rather than parochial, view of the field, encouraging cooperation both within and between institutions, by rewarding such cooperation and creating clinical and pre-clinical research in which talent could develop and establishing firm ties with leading institutions abroad which could nurture developments in Israel... We recommend that special funds be set aside to encourage cooperative programs in Psychobiology; that a small number of government sponsored grants for two year clinical research Fellowships be established; that funds be set aside to establish curricula for such training; that a small number of clinical research units be established; and the creation of a National Center for Applied Pharmacology, with a special reference to Neuropharmacology, be considered." A tentative time table was also set out."

Those of you who have read our reports and publications know how much has happened since we began. Through the tremendous efforts of the Directors, Professor Carmon at first, then Professor Moshe Abeles, to whom we owe so much, including the change in status from a Center for Psychobiology to the status of the National Institute for Psychobiology in Israel, and now Professor Bernard Lerer's distinguished leadership; through the devotion and patient, steady hard work of the Scientific Advisory Committee – on which there always was wide national representation; through the manifold contacts and relationships with scientists and organizations abroad, the Institute, from its humble beginnings, has now assumed high visibility on the international scene. The harvest has been rich, indeed; and, as the saying goes, we have reason to be truly thankful.

Since its inception, some 374 research grants have been funded, 62 Post-Doctoral Fellowships and three Senior Scientist Awards have been made. In 1988, to implement cooperation at a substantive, practical level, a special laboratory – the Smith Family Laboratory for Collaborative Research – was created. Professor Shaul Hochstein has been its distinguished Director since its inception. The premise of the Laboratory is simple. It provides special facilities and equipment not readily available in universities to guest scientists to carry out collaborative studies on a time-limited basis. The equipment – an electrophysiological recording facility, a facility for tissue culture, a small animal behavior laboratory and a psychophysics facility for human studies – allows an unusually broad range of studies in a space which is compact and which is in very high demand. No less than forty studies have been hosted by the Laboratory since its inception; the collaboration involving not only Israelis but also scientists from abroad. The Institute has supported some 20 national meetings and some 38 international symposia and meetings. It has developed fine relationships, has funded three Lectures in honor of Mr. Charles E. Smith and has been responsible for two special issues of the Israel Journal of Medical Sciences. Some 340 major publications have included articles, books and critical reviews. Scientists, who now occupy senior positions in Israeli Neuroscience; Psychobiology and Psychiatry (and Chairmanships of Departments), began their careers with the support of the Institute of Psychobiology. Israel is highly visible on the international scene. In short, we seem to have made it.

Like Jerusalem, Psychobiology is a city of many gates: One can enter it by way of Physics, or Chemistry, or Biology, or Experimental Psychology, or the study of Animal Behavior, or the study of Perception and Thought. It bears on both Illness and Well-beeing. One could well argue-even at this early stage – that Psychobiology provides a fine foundation for a Future Science of Man.

It is this broad perspective which Charles Smith grasped, as year by year, he allowed us to explain to him what we were doing. The Blessing he gave us twenty-five years ago is with us today as we embark on our work.

I would now ask you to rise as we honor his memory: "Blessed be the Memory of a Righteous Man."

REFERENCES:

Psychobiology in Israel. Report submitted to the Prime Minister's Office by Amiran Carmon, M.D., Daniel Dagan, Ph.D., Joel Elkes, M.D. Jerusalem,1974

Part Eleven

TWO FRIENDS

PAPERS

32. J. Elkes: Letter to Dr. Jonas Salk on his Eightieth Birthday. October 14, 1994
33. J. Elkes: A personal laboratory. Review of Norman Cousins' The Healing Heart: Antidotes to Panic and Helplessness.
    Reprinted from Saturday Review, September–October (pp. 55–57), 1983
34. J. Elkes: A tribute to Norman Cousins.
    Reprinted with the kind permission of the Fetzer Institute from Advances, The Journal of Mind-Body Health 7: 59-62, 1991

Jonas Salk and Norman Cousins were friends of Joel Elkes. Before accepting the appointment at Johns Hopkins, Joel Elkes was considering – and was being considered – for a Senior Fellowship at the Salk Institute. With Jonas Salk, he organized the first Symposium on the Neurosciences at the Salk Institute which later led to the formation of the Program in Neuroscience at the Institute, headed by Floyd Bloom (who had previously succeeded Elkes at the National Institute of Mental Health/St. Elizabeth's Center).

Norman Cousins, distinguished journalist and editor of the Saturday Review, and Joel Elkes served together on the Board of the Institute for Advancement of Health, founded by Eileen Growald. Norman Cousins was warmly supportive of Elkes' and Leah Dickstein's program on Health Awareness in Medical Students as developed at the University of Louisville (see Part Seven, Paper 20). He also supported the pioneering work of Joel Elkes' second wife, Josephine Rhodes, on Professional Peer Group Counseling in Rheumatoid Arthritis.

The letter to Jonas Salk (Paper 32) was sent to mark his eightieth birthday. The review of Norman Cousins' The Healing Heart (Paper 33), and the Obituary (Paper 34) convey their relationship.

LETTER TO DR. JONAS SALK
on His Eightieth Birthday, October 14, 1994

Jonas Salk
The Salk Institute
La Jolla, California

Dearest friend,

Thirty-five years later, the images are as lucid as the sunlit leaves on the tree outside my window.

1. It is '59 or '60 or '61, – we are in your room at the Carlton Hotel on K Street in Washington. Darrell and Peter are kidding around, while you and I sit on the edge of your bed, talking. You pull out an envelope and quickly sketch the layout of the future Institute. South Wing–North Wing; Science and Humanism conjoined. I say: "You're building a new kind of monastery, aren't you?" We talk of serving nature with mind and heart. You give me that faraway, double-take look which I have come to treasure.

2. We are on the bluff – the building site of the future Institute, – overlooking the Pacific. It is a marvelous windswept, sunny day. On the ground lie about ten or twelve slabs of concrete drying in the sun – samples of the facing of the Institute. You run and jump and skip from slab to slab, like a gazelle. Lou Kahn and I trying to keep up with you. "Should it be this or that or that one over there?" you cry out in your enthusiasm. A warm grey? Ochre? Paler? Darker? More dappled? More white? More veining? You are flushed with excitement. My jaw drops as I watch. "What a kid!" I mumble. "What toys!"

3. We are still in the temporary wooden building; the foundations of the Institute are being dug. You and I put together the first symposium on the Neurosciences, in the face of a good deal of grumbling. It is a good meeting. Leo Szilard nods in his chair – lucid questions bobbing up out of his sleep like marker buoys upon the sea.

My paper starts the afternoon session. My throat is dry. I speak on regional chemical fields in the brain, – of families of neuroregulatory substances affecting mood, thought, consciousness and behavior. I have written the word "awareness" on the board, and stress its central role. I draw devastating fire from some of those present. I give as good as I get. Then I look at you. You give me a wink.

So now, dearest friend, I wink back at you. Eighty, and still playing in the nursery of your life. Some kid, some toys! Joy is the heart's hormone. Your inner pharmacy is doing very nicely.

Love to you and yours,
Devotedly,

Joel Elkes

PAPER 33

A PERSONAL LABORATORY
The Healing Heart: Antidotes to Panic and Helplessness by Norman Cousins[*]

Joel Elkes

"I have already lived more than an average lifetime, but I want to continue to live long enough to see the establishment of a world under law and a planet made safe and fit for human habitation," said Norman Cousins, and he intends to keep his word. Cousins has traveled extensively and has met the leaders of his age, at times carrying critical messages on matters of public policy. To a devoted worldwide public he has brought his vision, clarity, and courage through his editorials for *Saturday Review*. (I wish collection of these editorials would be reprinted; *Present Tense* leaves the reader breathless with the scope and depth of his energy and enterprise.) His efforts exacted a price. In 1964 he was incapacitated by an illness affecting his muscles and joints. Fierce pain and a guarded prognosis by his physician forced him to look inward. He mobilized himself and his friends and called in King Mirth. The story of his recovery, as told to an astonished public in a famous article in the *New England Journal of Medicine* and subsequently in his book *Anatomy of an Illness*, is history.

In 1978 Cousins accepted a distinguished teaching post at UCLA. Success pursued him: Overcrowded speaking schedules, traffic, queuing, carrying luggage, no regular exercise, broken routines. Again his body reacted. On December 22, 1980, he suffered a massive heart attack. *The Healing Heart* recounts his recovery and the growth of a partnership between patient and physician. It extends an important message to patients, and to medicine.

Shortly after his attack, Cousins is wheeled into UCLA's Intensive Care Unit. Reading apprehension on the faces of Dean Mellinkoff and others there, he informs them in a clear voice that they are "looking at what is probably the darndest healing machine that has ever been wheeled into the hospital." During his first night among the ticking machines of the ICU, he wonders the obvious. Other thoughts come too: "Have I told those I love that I love them?" He remembers his father's last days. He dares not close his eyes for fear of exit. Then he laughs at his panic, asking himself what "a walking health exhibit like me is doing in an ICU?" He snaps on the TV, and makes it through the night. He has confronted the panic and begun a process of "taking charge."

There is not doubt about the diagnosis. Tests and symptoms indicate extensive damage to the heart wall. As before, Cousins makes his body a personal laboratory and befriends the society within his skin. He refuses morphine; he asks for a changes in the visiting routine to ensure rest. Gradually he improves. Later he wears a portable monitor and is encouraged by its readings. But then come the treadmill tests. He is "scared stiff" at *being* exercised, at an accel-

---

[*] Published by W.W. Norton, 288 pp
Reprinted from Saturday Review, September-October (pp. 55-57), 1983

erating pace, on a moving band over which he has no control. He tries to suppress his fear, but fails and has to stop. He tries again and cannot manage. The tests show beyond doubt the existence of atherosclerotic blockage. He accepts this finding, but inquires whether fear could not contribute to coronary spasm by further narrowing the flow through a partly obstructed artery. He finds evidence for this in the literature and takes it up with his physician. When Dr. Shine suggests an angiogram, which to Cousins carries the prospect of bypass surgery, Cousins has his doubts.

Their discussions are poignant and extraordinarily moving in this search for personal truth. Physician and patient, friend and friend, move from their perspective terrains of experience to the common ground of trust. Cousins again reads the literature on bypass surgery and the remarkable relief it affords in cases with severe pain. He notes that this pain is intermittent and highly susceptible to emotional influence. Dr. Shine again recommends angiography, but suggests that Cousins receive a second opinion. Cousins consults Dr. Cannom and decides to follow his own route. He establishes a disciplined routine to exercise and nourish his body, mind, and spirit. He walks; he eats the delicious salad meals set before him by his wife, Ellen; he returns to golf and tennis, music and photography. He ensures "time-out" and keeps his schedule rigidly within bounds. He embarks upon the construction of a separate study-library to house his papers and books. The beautiful circular structure stands on a hill for a reason other than the view: it forces him to climb the steps twice a day to get his reward.

His recovery is striking. Within six months he ventures onto the treadmill again, but on his own terms. He asks to be given control of the speed of the moving platform; to lift his spirits he brings tapes of the Bach Toccata and, for good measure, of Woody Allen. This time he passes the test.

He returns to his work, particularly his programs for cancer patients ("We Can Do") and for heart patients (CHEER), which include listening, sharing with the staff, and monitoring of the inner laboratory.

On the anniversary of his heart attack his colleagues plan a surprise party at his home. The prankster in him returns the compliment. He has Universal Studios make him up so that even his wife does not recognize the distinguished, bearded visitor at the door inquiring after Mr. Cousins. When the guest are assembled, the visitor strikes out on the organ. His daughter in the kitchen shrieks with the delight of recognition: "Daddy is home!"

This bare outline cannot remotely convey the warmth, humanity, and wisdom of this book. In telling his tale, Cousins educates. In sharing his feelings of helplessness, fear, and panic, he strikes at universals in us all. The book is about awareness, listening, trust, choice, and intention, and about the intelligent use of a benevolent, centering will. It is about communication and partnership between the healer and the healed. It addresses as complementary the art of medicine and the science of medicine, the person and the institution, and freedom of choice and professional responsibility. It affirms hope and belief as biologically constructive forces: not as blind faith, but as belief guided by knowledge and tempered by reason. It asserts that the quality of a person's life is the sum of the quality of his days.

At the core of the narrative is Cousins' relationship with himself and with his physicians. In their respective afterwords, his physicians – Drs. Shine, Hitzig, Cannom, and Fareed – attest to his extraordinary degree of acceptance and his willingness to communicate.

Words are medicine. According to Cousins, "It is no *whether* to tell the truth, but *how* to tell the truth that matters." Words do not figure in the pharmacopoeia, but as Dr. Lown points out in his splendid introduction, they can heal, maim, or kill. Good physicians, wherever they work, still take time to explain, explore, and reassure. Admittedly, this becomes harder as the health industry moves into higher gear. Yet, here the industry itself faces a strange and stubborn paradox that may well presage profound shifts.

The pattern of disease has changed radically over the past fifty years. The killers and maimers of old – diphtheria, typhoid, cholera, and polio – have been replaced by heart disease, hypertension, cancer, and stroke, with the mood and mental disorders following closely. There is strong suspicion that some may be "stress-related." Indeed, life itself – that is, our mode of life – may well emerge as the major pathogen in the Western world. Behavior can maim and probably kill.

The public may be more ready for this prognosis than the professionals. "Stress Management" is a brisk business, and shelf upon shelf of self-help books attest to a hunger for useful information. As Cousins points out, consumerism has reached medicine, and the public is going to medical school. The sad thing is that much of this information is biased, patchy, wrong, or plain dotty, and is purveyed for less-than-pure motives.

This new body of knowledge is lessening the contradiction of soma and symbol, or body and mind. The society within the skin is emerging as a magnificently coordinated system of communication, exquisitely in touch with the environment without. This communication is chemically mediated. The structure of many of mediators (neurotransmitters, neuromodulators, encephalins, hormones) is known. The brain is a regionally organized organ of communication. It is also an awesomely endowed endocrine gland, harboring a still poorly understood "inner pharmacy" capable of affecting basic sensations like pain and other key regulatory processes; the placebo effect may well have chemical correlates. The brain interacts with the body's defense system, the immune system, which is influenced profoundly by mental events and social circumstances. Neuropsychoimmunology has all the excitement in 1983 that psychopharmacology had thirty years ago. Biofeedback has provided understanding of the voluntary control of involuntary processes. Advances in cognitive psychology suggest that it is not events, but our perception of events that influences outcome – a sort of theory of the self-fulfilling prophecy. There are deep metabolic and hormonal shifts during states of relaxation and meditation. We are beginning to see the first outlines of a biology of loneliness and loss, and a biology of hope, intention, expectation, and belief – all old friends of *Homo sapiens*. When the place of behavior in medical practice and prevention is fully recognized, the effect may be comparable to the advent of antibiotics.

This is a story about self-communication and other-communication, from a master communicator. In a strange continuum, it leads from the society within the skin to the society without. It maintains that health is not only matter of psychology but a matter of attitudes and values. Values are at the heart of society. When values falter, a society is in danger; when *that* heart stops, a society dies. To Norman Cousins, personal health and social health are one. We can do no better than to give him the toast which he gave to himself in a twilight hour: "Be of good heart to your great heart!" and thank him for sharing this same great heart with us.

PAPER 34

A TRIBUTE TO NORMAN COUSINS*

Joel Elkes

We met at one of the early board meetings of the Institute for the Advancement of Health. Eileen Growald introduced us, suggesting that we might find common ground.

I still remember his opening remarks. The intense gaze, body bent forward across the table, tiny gestures emphasizing the cadences in his voice. The sentences flowed readily as he presented his argument. It was lucid, strong, simple – indeed, almost self-evident. The logic formed a sort of foreground to what he said. But resonating in the background, there was a muted passion and compassion which seized one by the throat. A wondrous combination of the light and the dark. This is Art, I thought. This man is an artist, whatever the world's patents of Norman Cousins. And just as I was fully absorbing what he had said, the expression across the table changed suddenly. Here was a pixie – a Disney dwarf – telling an apocryphal story about a car repairman and his landlady. Everybody convulsed: and as usual Norman had restored a sense of proportion to the proceedings. I wish I could remember the story.

In truth, I had met Norman long before I had met Norman. Some 25 years ago, while in Baltimore, a kindly physician friend had given me a copy of *Present Tense,* a collection of editorials from the *Saturday Review,* spanning some 40 years. My friend knew it was a fitting gift. For, ever since my coming to this country as a visitor in 1950, the editorials signed N.C. had been a sort of "guide to the perplexed" to me. In time, I came to regard them as the very conscience of international journalism. I hope Present Tense is reissued before long. It would, indeed, be thoroughly topical. To understand the present cataclysm, leaf through its pages, or through *Human Options*, Norman's autobiographical notebook. Read his reports on Hiroshima, Korea, Suez, Laos, the Congo. Let him guide you through the follies of the arms race. Meet him as he meets our masters – Churchill, F.D.R., Harry Truman, Eisenhower, MacArthur, Nehru, J.F.K., Lyndon Johnson, Gerald Ford. The panorama of an age flowing through one man into a single pen.

Many of these impressions were crowded in my mind as I listened to him that autumn morning, some ten years ago. I confess I was tongue-tied and awed.

For that day Norman was not talking about politics, but about a healing system at work in man, mysteriously activated by Hope, Intent, and Sense of Purpose. I knew he had come to it through facing the "anatomy" of his own illness. But, then, as a journalist he had also seen and understood the sickness of the planet, like few of his contemporaries. What was the "biology of hope" in individual and collective human affairs? How did it exert its beneficent effects? Which was the metaphor – person or planet? Were there, perchance, biological congruities

* Reprinted with the kind permission of the Fetzer Institute from Advances, The Journal of Mind-Body Health, 7:59-62, 1991.

running through person, group, and nation which, in our tribal passions, we had failed to understand? This is how our conversations began.

They continued, in a sort of Morse code, for the past nine years. I say "Morse" because there were long periods of silence – then, suddenly a message (we were both busy and at opposite ends of the continent). Altogether, we must have met some eight or ten times – three of them on occasions when I had the privilege of staying at his home, Eden Place. In retrospect, they were some of the most significant conversations of my life.

We found common ground in psychobiology. How does the billion-cell society within the skin converse with the society without? How are messages transcribed coded, stored, and evoked as precise electrochemical signals? How do the three communication systems within the skin – the nervous, the endocrine, and the immune systems – talk to each other? Is the immune system, as I facetiously suggested one day, a kind of "liquid brain"? Are pervasive electrical fields within the body evanescent embodiments of mind? Do Hope, Expectation, Intention, and Purpose have a molecular body of their own? Do we know most about the biology of depression because we have looked at it most intently? Do we know less about the biology of positive emotions because, being physicians preoccupied with pathology, we have looked less? Could there be a science of well-being, solidly documented by accepted methods of biomedical research? And what of the mounting relevance of this new body of knowledge to the training and personal well-being of physicians? What of its import in deepening the therapeutic alliance between physician and patient?

These and cognate subjects preoccupying many of us as we met under the aegis of the Institute for the Advancement of Health, cropped up again and again in our conversations. He was gracious and encouraging about our Health Awareness Program for incoming medical students at the University of Louisville and my wife Josephine's program on group work with rheumatoid arthritics. He told me much of his personal work with patients, and the deep satisfaction it gave him. When, much later, I saw his name as second author of two path-breaking papers in the *Archives of Psychiatry*, based on work inspired by his instinct and intuition, I was deeply moved, and wrote him immediately. A natural physician was Norman. The honorary M.D. degree from Yale, and the Schweitzer Medal from Johns Hopkins say it all.

Again and again, we returned to communication as the central problem of human biology. Here, evolution had given the society within the skin an advantage: for the precise and elegant mechanisms of molecular information transfer had been honed by evolution through some billions of years. But human society, with language barely 10,000 years-old? Should we wonder about the cacophony in our tribal Towers of Babel, the U.N., and CNN notwithstanding? Small wonder that the "physician as communicator" became Norman's central theme; small wonder that he put his immense talent as a communicator to the service of both person and planet.

In *Human Options,* he tells of the conversations between East and West that he initiated through the Dartmouth conferences, which have run for 30 years. In his little-known book, *The Improbable Triumvirate* (1972), he recounts the critical role he played in carrying important messages between President Kennedy, Pope John XXIII, and Nikita Krushchev – messages that decisively influenced the negotiations leading to the Nuclear Test Ban Treaty. He saw through the trappings of the Scientific Technological Elite as he probed the mortal dangers of the Military Industrial Complex. Yet he was awed by the sincerity and determination of two great generals – Eisenhower and MacArthur – to advance the cause of planetary peace. Albert Schweitzer's *My Life Is My Argument* applies as much to Norman Cousins as it does to

Schweitzer. Name one person who could have brought that enormous wealth of experience to the medical establishment. The University of California was indeed prescient in inviting him, and immensely fortunate to have him. All of us in the field have felt his steady, beneficent influence.

At no time was this more apparent than at the Arrowhead Conference (1988), which he and his colleagues put together with such infinite care. In retrospect, it may well prove to be a historic conference. For not only did it bring together a group to discuss the scientific foundations of the emerging field of neuropsychoimmunology, but, equally, the implications of what has come to be known as "Mind-Body Research" for the teaching and the practice of medicine. The pervasive theme of that conference, again, was communication. Dr. Herbert Weiner provided a searching and comprehensive paper on the subject. Many of the recommendations of that meeting are now being implemented through the task force which Norman constituted only a few years ago.

Yet, only a few weeks after the conference, I received Norman's *The Pathology of Power,* a book on which he must have been working at the very time he was preparing the Arrowhead Conference. If there be a book topical for today's news, it is this. If you wish to understand our global pathology and the addiction to power among the holders of power, read this book. As I write, my television screen brings the image of a blackened, terrified cormorant struggling through the oil slick released into the Persian Gulf by a ruthless despot. Both bird and tar are metaphors for our time. If Norman were there, he would have cried out in rage.

I saw him cry once. It was at the time when my wife, Jo, and I were staying with Ellen and him at Eden Place, some four years ago. Helping at breakfast, there was Shigeko Sasamori, his adopted daughter, one of the survivors of Hiroshima (a "Hiroshima Maiden"), whom Norman had brought to the states for plastic surgery. A schoolgirl at the time of the explosion, she had been badly burned on the scalp and. forehead; her fingers had been scorched to the knuckles as she had protected her eyes. But there she was that morning, helping Ellen and joking, humming as she worked. It so happened that Jo's rheumatoid arthritis was playing up badly as we sat down. "I will do some Shiatsu massage on you," said Shigeko and immediately set to work. Norman and I had been talking about a number of things, including the Holocaust. And suddenly, the synchronicity of it struck me. Here we were talking about one holocaust, while a survivor of that other "total burning" was healing my wife, digging the stumps of her scorched knuckles deeply into her back. I was overcome by the moment, and could not hold back the tears. As I turned to Norman, his eyes were moist. He just looked at me and we sat silent for a little while, and then proceeded with the day's business.

"Who Speaks for Man?" Norman asked in 1959. Not far organizations, tribes, nations, but for Man? I know no one quite like him; and, today, he is needed more than ever.

He was a vast continent of a man; and I was fortunate to catch a few glimpses of that continent at various times of day and season. We must see to it that his voice continues to be heard. At Louisville, we are founding two modest Norman Cousins scholarships to encourage students (medical and nonmedical) to carry forward what he began. Perhaps other places may wish to do the same. There should be candles for Norman in Places of Healing.

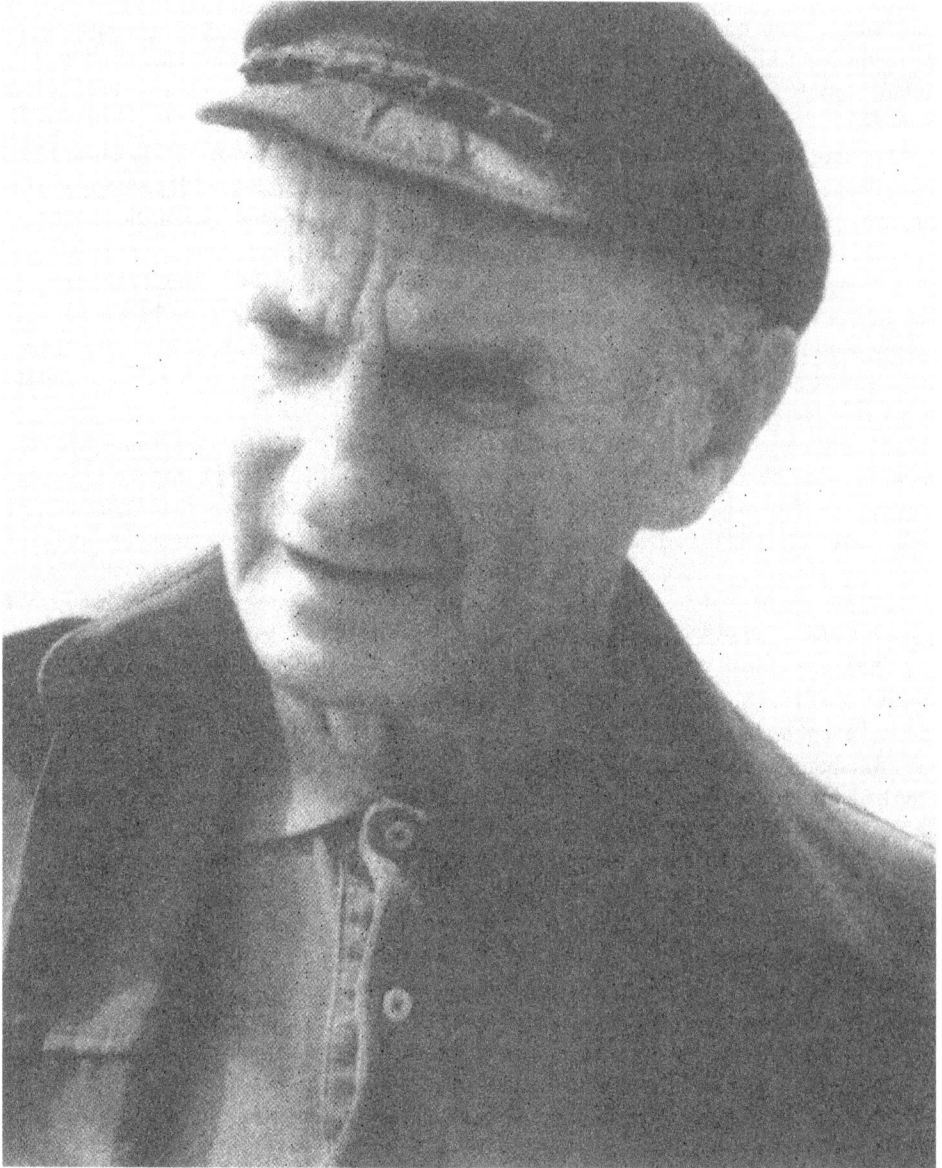

Part Twelwe

ON ART AND HEALING

A PROGRAM IN THE ARTS IN MEDICINE AT THE UNIVERSITY OF LOUISVILLE

Ever since his student days, Joel Elkes has been intrigued by the relation of the Arts to Healing. Their deep roots in history and the place of music, painting, dance, storytelling, and poetry in healing practices, irrespective of culture (Persia, Biblical Judea, Greece, Africa, and the Shaman rites of Native Americans come to mind) pose some obstinate questions. As a biologist, one asks, "Why this persistent connection?" "Do the Arts *work?*" and if they work, "How and Why?" At the present time, the Arts are well established in mental hospital settings, and in institutions for the care of the mentally retarded, and physically handicapped – all peripheral to medical education. Their place in a modern school of medicine and their use in teaching hospitals are less well established. Yet a reading of a rich and scattered literature – and also Joel Elkes' personal experience – suggest that the Arts can profoundly "move" a patient; and rapidly reach areas of personal functioning and emotional life inaccessible to traditional approaches. These therapies are non-verbal; they move beneath and beyond words. They can be very powerful, and, at their best, are deeply restorative and healing. Joel Elkes has seen this in his own work. It is this which spurred his interest in this area.

When Elkes was at Johns Hopkins he had the good fortune of finding a well equipped Art Therapy department, founded by Adolf Meyer, in the Henry Phipps Clinic which he headed. He made good use of this department in his treatment program, causing quite a stir among his collegues at the time. When he went to Louisville he was impressed by the extraordinary riches of talent in the city in music, drama, and the arts. He was also fortunate in finding that one of the leading schools for training Expressive Therapists in the United States, led by Dr. Vija Lusebrink, was in the University, and that Leah Dickstein, who was to become his key collaborator in the Student Health Awareness Program (see Part Seven, Paper 20) had organised an officially recognized Elective for students in the "Arts and Healing." Clearly, there were opportunities to establish a program for the Arts in Medicine in a major department in a School of Medicine and Elkes obtained funding to initiate this program as his overall effort to humanize the education of physicians. His aim was to introduce the "soft" Arts to the "hard" Sciences and bring about a meeting of two cultures – the culture of the Arts and of the Medical Sciences in a School of Medicine. The Head of the Department Dr. John Schwab, was most supportive.

Broadly stated, the objectives of the program were:

1. To introduce the practice and appreciation of the Arts as an accepted therapeutic modality into treatment settings.
2. To study and assess the effectiveness of such interventions by accepted methods of biomedical research.
3. To enhance the practice of art forms in health care personnel as an effective means of self-exploration.
4. To identify and attend to the special treatment needs of practicing artists which would enhance their personal wellbeing and creativity.
5. To develop educational programs to bring to the attention of the health community the place of the arts as an effective noninvasive therapeutic intervention.

A PERSONAL SORTIE INTO THE ARTS

Joel Elkes has dabbled in painting during his days in high school. He resumed it, to an extent, during World War II and his early days in Birmingham. However, he was never consistent in the matter; painting simply remained a spuriuos, though deeply meaningful, outlet.

An exhibition of Cezanne's watercolors at the Tate Gallery in London at the end of the war, got him painting more consistently, though, never, he estimates for more than about 5 percent of his time. A deeper shift occurred when, with his late second wife, Josephine Rhodes, he began spending summers in their home on Prince Edward Island, Canada. The house stood within two miles of the oldest lighthouse on the island.

The daily walks to the lighthouse and deep encouragement from Josephine did their inner work. The resulting paintings, all quite small, and executed in charcoal and watercolors, were the subject of a one-person Show at the Floyd County Museum near Louisville in 1993. Since then, Joel Elkes has tried to paint a little more consistently.

Since Josephine's death in March 1999, Elkes spends part of his summer at the Fetzer Institute, Kalamazoo, Michigan, staying at a cottage which the Institute has very generously put at his disposal. The cottage stands on a lake: and "the light on the lake continues its perennial challenge."

A brief extract from the 1996 catalogue conveys something of the "wherefore" and "why" of Joel Elkes" work. Paintings 1 to 14 are offered by way of illustration.

ARTIST'S STATEMENT[*]

Painting with my eyes has been with me all my life. One of the greatest pleasures I know comes from staring at objects, and listening into a conversation between the mundane and the mysterious. Translating this silent traffic into images is hard, and requires practice. In my own case, practice has been lacking; though, of late, it has increased somewhat.

I use watercolor, because water has a life of its own, and guides the brush into all kinds of unpredictable ventures. Mistakes, once made, endure: like life itself, one learns to live with them.

I find both white and charcoal congenial. White comprises all colors; it is also a color in its own right. Black reflects source, beginnings, and endings. In between lie the colors of life. Hence the title of this show.

I like staring at objects while I walk. In the summer, my walks take me from our house on Point Prim, Prince Edward Island, Canada to the oldest lighthouse on the island. There are stones, and fields, and wild flowers, shimmering waters, red soil, and fallen trees under huge Canadian skies. My paintings are mere footnotes to an unfathomable magic.

---

[*] Reprinted from the Catalogue of the Exhibition "The Light and the Dark." Works on Paper The Floyd County Museum, 1993

NAME INDEX

PHOTO INDEX

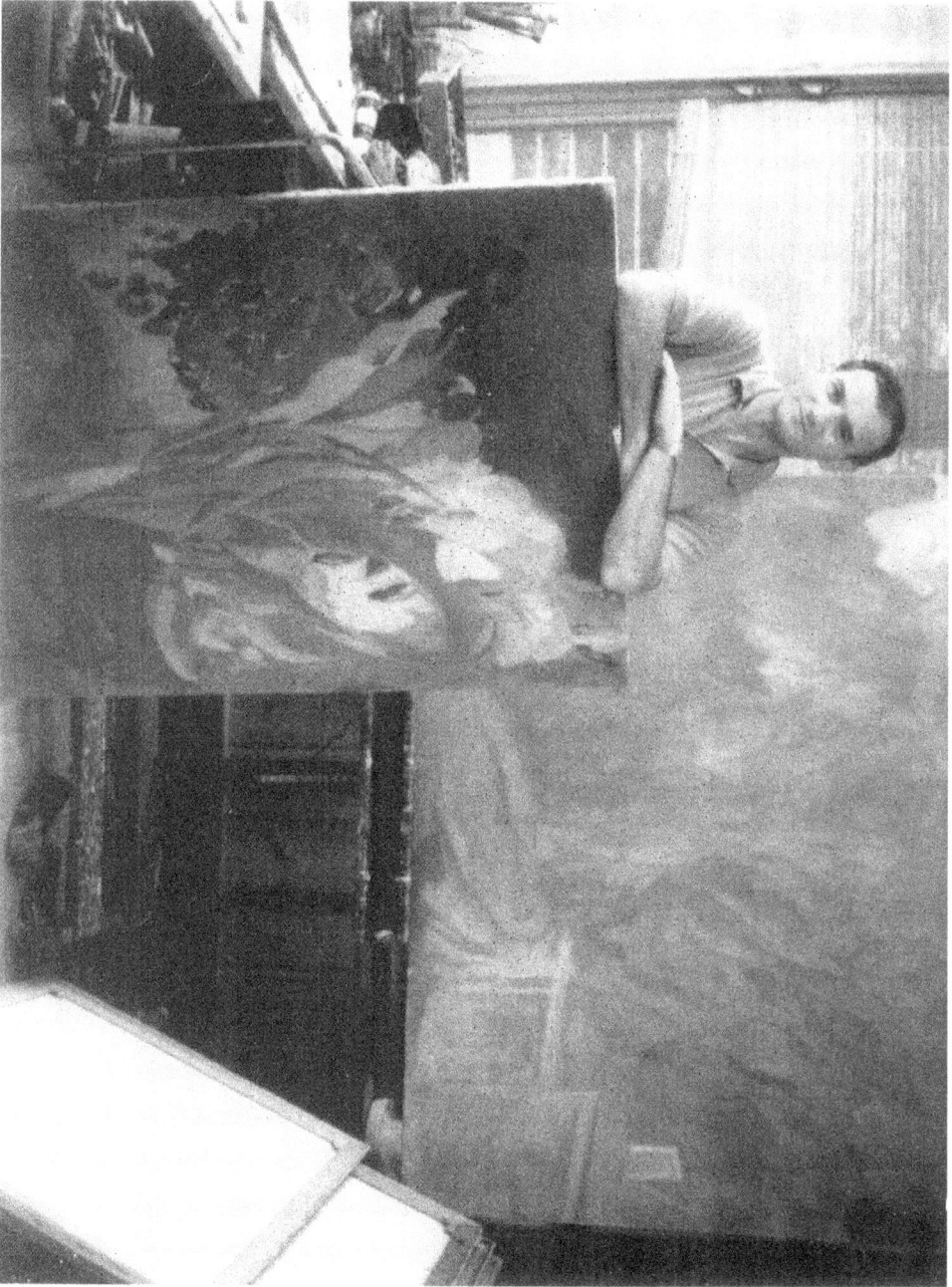

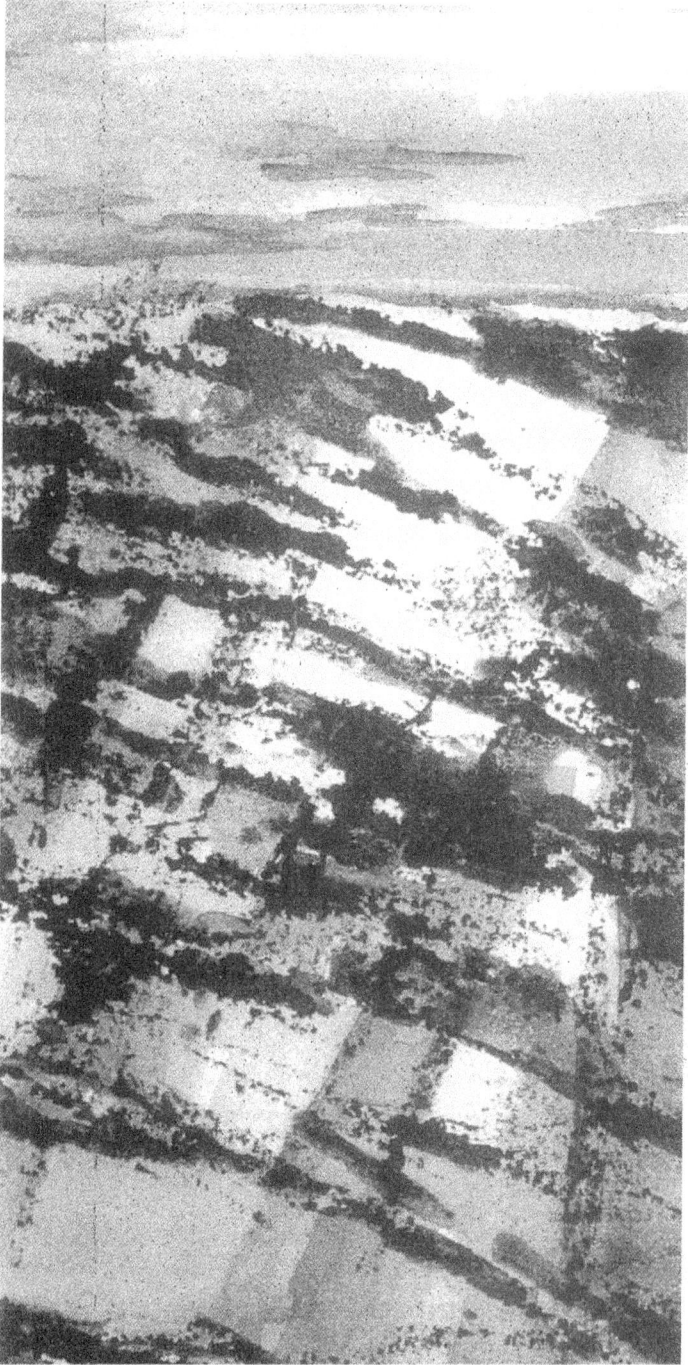

The Rocks at Joggins (1990)

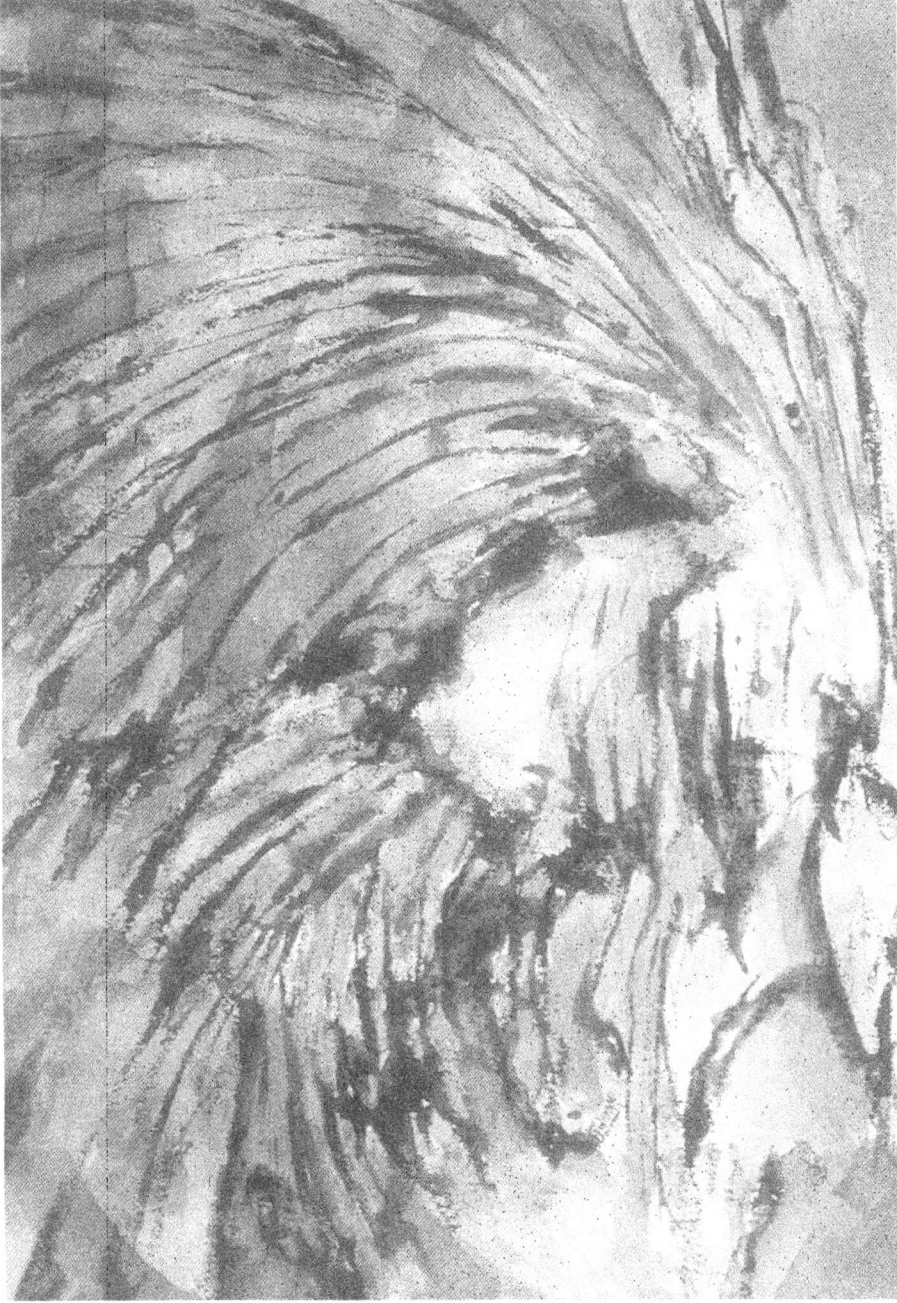

Patterns in Rocks (1989)

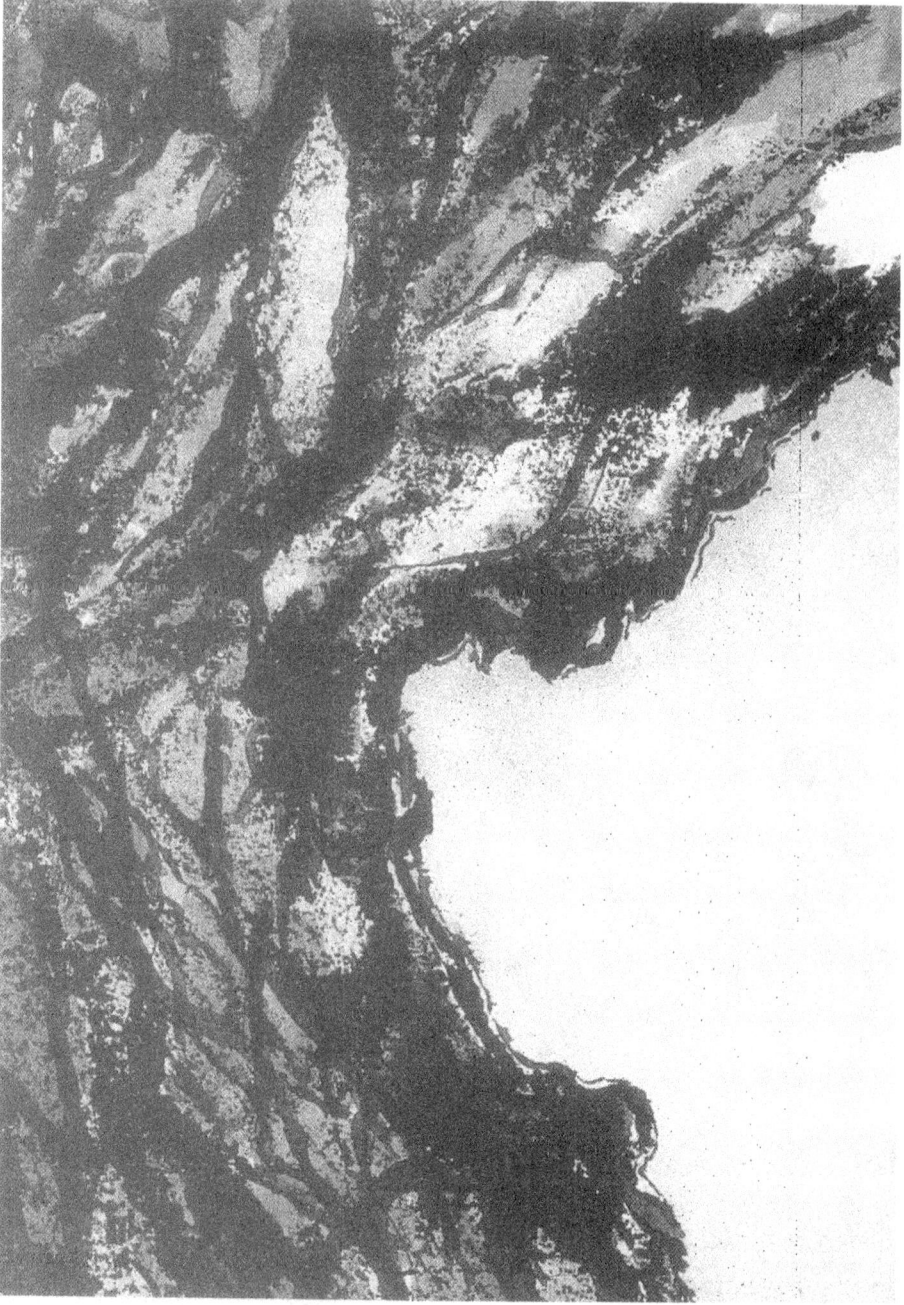

Pool and Rocks (1989)

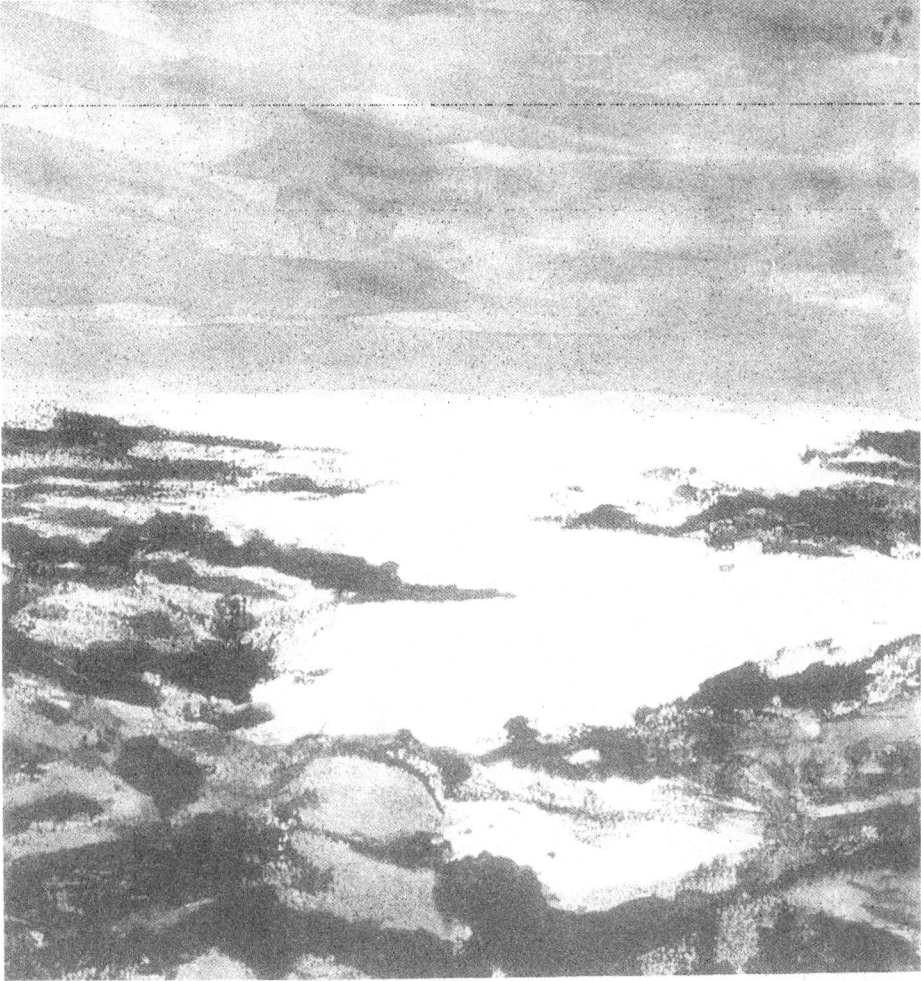

A Conversation (1988)

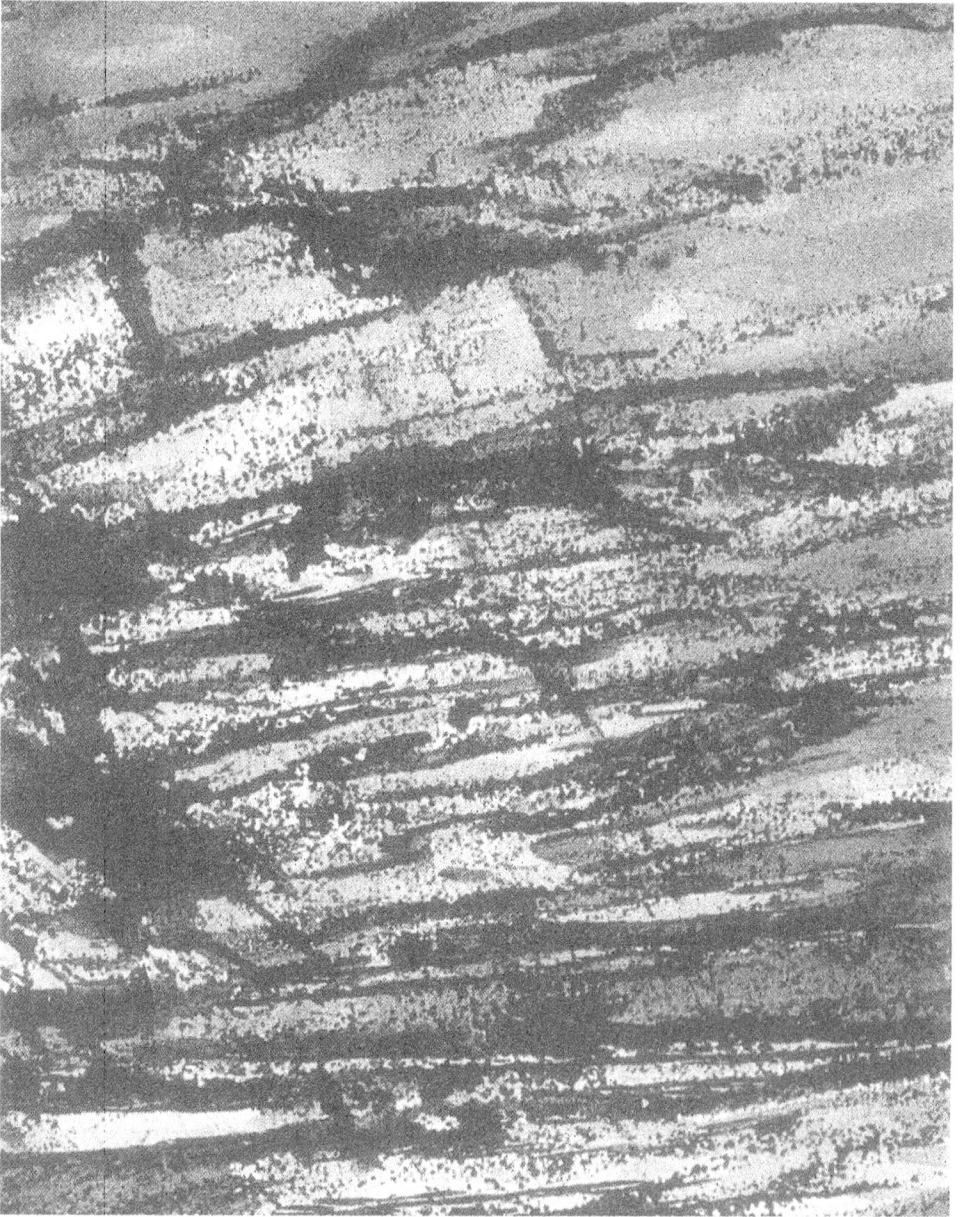

Shore Colors, Afternoon (1990)

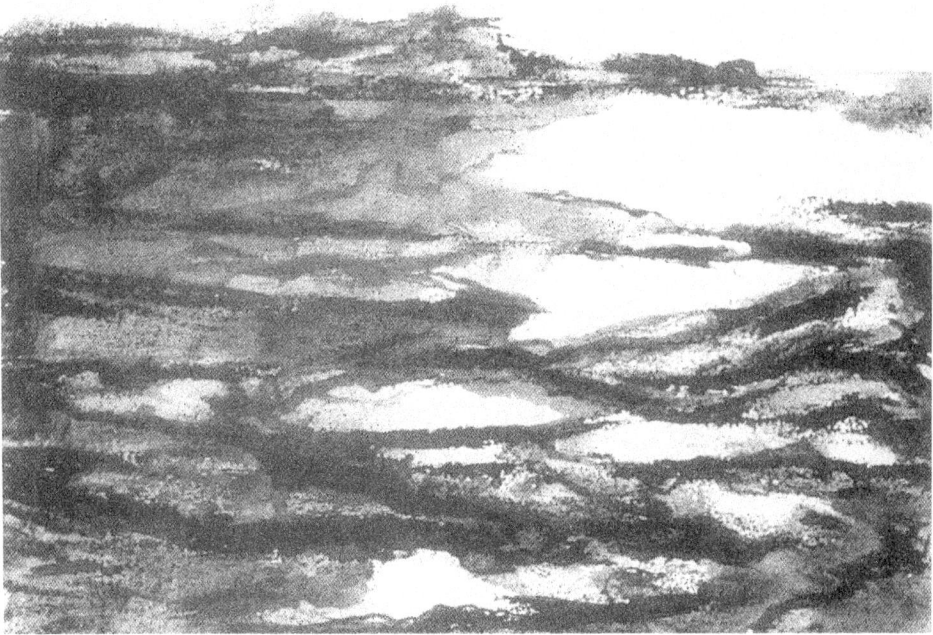

On my Walk (1990)

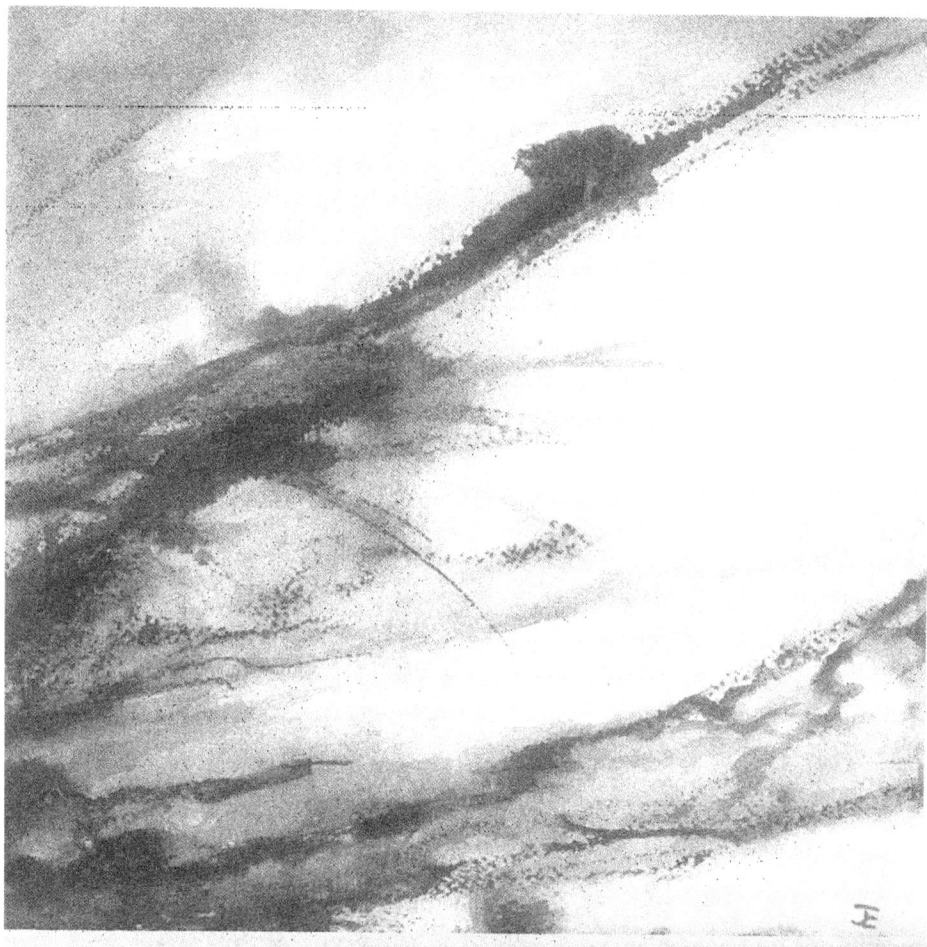

Tree Form (1992)

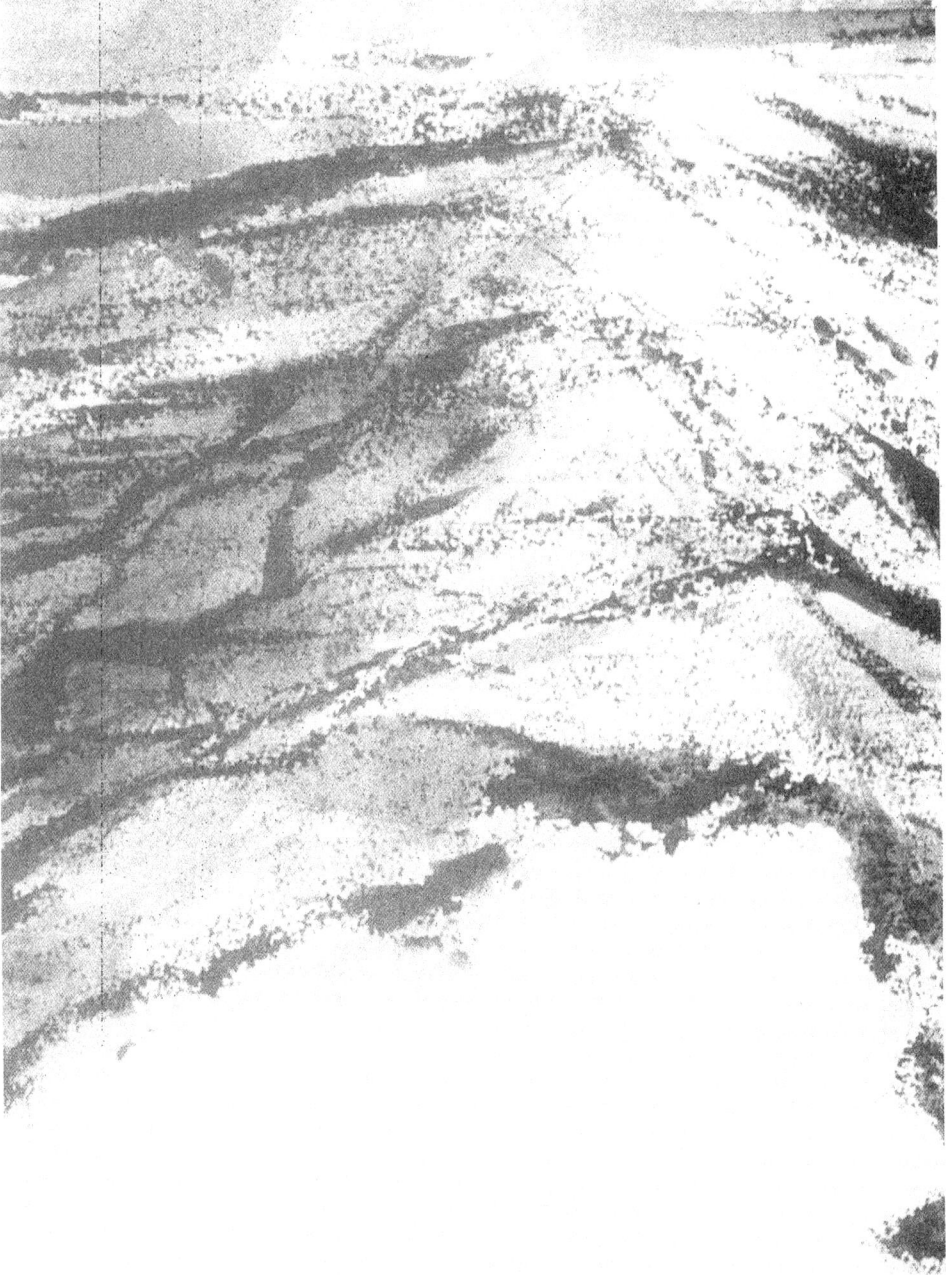

Pool and rocks II (1989)

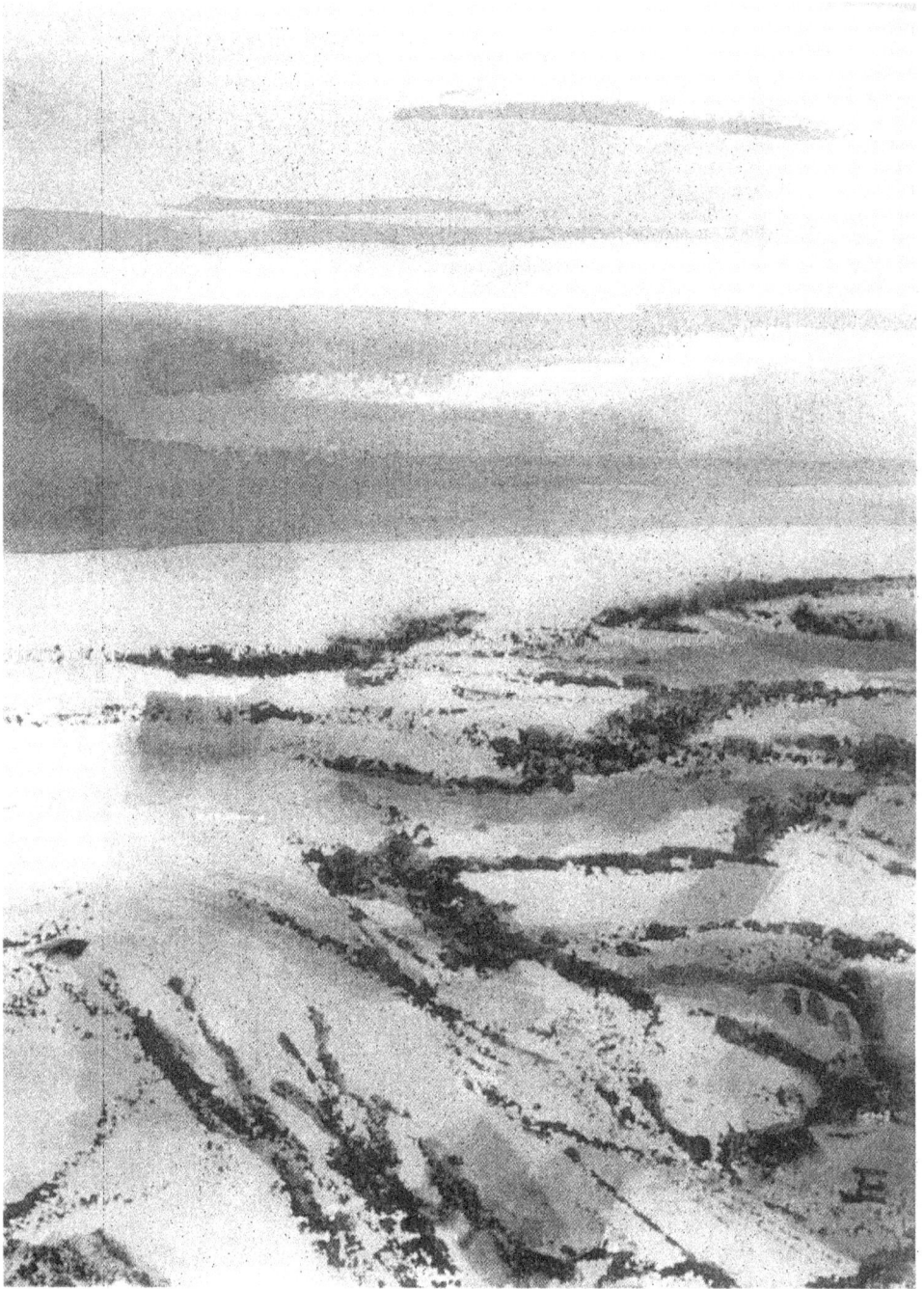

After the rain (1991)

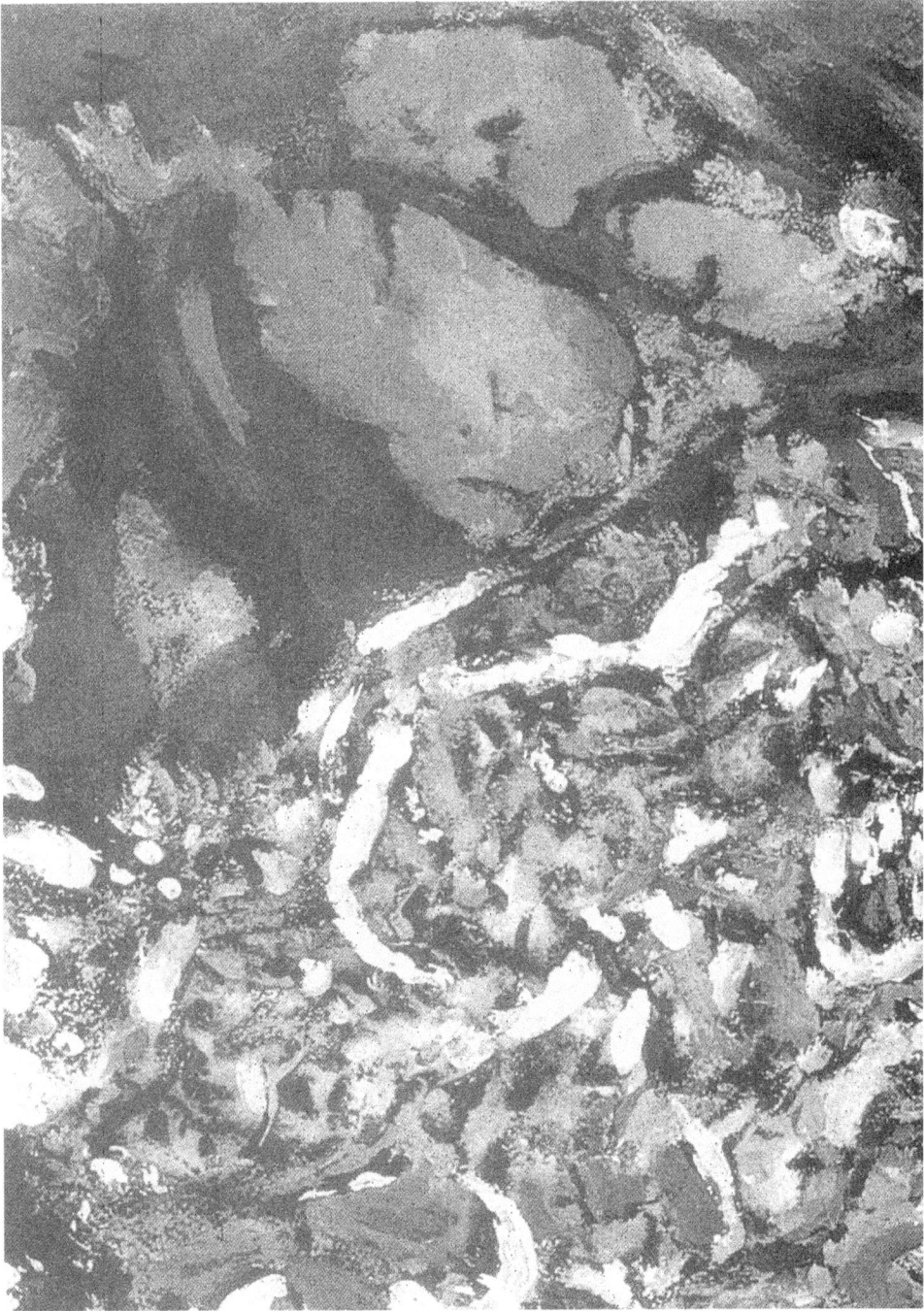

Forms by Shore (1990)

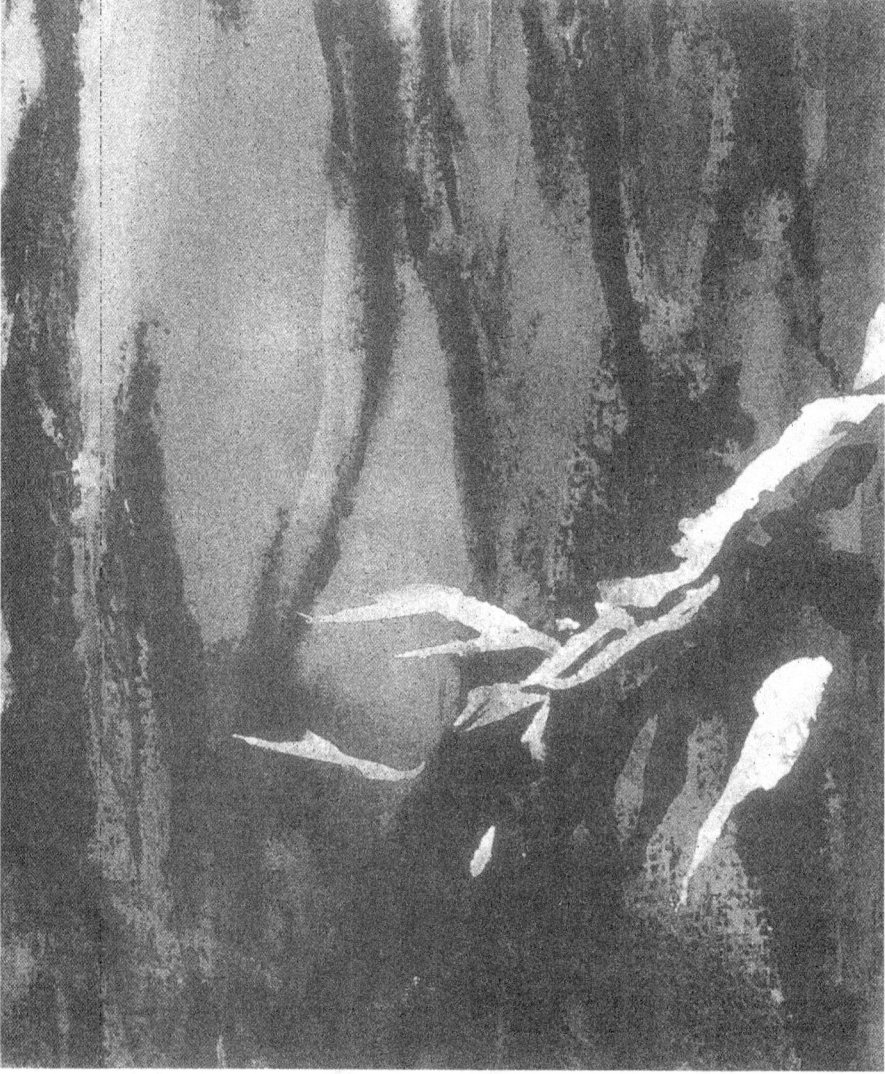

Dusk: Point Prim, P.E.I. (1990)

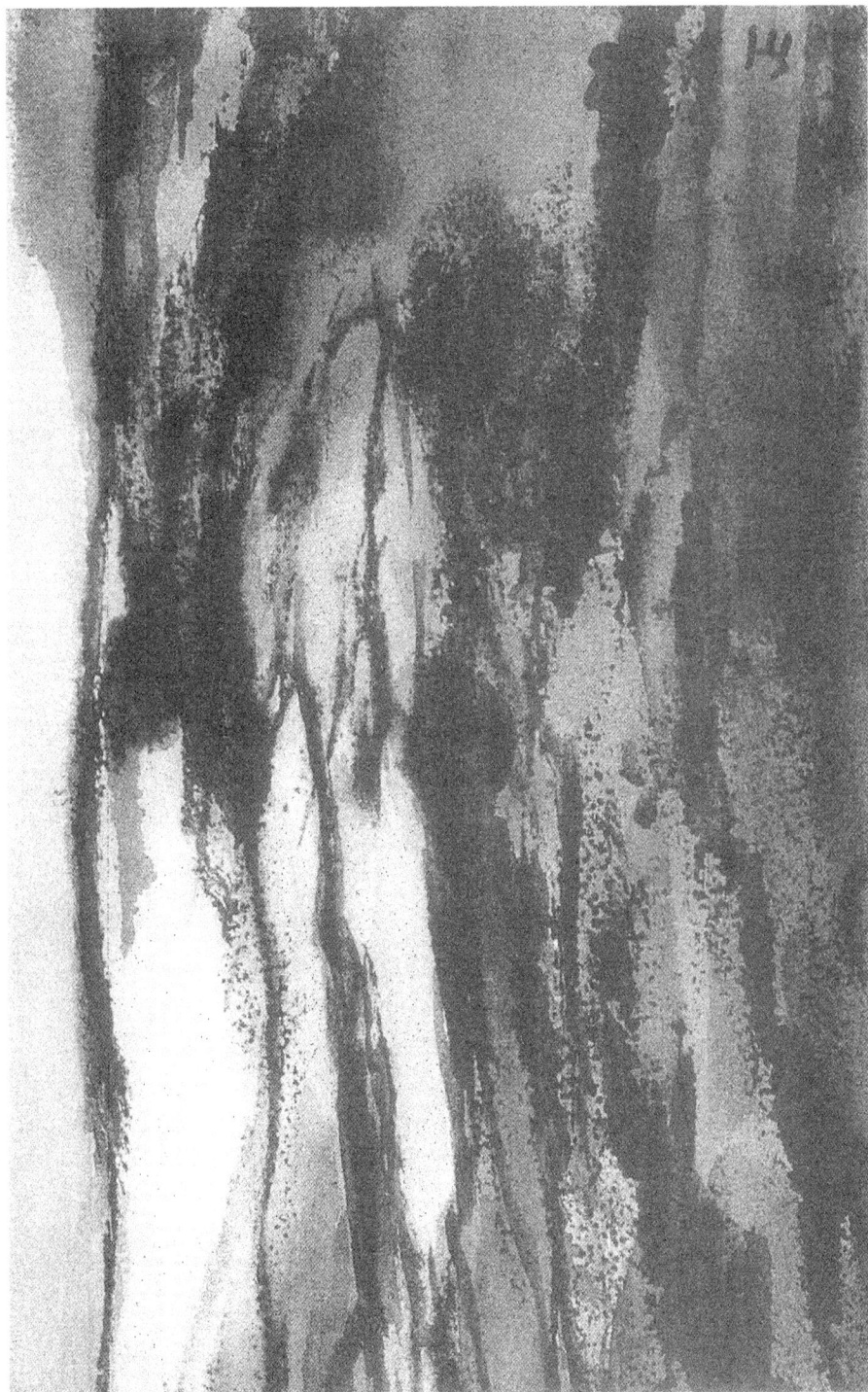

Rocks, Afternoon (1991)

Afternoon Light (1988)

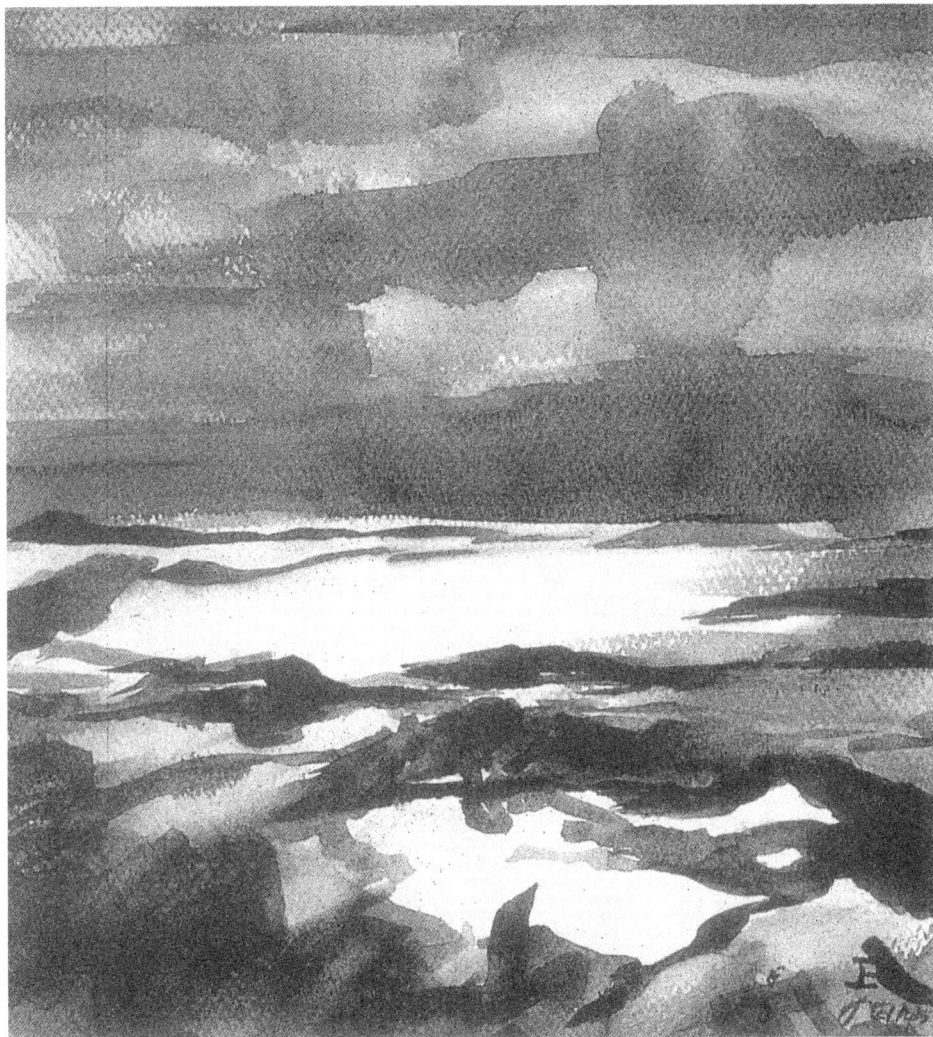

Play of Light, Afternoon (1992)

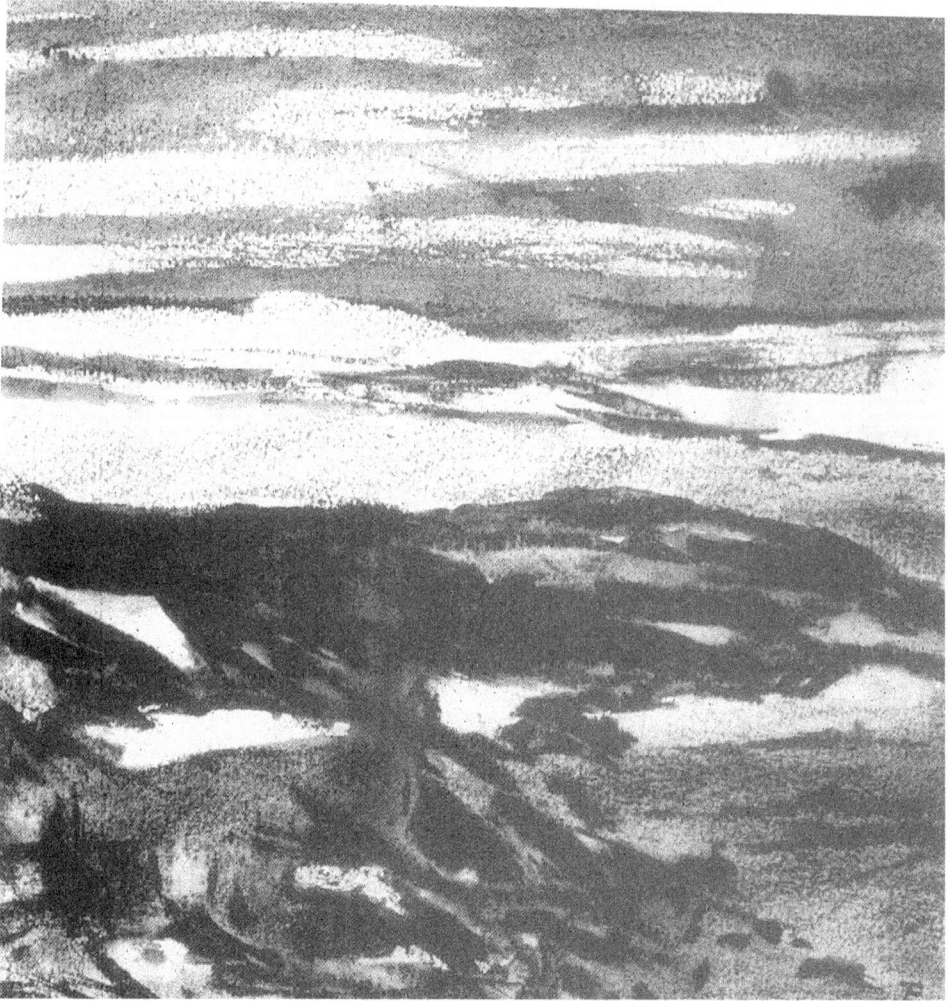

The Light and the Dark (1992)

www.ingramcontent.com/pod-product-compliance
Lightning Source LLC
Chambersburg PA
CBHW051201200326
41519CB00025B/6971